The Inherited Metabolic Diseases

For Churchill Livingstone:
Publisher: Timothy Horne
Project Editor: Dilys Jones
Indexer: Frank Wallis
Production Controller: Nancy Arnott
Sales Promotion Executive: Duncan Jones

The Inherited Metabolic Diseases

Edited by

John B. Holton BSc PhD ARCS FRCPath
Formerly Consultant Clinical Scientist,
Southmead Hospital, Bristol;
Senior Clinical Lecturer in Chemical Pathology,
University of Bristol, Bristol, UK

SECOND EDITION

CHURCHILL LIVINGSTONE
EDINBURGH LONDON MADRID MELBOURNE NEW YORK AND TOKYO 1994

CHURCHILL LIVINGSTONE
Medical Division of Longman Group UK Limited

Distributed in the United States of America by Churchill Livingstone Inc., 650 Avenue of the Americas, New York, N.Y. 10011, and by associated companies, branches and representatives throughout the world.

First edition 1987
Second edition 1994

ISBN 0-443-04497-X

British Library Catologuing in Publication Data
A catalogue record for this book is available from the British Library.

Library of Congress Cataloging in Publication Data
The Inherited metabolic diseases / edited by John B. Holton.
-- 2nd ed.
p. cm.
Includes bibliographical references and index.
1. Metabolism, Inborn errors of. I. Holton, J. B. (John B.)
[DNLM: 1. Metabolism, Inborn Errors. WD 205 155 1994]
RC627.8.154 1994
616.3'9042--dc20
DNLM/DLC
for Library of Congress 93–4001
CIP

The publisher's policy is to use **paper manufactured from sustainable forests**

Produced by Longman Singapore Publisher Pte Ltd
Printed in Singapore

Contents

Contributors

G. Michael Addison MA MB BChir MSc PhD
Consultant Paediatric Chemical Pathologist, Royal Manchester and Booth Hall Children's Hospitals, Manchester, UK

Peter J. Aggett MB FRCP DCH
Head of Department of Nutrition, Diet and Health, AFRC Institute of Food Research, Norwich; Honorary Consultant Paediatrician, Norfolk and Norwich Hospital, UK

Laurence Bindoff MSc MB BS MD MRCP
Lecturer in Neurology, Division of Clinical Neuroscience, The Medical School, University of Newcastle upon Tyne, Newcastle upon Tyne, UK

Colin H. Bolton BSc PhD
Lecturer in Biochemistry, University of Bristol, Department of Medicine, Southmead Hospital, Bristol, UK

Ronald A. Chalmers DSc PhD FRSC FIBiol MRCPath
Senior Lecturer in Paediatric Metabolism, St George's Hospital Medical School, London

D. B. Dunger MD MRCP DCH
Consultant Paediatrician, John Radcliffe Hospital, Oxford, UK

G. H. Elder BA MD FRCP FRCPath
Professor of Medical Biochemistry, University of Wales College of Medicine, Cardiff, UK

A. J. Grimes BSc PhD FRCPath
Emeritus Professor of Haematology, University of London, London, UK

J. B. Holton BSc PhD ARCS FRCPath
Formerly Consultant Clinical Scientist, Southmead Hospital, Bristol; Senior Clinical Lecturer in Chemical Pathology, University of Bristol, Bristol, UK

Alan C. Nicholls BSc PhD
Dermatology Research Group, MRC Clinical Research Centre, Harrow, UK

C. A. Pennock MD BSc FRCPath
Consultant Paediatric Chemical Pathologist, United Bristol Hospitals Health Care Trust; Senior Lecturer in Child Health, University of Bristol; Visiting Fellow, University of Bath, Bath, UK

R. J. Pollitt MA PhD MRCPath
Director, Trent Region Neonatal Screening Laboratory and Honorary Lecturer, University Department of Paediatrics, Children's Hospital, Sheffield, UK

Ruud B. H. Schutgens PhD
Clinical Chemist, University Hospital Amsterdam, Department of Pediatrics, Division of Pediatric Clinical Biochemistry, Amsterdam, The Netherlands

H. Anne Simmonds MSc PhD
Senior Lecturer, Purine Research Laboratory, United Medical and Dental Schools of Guy's and St Thomas' Hospitals, London, UK

Nicolas G. P. Slater MB FRCPath MRCP
Senior Lecturer and Honorary Consultant in Haematology, United Medical and Dental Schools, St Thomas' Hospital, London, UK

D. M. Turnbull PhD MD FRCP
Professor of Neurology, Division of Clinical Neuroscience, School of Neuroscience, The Medical School, University of Newcastle upon Tyne, UK

Linda A. Tyfield BSc MSc PhD DRCPath
Head, Section of Molecular Genetics, Department of Clinical Chemistry, Southmead Hospital, Bristol; Honorary Senior Fellow, Biochemistry Department, Bath University; Recognised Tutor, Institute of Child Health, University of Bristol, Bristol, UK

Ronald J. A. Wanders PhD
Biochemist, Associate Professor, University Hospital Amsterdam, Department of Pediatrics, Division of Pediatric Clinical Biochemistry, Amsterdam, The Netherlands

Preface to the second edition

The aims and format of this new edition remain the same as in the original but, not surprisingly, it has grown a little. The growth may be justified by developments that have occurred since the first edition, which can be put into two categories.

First are those increases in knowledge which have occurred within the subject areas included in the original book, and in almost all cases the major difference is information accruing on the diseases at the molecular genetic level. Unfortunately, we are only at the beginning in this development and often only a catalogue of known mutations at a gene locus is recorded. The era of rationalisation, classification and integration with knowledge about the phenotype, leading to deeper understanding of disease, has yet to come.

Secondly, two fields which were scarcely mentioned in the 1987 edition have developed to a point where they need to be the subject of a separate chapter. These are the peroxisomal and respiratory chain disorders.

Reference to McKusick's *Mendelian Inheritance in Man* continues, with the use of the 9th, 1990, edition in which 6 digit numbers were adopted for the first time.

Bristol 1993 J.B.H.

Preface to the first edition

For some time I have felt that there was a need for a book which filled a gap somewhere between the large, multi-author, *Metabolic Basis of Inherited Disease* of Stanbury and his colleagues and a variety of short, single author texts on the inherited metabolic diseases. Whilst it is to be hoped that the former will remain the standard reference work for those actively engaged in this field, it is rather daunting for those who are less committed yet still require a fairly comprehensive, accurate and up-to-date account of the subject. On the other hand, the subject has grown to such an extent that a single author can only write authoritatively on a small part of it, or give an overview illustrating general principles and describing representative diseases.

The object of this book is to be concise, but nevertheless comprehensive and accurate. It is hoped that it will be acceptable to the student but, also, with the use of the bibliography to such important practical aspects as diagnosis and treatment, that it will be a valuable alternative source of reference to all those more directly involved with the diseases. Twelve authors have written a chapter each on one of the accepted sub-divisions of the subject. Although none of these authors is likely to have first-hand experience of all the diseases within their chapter, they should be able to write critically in an area in which they are recognised to have a special expertise.

The production of this book has highlighted for me a number of problems which arise from the fact that there is no clear, systematic classification of the inherited metabolic diseases. The sub-divisions I have employed, which are in use widely, are not based on a uniform criterion. Some of the sections are concerned with diseases which all share a well-defined area of metabolism; but, more often, they include a heterogeneous collection of diseases which have in common only that abnormal metabolites which are excreted have similar chemical properties, conveniently linked because they can be investigated by the same analytical techniques. Other sections describe disorders in which the primary defects are in the same tissue, type of cell or subcellular organelle.

The practical difficulties that arise because of the above method of subdividing the inherited metabolic diseases, are, firstly, that a disorder may be reasonably classified into two or more sections; secondly, some disorders do not fit conveniently into any section and tend to get omitted; and thirdly, a chapter may cover groups of diseases with very little in common other than, for example, that they are all diagnosed by the use of gas chromatography. In this last situation, in particular, it is extremely difficult to write a concise account of the diseases within such a group. Unfortunately, it seems that alternative methods of classification involve many more subdivisions, or are based on even more arbitrary criteria.

It should be noted that, in common with many other publications in human genetics, throughout the book diseases have been cross-referenced to the 'Catalogs of autosomal dominant, autosomal recessive and X-linked phenotypes' of McKusick (McKusick V 1983 *Mendelian Inheritance in Man*, 6th edn. John Hopkins University Press, Baltimore), although there were a few recently described conditions where this was not possible. This has two main purposes. Firstly, it is a further means of identifying and distinguishing a specific disease. This may be useful when several variant or closely related forms exist. Secondly, it gives access to an additional bibliography on each condition. In particular, references to the original descriptions of a disease may usually be found in McKusick.

Also, I would like to acknowledge a debt of real gratitude to the contributors, who have all had to face the difficult challenge of how to approach their task; what to put in and what to leave out. Finally, I would like to thank Miss Iris Lynn who typed my manuscript and re-typed parts of many others.

Bristol, 1987 J. B. H.

1. Introduction

J. B. Holton   L. A. Tyfield

The father of the subject of this book, inherited metabolic diseases, is, unquestionably, Archibald Garrod. In a series of lectures delivered at the beginning of the present century[1], Garrod documented 4 conditions which were clearly inherited and had a notable biochemical abnormality. He attributed the cause of these 'inborn errors of metabolism' to a block in a specific metabolic pathway, subsequently seen to be a consequence of an enzyme deficiency. Garrod's hypothesis was correct in 3 out of the 4 disorders, namely alkaptonuria, pentosuria and albinism. In the other, cystinuria, it was shown almost 50 years later that the defect was not a block in a metabolic pathway but rather in a membrane transport protein which causes decreased intestinal absorption and renal tubular reabsorption of cystine, lysine, ornithine and arginine.[2]

Garrod's work provided some insight into the genetic control of the synthesis of all proteins. In theory, mutations can occur in every gene in the genome with consequent abnormalities in the proteins which they encode. Because the functions of proteins are multifarious, the disorders which are a consequence of mutations at individual gene loci are equally diverse in nature. In the present context, the classification of disorders as 'inherited metabolic diseases' is of more pragmatic than academic interest and so, in the interests of keeping this book to a reasonable size, a more traditional view is taken.

In this introduction, the mechanisms of normal and abnormal genetic control of protein synthesis are discussed, followed by a consideration of the wide diversity of effects on protein structure and function. The effects on enzyme proteins will be emphasised; however many of the mechanisms would apply equally to the variation that is found in non-enzymic proteins.

GENETIC MECHANISMS OF INHERITED DISORDERS

It is beyond the scope of this book to provide details of the organization and regulation of human genes. Nevertheless, some of the key features of the structure of genes and of the transcription and translation processes are mentioned, with the aim of providing some understanding of the underlying defects causing the metabolic disorders that are discussed. The interested reader who wishes to have information in greater depth is referred to other appropriate texts.[3]

Gene structure

DNA consists of two chains of deoxyribonucleotides which are coiled in a helical fashion and which are arranged sterically so that they are antiparallel or, more simply, they run in opposite directions. The deoxynucleotides are made up of deoxyribose, phosphate and one of four bases, adenine (A), guanine (G), cytosine (C) and thymine (T). Because of their particular shapes, the alpha helical structure is maintained by A on one strand always pairing with T on the other, and G always pairing with C. Genetic information is encoded by the order of the bases; it is a triplet non-overlapping code in which 3 bases, called a codon, determine a particular amino acid. Because there are only 20 naturally occurring amino acids and 64 possible codons, the genetic code has become degenerate, some amino acids being determined by more than one codon (Table 1.1). The greatest variability is usually seen in the last base in the triplet.

Structural genes contain several elements, some of unknown function and others that are essential for correct transcription and processing of the mRNA transcript or for translation into protein. Many of these sequences are given in Figure 1.1. Almost all mammalian genes carry sequences of unknown function called introns which are interspersed along their length with the coding regions, or exons. The number and size of the introns vary

Table 1.1 The genetic code

1st position (5' end)	2nd position				3rd position (3' end)
	U	C	A	G	
U	Phe	Ser	Tyr	Cys	U
	Phe	Ser	Tyr	Cys	C
	Leu	Ser	STOP	STOP	A
	Leu	Ser	STOP	Trp	G
C	Leu	Pro	His	Arg	U
	Leu	Pro	His	Arg	C
	Leu	Pro	Gln	Arg	A
	Leu	Pro	Gln	Arg	G
A	Ile	Thr	Asn	Ser	U
	Ile	Thr	Asn	Ser	C
	Ile	Thr	Lys	Arg	A
	Met	Thr	Lys	Arg	G
G	Val	Ala	Asp	Gly	U
	Val	Ala	Asp	Gly	C
	Val	Ala	Glu	Gly	A
	Val	Ala	Glu	Gly	G

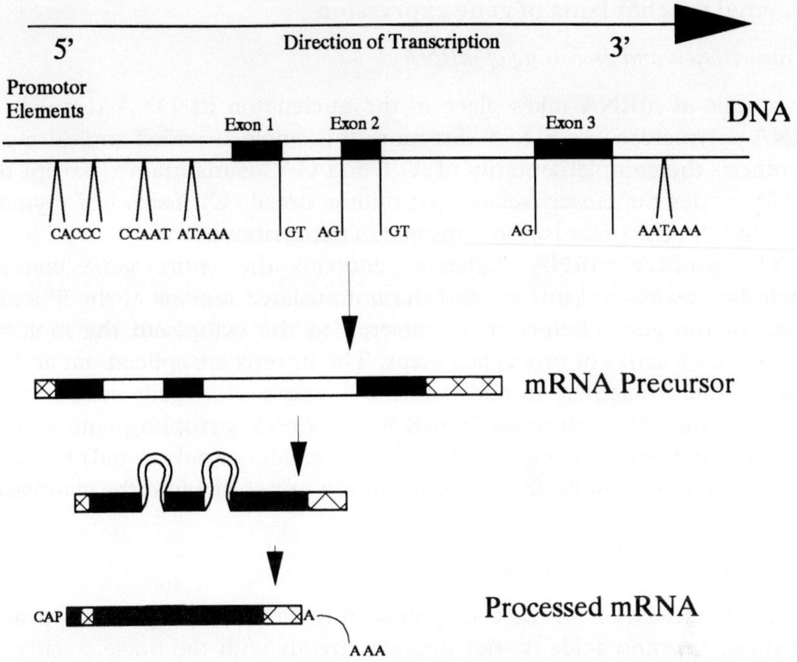

Fig. 1.1 The structure of a gene and the processing of its mRNA transcript.

from gene to gene. In all mammalian genes the dinucleotides GT and AG are found at the 5' and 3' ends of the introns and, in addition, there are highly conserved consensus sequences in the introns close to these dinucleotides. All of these sequences are essential to the correct processing of the precursor mRNA molecule, when introns are spliced out and the transcribed exons joined together. It is important to appreciate that an exon/intron boundary does not always occur at the end of a complete coding triplet. It is just as likely that the exon/intron junction occurs after the first (or second) base of the codon with the second (or third) base beginning the next exon. It is only after the intron is spliced out and the two exons brought together that the codon triplet is complete. This has enormous implications when a genetic disorder can be caused by large deletions whereby multiples of whole exons are missing.

At the 5' and 3' ends of genes there are specific triplets which determine the initiation and termination of protein synthesis on mRNA molecules. There are also sequences of varying lengths at both ends which determine the structure of non-translated regions of mRNA. At the 5' end these regions are involved in the regulation of mRNA transcription. Because of this, they are called promoters or upstream promoter elements and are regions of DNA to which RNA polymerases bind to initiate transcription.

Normal mechanisms of gene expression

Transcription and processing of mRNA

Synthesis of mRNA takes place in the nucleus on its DNA template by RNA polymerase in a 5' to 3' direction. It is single-stranded and during its synthesis the complementarity of A–T and G–C is maintained except that RNA carries the closely related pyrimidine uracil (U) instead of thymine. In addition, the sugar is ribose instead of deoxyribose.

The primary mRNA transcript contains the entire gene complex including exons and introns and the untranslated regions at the 5' and 3' ends of the gene. Before it is delivered to the cytoplasm the molecule undergoes a series of processing steps. The introns are spliced out and the exons joined together. In addition, the 5' end is essentially sealed by the addition of a *CAP* structure which forms a 5'–5' pyrophosphate linkage, and at the 3' end a string of adenylic acid residues (poly A tail) is added. These serve to stabilise the molecule during its passage into the cytoplasm.

Translation of mRNA into protein

Once the mRNA is in the cell cytoplasm it acts as a template for protein synthesis. Amino acids do not interact directly with the nucleic acids but are brought to the mRNA by another type of RNA molecule, transfer RNA or tRNA. There is a specific tRNA for each amino acid. Protein synthesis takes place on the ribosomes which consist of 2 ribonuclear protein subunits. Protein synthesis begins when a ribosome binds to the region of the initiation codon AUG and when an initiator tRNA pairs with this codon. Chain elongation occurs in a 5'–3' direction until a specific termination codon is reached (UAA, UAG or UGA) and the completed peptide is released as the complex of ribosomes, mRNA and tRNAs fall apart.

Molecular pathology of single gene disorders

The underlying cause of single gene disorders must be present in the DNA of the gene involved. Fundamentally, there are only three types of mutation within a functional gene: single base pair substitutions, and insertions or deletions of individual bases or larger segments of DNA. There are, however, some subtle variants within these more general classifications. For example, one type of disease-causing mutation which has been described recently is the amplification (rather than the insertion) of unstable nucleotide repeat sequences. Within 1 year of the first description of an unstable trinucleotide repeat as the underlying molecular defect in the fragile X syndrome[4,5], this type of mutation has also been identified as the cause of two other genetic disorders[6,7]. These unstable sequences have been found in the 5' and 3' non-coding regions of the gene in two disorders and within the coding region in the third. Undoubtedly more descriptions of this type of molecular defect will follow. Sometimes there are more extensive defects involving major rearrangements that lead to the formation of fusion genes, but strictly speaking these are combinations of insertions and deletions of large segments of a gene or genes. The primary effect of the mutations can be at any level in the regulated flow of information, from transcription into mRNA to translation into the protein product. Their secondary effect is manifest either in the synthesis of a structurally abnormal protein or in the reduced synthesis or absence of a particular protein product.

Single base pair substitutions

The effects of single base pair substitutions or point mutations are numerous and depend on their type and where they occur within the gene. Point mutations at important sequences within the promoter region of a gene can reduce transcription into mRNA or affect the initiation of protein synthesis. If a point mutation occurs within an exon it can cause the substitution of one amino acid for another (a mis-sense mutation) thereby affecting the function or stability of the protein. Alternatively, a single base substitution in an exon can change a triplet which normally encodes an amino acid into a *STOP* codon (a non-sense mutation) so that a truncated and unstable protein is made. Equally a point mutation could change the *STOP* codon into one which encodes an amino acid. The mRNA would continue to be read, incorporating additional amino acids until another *STOP* codon is reached and the result would be the synthesis of a larger protein.

Some disease-causing point mutations are also found in introns within the consensus sequences at or near splice sites with the result that the precursor mRNA molecule is incorrectly processed before being transported to the cytoplasm. The final effect on the protein structure or protein synthesis depends on whether the mutation is at the splice site beginning or ending an intron, and on whether the mutation ultimately disrupts the reading frame (the coding triplet) of the rest of the mRNA molecule. Occasionally mutations within introns can lead to the formation of an additional, new splice site. This *cryptic* splice site may be used preferentially to the normal one and so the mRNA will contain additional nucleotides. If the reading frame is maintained (that is, the additional number of bases is a multiple of 3) a protein with additional amino acids will be synthesised. If the *cryptic* splice site functions less efficiently than the normal one, both splice sites may be used and two processed mRNA molecules will appear in the cytoplasm.

It has been suggested within the last few years that the dinucleotide sequence CpG is highly mutagenic, having a mutation frequency about 42 times greater than that of random mutation within the mammalian genome.[8] (Presumably the dinucleotide sequence is depicted showing the phosphate bond between them in order to differentiate between C–G base pairing on opposite DNA strands.) At these dinucleotide sequences cytosine very often carries a methyl group at its position 5 and spontaneous deamination of 5-methyl cytosine results in the formation of thymine. This would result in a C–G base pair becoming a T–A base pair with any of the potential consequences mentioned above, depending on the site of the mutation.

Insertions or deletions

If an insertion or deletion of sequences of DNA is not a multiple of 3 base pairs the reading frame of the mRNA molecule distal to the site of the mutation will be disrupted. As a result the amino acid sequence will be different from the point of the mutation, and alternative splice sites or premature stop codons created so that a truncated and unstable or functionally inactive protein is synthesised. The phenotypic consequences of such a mutation will depend on whether it has occurred early or late in the gene sequence.

If the reading frame is maintained a milder clinical phenotype sometimes may be observed. However, this depends entirely on the site of the insertion or deletion in relation to the structure and function of the protein.

Structural variants caused by more extensive defects in genes include major rearrangements that lead to the formation of fusion genes which encode novel protein products.

As an increasing number of mutations are being identified at the molecular level for many disorders, a convention has been adopted to describe the site, and, when they occur in coding sequences, the effect of the mutation in the protein sequence. An explanation of some of the more common types of mutations described in this book is offered. The nomenclature uses single letters to characterise each amino acid and these are listed in the Appendix. When a mutation results in the substitution of one amino acid for another in the protein molecule, the first letter denotes the amino acid in the normal protein, the number following this is its position within the protein and the last letter denotes the amino acid which has been substituted. Thus, a mutation written as R408W describes the alteration of the normal amino acid arginine (R) to tryptophan (W) at position 408 of the protein molecule. This does not identify exactly the single base substitution in the gene, but this could be established easily from tables of the genetic code (Table 1.1). If the mutation changes an amino acid to a stop codon, the letter X is used so that R408X describes the alteration of arginine (R) to a stop codon at amino acid position 408 of the protein molecule. A deletion of a single amino acid is described by the Greek letter delta preceding the letter for the amino acid. The most common mutation for cystic fibrosis in caucasians is thus described as ΔF508 – a deletion of the amino acid phenylalanine at position 508 of the CFTR protein.

Unfortunately the delta symbol is also sometimes used to describe the size of the expanded fragment in disorders which are caused by amplification of an unstable nucleotide repeat. It would be obvious from the context, whether the symbol denotes an amplification or a deletion.

Mutations within introns are described by the letters IVS (for intervening sequence) followed by the intron number and then by the lower case letters nt (for non-translated) followed by another number which describes the nucleotide position within the intron. Thus, IVS12nt1 describes a mutation at the first untranslated nucleotide in intron 12 and so is a mutation in a splice site. IVS10nt546 describes a mutation at the untranslated nucleotide position 546 in intron 10 of the gene. This nomenclature does not identify the consequences of the mutation on the protein molecule and so an explanation is usually needed.

Characterising specific mutations

Within any single genetic disorder the clinical phenotype can be caused by several different mutations at the same gene locus. Except for sickle cell anaemia, this allelic heterogeneity is almost certainly the rule rather than the exception, although for a particular genetic disorder, one or two mutations may predominate in any individual population or race. For autosomal recessive disorders, affected individuals are often compound heterozygotes in that they carry a different mutation at the same gene locus on each homologous chromosome.

The advent of automated gene amplification has revolutionised the ability to characterise mutations at individual loci. The technique, called the polymerase chain reaction (PCR), generates several million copies of a segment of a gene in an automated thermocyclic reaction. A large variety of techniques are now available to characterise the mutations in the amplified product. The specific technique to be used will depend on whether samples are being tested for individual mutations that have been previously characterised, or whether they are being screened for a collection of mutations which may or may not have been identified already.

EXPRESSION OF THE MUTANT GENE

The variety of effects a gene mutation has on the protein end-product has already been alluded to: a mutation within a sequence that regulates gene expression or controls the correct processing of the primary mRNA transcript could result in a complete lack of synthesis of the protein. In other instances, a mutation might result in a protein of normal structure and function being synthesised but in reduced amounts. Another possibility is that a protein of abnormal structure is synthesised and this affects the binding of the protein to its substrate or cofactor, the protein's stability, or its ability to bind with other polypeptides or structural components.

Sometimes, it is possible to determine whether the synthesis or the function of a protein is affected in an individual patient by reacting abnormal cells or tissues with an antibody raised to the normal protein, and determining whether there is any cross-reacting material (CRM) with the antibody. If the reaction is CRM+, a modified protein is being produced which has retained antigenic properties. CRM– could mean that no protein is being synthesised or that a protein is being produced but which is sufficiently modified that it no longer reacts with the antibody. Decreased but measurable levels of a protein could be the result of reduced synthesis of a structurally normal polypeptide, or of the synthesis of an unstable molecule.

Extension of the 1 gene – 1 polypeptide concept

In recent years, the *1 gene – 1 enzyme* hypothesis originally proposed by Beadle and Tatum[9] has been modified to *1 gene – 1 polypeptide*, and although this basic tenet holds for most genes an increasing number of exceptions to the rule are being reported.

There are examples where one gene encodes more than one peptide, sometimes with varying functions. For instance, in the case of neuropeptides and muscle proteins, differential splicing of mRNA enables one gene to encode different proteins in different tissues. In the condition known as orotic aciduria, it appears that two enzymes with different functions (orotic acid phosphoribosyl transferase and oritidine 5-monophosphatase) are encoded by one gene. Yet another example is in the modification in the pre-mRNA of apolipoprotein B when a cytosine is converted to a uridine thereby creating a stop codon. The result is that two functional apoproteins, one shorter than the other (B-48 as opposed to B-100) are synthesised on the same gene. Probably the best known example is in the synthesis of a million or so discrete immunoglobulins. Only a few genes in the human genome are involved but for each immunoglobulin a unique DNA is produced as a result of rearrangements prior to transcription.[10]

Although the concept of 1 gene – 1 polypeptide still applies, it is also now well established that some enzymes or structural proteins function only when they are an aggregate of more than one polypeptide, each of which is encoded by a gene at a different locus. An appreciation of this is sometimes essential to understanding the phenotypic effects in some inherited metabolic or structural disorders. A well established example is that of the lysosomal enzymes, hexosaminidase A and B, which each consist of two polypeptide subunits, alpha and beta, which are encoded at two separate loci. The A enzyme consists equally of alpha and beta subunits whereas the B enzyme contains only beta subunits. Thus, the gene for the beta subunits is involved in the synthesis of two distinct enzymes (A and B) and the synthesis of the A enzyme requires two independent genes. Although mutations in the alpha or beta subunits are distinguishable by molecular genetic or biochemical means, the consequent clinical conditions are almost identical. However, for family counselling and establishing carrier status by molecular genetic techniques, it is essential to know which locus is involved.

When a functional protein is composed of different protein subunits in varying proportions, the clinical phenotype resulting from mutations at one or other gene locus become even more complex. The enzyme phosphofructokinase (PFK), for example, is a tetramer composed of three kinds of subunit encoded by three separate genes. Muscle expresses only the M subunit gene and so its PFK has the structure M4. Erythrocytes synthesise approximately equal amounts of M and L subunits thereby giving five isoenzymes and the F type is found in fibroblasts, brain, platelets, lymphocytes and kidney. Two PFK-deficiency diseases exist, one involving a mutation at the M subunit locus (p. 36) and another at the L subunit locus (p. 536). The site of the mutation will determine which cells are predominantly affected. Another example is in the variety of clinical phenotypes seen in the type 1 collagen disorders. Type 1 collagen is composed of three subunits encoded at two different gene loci and mutations at either locus can lead to phenotypes varying from very mild to early lethal in the heterozygous or homozygous state. Explanations for this have been provided by the concept of *included* (inc) or *excluded* (exc) mutants.[11] In *excluded* phenotypes, the mutation may disrupt the protein structure to such an extent that incorporation of the product of the mutant allele into collagen molecules is prevented. Thus, only normal molecules will be produced, albeit in a reduced amount and so the associated phenotype is less severe. In *included* phenotypes, the incorporation of an abnormal chain results in an abnormal collagen molecule which is then structurally and functionally abnormal, thereby resulting in a more severe phenotype.

Situations also arise whereby one single gene mutation leads to multiple enzyme deficiencies. In some conditions, this arises through a defect in the synthesis of a cofactor which is involved in more than one enzymatic reaction. Vitamin B_{12}, or cobalamin, for example, is the precursor for two active cofactors, adenosyl and methyl cobalamins, which themselves are required by two separate enzymes. Three distinct gene mutations are known which affect the synthesis of both cofactors, and hence, the activity of both enzymes. In other conditions, a mutation at a single gene locus affects a group of enzymes which all function within a single subcellular organelle. This can happen either by the integrity of the organelle being affected as in the peroxisomal disorders (p. 249) or by an effect on the targeting of the group of enzymes to the organelle. In l-cell disease (p. 236), a number of hydrolases are deficient in the lysosome where they normally function. The defect in this disorder lies in the enzyme that attaches an identity marker, mannose phosphate, to the hydrolases, which targets them to the lysosome.

PATHOGENESIS

One of the main incentives for studying a rare inherited metabolic disease is to elucidate the disease processes at the molecular level, with the hope that ultimately this leads to the understanding of pathogenic mechanisms in general. Unfortunately there has been only limited progress in this area, the main reasons being restriction on the use of humans in experimentation and, very often, the absence of a close animal model for the disease. Hypotheses abound, but rarely can they be tested.

Discussions of pathogenic mechanisms usually divide into a consideration of enzyme and non-enzymic protein abnormalities. Fewer non-enzymic defects are recognised at the moment, but generally the mechanisms by which they cause disease are more apparent. For example, disorders of the globin chains are seen to have a direct effect on the oxygen-transporting ability of haemoglobin, or sometimes, on the maturation and stability of the red cell (p. 554). Abnormalities of proteins involved in the red cell cytoskeleton likewise affect red cell function and stability in a way which is quite easy to comprehend (p. 523).

Regarding enzymic defects, the work of Garrod postulated that the pathogenesis is related to the metabolic imbalance which it causes. Figure 1.2 shows the possible metabolic distortions which can occur. There are some diseases in which the relationship between the metabolic abnormality and clinical signs is readily apparent. In glycogen storage disease Type 1, for example, the deficiency of glucose-6-phosphatase leads to a failure to

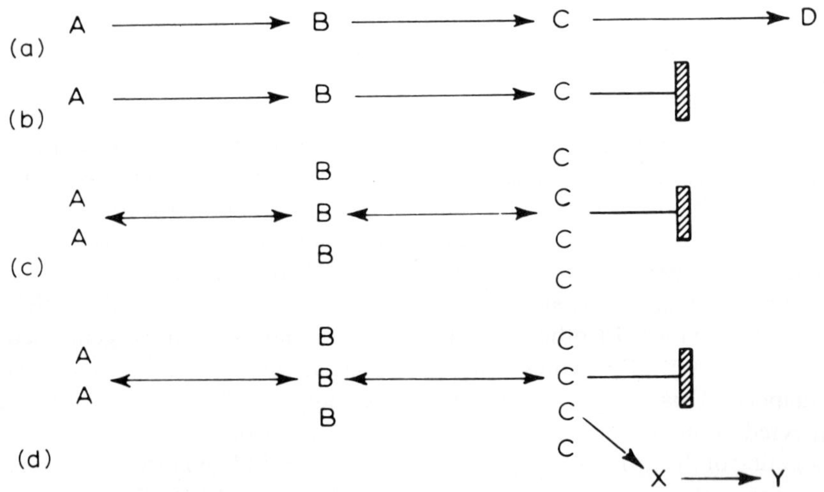

Fig. 1.2 The consequences of a metabolic block. (**a**) A hypothetical pathway synthesising D from A through intermediates B and C. (**b**) The block between C and D may lead to a failure to form the end-product; (**c**) with a possible accumulation of precursors prior to the block, and (**d**) the formation of unusual metabolites.

release the enzyme product, glucose, from the liver and hypoglycaemia is a direct consequence. The same defect causes an accumulation of glycogen in the liver which results in histological changes and hepatomegaly (p. 26). In the congenital adrenal hyperplasias, the cortisol synthetic pathway is affected and the end-product is deficient with the result that an Addisonian crisis can ensue (p. 421). Thus the symptoms of the disease may be explicable at a biochemical level although the explanation may be more complex at the molecular level.

Many complexities are apparent in some disorders which have been researched for the longest time. It has been known for some time that phenylketonuria is characterised by a large accumulation of phenylalanine in the body and, secondarily, by the abnormal production and excretion of phenylalanine metabolites. There is a clear correlation between the degree of exposure to phenylalanine and the reduction in IQ[12], but the direct cause of the neurological damage is unclear. Evidence from in vitro experimental systems offer mechanisms whereby either the hyperphenylalaninaemia or the secondary metabolites could be the cause of the brain damage, and both hypotheses would be consistent with the clinical data. Galactosaemia is another disease in which there are more questions raised than answers given with regard to its pathogenesis (p. 37).

In metabolic pathways involving negative feedback control (Fig. 1.3), failure to synthesise the end product because of an enzyme defect has direct consequences within the same metabolic pathway. In the autosomal dominant disorder acute intermittent porphyria (AIP) the biochemical and clinical consequences of incomplete negative feedback control are well

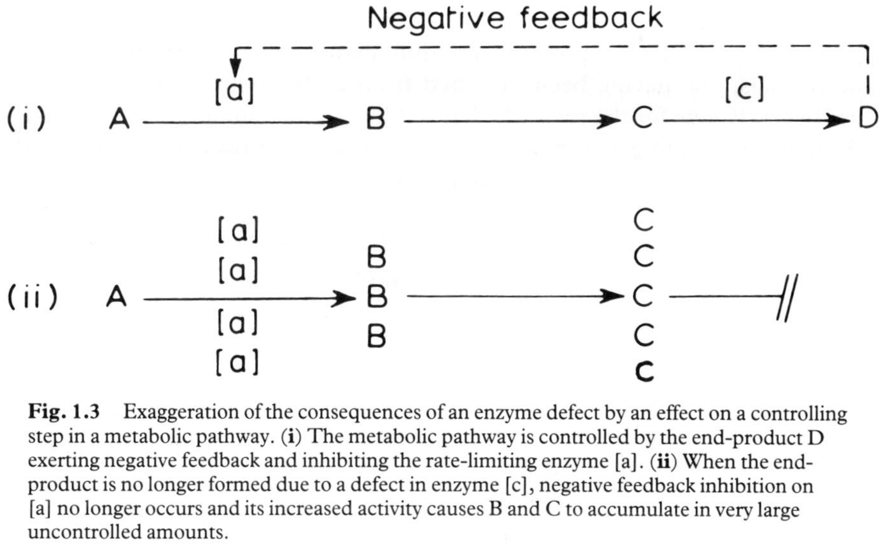

Fig. 1.3 Exaggeration of the consequences of an enzyme defect by an effect on a controlling step in a metabolic pathway. (**i**) The metabolic pathway is controlled by the end-product D exerting negative feedback and inhibiting the rate-limiting enzyme [a]. (**ii**) When the end-product is no longer formed due to a defect in enzyme [c], negative feedback inhibition on [a] no longer occurs and its increased activity causes B and C to accumulate in very large uncontrolled amounts.

illustrated. The mutation is in the locus encoding porphobilinogen (PBG) deaminase which is on the haem synthetic pathway. An enzyme earlier in the pathway, delta aminolaevulinic acid (ALA) synthase, is rate-limiting and its activity is controlled by negative feedback depending on the size of the free haem pool. In the affected heterozygotes, who have about 50% of normal enzyme activity, adequate haem synthesis is usually maintained, but in certain circumstances, such as on administration of barbiturates or oestrogens, increased demands are made on the haem pool for the synthesis of cytochrome P_{450} which is used to metabolise the drugs. Haem depletion stimulates ALA synthase and the increased flux of metabolites through the pathway overwhelms the compromised PBG deaminase. ALA and PBG, in particular, accumulate and these are linked with the appearance of acute symptoms of AIP.

PATTERNS OF INHERITANCE

Many of the diseases that are discussed in this book follow a Mendelian form of transmission in families and they can be classified according to whether they are inherited in an autosomal recessive, autosomal dominant or X-linked manner. However, when there is an apparent divergence from Mendelian inheritance, additional factors and concepts have to be taken into account and some of these will be discussed below. The simplest forms of transmission of monogenic disorders are shown in various hypothetical pedigrees given in Figure 1.4.

Autosomal transmission

Most of the inherited metabolic diseases are determined by mutations in genes at a single locus on one of the 22 pairs of autosomes. Two mutant genes are required to produce the full clinical phenotype in affected individuals, one having been inherited from each parent who themselves are heterozygous for the mutant allele. Although the mutant gene is passed from generation to generation, the heterozygous state usually produces no clinical effects and there is often no previous family history of the disorder. At each conception the parents have a 25% chance of having an affected child, and males and females are equally affected. Without a family history of a particular genetic disorder, the background risk of any couple having affected offspring is defined by the Hardy–Weinberg equilibrium, $p^2 + 2pq + q^2$, where p and q are the frequencies of the normal and mutant alleles in the population. The frequency of homozygous affected individuals (q^2) is usually known and so with this information it is possible to determine the frequency of heterozygote carriers (2pq). The frequency of matings between heterozygotes, and thus of couples at risk of having an affected child, is 2pq x 2pq. The risk of a recessive disorder occurring is greatly increased if there is parental consanguinity.

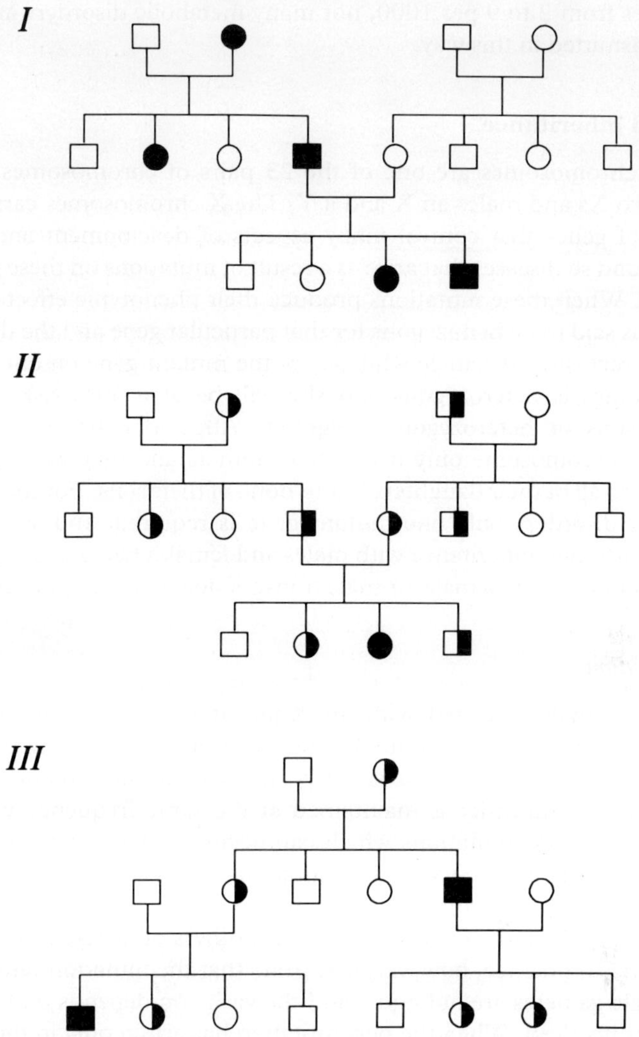

Fig. 1.4 Hypothetical pedigrees illustrating different forms of monogenic inheritance; squares – males, circles – females, filled – affected individuals, half-filled – carriers. Pedigree I, autosomal dominant inheritance; II, autosomal recessive inheritance; III, X-linked inheritance. In I and II, males and females are equally affected; in III, normally only males are affected (but see text).

When the full spectrum of biochemical abnormalities, and the disease itself, is expressed in the heterozygotes, the condition is autosomal dominant. The abnormal allele is transmitted to one in two of the offspring regardless of sex and so males and females are equally affected. Unlike autosomal recessive disorders in which affected individuals usually occur in a single sibship, autosomal dominant disorders can often be traced through many generations. Although the frequency of dominantly inherited disorders varies from 2 to 9 per 1000, not many metabolic disorders are known to be transmitted in this way.

X-linked inheritance

The sex chromosomes are one of the 23 pairs of chromosomes, females having two Xs and males an X and a Y. The X chromosomes carry a large number of genes that control many aspects of development and cellular function and so diseases that arise as a result of mutations on these genes are X-linked. When these mutations produce their phenotypic effect only in a male, he is said to be hemizygous for that particular gene and the disorder is X-linked recessive. A female who carries the mutant gene on one of the X chromosomes is heterozygous and she will be at a 50% risk of having affected sons or heterozygous daughters. Affected males can inherit a mutant X chromosome only from their mothers and they would pass the mutation to all of their daughters but to none of their sons. For the X-linked dominant disorders only one mutant gene is required, and so there is a vertical pattern of inheritance with males and females being equally affected although, once again, a male-to-male transmission would not be seen.

New mutations

Mothers of males affected with an X-linked recessive disorder are not necessarily carriers of the mutant gene themselves. Especially with those disorders in which males are so severely affected that they do not reproduce themselves, the disorder is maintained at the same frequency within the population by new mutations which can occur during either oogenesis or spermatogenesis. In theory, if the mutation rate (μ) is equal in male and female gametes, the proportion of new mutations among affected males would be 1 in 3, and so two out of three mothers of affected males would be carriers. In practice, however, it appears that the mutation rates in male and female gametes are not equal and the variation depends on the particular locus involved. When the new mutation has arisen only in the affected son, there is no increased risk to his mother or to his sisters of having further affected sons.

Germinal mosaicism

The assumed background risk of the mother of an affected son can sometimes be modified upwards or downwards by the use of biochemical or molecular genetic tests. Occasionally, DNA analysis has indicated that the peripheral leukocytes do not carry the mutation and yet there is multiple transmission of a mutant allele to affected offspring. This can be accounted for by germinal (or gonadal) mosaicism whereby the mutation is found in a proportion of the mother's germ cells (ova) but is not present in her somatic cells. The mutation would have arisen in the mother's germ cells in embryonic life at some stage after differentiation and specialisation. The proportion of germ cells affected depends on when the mutation had occurred, and so under these circumstances it is often difficult to establish the risk of a woman having further affected offspring. At the dystrophin locus it has been estimated that the risk of germinal mosaicism might be as high as 15%.

Mitochondrial inheritance

Mendelian inheritance describes the transmission of genes encoded by chromosomes in the nucleus of cells. Perhaps because their progenitors were separate organisms, mitochondria, which reside in the cytoplasm of cells, also carry their own DNA. Unlike sperm, ova contain a considerable amount of cytoplasm and as a result mitochondrial DNA (mtDNA) is only maternally inherited.

The size of the mitochondrial genome is tiny compared to the nuclear genome, consisting of only 16 569 individual base pairs in a single, continuous double-stranded loop. In addition to encoding the RNA for its ribosomes and 22 tRNAs, mitochondrial DNA encodes 13 proteins which are subunits in the respiratory chain.

It is now known that some disorders are caused by mutations in the mitochondrial genome but there can be wide variation in the severity of expression of mtDNA-linked changes. This is probably because each mitochondrion contains between four and ten copies of the mtDNA genome and there are many mitochondria per cell. When a cell divides, mitochondria are randomly assigned to the daughter cells and so, although a mutation may be present in the mtDNA somewhere in the cell, it can be far outnumbered by the normal, non-mutated copies that are also present. The clinical changes may not be manifest until the mutation has spread to a sufficient number of mitochondria.

Point mutations can be transmitted from generation to generation but deletions are sporadic. Both males and females are equally affected and because mtDNA is only maternally inherited there will be no affected offspring of affected males.

Divergence from expected patterns of inheritance

Divergences from expected patterns of inheritance are most apparent when only one mutant gene is needed to produce the phenotypic effects in an individual.

Females affected by X-linked disorders

Occasionally females show, to varying degrees, all the signs of being affected by an X-linked recessive disorder. This would arise if a female were homozygous for a mutant gene, one having been inherited from each parent as in the case of an autosomal recessive disorder. However, it would be expected that the father of the affected female was also clinically affected and that his life expectancy and reproductive fitness had not been significantly reduced.

When an affected female is not homozygous for a mutant gene on the X chromosome, the effects of X-chromosome inactivation, a concept which was first postulated by Mary Lyon in the early 1960s must be considered. X-inactivation (also called Lyonization) is the strictly cis-limited inactivation of many, but not all, genes on one of the two X chromosomes in somatic cells of mammalian females during early embryonic development. The mechanism of inactivation is unknown except that DNA methylation is involved. It is almost certain that this process is controlled by a gene called *XIST* which is situated on the proximal long arm of the X chromosome and is transcribed only on inactive chromosomes.

X-inactivation results in dosage equivalence between females and males of the genes on the X chromosome. Some genes escape X-inactivation and most of these are in the pseudoautosomal regions at the distal ends of the short arms of the X and Y. However, it is now known that other regions of the X chromosome also escape inactivation and it is likely that these regions carry genes which have a counterpart on the Y. The process is usually random, resulting in two populations of somatic cells of about equal size, so that the result of inactivation is that the female is a mosaic of cells. Once inactivation has occurred in embryonic life, all descendants of that cell have the same inactive X chromosome.

When both alleles at a gene locus are the same, the two populations of cells are the same with regard to that particular gene function. However, in the heterozygote female, one population of cells will be expressing one allele and the other population of cells the other allele, as if she were a mixture of cells from a hemizygous affected male and a normal male. With random X-inactivation a heterozygous female would have approximately equal numbers of normal and affected cells. However a small proportion of heterozygous women have either a great excess of normal cells, or of defective cells and it is in the latter situation that clinical manifestations are likely to occur. Provided the normal cells do not correct the defective cells (by means of a diffusible enzyme, for example) or provided they do not always outgrow them during development, variation in the X-inactivation process can lead to variation in the clinical manifestion of the gene between heterozygous females.

Genomic imprinting

It is becoming increasingly evident that mutations in some parts of the genome function differently depending on whether they come from the mother or the father. The term 'genomic imprinting' is now used to describe this differential expression of genetic material at the chromosomal or allelic level depending on its parental origin. The exact mechanism of genomic imprinting is not known but it probably involves a process which modifies the nuclear DNA in somatic cells by tagging genes or segments of chromosomes with varying degrees of methylation. As for the inherited disorders of metabolism, which are invariably inherited in an autosomal recessive fashion, differences in phenotypic expression between affected individuals undoubtedly result from different combinations of mutations within the gene locus rather than genomic imprinting. However, at loci where there are genes involved in the regulation of cell growth, genomic imprinting may be another important mechanism which adds an increased flexibility to their control and expression.

Reduced penetrance, variable expressivity and anticipation

In disorders inherited in an autosomal dominant or X-linked fashion, individuals who are obligate carriers of the mutant gene very often show sparse or no clinical symptoms. In other situations, affected siblings may show variation in the clinical expression of the mutant gene, with one being more severely affected than the other despite the fact that they have inherited the same mutant gene from their parent. The identification of unstable and expandable trinucleotide repeat sequences as the underlying molecular pathology in four separate disorders (fragile X, and spinal and bulbar muscular atrophy, which are X-linked, and myotonic dystrophy and Huntington's disease which are autosomal dominant) helps to explain these clinical findings as well as the phenomenon of genetic anticipation. This refers to the fact that as a mutant gene is passed through successive generations there appears to be an earlier onset and an increased severity of the clinical phenotype in affected individuals.

Near to or within these genes there are sequences consisting of trinucleotide repeats. In the normal population, the copy number is variable but is contained within a specific limit (between 5 and about 35 for myotonic dystrophy), and is inherited in a stable fashion from generation to generation. Some individuals carry an increased copy number on one chromosome (between 50 and about 100 repeats for myotonic dystrophy) and this is referred to as a premutation. With very small increases these people may be totally asymptomatic but with larger increases in the premutation range they may manifest very mild symptoms of the disorder. Within this premutation range, the sequence is unstable and has a tendency to increase as it is passed through successive generations. A very large increase in the copy number (sometimes to several thousand) is associated with the increased severity and earlier age of onset of the clinical phenotype. The size of the expansion can vary from one meiosis to another and so a carrier of a premutation can have several children with varying degrees of expressivity of the disorder, depending on the size of the expanded fragment that they have inherited. The underlying cause of the expansion from a normal range to a premutation range has yet to be elucidated but it is thought that an imperfect trinucleotide repeat sequence is more stably inherited than a perfect one.

In vitro expression analysis and genotype/phenotype correlations

The first evidence for an association between a single base substitution and a clinical phenotype is usually obtained through genetic studies: that is, the observed mutation is never observed on a large number of normal alleles and it segregates only with the disease phenotype in family pedigrees. However, in order to verify the effect of a single base substitution on protein function, additional evidence is required. It has already been mentioned that when a protein is normally synthesised in readily accessible fluid or tissue, the presence or absence of antibody cross-reacting material (CRM+ or CRM–) in a patient's sample can help to establish whether the mutation affects the synthesis of the relevant protein. Unfortunately when the protein is expressed only in less accessible tissue such as liver or brain, alternative strategies must be used. In vitro expression analysis is a valuable technique which can demonstrate the effect of an observed single gene alteration on protein function.

In this technique, site-directed mutagenesis is used to introduce the mutation into an otherwise normal cDNA sequence which is incorporated into an expression vector. Normal and mutant constructs are then separately introduced into cultured cells and, following incubation, the levels of mRNA, immunoreactive protein and functional activity are compared. Thus, this provides a mechanism for confirming that the sequence change is, indeed, a mutation and for determining whether the mutation primarily affects the synthesis of mRNA, the synthesis of the protein molecule or the function of the protein.

While useful for providing further evidence for an association between a particular gene alteration and the clinical phenotype, expression analysis is not without limitations, and some degree of caution must be used if studies of different mutations at the same locus are being used to establish a genotype/phenotype correlation. For example, the levels of residual enzyme activity obtained in expression studies are often significantly higher than those obtained from biopsied tissue specimens and so in vitro studies cannot be used to assess absolute in vivo activities. For those genetic disorders which are highly heterogeneous, the situation can be complicated further by the fact that an affected individual is likely to bear two different mutant alleles and thus a mixture of protein species. A simple average of the in vitro levels of enzyme activity associated with the proteins produced by each mutant allele does not give an exact measure of in vivo activity;

nevertheless, this rudimentary formula appears to allow a qualitative correlation to be drawn between 'predicted enzyme activity' and severity of the clinical phenotype.[13]

In addition to this, gene dosage or negative allelic complementation might affect the manifestation of genotype in vivo. For example, when the functional enzyme is a dimer of two identical protein subunits, the synthesis of two protein species in an individual who is a compound heterozygote for two different mutations would result in three types of functional (or non-functional) enzyme. The contribution of each unit to overall enzyme activity in vivo depends on whether either mutation affects protein stability or the rate of protein synthesis. Detailed examination of allelic complementation awaits the development of more sophisticated expression systems which are capable of producing equivalent amounts of different mutant peptides.

One final limitation is the fact that expression studies of a single mutant gene do not take account of the effects of other genes and environmental factors that might be important determinants of the protein's function or of substrate homeostasis.

Despite these considerable drawbacks, expression analysis appears to provide extremely useful genotype/phenotype correlations when sufficiently large numbers of patients of widely differing phenotypes are examined.

REFERENCES

1. Garrod A E 1908 Inborn errors of metabolism (Croonian Lectures). Lancet 2:1, 73, 142, 214
2. Dent C E, Rose G A 1951 Amino acid metabolism in cystinuria. Quarterly Journal of Medicine 20:205
3. Watson J D, Hopkins N H, Roberts J W, Steitz J A, Weiner A M 1988 Molecular biology of the gene, 4th edn. The Benjamin/Cummings Publishing Co, California
4. Oberle I, Roussear F, Heitz C, Devys D, Hanauer A, Boue J, Bertheas M F, Mandel J L 1991 Instability of a 550-base pair DNA and abnormal methylation in fragile X syndrome. Science 252:1097–1102
5. Verkerk A J, Pieretti M, Sutcliffe J S, Fu Y H, Kuhl D P, Pizzuti A, Reiner O, Richards S et al 1991 ldentification of a gene (FMR-1) containing a CGG repeat coincident with a breakpoint cluster region exhibiting length variation in fragile X syndrome. Cell 65:905–914
6. LaSpada A R, Wilson E M, Lubahn D B, Harding A E, Fischbeck K H 1991 Androgen receptor gene mutations in X-linked spinal and bulbar muscular atrophy. Nature 352:77–79
7. Harley H G, Brook J D, Rundle S A, Crow S, Reardon W, Buckler A J, Harper P S, Housman D E, Shaw D J 1992 Expansion of an unstable DNA region and phenotypic variation in myotonic dystrophy. Nature 355:545–6
8. Cooper C N, Youssoufian H 1988 The CpG dinucleotide and human genetic disease. Human Genetics 78:151–155
9. Beadle G W 1945 Biochemical genetics. Chemical Reviews 37:15
10. Butler J L, Cooper M D, 1989 Antibody deficiency diseases. In: Scriver C R, Beaudet A L, Sly W S, Valle D (eds) The metabolic basis of inherited disease, 6th edn. McGraw–Hill, New York, p 2687–2688
11. Sykes B 1985 The inherited genetics of collagen. BioEssays 3:112–117

12. Smith I, Beasley M G, Ades A E 1990 Effect on intelligence of relaxing the low phenylalanine diet in phenylketonuria. Archives of Disease in Childhood 65:311–316
13. Okano Y, Eisensmith R C, Guttler F, Lichter-Konecki U, Konecki D, Trefz F K, Dasovich M, Wang T, Henriksen K, Lou H, Woo S L C 1991 Molecular basis of phenotypic heterogeneity in phenylketonuria. New England Journal of Medicine 324:1232–1238

Appendix 1 Amino acids

Amino Acid	Three letter symbol	One letter symbol
Alanine	Ala	A
Arginine	Arg	R
Asparagine	Asn	N
Aspartic acid	Asp	D
Asparagine or Aspartic acid	Asx	B
Cysteine	Cys	C
Glutamine	Gln	Q
Glutamic Acid	Glu	E
Glutamine or Glutamic Acid	Glx	Z
Glycine	Gly	G
Histidine	His	H
Isoleucine	Ile	I
Leucine	Leu	L
Lysine	Lys	K
Methionine	Met	M
Phenylalanine	Phe	F
Proline	Pro	P
Serine	Ser	S
Threonine	Thr	T
Tryptophan	Trp	W
Tyrosine	Tyr	Y
Valine	Val	V

2. Disorders of carbohydrate metabolism

D. B. Dunger J. B. Holton

INTRODUCTION

The major dietary carbohydrates, starch, sucrose, and lactose are hydrolysed in the gut. The free monosaccharides glucose, fructose and galactose are then absorbed and reach the liver via the portal circulation, where they are rapidly utilised. Glucose is phosphorylated within the hepatocyte to glucose-6-phosphate by glucokinase. The hexose sugars, fructose and galactose are also taken up by the hepatocyte and enter the pathways of carbohydrate metabolism as triose sugars and glucose-1-phosphate respectively (Fig. 2.1).

Carbohydrate metabolism in the liver is primarily concerned with the maintenance of plasma glucose homeostasis. Glucose may be generated by the breakdown of stored glycogen, the uptake and metabolism of dietary carbohydrate, and gluconeogenesis whereby amino acids, glycerol and lactate are metabolised via a reversal of the glycolytic sequence.

Glucose-6-phosphate occupies a central position in carbohydrate metabolism, for there are five direct pathways for its metabolism:

1. Synthesis of glycogen
2. Glycolysis to yield either lactic acid or, through acetyl CoA and the Krebs cycle, to yield CO_2
3. Release as free glucose
4. Via the pentose cycle with production of NADPH and CO_2
5. Glucuronate formation.

Curiously the first defect of carbohydrate metabolism to be identified, pentosuria, which is the result of an enzyme defect affecting the last of these pathways, glucuronate formation, proved to be the least clinically important. Essential pentosuria (McKusick 260800) first described by Salkowski and Jashrowitz in 1892[1], is the result of a defect in the glucuronic acid oxidation pathway. It has an incidence of 1:40 000, and occurs primarily in those of Jewish race, being inherited as an autosomal recessive. Apart from the diagnostic confusion with diabetes mellitus it has no clinical significance.

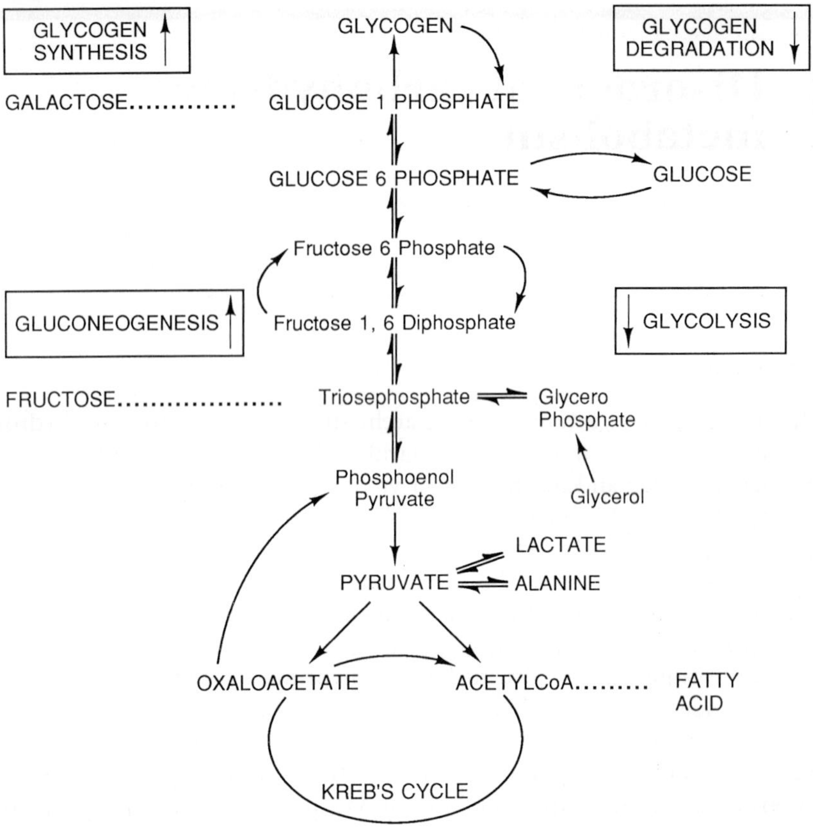

Fig. 2.1 The major pathways of carbohydrate metabolism.

Since the early description, inborn errors involving all of the major pathways of carbohydrate metabolism have been discovered and these will be surveyed in the following chapter.

DISORDERS OF GLYCOGEN METABOLISM

The first description of a child with an apparent defect of glycogen mobilisation appeared in 1928 and the hepatic form of glycogen storage disease (GSD) was identified by Von Gierke the following year. Four years later Pompe described a patient where the glycogen accumulation was principally in the heart, and in 1951 McArdle reported a condition presenting in adult life with excess glycogen deposition in skeletal muscle. Hepatic glucose-6-phosphatase deficiency (Von Gierke's disease) was the first enzyme defect to be identified and there followed identification of many other defects of glycogen metabolism.

Normal glycogen metabolism

Glucose is stored as glycogen, a high molecular weight polysaccharide, present in many cells, but principally found in the liver and muscle. It has a branched structure being composed of glucose residues linked by (1–4) bonds to form long chains, which are branched every 12–18 residues by the inclusion of a (1–6) linkage (Fig. 2.2). The precursor for glycogen synthesis is glucose-1-phosphate which is in equilibrium with glucose-6-phosphate (Fig. 2.1). Glucose-1-phosphate is converted to uridine disphosphoglucose (UDPglc) by a specific pyrophosphorylase. In a second reaction, catalysed by glycogen synthetase (EC 2.4.1.21), the glucose residue from UDPglc is attached to a glycogen primer through a (1–4) bond, lengthening the glucose chain. The branch points of the glycogen molecule are incorporated by the action of the branching enzyme (amylo (1–4), (1–6) transglucosidase, EC 2.4.1.18).

Glycogen degradation is mediated through two enzyme systems: phosphorylase and the debrancher (amylo-(1–6)-glucosidase). The enzyme phosphorylase (EC 2.4.1.1) exists in two forms, one active and the other inactive. The activation of phosphorylase is complex and involves several steps. It is initiated by glucagon and adrenaline which cause the release of a second messenger, cyclic (3'5')-adenosine monophosphate, from the cell membrane. This in turn activates a series of enzymes including a specific phosphorylase kinase (EC 2.7.1.38) which result in the conversion of phosphorylase from its inactive to its active form (Fig. 2.3). Once activated, phosphorylase cleaves the (1–4) bonds of glycogen releasing glucose-1-phosphate but it does not hydrolyse the (1–6) bonds and stops along the straight chains four glucose residues from the branch points. The debrancher enzyme (EC 3.2.1.33, transferase 2.4.1.25) is necessary for

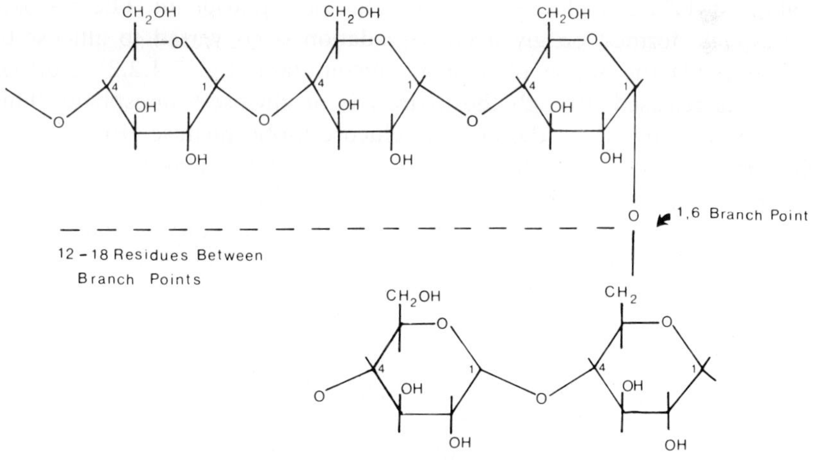

Fig. 2.2 The structure of glycogen.

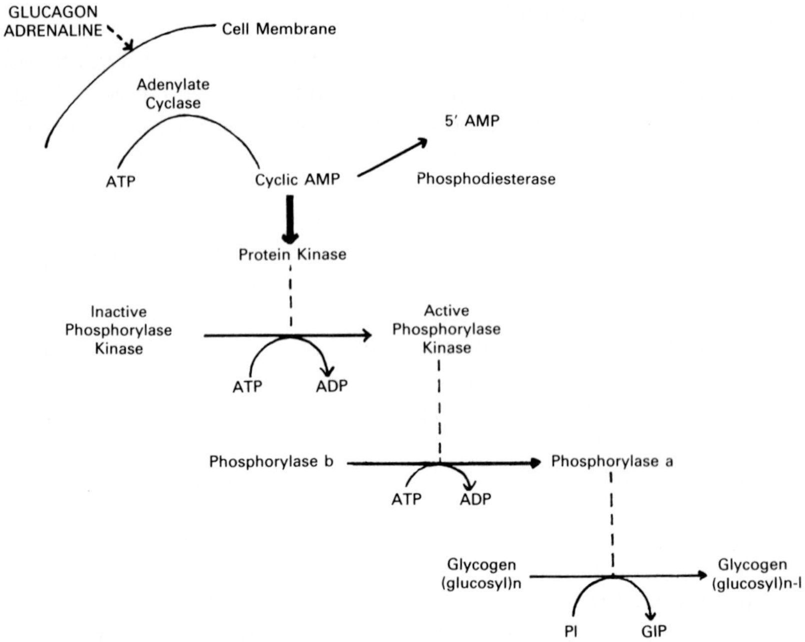

Fig. 2.3 A schematic representation of the phosphorylase cascade.

glycogen breakdown to proceed. Three glucose residues are transferred from the side-chain to the main chain by the transferase that forms part of the debrancher enzyme, leaving one glucose residue which is linked by a (1–6) bond. This is then hydrolysed by the debrancher, amylo-(1–6)-glucosidase. Sequential degradation of glycogen results in the production of about 8–12% free glucose and 90% glucose-1-phosphate. The glucose-1-phosphate formed on glycogen degradation is converted to glucose-6-phosphate via the action of phosphoglucomutase (EC 5.4.2.2). Further glucose is released through the hydrolysis of glucose-6-phosphate. This reaction is catalysed by the enzyme glucose-6-phosphatase (EC 3.1.3.9) which is found only in the liver, kidney and intestinal mucosa.

Glucose-6-phosphatase activity plays a central role in the regulation of blood glucose levels, and its molecular structure and regulation are complex. Glucose-6-phosphatase has been shown to comprise at least five different polypeptides.[2] The catalytic subunit of glucose-6-phosphatase is situated in the lumen of the endoplasmic reticulum and is associated with a calcium-dependent regulatory protein (Fig. 2.4). In addition there are at least three transport proteins, T1, T2 and T3 which transport glucose-6-phosphate, phosphate (and pyrophosphate) and glucose, respectively, across the endoplasmic reticulum membrane. Glucose-6-phosphate enters the lumen of the endoplasmic reticulum on a transport protein (T1); it is then

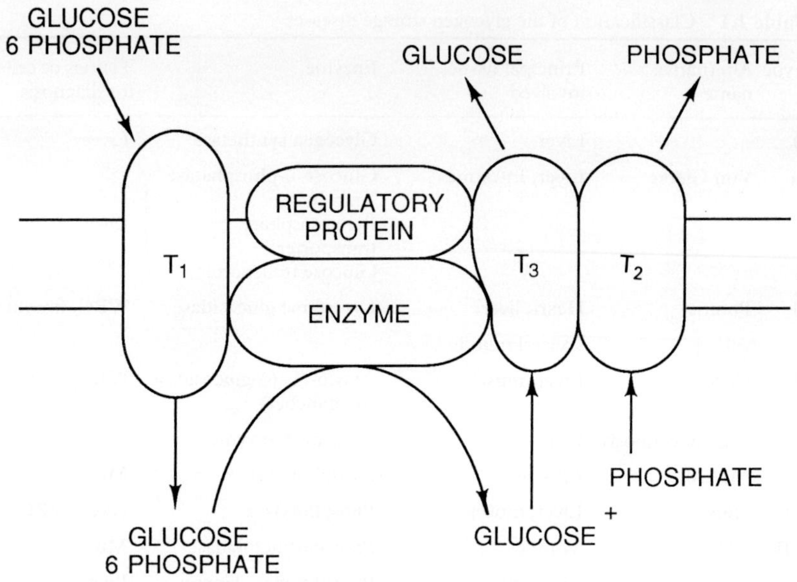

Fig. 2.4 A schematic model for the molecular organisation of hepatic microsomal glucose-6-phosphatase complex. (After Burchell[2].)

hydrolysed by the glucose-6-phosphatase enzyme. The transport proteins T2 and T3 return the products, glucose and phosphate, to the cytosol.

Hepatic glycogen functions as a reserve of glucose which is utilised during fasting. Glycogen synthesis and degradation are finely regulated by a number of substrate cycles and a variety of endocrine stimuli including insulin, adrenaline and glucagon[3].

Classification of the glycogen storage disorders

The classification of the glycogen storage diseases is confusing as the conditions were numbered in the order that they were first described and the various forms of Type I have only recently been elucidated. The classification shown in Table 2.1 is based on specific enzyme defects, but it also takes into account the tissues that are affected. Type VIII has been excluded because as yet no enzyme deficiency has been demonstrated in those children who have cerebral deposition of glycogen.[4] Discussion of Type II (Pompe's disease) where the defect is of lysosomal glucosidase is more appropriately reserved for the chapter on lysosomal disorders (Ch.5).

Although several of these conditions affect both hepatic and muscle glycogen, it is convenient to distinguish those disorders where the liver is principally affected from those where the primary defect is in muscle glycogen metabolism.

Table 2.1 Classification of the glycogen storage diseases

Type	Alternative name	Principal tissues involved	Enzyme	Tissues or cells for diagnosis
O		Liver	Glycogen synthetase	Liver
Ia	Von Gierke	Liver, Intestine	Glucose-6-phosphatase	Liver
b			Translocase	Liver
c			Pyrophosphate transporter	Liver
d			Glucose transporter	Liver
II	Pompe	Heart, liver, skeletal muscle	Lysosomal glucosidase	WBC, fibroblasts
III	Cori	Liver, muscle	Amylo-(1–6)-glucosidase (debrancher)	WBC, liver
IV	Amylopectinosis	Liver	Branching enzyme	Liver
V	McArdle	Muscle	Phosphorylase	Muscle
VI	Hers	Liver, muscle	Phosphorylase	Liver, WBC
VII		Muscle	Phosphofructokinase	Muscle, RBC
IX		Liver, muscle	Phosphorylase kinase	Liver, RBC

HEPATIC GLYCOGEN STORAGE DISEASES

The overall frequency of the hepatic glycogen storage diseases is approximately 1:60 000 live births. Type I with an incidence of 1:200 000 was thought to be the most common form, but the defects of phosphorylase kinase (Type IX) which are often asymptomatic may be more frequent than was previously suspected.[5]

The enzyme defects and their clinical presentation

Glucose-6-phosphatase

Glucose-6-phosphatase deficiency (Type Ia or Von Gierke's disease McKusick 232200) classically presents in early infancy with hepatomegaly, fasting hypoglycaemia and recurrent acidosis. However, it has long been recognised that there are children who are clinically and biochemically indistinguishable from Type Ia but have normal glucose-6-phosphatase activity in the liver.[6] It has since been discovered that freezing of liver biopsy specimens prior to enzyme assay disrupted the complex subunit structure of glucose-6-phosphatase activity in the hepatocyte. Recent improvements in both conventional glucose-6-phosphatase microassay techniques and transport assays in both intact and disrupted microsomes have permitted the identification of a number of additional disorders. These include Type Ib, a defect of the transport protein T1, (McKusick 232220), and Type Ic a deficiency of the pyrophosphate transport protein

(McKusick 232240). Other possible defects include a deficiency of the glucose transporter (T3) and of the 21 KDa regulatory protein.

The clinical features of these various forms of Type I are very similar and can be considered together although there is considerable variation in the severity of the clinical presentation. In its most severe form it may present within the first few days of life with profound hypoglycaemia and acidosis. On the other hand it may present in later childhood with short stature and hepatomegaly. Abnormal bleeding, usually epistaxis may occur and gastrointestinal symptoms such as intermittent diarrhoea, vomiting and failure to thrive are surprisingly common.

The infants are short, with decreased muscle mass, and a protuberant abdomen due to massive hepatomegaly. Adipose tissue around the face may be increased: the so called 'doll-like' facies. There is no splenomegaly and there are no signs of cirrhosis. Renal enlargement may be noted on ultrasound examination. Xanthomata and lipaemia retinalis have been reported but are very rare.

In most respects, patients with Type Ib and Ic are indistinguishable from those with Type I although they do tend to present with a severe form of the disease. Recurrent bacterial infections due to abnormalities of neutrophil mobility and neutropenia, have been described in Type Ib but not in Type Ia. Vitamin D-resistant rickets and a Fanconi syndrome have also been reported, but again, probably only in Type Ib.

All of these conditions are inherited as autosomal recessives.

Amylo-(1–6)glucosidase, the debranching enzyme (Type III)

The majority of children with deficiency of the debranching enzyme amylo-(1–6)-glucosidase (McKusick 232400), present within the first year of life with fasting hypoglycaemic convulsions and hepatomegaly, although a few will be diagnosed in later childhood when they are investigated for short stature and the protuberant abdomen and hepatomegaly are noted. As in Type I, diarrhoea may be a common symptom at presentation. Type III is inherited as an autosomal recessive.

Hepatic phosphorylase and phosphorylase kinase (Type VI and IX)

Low activity of phosphorylase in the liver was first reported in 1959 but the deficiency was not complete and it was not possible to decide whether the primary defect was of the phosphorylase or the kinase. Improved methodology has enabled recognition of several enzyme defects of the phosphorylase complex.[7]

Clinically, these patients have a very mild disease. Hypoglycaemia occasionally occurs in patients with phosphorylase deficiency but not in phosphorylase kinase deficiency. Hepatomegaly develops slowly and may only be noted as an incidental finding. Muscular hypotonia may be present.

Although growth delay may be evident at diagnosis, catch-up occurs during childhood. There has been one report of two children with phosphorylase kinase deficiency who developed nodular cirrhosis with portal hypertension in later childhood.[7]

Phosphorylase kinase deficiency is by far the commonest defect of the phosphorylase cascade and it is inherited as an X-linked recessive (Type IXb, McKusick 306000), or more rarely as an autosomal recessive (Type IXa, McKusick 261750). The deficiency of phosphorylase itself (Type VI, McKusick 232700) is inherited as an autosomal recessive.

Glycogen synthetase deficiency (Type 0)

Children with glycogen synthetase deficiency (McKusick 240600) present during the first year with hypoglycaemic convulsions after fasting. Ketosis is evident but the patients do not have hepatomegaly or any of the other features characteristic of the hepatic glycogen storage disorders. Glycogen synthetase has been reported in twins and an unrelated girl, and is probably inherited as an autosomal recessive.

Amylo-(1–4),(1–6)-transglucosidase, the branching enzyme (Type IV)

Type IV is probably the rarest form of hepatic glycogen storage disease (McKusick 232500). Infants with the condition are normal at birth, but develop failure to thrive, hepatomegaly and splenomegaly within a few months. Hypotonia, muscular atrophy and absent reflexes may be noted. Cirrhosis and portal hypertension follow, and death usually occurs within 2 years unless liver transplantation is undertaken. Heart dilatation with polysaccharide accumulation has been reported and death can occur from tamponade and cardiac failure. The diagnosis can be made by examination of leucocytes which contain an abnormal polysaccharide, or at liver biopsy. The enzyme defect is inherited as an autosomal recessive.

Pathophysiology

The pathogenesis of the various types of glycogen storage disease can be predicted in part from the site of the enzyme defects.

Glucose-6-phosphatase activity is essential for the normal release of hepatic glucose, irrespective of whether it is the product of glycogenolysis or gluconeogenesis. Further, the metabolism of the other hexose sugars, fructose and galactose will not result in the release of free glucose in the absence of the enzyme. Glucose production rates range between 30–100% of normal[8] and fasting hypoglycaemia is a common finding in Type I.

During fasting, the humoral response to hypoglycaemia (glucagon and adrenaline) results in activation of phosphorylase and hepatic glycogenolysis. The resulting glucose-6-phosphate is metabolised via glycolysis to lactate. Gluconeogenic activity is also increased and there is recycling between lactate and glycogen; however, overall there is net production of lactate by the liver and an increase in blood lactate concentrations.[9]

The increase in glycerol, acetyl CoA and NADH generated by the increased flux of the glycolytic pathway contributes to an increased rate of triglyceride and cholesterol synthesis. Serum cholesterol concentrations are elevated in Type I. Hypoglycaemia will also lead to an increase in the mobilisation of peripheral lipid stores with a rise in circulating free fatty acids. Clearance of chylomicra and very low density lipoprotein (VLDL) is also impaired because of reduced activities of hepatic and extrahepatic lipoprotein lipase.

Plasma urate levels are elevated in Type I. This was originally attributed to competitive inhibition of urate excretion by lactate; however an increased rate of purine synthesis is probably a more important contributory factor. The mechanisms leading to increased purine synthesis are not clear, but raised levels of glutamine and depletion of hepatic nucleotides[10] may be important in this respect and similar metabolic abnormalities in other carbohydrate disorders will be described in later sections of this chapter.

The abnormal bleeding in Type I is thought to be due to a defect of platelet adhesiveness secondary to hypoglycaemia. The gastrointestinal symptoms are only partially understood. There does not appear to be any intolerance to mono- or disaccharides or to fat, but impaired glucose absorption has been demonstrated which might contribute to the pathogenesis of the diarrhoea. The vomiting and failure to thrive are probably related to recurrent acidosis.

The enzyme defects in the other two major forms of hepatic GSD (Type III and defects of the phosphorylase cascade) impair breakdown of glycogen, but do not interfere with glucose synthesis via gluconeogenesis. This is undoubtedly one explanation for the generally less severe hypoglycaemia and clinical presentation of these conditions. Fasting lactate concentrations are normal in Type III although they may be raised after a carbohydrate meal. Fasting lactate in Type IX may be normal or only very slightly raised. Ketonuria is a common finding in both conditions and fasting ketone concentrations in the plasma are elevated whereas they are low in Type I. Concentrations of urate and cholesterol may be slightly elevated in Type III, but they are frequently normal in disorders of the phosphorylase complex.

The growth delay which occurs in the hepatic glycogen storage diseases is not completely understood.[11] A number of endocrine abnormalities have been described including low levels of insulin and insulin-like growth factor-1, together with normal or elevated growth hormone, and raised cortisol concentrations. It has been suggested that growth delay may be part of an hormonal adaptation to the failure to maintain normal glucose homeostasis[12], although chronic acidosis and disordered calcium metabolism may also be important.

Diagnosis

A diagnosis of hepatic glycogen storage disease is usually suggested by the finding of hypoglycaemia and hepatomegaly. The standard fasting glucagon test (20 μg/kg i.m.) is useful in this situation although it is important to remember that there may be considerable variation in the response (Fig. 2.5). A normal test response is defined as a rise in blood glucose of more than 2 mmol/1 or 50% over the fasting level. Some children with Type I have a normal response to glucagon, but lactate levels are invariably elevated during the test.

The glucagon test should not be carried out in children who clearly have severe fasting hypoglycaemia or severe lactic acidaemia, and alone it will not necessarily differentiate between the various types of hepatic glycogen storage disease.

The type of glycogen storage disease may be evident from clinical history alone, but there are a few additional biochemical pointers which may be of help. Whereas lactate concentrations may be slightly elevated in Type IX, they are normal except after a carbohydrate meal in Type III, and significant lactic acidaemia either fasting or during the glucagon test always points to Type I. The only other differential diagnoses are the disorders of gluconeogenesis. High plasma concentrations of urate and blood lipids usually indicate Type I, but cholesterol concentrations may be quite high in Type III.

In the past, a variety of loading tests have been recommended for the further differentiation of the various types of hepatic glycogen storage disease. These include: the oral glucose tolerance combined with a postprandial glucagon test[13]; intravenous glucose[14] or fructose tolerance tests and glycerol loading tests[15]. However, these tests may be technically difficult and distressing in young infants and do not always give clear results. Ultimately the diagnosis must be established by enzymology, and for Type III, VI and IX, this is possible by examination of peripheral blood cells. The approach outlined in Figure 2.6 offers a simple and reliable guide to the diagnosis of the common forms of hepatic glycogen storage disease.

The definitive diagnosis of Type I glycogen storage disease can only be made by liver biopsy. Differentiation between the various types of defects requires a complete kinetic analysis of the glucose-6-phosphatase activity with at least two substrates in both the intact and fully disrupted microsomes (i.e. in fresh and frozen liver biopsy material).

The diagnosis of Type III can also be made at liver biopsy but it is more

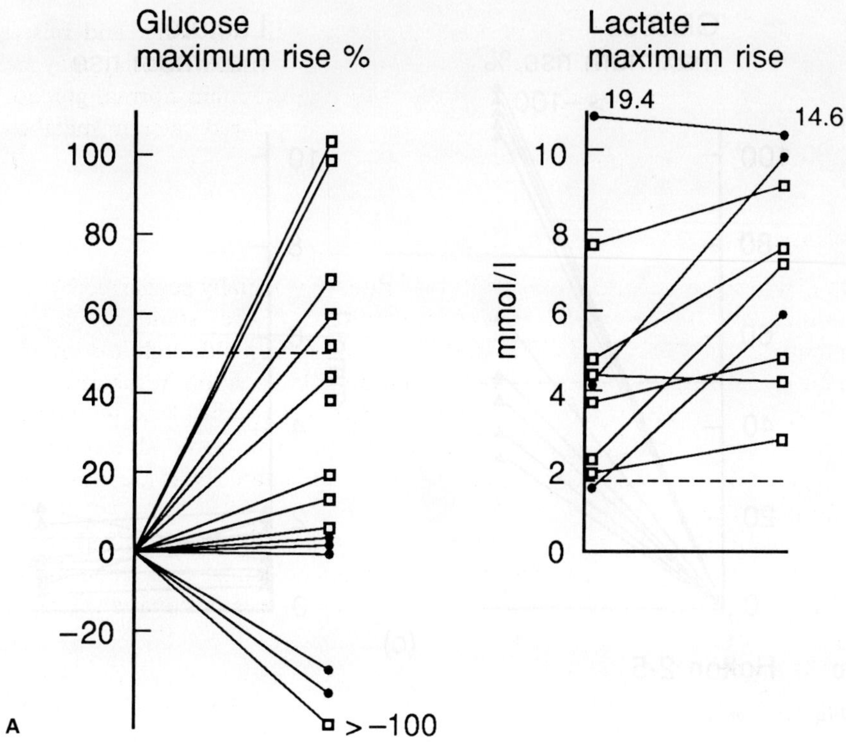

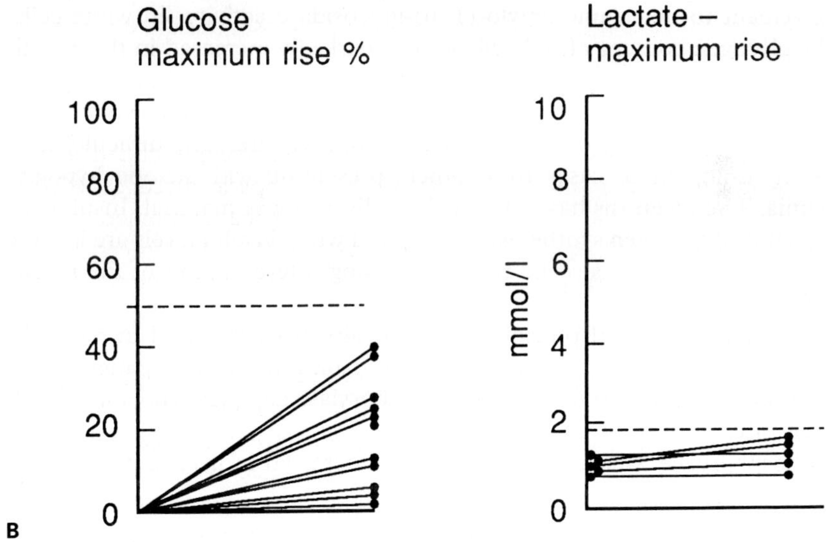

Fig. 2.5 Maximum change in blood glucose and lactate during fasting glucagon tests in patients with: **A** Type 1A (□) and Type IB (•), **B** Type III, and **C** Type IX hepatic glycogen storage disease.

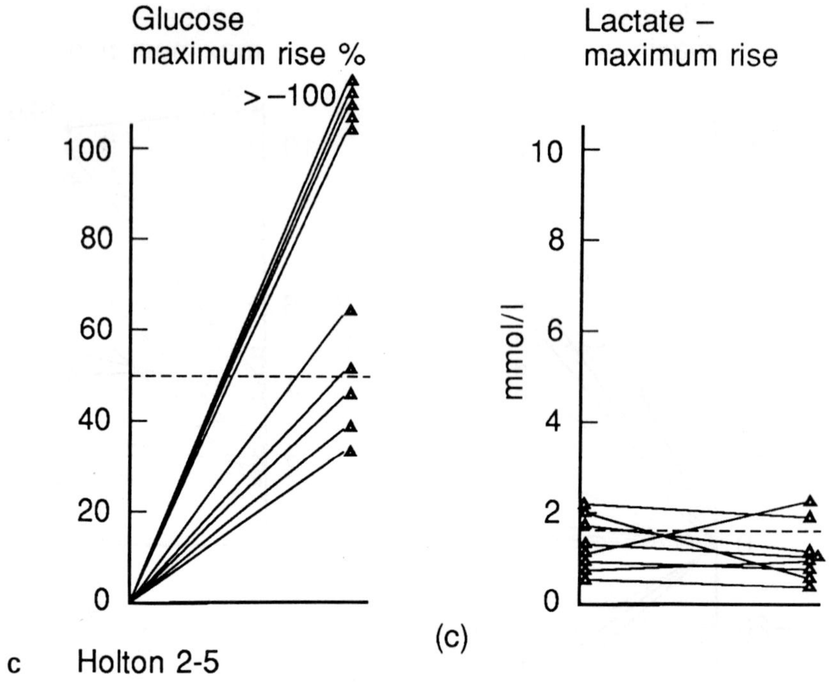

Fig. 2.5 *contd.*

convenient to determine amylo-(1–6)-glucosidase activity in white cells. The glycogen content of red cells is also markedly increased in this condition[16].

Phosphorylase deficiency has been diagnosed in liver and white blood cells. True deficiency of this enzyme is probably rare. The difficulty is in distinguishing these cases from others presenting with ketotic hypoglycaemia. The diagnosis has to be made on liver biopsy material. Insulin is a regulator of glycogen synthetase activity and when insulin levels are low the enzyme activity may also be reduced making interpretation of the results difficult.

Partial deficiency of phosphorylase has also been reported in red cells, with normal activity in liver, and there remain a number of patients with reduced activity of enzymes of the phosphorylase complex who are difficult to classify.[7]

Phosphorylase kinase deficiency can be detected in liver and red blood cells.

Treatment

Children with Type I glycogen storage disease require continuous enteral

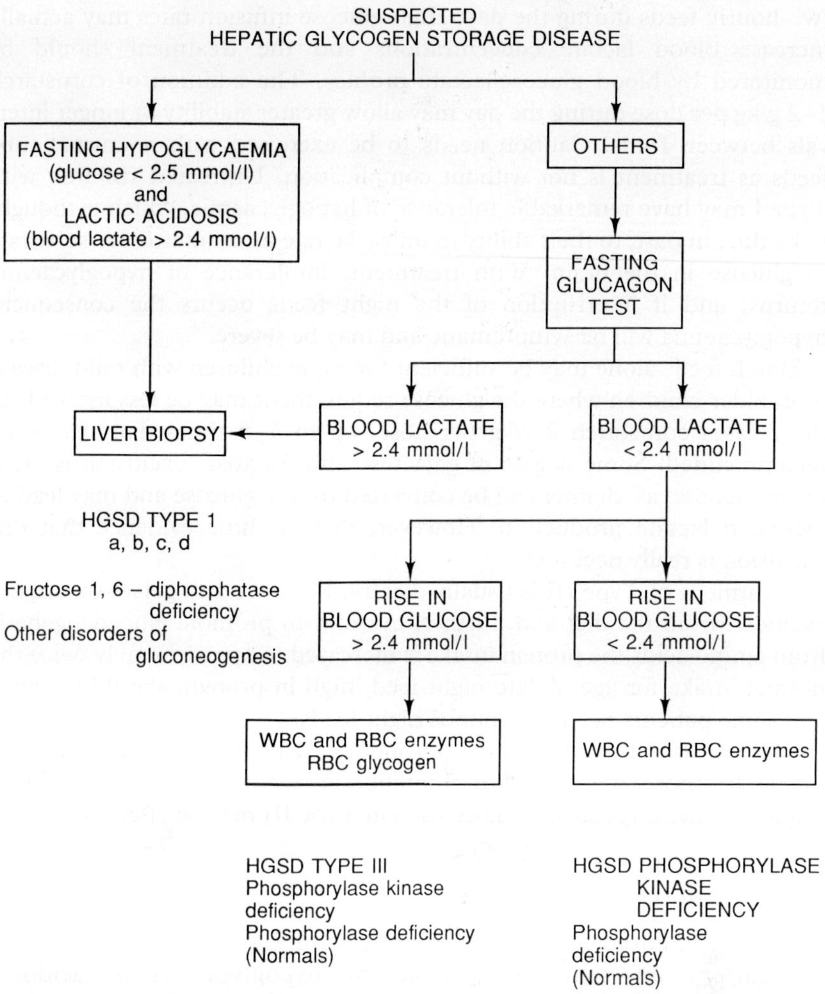

Fig. 2.6 A scheme for establishing the diagnosis of hepatic glycogen storage disease (HGSD).

glucose in quantities which equal or even exceed the normal hepatic glucose production rate (0.25–0.5 g kg^{-1} h^{-1}, or 8–9 mg kg^{-1} min^{-1}).[17] Other forms of treatment such as frequent carbohydrate feeds, diazoxide or portocaval anastamosis fail to correct the acidosis, hyperlipidaemia, hyperuricaemia and growth delay which contribute to the morbidity of this condition.

The glucose can be provided either as a combination of frequent glucose drinks by day with nasogastric tube feeds at night or as frequent starch feeds alone. Nasogastric night feeds are usually necessary in small infants where hypoglycaemia is a common feature. The polymer Caloreen is given at a rate of 0.5 g kg^{-1} h^{-1} overnight and, in the same quantities, as hourly or two-hourly feeds during the day. High glucose infusion rates may actually increase blood lactate concentrations and the treatment should be monitored by blood glucose/lactate profiles. The addition of cornstarch 1–2 g/kg per dose during the day may allow greater stability or longer intervals between feeds. Caution needs to be exercised with nocturnal tube feeds as treatment is not without complication. Untreated children with Type I may have remarkable tolerance of hypoglycaemia, which is thought to be due, in part, to their ability to utilise lactate as an alternative substrate to glucose in the brain. With treatment, intolerance of hypoglycaemia returns, and if interruption of the night feeds occurs the consequent hypoglycaemia will be symptomatic and may be severe.[18]

Starch feeds alone may be sufficient for some children with mild disease or in older children where the glucose requirement may be less marked. In these cases cornstarch 2 g/kg per dose, up to 4–5 times daily has been recommended. Some degree of galactose and fructose exclusion is often recommended as neither can be converted to free glucose and may lead to increased lactate production. However, there is little evidence that this exclusion is really necessary.

Treatment of Type III is usually dietary. Fructose and galactose are not excluded from the diet and, further, in order to promote gluconeogenesis from amino acids the protein intake is increased to approximately twice the normal intake for age. A late night feed, high in protein, should be given and some patients need continuous night feeds.

Children with disorders of the phosphorylase complex rarely need treatment. In those who are symptomatic, or whose growth is seriously impaired, measures such as those used in Type III may be effective.

Outcome of treatment

Untreated children with Type I may die during infancy or later from intercurrent infections complicated by hypoglycaemia or acidosis. However, there is considerable variation. Survival beyond adolescence is associated with adaptation to the disease and amelioration of the symptoms. Successful pregnancies in patients with Type I have been reported. Severe growth delay usually occurs and sexual maturation is delayed. Gout and uric acid nephropathy may develop and there have been an increasing number of reports of hepatic adenomata. Furthermore, there have been reports of hepatocellular carcinoma developing in patients thought to have benign adenomata, but this appears to be very rare.

Satisfactory treatment of Type I results in improvements in growth, a reduction in liver size and correction of the metabolic abnormalities, and hepatic adenomata may be prevented. However, intensive treatment may not improve all the biochemical abnormalities. Urate levels remain elevated and treatment with allopurinol is often necessary. High low-density lipoprotein (LDL) and low high-density lipoprotein (HDL) cholesterol and hypertriglyceridaemia levels may persist, even in children treated with nocturnal nasogastric tube feeds, and patients may remain at risk of developing atherosclerosis in later life. With longer survival and surveillance into adult life, it has also become clear that patients with Type I may also develop renal disease. Following a 'silent' period, characterised by glomerular hyperfiltration and microalbuminuria, progression to hypertension and chronic renal failure may occur in adult life.[19] The effects of intensive therapy on this progression have not yet been determined.

Treatment of Type III is generally successful; with adolescence the hepatomegaly becomes less pronounced and catch-up growth occurs, although sexual maturation may be delayed. The associated myopathy is generally mild, although occasionally it may be severe and the cardiomyopathy does not improve with intensive treatment. Rarely, cirrhosis requiring portal diversion, or milder degrees of hepatic fibrosis, may develop.

THE MUSCLE GLYCOGEN STORAGE DISEASES

The muscles are affected in the previously described Types III, VI and IX glycogen storage diseases and the resulting myopathy may be quite severe in Type III. There are two conditions, Type V (McArdle) which is a defect of muscle phosphorylase and Type VII, where the enzyme phosphofructokinase is deficient, which primarily affect skeletal muscle.

In contrast to hepatic glycogen, muscle glycogen functions solely as a fuel reserve for ATP generation during muscle contraction and does not contribute to maintaining plasma glucose homeostasis. Glycogen synthesis and degradation in muscle involve similar pathways to those found in liver but isoenzymes are present. The activation of phosphorylase is controlled by changes in the concentrations of ATP, AMP and adrenaline. Generally, muscle glycogen is oxidised when supplies of glucose and fatty acids are low, to provide additional energy, but under conditions where oxygen is lacking glycogen can be degraded to lactate by glycolysis. Phosphofructokinase (EC 2.7.1.11), the enzyme which catalyses the conversion of fructose-6-phosphate to fructose 1:6-diphosphate, is important in the regulation of glycolysis in muscle.

Muscle phosphorylase deficiency (Type V)

Deficiency of muscle phosphorylase or McArdle's disease (McKusick 232600) usually presents in adult life and symptoms in childhood are rare. During the teenage years the only symptom is muscle fatigue particularly after strenuous exercise. With early adult life progressive weakness develops associated with cramping pains, and myoglobinuria may occur. No muscle wasting is noted until the 4th or 5th decade. Hepatomegaly is absent and the cardiovascular system is normal. Fasting hypoglycaemia does not occur.

The diagnosis can be confirmed by muscle biopsy. The activity of phosphorylase is reduced and the glycogen content is either elevated or at the upper limit of normal. Muscle phosphorylase deficiency is inherited as an autosomal recessive.

Phosphofructokinase deficiency Type VII

The clinical presentation of this disease (McKusick 232800) is identical to that seen in McArdle's disease although one child has been described who presented in infancy and died, aged 6 months, of respiratory failure.

Muscle phosphofructokinase is a different isoenzyme from that found in the liver. Erythrocytes have approximately half of each form and in affected individuals levels are reduced by 50%. Absence of the muscle isoenzyme may be confirmed in muscle biopsy specimens.

Pathophysiology

Resting muscle derives its energy mainly from the oxidation of glucose and fatty acids. The requirement for ATP may increase 100-fold during strenuous exercise and the demand exceeds the supply of substrates from the blood, despite increases in blood flow. Glycogenolysis occurs under these circumstances, supplying substrate for oxidation or anaerobic metabolism to lactate.

Deficiency of the phosphorylase results in an inability to catabolise glycogen, limiting the availability of this important source of substrate. The phenomenon of 'second wind' is often described in McArdle's disease, where continued exercise actually leads to a lessening of symptoms. It has been suggested that this results from changes in blood flow and increased availability of alternative substrates such as free fatty acids.

Diagnosis

Ischaemic exercise in patients with Type V and VII fails to produce a rise in blood lactate. During attacks myoglobinuria may be noted and lactate dehydrogenase, aldolase and creatinine kinase levels may be elevated in the blood. The reduced tolerance of exercise can be demonstrated by getting the patient to squeeze a rubber ball while a blood pressure cuff is inflated to above systolic but this test can be very painful. Nuclear magnetic resonance may offer an alternative aid to diagnosis. Phosphorus nuclear magnetic resonance (^{31}P NMR) permits non-invasive measurements of intracellular pH, ATP and phosphocreatine. McArdle's patients differ from normal in having no fall in intramuscular pH and an excessive reduction in phosphocreatine in response to exercise.[20]

Treatment

Avoidance of strenuous exercise is usually the only recommended treatment. Improving the availability of substrates with dietary glucose and fructose supplementation has been attempted, and drugs which increase blood flow to the muscles have been tried but have not proved to be consistently effective.

DISORDERS OF GALACTOSE METABOLISM

There are three clinically significant disorders of galactose metabolism which are due to deficiencies of galactokinase (EC 2.7.1.6), galactose-1-phosphate uridyl transferase (transferase, EC 2.7.7.10) and uridine diphosphate galactose-4-epimerase (epimerase, EC 5.1.3.2.).[21] There is, also, a variant of epimerase deficiency in which the defect is expressed mainly in erythrocytes with no reported clinical abnormality.

Normal galactose metabolism

The metabolism of galactose fulfils two main purposes. First, galactose is converted to glucose-1-phosphate (glc-1-P) which is then utilised by the normal metabolic pathways of this compound. Thus, galactose, derived from the lactose in milk and milk products, becomes available as an energy source. This is particularly vital in the infant and young child. Secondly, galactose must be incorporated into glycoproteins, glycolipids and other complex polysaccharides, which are collectively termed galactosides. The galactosyl donor for galactoside synthesis is uridine diphosphate galactose (UDPgal).

The metabolism of galactose to glc-1-P involves the Leloir, or main, pathway (Fig. 2.7), which is most active in the liver although present in erythrocytes and other cell types. Galactose is phosphorylated to galactose-1-phosphate (gal-1-P) by the specific kinase, galactokinase. The gal-1-P then takes part in a transferase reaction with UDPglc, the products of which are UDPgal and glc-1-P. At this point there has been no actual conversion of galactose to a glucose moiety, and this is achieved through the action of the third enzyme, epimerase, which inverts the H and OH groups at position C4 of the galactosyl group of UDPgal. The UDPglc formed may be utilised in the transferase reaction and the net effect of the Leloir pathway is then the conversion of galactose to glc-1-P with the expenditure of 1 molecule of ATP. In some circumstances the UDPglc produced from UDPgal may be converted to glc-1-P by the action of pyrophosphorylase (Fig. 2.8), and UDPglc synthesised from glc-1-P by

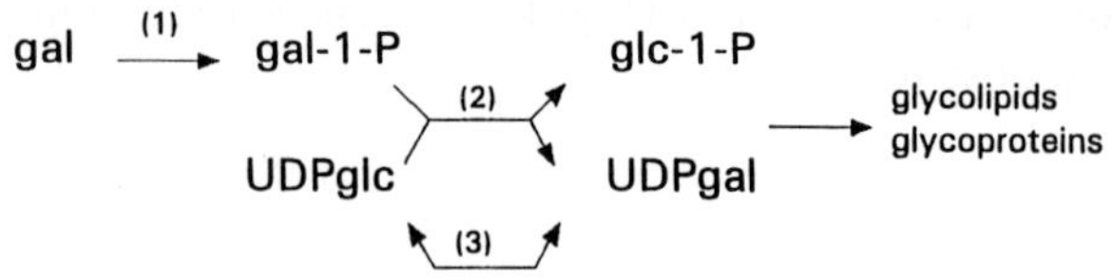

Fig. 2.7 The Leloir or main pathway of galactose metabolism to glc-1-P. Enzymes: (1) galactokinase, (2) galactose-1-phosphate uridyl transferase, (3) uridine diphosphate galactose-4-epimerase. UDPgal may be incorporated into glycolipids and glycoproteins (galactosides).

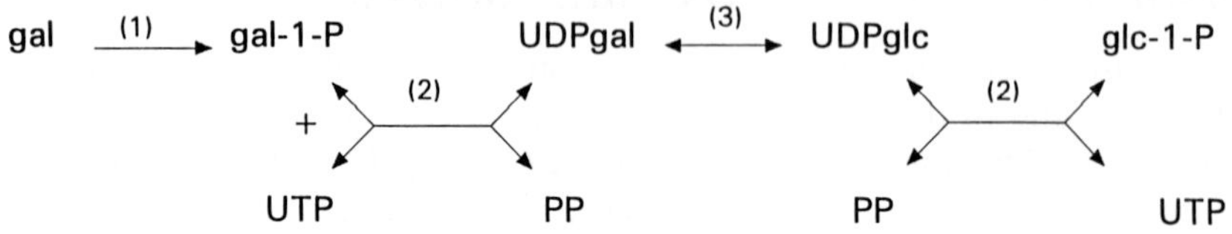

Fig. 2.8 The pyrophosphorylase pathway, described originally as an alternative means of metabolising gal to glc-1-P but the individual enzymes may have more significance in other ways (see text). Enzymes: (1) galactokinase, (2)pyrophosphorylase, (3) uridine diphosphate galactose-4-epimerase.

pyrophosphorylase may be used to prime the transferase reaction, particularly to initiate the metabolism of a galactose load.

UDPgal, the galactosyl donor, may be synthesised from dietary galactose as a normal result of galactokinase and transferase activity (Fig. 2.7). However, until recently, it was assumed that, in the absence of dietary galactose or of galactokinase or transferase activity, UDPgal levels could be maintained by the metabolism of glc-1-P through the pyrophosphorylase pathway in reverse (Fig. 2.8). Reports of low UDPgal concentrations in the erythrocytes, cultured skin fibroblasts and liver of galactosaemic patients[22] have suggested that this assumption may be incorrect, but there remains some controversy on this matter (see later).

Two other minor routes of galactose metabolism may become important in situations in which galactose accumulates (Fig. 2.9). It may be reduced by a non-specific aldose reductase to galactitol. This substance is implicated in the formation of cataracts associated with galactosaemia. Secondly, increased urinary excretion of galacturonic acid, an oxidative product of galactose, is found also in galactosaemia.

Enzyme defects

Galactose-1-phosphate uridyl transferase

Deficiency of transferase, or classical galactosaemia (McKusick 230400),

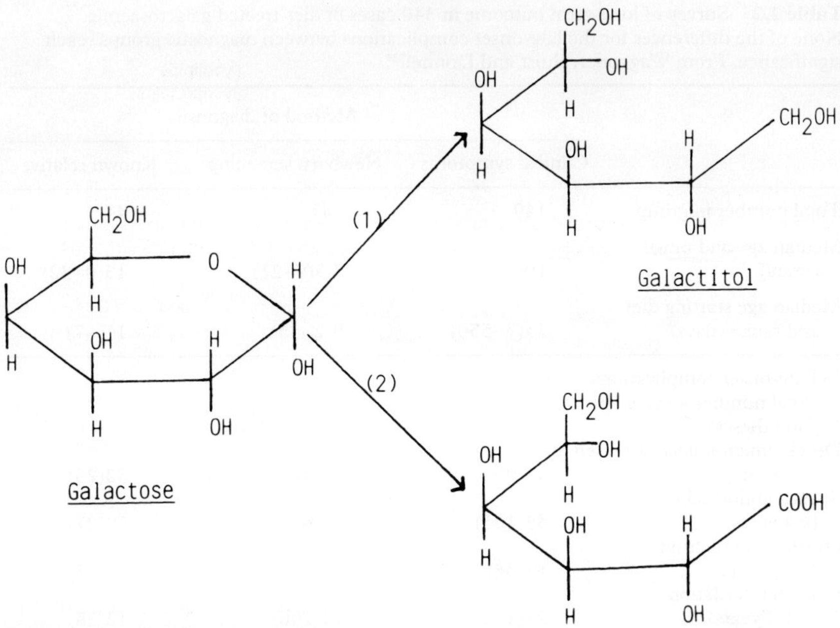

Fig. 2.9 Minor pathways of galactose metabolism by non-specific aldose reductase (1) to galactitol and by aldehyde dehydrogenase (2) to galactonic acid.

was the first recognised disorder of galactose metabolism and is the most common. Affected infants appear normal at birth and, typically, become ill in the second week of life. In a recent study in the UK[23], the presenting features in decreasing order of frequency, were jaundice, failure to thrive, hepatomegaly and liver failure, vomiting, cataracts, splenomegaly, septicaemia and urinary tract infection. Hypoglycaemia, glycosuria and aminoaciduria are other recognised signs of the acute illness. If the disease is severe, undiagnosed and untreated, death may ensue. Some cases follow a more chronic course; diagnosis may be delayed for some months and, if the child survives, mental retardation of varying severity is a long-term complication.

In almost all cases the early signs and symptoms of the disease resolve rapidly on the introduction of a galactose-restricted diet and for many years the outlook was thought to be good. However, it is now recognised that there are long-term complications in patients on treatment. An international survey of 340 cases[24] has documented a high incidence of developmental delay, speech abnormality and growth retardation, with ovarian dysfunction in females (Table 2.2). The incidence of these complications does not seem to be related to the time of diagnosis and commencement of treatment. Three studies have shown a falling IQ with age. The performance of preschool children may appear satisfactory but one study found

Table 2.2 Survey of long-term outcome in 340 cases of diet-treated galactosaemia. None of the differences for the late-onset complications between diagnostic groups reach significance. From Waggoner, Buist and Donnell[24]

	Method of diagnosis		
	Clinical symptoms	Newborn screening	Known relative
Total number in group	149	147	44
Median age and range (years)	10(0–38)	3.5(0–21)	13(0–32)
Median age starting diet and range (days)	25(3–550)	9(2–45)	1(1–7)
% Late-onset complications (total number assessed in parentheses)			
Developmental delay assessed at (≥ 6 years)	45(95)	36(36)	32(25)
Speech abnormality (≥ 4 years)	53(105)	57(63)	70(27)
Ovarian dysfunction (≥ 12 years)	87(38)	80(5)	80(15)
Growth retardation (≥ 1.5 years)	21(126)	14(106)	12(28)

that by the age of 12 years 83% of children had an IQ less than 85. Originally it was thought possible that these findings might be an artefact of the use of different IQ tests over the period of the longitudinal studies, but there is now enough data to make this seem improbable. Progressive neurological abnormality is a feature in a small proportion of patients.

Transferase deficiency is inherited as an autosomal recessive condition. Classically affected individuals are homozygous for the so-called galactosaemia allele with transferase activity in all tissues examined varying from zero to only a few percent of the level in control subjects. Estimates of the incidence of the disease have varied widely from 1:35 000 to 1:200 000. A mean incidence of 1:62 000, based on newborn screening in parts of North America, Europe and Asia, should represent a close approximation of the true incidence in these populations. However, recent attempts to ascertain all cases of galactosaemia in the UK and the Republic of Ireland have shown incidences of 1:42 000 and 1:26 000 in the respective populations.[23]

A number of other mutant alleles exist which are associated with characteristic transferase activities varying from 1 to 140% of normal (Table 2.3). These variants may be distinguished from the galactosaemia allele by their activity, electrophoretic mobility and stability. Individuals who are homozygous for some of the variant alleles and others, who are compound heterozygotes for a variant and the galactosaemia allele, may have some of the clinical symptoms associated with classical galactosaemia. The most

Table 2.3 Variant alleles of the tranferase gene and their effect. (Enzyme activities are measured in erythrocytes except where stated)

Variant allele	Homozygote transferase activity as percentage of normal mean	Clinical symptoms: Homozygotes	Clinical symptoms: Compound heterozygotes with galactosaemia allele
Galactosaemia	0 to few (also in liver, slightly higher in fibroblast)	Yes	—
Negro	0 (up to 10 in liver)	Yes	Yes
Duarte	About 50	No	Possibly in neonates
Rennes	7–10	Yes	Yes
Indiana	0–40	?	Yes
Münster	About 30	Yes	Yes
Berne	About 40	?	?
Chicago	About 25 (also in fibroblasts)		Yes
Los Angeles	100–140	No	No

common variant is determined by the Duarte allele with an estimated frequency of carriers in the population of 8–13%. This is 10 times higher than that of the galactosaemia allele.

The transferase gene has been mapped to chromosome 9p13 and a 1.4 kb cDNA has been cloned, coding for a 43 kDa protein. A number of mutant alleles have been identified in patients with classical galactosaemia, but one of them, a substitution of arginine for glutamine at amino acid position 188 in the transferase molecule, has been found with a frequency of about 67% in a North American population[25].

Galactokinase

The salient feature of galactokinase deficiency (McKusick 230200) is the development of bilateral nuclear cataracts in early infancy. There are none of the other acute features associated with transferase deficiency. Pseudotumour cerebri has been described in a few cases, as it has been in transferase deficiency also.[26] The occurrence of this complication is so low that it is not possible to be certain of a causal relationship to the galactose disorders, but it has been suggested that it may be a consequence of galactitol accumulation and osmotic swelling in the brain. Retarded development in some earlier untreated cases has been ascribed to the handicap of their total blindness, rather than to a primary effect of the metabolic disorder, but the true outcome of the defect may only be apparent if a large study is set up, as it was in transferase deficiency.

The enzyme defect may be demonstrated easily in red cells or skin fibroblasts in which the activity is essentially zero. However, when [^{14}C] galactose was administered to patients 5% of the label appeared in expired

CO_2. This indicated that a little enzyme activity is present in some body tissue(s). A variant enzyme found exclusively in Black populations has about 30% of normal activity in red cells.

The galactokinase gene is located on chromosome 17 (17q21–22) and the defect is inherited as an autosomal recessive. In Switzerland, where the disorder was first recognised, the incidence has been estimated to be 1:40 000. Other indications, including newborn screening data from North America, are of a much lower occurrence rate.

Epimerase

Defects of epimerase (McKusick 230350) are the most recent galactose disorders to be described, and two distinct forms can be defined. The first was discovered in 1971 in infants who were positive in a galactosaemia screening programme. The method employed detected raised levels of galactose and gal-1-P. Subsequent investigations proved that the red cell transferase was normal, but the epimerase was deficient. The ability of the whole body to metabolise galactose was not significantly affected, however, and follow-up of these cases suggests that the disorder is completely benign, with no change in red cell morphology or function even.

The second form of epimerase deficiency was first described in 1981 in a newborn infant presenting with a clinical picture similar to that of classical galactosaemia.[27] Red cell epimerase was shown to be absent. Only one other patient with this acutely presenting form has been reported.[28] Together, the patients have shown all the signs and symptoms of classical galactosaemia, including jaundice, vomiting, failure to thrive and septicaemia, with the typical liver, renal tubular and eye abnormalities. These early features resolve on the introduction of a restricted galactose diet (see later), but the long-term follow-up of the cases has shown sensorineural deafness and mild mental retardation in both, but no evidence of ovarian dysfunction. It is possible that the learning problems are secondary to the severe deafness.

Laboratory investigations in the earlier, benign, form of epimerase defect showed that the variant enzyme was relatively unstable and had a high K_m for its cofactor NAD^+. It was presumed that the long lifespan of the red cell, combined possibly with an unfavourable NAD^+/NADH ratio, leads to a decline of its epimerase activity. Apart possibly from circulating lymphocytes, other cells, notably liver and skin fibroblasts, had normal enzyme levels. In the second, more severe defect, epimerase activity is undetectable in erythrocytes and skin fibroblasts. Liver was shown to have 10% of the epimerase activity of controls and this enzyme was indistinguishable from normal in respect of pH optimum and its K_m for UDPgal and NAD^+.[29] This would be consistent with a structural change in the enzyme affecting only its stability.

Evidence would suggest that both forms of epimerase deficiency are inherited as autosomal recessive conditions, the gene being located on chromosome 1. Both of the acutely presenting patients were the products of consanguineous marriages of Pakistanis. The incidence of the benign form was found to be 1:46 000 as a result of galactosaemia screening in Switzerland and Liechtenstein, although moderate increases in galactose and gal-1-P may not always be detected. The incidence of the severe form would appear to be extremely low, but it is possible that cases are dying because they occur most frequently in countries where the diagnosis would not be made and treatment instituted.

Pathophysiology of the enzyme defects

Biochemistry

The accumulation of precursor compounds and excretion of abnormal amounts of metabolites in the three enzyme defects of galactose metabolism can be predicted from the blocks in the Leloir pathway.

In *galactokinase* deficiency, the defect in the first stage in galactose metabolism leads to profound galactosaemia and galactosuria in patients on a normal diet. Significant amounts of galactose are metabolised to galactitol which accumulates within body fluid compartments, particularly the eye lens. This is considered to be relevant to the mechanism of cataract formation and, possibly, other pathological processes. The possible importance of the Leloir pathway in UDPgal synthesis has been mentioned but there is no evidence of UDPgal deficiency in galactokinase deficiency. This could be because of residual activity in the enzyme, at least in some tissues.

Transferase deficiency leads to an accumulation of the immediate precursor, gal-1-P, but also of galactose. The expansion of the galactose pool results in galactitol accumulation, as in galactokinase deficiency. Galactose is distributed throughout intra- and extracellular fluid and is readily excreted by the kidney. Gal-1-P, on the other hand, accumulates intracellularly and its loss from the cells is slow. Newly diagnosed galactosaemic infants when put on a galactose-free diet have high gal-1-P levels for the next 10–15 days, reflecting the large accumulation of the metabolite and its slow clearance. If older galactosaemic children on a well controlled galactosaemic diet are given a small dose of galactose, raised gal-1-P concentrations persist for at least 24 h.

The build up of abnormal metabolites in transferase deficiency has been shown to occur in the fetus as early as 21 weeks gestation (Table 2.4). The concentration of erythrocyte gal-1-P was equivalent to that in children diagnosed with severe signs of disease and liver concentrations of galactose, gal-1-P and galactitol were 20–50% of levels in infants dying of galactosaemia. High gal-1-P concentrations have been found also in the cord blood of galactosaemic infants.

When transferase-deficient patients are given a galactose-restricted diet,

Table 2.4 Concentration of galactose and its metabolites in liver and erythrocytes of a fetus with transferase deficiency

	Transferase-deficient fetus	Controls (n = 2)
Liver (μmol/kg wet tissue)		
Galactose	277	0
Galactose-1-phosphate	115	0
Galactitol	247	0
Erythrocytes (μmol/1 packed erythrocytes)		
Galactose-1-phosphate	990	0

red cell gal-1-P levels fall from the very high pretreatment levels, but remain significantly higher than normal reference values for an indefinite time. Also, the galactosaemic infants of mothers who have been on a low galactose diet during pregnancy still have high cord blood gal-1-P concentrations. Two explanations have been made for these observations. The first postulates the de novo synthesis of gal-1-P from glc-1-P via the pyrophosphorylase pathway (Fig. 2.8). This proposal was supported by a study of a newborn galactosaemic infant who was given only intravenous glucose for the first 24 h of life, but whose gal-1-P rose significantly between 5 and 24 h of age.[30] The second proposal is that gal-1-P is synthesised from free galactose which is generated from the turnover of tissue galactosides or is present in small amounts in the diet.[31] The galactoside source could only explain, by itself, a short-term increase in gal-1-P levels, but could provide an alternative explanation for the rise in the newborn baby. On the other hand, the presence of free galactose in a supposedly galactose restricted diet is now established, as it has been shown that there are many other sources of free galactose than the conventional ones of milk and milk products.[32]

The possibility of UDPgal depletion in transferase deficiency was mentioned previously and it was indicated that there is some controversy about this matter. Early reports claimed that patients with no measurable transferase activity had, on average, only 40% of control levels of red cell UDPgal.[22] A small proportion of patients who had up to 1% enzyme activity, but who may still have had a severe presentation in the newborn period, had normal erythrocyte UDPgal concentrations. It appeared that these patients were less at risk of long-term complications of the disease. Unfortunately subsequent studies, using different techniques for assaying UDPgal, have found much lower levels of the metabolite in control patients' red cells and a less clear cut difference between transferase-deficient patients and controls.[33] UDPgal deficiency in galactosaemia remains a very interesting possibility, although its clinical significance needs to be established. It is probable that the erythrocyte would show the deficiency less clearly than cells actively synthesising galactose-containing macromolecules.

In the benign form of *epimerase* deficiency erythrocyte gal-1-P levels may be increased, at least in the newborn, but the overall capacity to metabolise galactose in the body is little affected and galactosaemia and galactosuria is not a feature. In the more severe form of this enzyme deficiency the untreated patient does have marked galactosaemia, galactosuria and increased gal-1-P in red cells. On a galactose-restricted diet these biochemical signs disappear and, contrary to the findings in transferase deficiency, gal-1-P is completely normalised.[27] This last observation is consistent with either of the hypotheses elaborated earlier to explain the persistently raised erythrocyte gal-1-P levels in transferase-deficient patients, because de novo gal-1-P synthesis via the pyrophosphorylase pathways requires active epimerase but, also, small amounts of galactose are more likely to be metabolised through to UDPgal rather than gal-1-P in epimerase deficiency.

Figure 2.10 shows that in a patient with the generalised epimerase defect small amounts of galactose are preferentially converted to UDPgal. With increasing supplements to the restricted diet (1,2 and 4 g per day) UDPgal levels reached a maximum level with the smallest dose, whilst gal-1-P rose linearly with increasing galactose intake. The possible explanation for these

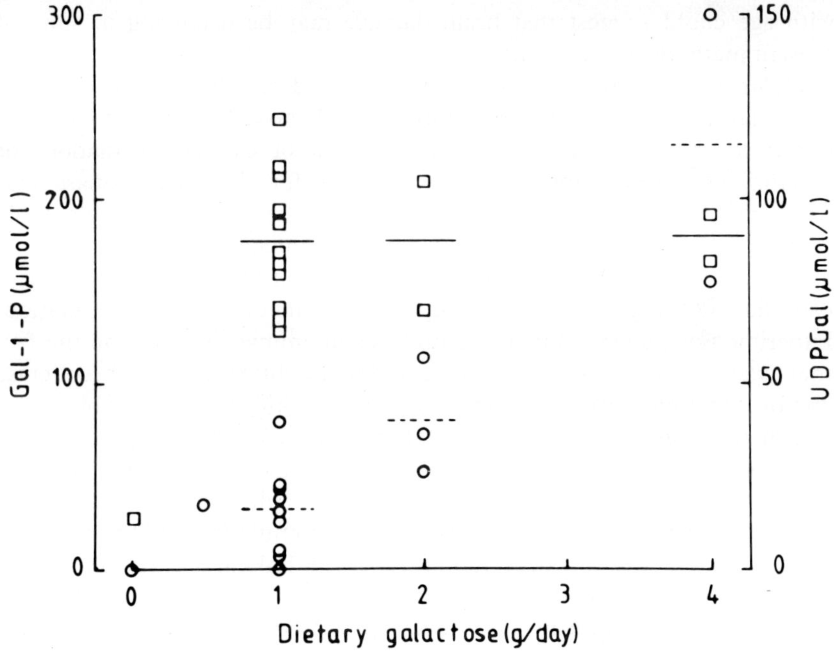

Fig. 2.10 Accumulation of galactose metabolites in a child with uridine diphosphate galactose-4-epimerase deficiency given varying galactose supplements; o – level of gal-1-P in packed red cells, (---) – Mean levels of gal-1-P at the same galactose intake, □ – Level of UDPgal in packed red cells, (—) – Mean level of UDPgal at the same galactose intake.

findings is that at the lowest levels of galactose intake gal-1-P is metabolised to UDPgal by transferase, the UDPglc cofactor required being synthesised from glc-1-P by pyrophosphorylase, or from UDPgal by some residual epimerase activity. When the flux of galactose becomes greater, the availability of UDPglc becomes limiting and gal-1-P then accumulates.

Pathogenesis

The main tissues involved in the diseases of galactose metabolism are those of the lens, liver, kidney, brain and ovary. The metabolites which have been implicated in the disease mechanisms are galactitol, galactose-1-phosphate and UDPgal and each of these will be discussed below. A fundamental question to be answered is when tissue damage occurs. As mentioned earlier galactitol and gal-1-P accumulate in the transferase-deficient fetus and prenatal damage is therefore a distinct possibility. Very early cataracts and liver dysfunction, together with fetal abnormalities associated with experimental galactose toxicity in pregnant rats, support this hypothesis. There is no evidence, however, that the time which elapses from birth to diagnosis and treatment is critical in determining long-term outcome in this condition.[24] On the other hand, the progressive deterioration in IQ with age could suggest that brain damage may be occurring in spite of present methods of treatment.

Galactitol accumulation has been associated mainly with the cataracts which are a feature of all three forms of galactose disorder. It has been suggested that there is some increased risk of cataract formation for heterozygotes and compound heterozygotes for the galactokinase and transferase deficiency alleles.[34] The lens may be particularly vulnerable because it has a high concentration of aldose reductase.

The causation of cataract formation by galactitol has been related to osmotic swelling consequent upon the metabolite accumulation. Experimental evidence for this hypothesis in animals is based on the fact that cataract formation can be prevented by inhibitors of aldose reductase and by direct measures to stop the osmotic swelling. Many other biochemical changes have been found in the affected lens, which may be secondary to galactitol accumulation. One of the most important is a deficiency of myo-inositol. This substance is involved in phospholipid metabolism and many other aspects of cell function. Polyol accumulation and myo-inositol depletion might also be a common mechanism linking diabetic and galactose disorder cataracts. In addition, myo-inositol depletion and deranged phospholipid metabolism have been proposed as the mechanism of diabetic neuropathy and of the mental retardation in galactosaemia.[35] Interesting though this last hypothesis is, it is difficult to explain why mental retardation is not perceived as a feature of galactokinase deficiency.

Galactose-1-phosphate at increased levels has been seen as the probable cause of the acute toxic features of both transferase and epimerase deficiency, involving the liver and kidney in particular. This is because the biochemical abnormality occurs in these conditions, but gal-1-P is not increased in galactokinase deficiency which does not have any neonatal manifestations apart from cataracts. The resolution of the acute signs in transferase and epimerase deficiency on the introduction of a galactose-restricted diet appears to parallel the fall in red cell gal-1-P concentration. Direct evidence of gal-1-P involvement in the disease processes is lacking, however. It inhibits a number of enzymes involved in glucose metabolism in vitro, but similar effects cannot be demonstrated in the intact animal. An alternative mechanism has been proposed in which energy depletion arises because of the trapping of ATP in gal-1-P, because this compound cannot be metabolised further in transferase deficiency and in the acute phase of epimerase deficiency. Animal model systems in which liver necrosis is induced by galactose analogues would seem to support the futile metabolism hypothesis.[36]

UDPgal is a cofactor for galactoprotein and galactolipid synthesis and its depletion might lead to abnormal synthesis of these macromolecules. In the first full report of reduced erythrocyte UDPgal concentration in transferase-deficient patients it was claimed that this correlated with ovarian dysfunction. The ovary contains large amounts of bound galactose and it was postulated that this organ, in particular, might be at risk of UDPgal deficiency. However, galactolipids have important functions in the central nervous system and, therefore, UDPgal depletion might be the cause of mental impairment also.

In addition to the erythrocyte, reduced UDPgal concentrations have been reported in liver and skin fibroblasts in transferase-deficient patients. More significantly, perhaps, two independent studies have found evidence that galactose incorporation into galactoprotein is reduced in transferase-deficient skin fibroblast cultures.[37,38] These experiments support the hypothesis that UDPgal depletion is a mechanism for pathological changes in galactosaemia. The major doubt currently arises from a dispute about the original methods used to measure UDPgal, although a smaller, but significant, reduction in erythrocyte levels has been confirmed by a different and well-validated technique and, interestingly, a similar change was found in non-galactosaemic patients on galactose-restricted diets.[33]

Epimerase deficiency is unique in having UDPgal accumulation when galactose is being metabolised in moderate amounts. The pathological significance of this is unclear, although the futile production of this compound is more costly in energy terms than gal-1-P in transferase deficiency. It is conceivable that UDPgal production in excess may cause a clinical sign which is unique to epimerase deficiency, sensorineural deafness for example.

Treatment

The treatment of all clinically important galactose disorders is to exclude galactose from the diet. In the case of galactokinase and transferase deficiencies this restriction is made as complete as possible. Milk and all milk products must be excluded. Uncertainty exists about the need to exclude galactose in α-linked galactosides, for example in offal, soya and vegetables. There is conflicting evidence on whether galactose in this form is absorbed by man and whether it affects erythrocyte gal-1-P levels in transferase deficiency. As a precaution it has been recommended that these foods are excluded in early life. Recently, it has been shown that free galactose is present in significant amounts in some fruits and vegetables and it must be concluded that diet has been less strict than imagined.[32]

As mentioned previously, erythrocyte gal-1-P levels remain above normal in transferase-deficient patients on a diet and it is now appreciated that galactitol is raised in both transferase and galactokinase deficiency in spite of the galactose restriction. Endogenous and exogenous sources to explain this have been discussed earlier. There has been a long understanding, though based purely on empirical reasoning, that gal-1-P levels should be controlled below 150 μmol/l of packed red cells. A small proportion of patients exceed this level in spite of careful attention to the diet, particularly during the first year or so of life. The reason for this has not been elucidated, although it appears that the same patients have higher galactitol levels.[39]

It was suggested originally that galactose supplements were necessary in treating epimerase deficiency in order to allow some generation of UDPgal from the Leloir pathway, synthesis via the pyrophosphorylase route being impeded by the block at the epimerase stage. Subsequent work has suggested that the epimerase deficiency is not complete and, therefore, normal UDPgal levels should be maintained on the restricted diet used in the other defects.

In view of the poor long-term outlook in galactosaemia, other, or additional, methods for treating the condition need to be sought. Possible approaches can be proposed, but have not been put to the test apart from the possible enhancement of UDPgal levels by administration of uridine. Claims have been made that this is metabolically effective and that it has a beneficial effect on intellectual development.[40] However, there is some scepticism regarding these claims and the fundamental work on which this therapeutic approach is based. It is premature to use uridine therapy except in a controlled trial.

Female patients who develop ovarian dysfunction require hormone replacement treatment. Gonadotrophin and oestrogen levels should be assessed from 6 months of age onwards; by this means it may be possible to predict which of the patients will develop early ovarian failure. Treatment of ovarian failure should not be delayed since oestrogen deficiency may result in a loss of bone mineral content. Patients have been treated from the age of 16 years who have primary or secondary amenhorrhoea, plasma FSH levels increased above 40 mIU/ml for a period of 3 months or more and urinary oestradiol excretion less than 20 pg/ml.[41] The regime should include oestrogen and progestin, with the level of the former hormone being less than that included in birth control pills.

Biochemical diagnosis

The primary investigation in all patients suspected of having a galactose disorder is usually to measure the urine total reducing substances and, if this is positive, chromatographic methods are then used to demonstrate which reducing sugar is responsible. A number of errors can arise in the use of these simple methods. First, babies who have already developed the acute signs of a galactose disorder, vomiting and poor feeding in particular, may not be taking in and, thus, excreting galactose. If this possibility is suspected an enzyme diagnostic test is indicated. Even infants with very little in the way of galactosaemic signs, and who may appear to be feeding normally, may test negative for reducing substances in urine passed a few hours after the last milk feed. Secondly, it is well recognised that non-laboratory staff confuse methods which measure urine glucose specifically (Clinistix) and those which measure total reducing substances (Clinitest). Obviously, the former will give a false negative result for galactosaemia. Thirdly, the urine of normal neonates frequently contains small amounts of galactose (usually associated with lactose) which produces false positive tests for the galactose disorders. This is not of real concern, providing further tests are made to confirm the diagnosis.

Although it is standard practice to put a baby on a galactose-restricted diet on the basis of preliminary urine investigations, the diagnosis should be confirmed as soon as possible using a definitive method. Cases still arise where the patient has been on a diet for many years without this confirmation being carried out, and when the diagnosis is finally checked a negative result is obtained. The possibility that galactose restriction may be harmful emphasises the importance of not allowing this to occur. A diagnosis can be confirmed by measuring the red cell enzyme activity. The most commonly occurring, acutely presenting disorder, transferase deficiency, can be assayed by the very simple Beutler assay.[42] In this method red cells are incubated with gal-1-P, UDPglc and $NADP^+$. In the presence of normal transferase glc-1-P is generated and converted sequentially to glc-6-P and 6 phosphogluconate using the red cells' phosphoglucomutase and glucose-1-phosphate dehydrogenase respectively. The last reaction is accompanied by reduction of $NADP^+$ to NADPH and the final product is detected by fluorescence under UV light, the reaction mixture being spotted onto filter paper. The absence of transferase prevents the whole series of reactions and no fluorescence is seen within a specific time period. The Beutler test seems to be liable to fairly frequent errors unless carried out with meticulous care. Probably the most common problem is false positive results caused by the use of blood anticoagulated with EDTA, when magnesium, necessary for activity of some of the enzymes involved, is chelated.

Strict quantification of transferase in red cells is possible by a number of methods and these are capable of distinguishing not only galactosaemic patients but also heterozygotic and normal.[43] Homozygotes and compound heterozygotes of the Duarte variant can usually be differentiated. The same distinctions can be achieved by enzyme assay on cultured skin fibroblasts and amniotic fluid cells, the latter making prenatal diagnosis available. The necessity for prenatal diagnosis has been suggested for many years now, although it is rarely carried out in practice. Prenatal diagnosis is possible also by transferase assay in chorionic villus[44] and by galactitol measurement in amniotic fluid supernatant in the first or second trimester.[45] Prenatal diagnosis using enzyme assay on cultured amniocytes for the galactokinase and epimerase defects is available, although justification for the former might be questioned.

Newborn screening is carried out fairly widely in North America but not particularly so in European countries. This is partly because the case for screening is not universally accepted. Although it should ensure complete detection of all affected patients, some are found to have died before the screening result is available. Cord blood can be used in order to obtain the earliest possible result, but this requires quite difficult organisation, completely separate from the other neonatal screening programmes. Other contraindications are the low frequency of the conditions and the uncertain benefit of early treatment in respect to long-term outcome. Early screening programmes utilised the Beutler enzyme method, but a microbiological assay (Paigen)[46], which detects increased galactose and gal-1-P, and therefore is capable of picking up all three enzyme defects, is now used more frequently. One other complication of screening for galactosaemia is that it detects some compound heterozygotic individuals for the Duarte and classical galactosaemic alleles, who may have raised gal-1-P levels and have been reported to sometimes show toxic signs in the neonatal period.[47] Although there is no evidence that any harm comes to the infants with this genotype, some treatment centres place the patients on a galactose-restricted diet for a period of up to 1 year.

DISORDERS OF FRUCTOSE METABOLISM AND RELATED PATHWAYS

There are two enzyme deficiency disorders in the specific pathway by which fructose is converted into glucose intermediary metabolites. The first of these, known as essential fructosuria, was described as early as 1876, although it is a completely benign condition. The clinically significant hereditary fructose intolerance was first reported in 1956. Discussions of fructose intolerance also usually include the deficiency of fructose 1:6 bisphosphatase, an enzyme which is not involved in fructose metabolism as such but is a key enzyme in gluconeogenesis. In common with other defects in the gluconeogenesis pathway, there is an unfavourable response to fructose ingestion and there may be some diagnostic confusion with hereditary fructose intolerance. In addition, there will be brief mention of a disorder of sorbitol dehydrogenase, the enzyme which can generate fructose from sorbitol and may be associated with congenital cataracts and of glycerate kinase deficiency which leads to the excretion of D-glyceric acid.

Normal fructose metabolism

Free fructose is a major constituent of many fruits and vegetables and of honey. Fruits and vegetables also contain sorbitol, which is readily converted to fructose by sorbitol dehydrogenase (Fig. 2.11). Fructose is the major carbohydrate and energy source in seminal fluid and is synthesised from glucose in the male by the accessory glands of the reproductive tract. The pathway from glucose to sorbitol, catalysed by aldose reductase, and then through to fructose, is not operative in other tissues. Free fructose has been used widely as a sweetener and as an energy source in parenteral nutrition. This practice may be harmful to people with normal fructose metabolism, as well as those with an inherited disorder and, therefore, it has been discouraged.

In many individuals the major source of fructose is sucrose, and fructose intolerance is first evident when this disaccharide is introduced to the diet. Fructose in the trisaccharide rafinose and the tetrasaccharide stachiose is not thought to be absorbed because they are not hydrolysed in the intestine, but small amounts of the fructose contained in inulin may be available.

Absorbed fructose is metabolised mostly by the liver (75%) with the kidney and intestine accounting for 20 and 10% respectively. The major route of fructose metabolism is shown in Fig. 2.11. First, it is rapidly phosphorylated to fructose-1-phosphate, catalysed by fructokinase. ATP is the main phosphoryl donor, but GTP can also be utilised. Fructokinase has a particularly high K_m and V_{max} for fructose. Fructose-1-phosphate is then split by aldolase B to glyceraldehyde and dihydroxyacetone phosphate. Aldolase B also catalyses the splitting of fructose 1:6 bisphosphate to glyceraldehyde-3-phosphate and dihydroxyacetone phosphate. Glyceraldehyde is converted to glyceraldehyde-3-phosphate using triokinase, preferentially with ATP as phosphoryl donor, although GTP may be used. Dihydroxyacetone phosphate, also, is converted to glyceraldehyde-3-phosphate, by the action of triose phosphate isomerase. The glyceralde-

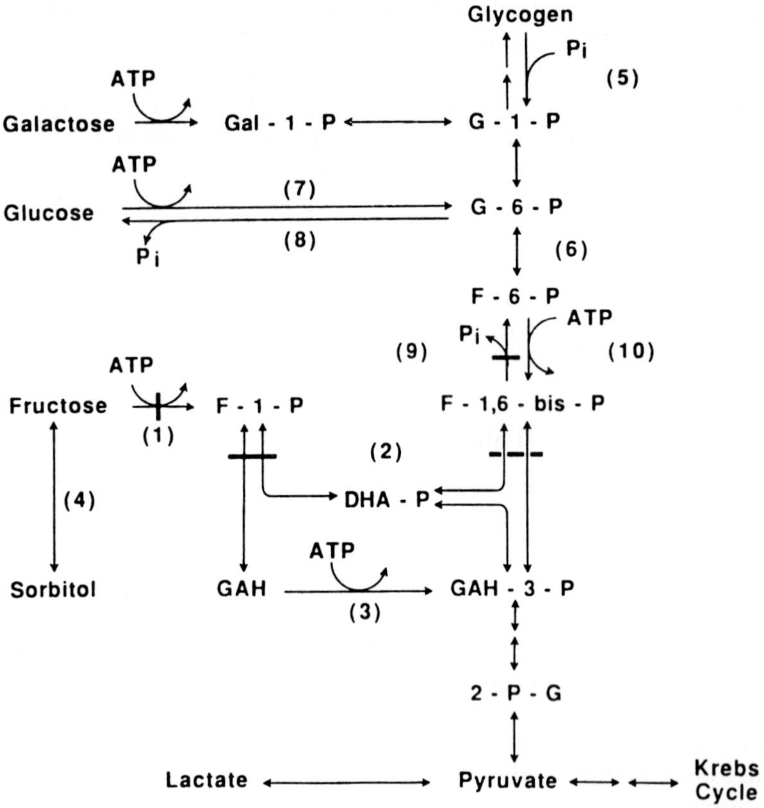

Fig. 2.11 Pathways of fructose metabolism in the liver. DHA – dihydroxyacetone, G – glucose, GAH – D-glyceraldehyde, F – fructose, P – phosphate, 2P-G – 2-phosphoglycerate. Enzymes: (1) fructokinase, (2) aldolase, (3) triokinase, (4) sorbitol dehydrogenase, (5) glycogen phosphorylase, (6) phosphohexose isomerase, (7) glucokinase, (8) glucose-6-phosphatase, (9) fructose-1,6-bisphosphatase, (10) phosphofructokinase. The aldolase-B-defect (HFI) is shown by both the solid and dotted bars. Fructokinase and fructose-1,6 bisphosphatase deficiencies are shown by solid bars.[49]

hyde-3-phosphate so formed may be incorporated into the glycolytic pathway to pyruvate, or, by aldolase B acting in the reverse direction from that previously described, it can be fed into the gluconeogenic pathway.

Aldolase is a key enzyme in fructose metabolism and exists in three isoenzyme forms A, B and C, present in muscle, liver and brain respectively. Table 2.5 (p. 61) compares the V_{max} for fructose 1:6 bisphosphate with that for fructose-1-phosphate in the three isoenzymes. V_{max} for the former substrate is similar in all three, but for fructose-1-phosphate it is much higher for the liver enzyme. It follows, that fructose-1-phosphate, and hence free fructose, is only metabolised in substantial amounts in liver. Each isoenzyme contains four identical subunits, but the type of subunits differs from one form of enzyme to another. The form of fructaldolase also changes during development; human fetal liver having a higher activity ratio than is typical of adult liver enzyme.[48]

Alternative pathways for the metabolism of fructose have been proposed as follows[49]:

1. Utilisation of glyceraldehyde by reduction to glycerol, catalysed by alcohol dehydrogenase or aldose reductase, followed by phosphorylation to glycerol-3-phosphate (glycerol kinase) and oxidation to dihydroxyacetone phosphate (α-glycerophosphate dehydrogenase).

2. Oxidation of glyceraldehyde to D-glycerate (aldehyde dehydrogenase) and phosphorylation to 2-phosphoglycerate (glycerate kinase).

3. Direct conversion of fructose-1-phosphate to fructose 1:6 bisphosphate without being split by aldolase.

4. Metabolism of fructose to fructose-6-phosphate by hexokinase in muscle or adipose tissue.

The above pathways are of doubtful significance in absolute terms and the aldolase pathway remains the most important route of fructose metabolism, as demonstrated by the seriousness of its deficiency. Pathway 2 however may be invoked in explaining the rare disorder D-glyceric aciduria that is described later.

Enzyme defects

Fructokinase (EC 2.7.1.4)

Fructokinase, was one of the earliest inherited metabolic disorders to be described and was called essential fructosuria (McKusick 229800). The most important site of the enzyme is the liver and the absence of activity in this organ in individuals with the disorder has been demonstrated by direct assay. It is likely that such individuals also have a deficiency of the enzyme in intestine and kidney cortex, the other tissues in which it is normally found.

As previously stated, fructokinase deficiency appears not to cause clinical symptoms and is usually found incidentally when the urine is tested for reducing substances as a screen for diabetes. A clinical history and the demonstration of fructose by further laboratory tests should reveal the correct diagnosis. It is probable that only a small proportion of cases of this condition are diagnosed, but it is thought to be rare and an incidence of 1:130 000 has been estimated. In some large published series there is a preponderance of Jews. The inheritance is autosomal recessive.

Fructaldolase (EC 2.1.2.13)

Fructaldolase deficiency, or hereditary fructose intolerance (HFI), is the most significant of the disorders of fructose metabolism (McKusick

229600). The enzyme deficiency has been demonstrated in liver, kidney cortex and intestinal mucosa, tissues in which fructaldolase B isoenzyme usually predominates. However, the liver is the main site of fructose metabolism and here the activity of the enzyme with fructose-1-phosphate as substrate is reduced to 15% or less of normal in HFI.

The appearance of clinical symptoms in HFI is completely dependent on the ingestion of fructose and, therefore, will be delayed so long as the infant is breast-fed and given no sucrose-containing drinks. The condition tends to present more severely the earlier the exposure to fructose. The clinical picture includes both acute episodes which follow immediately after exposure to large amounts of fructose and a chronic course which occurs as the result of protracted feeding of more moderate amounts of the compound. The former are characterised by sweating, trembling, nausea, vomiting, lethargy and coma, symptoms attributable to hypoglycaemia. They can end in death if the diagnosis is not made and the patient treated appropriately. The most frequent features of the longer-term presentation are poor feeding, vomiting, failure to thrive and, less commonly, drowsiness, crying, jaundice, haemorrhages, abdominal distention, irritability and diarrhoea. Clinical examination usually shows trembling, jerks, shock and hepatomegaly; renal tubular syndrome, ascites, splenomegaly and oliguria are frequent findings. In one large series about half the children had a blood picture suggesting disseminating intravascular coagulation.[50]

It is interesting that in many cases the clinical course has been modified because the patients, or their parents, realise that certain foods are harmful and, thus, to be avoided. In patients displaying minimal symptoms there is usually a total lack of dental caries due to the avoidance of sucrose-containing foods. So remarkable is this that the diagnosis may arise from a dental examination. Variation in the clinical severity of the condition may be due also to heterogeneity in the enzyme deficiency.

HFI is an autosomal recessive condition with the majority of published cases being from Europe and North America. In Switzerland, where there is much interest in the disease, an incidence of 1:20 000 has been quoted. However this is no doubt an underestimate, as it is probable that many cases die without a diagnosis being made, or escape medical attention because of the intuitive restriction of fructose.

Considerable heterogeneity in the enzyme defect between patients has been demonstrated by different residual activity levels, varying *Km* values for fructose-1-phosphate, immunological cross-reaction methods, antibody activation and heat inactivation studies.[51] The heterogeneity of the enzyme defect has been supported by molecular genetic studies. The gene has been localised to chromosome 9q21.3–q22.2, its cDNA encoding a protein of 364 amino acids. So far four point mutations have been described which appear to have a widespread distribution and four deletions which appear to be specific to particular families.[52]

Fructose 1:6 bisphosphatase (EC 3.1.11)

The deficiency disorder of this enzyme (McKusick 229700) was described in 1970. It is probable that prior to this patients were misdiagnosed as other metabolic defects, including HFI. However, in the more recently delineated condition there is a less marked history of fructose intolerance, although in certain circumstances this monosaccharide precipitates or exacerbates the clinical condition. The enzyme deficiency has been demonstrated in liver, jejunum and kidney cortex. Muscle contains a fructose 1:6 bisphosphatase which is under different genetic control.

About half the recorded cases of the condition present early in the neonatal period[53], the main features comprising metabolic acidosis and hypoglycaemia together with hyperventilation, shock apnoea, trembling, lethargy, convulsions and loss of consciousness. The metabolic acidosis is due to accumulation of lactic acid, compounded by the effects of ketosis. The presentation of the remainder is divided more or less equally between the periods up to and after 6 months of age. The crisis in these groups often seems to be precipitated by fasting and, particularly in the oldest children, by infection. Between crises the most frequent abnormality is hyperventilation and lactic acidosis. Hepatomegaly and muscular weakness are the most persistent findings on clinical examination. The signs regress post crisis but may be precipitated again by fructose ingestion.

On the basis of the number of known cases this is a rare disorder. The frequent existence of early deaths in older siblings of known cases of the disease indicates that children may die undiagnosed. The inheritance is clearly autosomal recessive.

A possible variant form of fructose 1:6 bisphosphatase has been described in a 20-year-old mother and her 13-month-old daughter. There was evidence of hypoglycaemia in these patients but their condition was less severe. In the mother the main features were emotional lability, dizziness and fatigue, while the daughter suffered periods of unresponsiveness and confusion.[54]

Sorbitol dehydrogenase (EC 1.1.1.14)

Investigation of patients with congenital cataracts has revealed two families in which both cataracts and red cell sorbitol dehydrogenase deficiency occur (McKusick 182500). Deficient subjects had 20–25% of mean normal enzyme activity, with other members being affected to a lesser extent. The mode of inheritance of the enzyme deficiency was not apparent, however.

It is tempting to postulate that sorbitol dehydrogenase deficiency in the eye lens would lead to sorbitol accumulation, osmotic swelling and cataract. Increased lens sorbitol is one explanation for cataract formation in patients with diabetes mellitus. Unfortunately, within one of the families reported there was not an exact concurrence between the presence of cataracts and reduced enzyme activity.[55] There must be some doubt about a causal relationship between sorbitol dehydrogenase deficiency and cataract formation on the basis of the data available at present.

Glycerate kinase

The condition of D-glyceric aciduria has been described in five children, presenting soon after birth. In one, the features included tachypnoea, tachychardia, refusal to feed and a metabolic acidosis requiring permanent bicarbonate treatment. There were moderate degrees of motor and developmental delay. The remaining children presented with hypotonia, myoclonic jerks, seizures and hyperglycinaemia; developmental delay was a feature in these cases, also. The clinical features and hyperglycinaemia suggested that the disorder could be due to glycine cleavage enzyme deficiency (Ch. 3, p. 100) but this has been excluded. In several patients D-glyceric acid excretion and plasma D-glyceric acid levels were shown to be increased following a fructose load. The enzyme defect was ascribed to D-glyceric acid kinase [56] (see alternative pathway 2, p. 53). The D-glyceric aciduria might be expected as the result of other enzyme defects in the fructose pathways, and in view of the heterogeneous presentations other possible causes of the metabolic disorder may exist. It is notable that in one patient there was a reduction in D-glyceric acid excretion and some clinical improvement on a restricted fructose intake.

Pathophysiology of the enzyme defects

The practice of using fructose in parenteral nutrition has led to the realisation that the perceived advantage, rapid utilisation as a carbohydrate source, is the factor which may cause serious toxic effects in normal subjects. Extensive studies in humans and animals have provided explanations for this problem in normal individuals and to a large extent has provided the basis for understanding the abnormalities in HFI.

The life-threatening feature of fructose administration in normals is believed to be the severe metabolic acidosis due to lactate accumulation. The lactic acidosis produced with intravenous fructose is several times greater than if an equivalent amount of glucose is used. The greater lactate production from fructose appears to be caused by a number of factors, which include:

a. a tenfold higher V_{max} of fructokinase compared to glucokinase
b. phosphofructokinase, the main regulator of glycolysis is bypassed when fructose enters the pathway
c. fructose-1-phosphate stimulates pryuvate kinase, one of the minor regulators of glycolysis.

The other basic abnormal observations following fructose infusion are increased serum magnesium and increased uric acid in serum and urine. These changes are consequent upon a depletion of liver ATP, GTP and inorganic phosphate (Pi) which is secondary to an accumulation of fructose-1-phosphate. The reason for the accumulation of fructose-1-phosphate has been controversial[49], but may well be the result of a greater capacity to take up fructose into the hepatocyte and metabolise it by fructokinase and aldolase B than to metabolise the products further by triokinase and the glycolytic and gluconeogenic pathways. The principal accumulated product is fructose-1-phosphate and the direct result of this is depletion of ATP, GTP and Pi. ATP chelates Mg^{2+} strongly in liver. Depletion of ATP in liver leads to a loss of the metal ion from the tissue and an increased concentration in serum. The depletion of GTP and Pi, on the other hand, are the causes of a destabilisation of the adenine pool which leads to conversion of adenine and its derivatives to uric acid overproduction. GTP and Pi are known to be involved in maintaining AMP deaminase in an inhibited state where it usually operates at only 5% of its full activity. The reduction in liver GTP and Pi causes a relatively inappropriate loss of the adenine nucleotide pool (Fig. 2.12).

In essential fructosuria a fructose load causes a greater and more sustained rise in blood fructose compared to normal. However, there are no subsequent metabolic sequelae since the fructose is not metabolized to fructose-1-phosphate, which is the mediator of the abnormal responses to fructose administration. This lack of metabolic response is compatible with the absence of clinical consequences of the disorder.

The situation in HFI may be seen as an exaggeration of the normal response to fructose, with the accumulation of fructose-1-phosphate being more absolute due to the deficiency of aldolase B activity and particularly significant in those tissues normally having a high concentration of the enzyme. The predominant responses to fructose intake are demonstrated in Fig. 2.13: reduced serum magnesium, Pi and glucose, and increased uric acid and fructose.[57] Relative inhibition of fructokinase can explain the fructosaemia and fructosuria when the monosaccharide is fed, or administered. In spite of the block in fructose metabolism, less than 20% of a load is excreted unchanged. It is presumed that the remainder is utilised in tissues containing the other aldolase isoenzymes, like muscle and adipose tissue.

The fall in blood glucose is more profound following fructose administration in HFI patients compared to normals and hypoglycaemia is the main clinical consequence when the toxic monosaccharide is available in the diet. It is suggested that this results from a block in glycogenolysis, an inhibition of gluconeogenesis and possible stimulation of glucose uptake into tissues. The other important clinical abnormalities, in liver and kidney function, would be the expected consequence of a lack of energy-providing compounds, because of the primary depletion of ATP and GTP, and secondarily, the effect of the losses from the adenine pool. There are

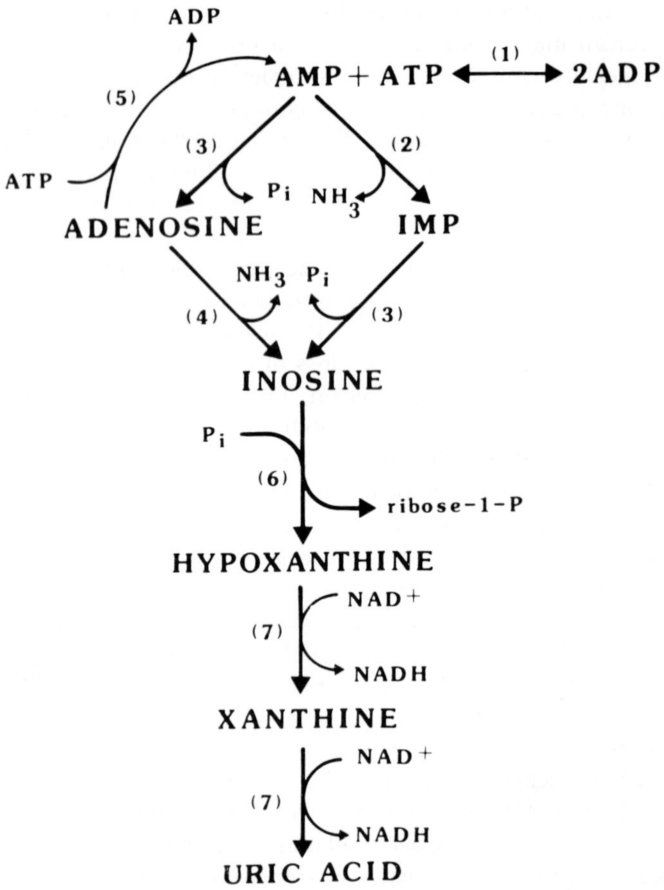

Fig. 2.12 Pathways of purine catabolism in the liver. Enzymes: (1) Adenylate kinase, (2) AMP deaminase, (3) Cytosolic 5'-nucleotidase, (4) adenosine deaminase, (5) adenosine kinase, (6) purine nucleoside phosphorylase, (7) xanthine dehydrogenase (oxidase).[53]

obvious similarities to the situation in galactose-1-phosphate uridyl transferase deficiencies (p. 43).

The predominant effect of fructose 1:6 bisphosphatase deficiency is an inability to maintain blood glucose levels on prolonged fasting when glycogen stores have been depleted, due to the block in gluconeogenesis (Fig. 2.14). In such a crisis, which may be life-threatening, there is a pronounced lactic acidosis because of the block in gluconeogenesis, and a marked ketosis because of the added use of fatty acids as an energy source. As expected from the position of the metabolic block, the hypoglycaemia is relieved by glucose or galactose, but not by fructose, glycerol, alanine or dihydroxyacetone. The main effect of giving substrates for gluconeogenesis is to cause more lactic acidosis and plasma bicarbonate depression.

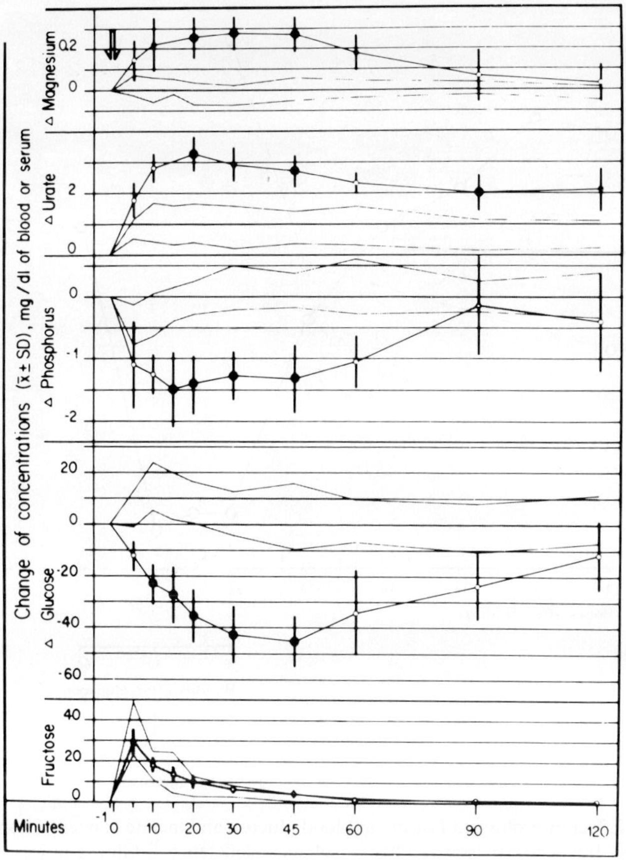

Fig. 2.13 Changes in blood concentration of fructose, glucose, phosphorus, urate and magnesium following an intravenous fructose load (200 mg/kg body weight) in 10 children with HFI and 16 control children.[57] The area between the faint lines represents the ± 1 SD limits for the controls. The vertical bars show the ± 1 SD range for the patients. Patient means indicated as a solid circle show that there is a significant difference from the control group. To convert mg/dl to SI units (mmol/l) multiply by the following factors: glucose and fructose, 0.06; phosphorus, 0.32; urate 0.06; magnesium, 0.41.

Although there is no particular clinical history of fructose intolerance in patients with fructose 1:6 bisphosphatase deficiency, it is well established that ingestion of large amounts of fructose may precipitate a hypoglycaemic crisis, although the actual fall in blood glucose is less severe than in HFI. The fructose load is cleared at normal rates from the blood and it is postulated that the effect on blood glucose is a consequence of the accumulation of fructose-1-phosphate, which occurs normally following fructose ingestion. As mentioned earlier, there is a block in glycogenolysis which can be ascribed to fructose-1-phosphate inhibiting liver phosphorylase A, combined with the depletion of Pi which is a substrate for this enzyme.

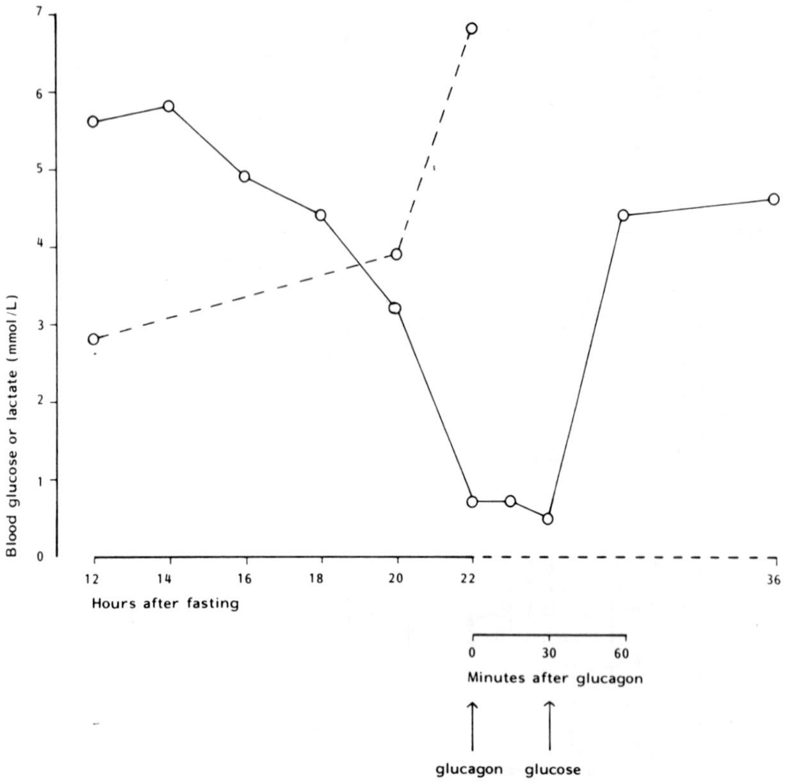

Fig. 2.14 Effect of prolonged fasting on blood glucose and lactate concentrations in a 17-month-old boy with fructose-1-6-bisphosphatase deficiency.[59] Glucagon was given after 22 hours. o—o – glucose, o---o – lactate.

This effect on glycogenolysis is critical in the presence of the permanent defect in gluconeogenesis.

Diagnosis

Fructosaemia and fructosuria in a patient in whom fructose intolerance is not a feature is indicative of essential fructosuria. The diagnosis may be supported by an oral fructose load test at a dose of 1 g/kg body weight up to a maximum of 50 g. A pronounced and prolonged rise in blood fructose with no response in blood glucose, or in other metabolites normally affected by fructose administration, is confirmation of the diagnosis.

HFI is usually suspected because of its clinical presentation, by a dietary history, the finding of fructosuria and fructosaemia and a favourable response to removal of fructose from the diet. It should be remembered, however, that, as in galactosaemia, the monosaccharide concerned may not be excreted if some hours have elapsed following the last possible ingestion of fructose. In a vomiting child it may be difficult to be sure when significant amounts of fructose had last been taken. Fructosuria must be confirmed by specific chromatographic methods. Unless the facts point clearly to HFI it is important to consider that a number of other inherited metabolic diseases have a similar clinical presentation, including tyrosinosis, some glycogenoses and galactosaemia. Hepatitis, liver cirrhosis and tumours, septicaemia and intrauterine infections may also have features in common with HFI.

Further confirmation of the diagnosis of HFI may be obtained with a fructose load test or tissue biopsy for enzyme tests. The former should only be done when the patient has been on a fructose-free diet for several weeks and is in a stable condition. Because of the untoward effects of an oral load, the fructose should be given intravenously with a dose of no more than 200 mg/kg body weight. Blood fructose, glucose, serum Pi, magnesium and uric acid are the main measurements to be made. The abnormal responses in HFI were described in the previous section and are shown in Fig. 2.13.

Tissue aldolase assays are usually performed on liver biopsy, although intestinal biopsies are an alternative.[58] It is usual to use both fructose 1:6 bisphosphate and fructose-1-phosphate as substrates in the assay and, as mentioned previously, the loss of activity is greater with fructose-1-phosphate in HFI, so that the ratio of activity with the two substrates, which is usually 1, is increased (Table 2.5). Diagnostic confusion with some liver diseases is possible, when liver biopsy is used, and with malabsorption states when intestinal biopsies are employed. Unfortunately aldolase activity in more accessible cells, leukocytes and skin fibroblasts, is not of the B isoenzyme.

Fructose 1:6-bisphosphatase deficiency should be considered in an infant presenting with hyperventilation, convulsions, coma, hypoglycaemia, ketosis and acidosis and in older children with hypoglycaemia triggered by fasting or infection. The acidosis is due to lactic acid. A very similar presentation and findings may be associated with deficiencies of glucose-6-phosphatase (p. 26), pyruvate carboxylase (p. 191), pyruvate dehydrogenase (p. 188) and phosphoenol pyruvate carboxykinase (p. 190), and it may be difficult to exclude these. The presentation of some organic acidurias due

Table 2.5 The three isoenzyme forms of fructaldase, their tissue distribution and activity ratios (rate with fructose 1:6-bisphosphate/rate with fructose-1-phosphate)

Type	Tissue	Activity ratio
A	Muscle	50
B	Liver	1
C	Brain	5–10

to branched chain amino acid or fatty acid metabolic disorders (p. 126) may also overlap with that of fructose 1:6 bisphosphatase deficiency. A fasting test (Fig. 2.14) and a lack of glycaemic response to fructose, glycerol, alanine and dihydroxyacetone may help to support the diagnosis[59], but these should not be carried out until the child is in a stable condition, and careful monitoring is required.

The enzyme deficiency may be confirmed in liver or jejunal biopsies.[60] Variable results have been reported of assays using leukocyte preparations and this seems due to the very low activity of fructose 1:6-bisphosphatase in these cells. On the other hand, cultured peripheral lymphocytes exhibit good activity and may be of diagnostic use.

Treatment

The essential treatment for *HFI* is immediate and lifelong removal of all sources of fructose from the diet. All signs and symptoms should disappear rapidly on this diet, apart from hepatomegaly which, for some reason, may persist for months or years. It is possible that fructose exclusion is not absolute in some of these cases and this is something to investigate. A severely ill child may require additional supportive measures at first, including the infusion of fresh frozen plasma and exchange transfusion. However, death is not always prevented, particularly when liver failure is well advanced before diagnosis. There is a suggestion that very early ingestion of fructose is more likely to result in liver cirrhosis.

The importance of strict dietary control throughout childhood is apparent from a report of growth retardation in some children with HFI who showed no other signs of chronic fructose intolerance.[61] More rigorous fructose restriction led to dramatic acceleration of growth.

The management of crises in *fructose 1:6 bisphosphatase deficiency* requires the administration of glucose and bicarbonate in order to correct the hypoglycaemia and acidosis. The most important features of the long-term management are frequent meals and avoidance of long fasts. This is very important when the patient has a febrile illness, and parents should be given specific instructions on how to manage these periods and given emergency regimes for this purpose. In addition, sources of fructose should be retricted because crises may be induced by ingestion of small amounts of this sugar, and a low fat, high carbohydrate diet has been recommended.[62]

REFERENCES

1. Hiatt H H 1978 Pentosuria. In: Stanbury J B, Wyngaarden J B and Fredrickson D S (eds) The metabolic basis of inherited disease, 8th edn. McGraw–Hill, New York, ch 5
2. Burchell A 1990 Molecular pathology of glucose-6-phosphatase. FASEB Journal 4:2978–2988

3. Newsholme E A, Start C 1973 Regulation of metabolism. John Wiley and Sons, Chichester
4. Hug G, Garancil J C, Schubert W K, Kaplan S 1966 Glycogen storage diseases, Types II, III, VII and IX. American Journal of Diseases of Children 111:457–474
5. Sidbury J B 1965 The genetics of the glycogen storage diseases. Progress in Medical Genetics 4:32–58
6. Spencer Peet J, Norman M E, Lake B D, McNamara J, Patrick A D 1971 Hepatic glycogen storage disease: clinical and laboratory findings in 23 cases. Quarterly Journal of Medicine 40:95–114
7. De Barsy Th, Lederer B 1980 Type VI glycogenosis: identification of subgroups. In: Burman D, Holton J B, Pennock C A (eds) Inherited disorders of carbohydrate metabolism. MTP Press, Lancaster, pp 369–380
8. Collins J E, Bartlett K, Leonard J V, Aynsley-Green A 1990 Glucose production rates in type I glycogen storage disease. Journal of Inherited Metabolic Disease 13:195–206
9. Sadeghi-Nejad A, Presente E, Binkiewicz A, Senior B 1974 Studies in Type I glycogenosis of the liver: the genesis and disposition of lactate. Journal of Pediatrics 85:49–54
10. Greene H L, Wilson F A, Hefferan P et al 1978 ATP depletion a possible role in the pathogenesis of hyperuricaemia in glycogen storage disease Type I. Journal of Clinical Investigation 62:321–328
11. Leonard J V, Dunger D B, Preece M A 1984 Patterns of growth in the hepatic glycogenoses. Archives of Disease in Childhood 59:657–660
12. Dunger D B, Holder A T, Leonard J V, Okae J, Preece M A 1982 Growth and endocrine changes in the hepatic glycogenoses. European Journal of Pediatrics 138:226–230
13. Fernandes J, Koster J F, Grose W F A, Sogedrager N 1974 Hepatic phosphorylase deficiency. Its differentiation from other hepatic glycogenoses. Archives of Disease in Childhood 49:186–191
14. Schwartz R, Ashmore J, Rendold A E 1957 Galactose tolerance in glycogen storage disease. Pediatrics 19:585
15. Senior B, Loridan L 1968 Studies of liver glycogenosis with particular reference to the metabolism of intravenously administered glycerol. New England Journal of Medicine 279:958–965
16. Sidbury J B, Cornblath M, Fisher J, House E 1961 Glycogen in erythrocytes of patients with glycogen storage disease. Pediatrics 27:103–111
17. Fernandes J, Leonard J V, Moses S W, Odievre M, Di Rocco M, Schaub J, Smit G P, Ullrich K, Durand P 1988 Glycogen storage disease: recommendations for treatment. European Journal of Pediatrics 147:226–228
18. Stanley C A, Mills J L, Baker L 1981 Intragastric feeding in Type I glycogen storage disease. Factors affecting the control of lactic acidaemia. Pediatric Research 15:1504–1508
19. Chen Y T, Coleman R A, Scheinman J I, Kolbeck P C, Sidbury J B 1988 Renal disease in type I glycogen storage disease. New England Journal of Medicine 318:7–11
20. Ross B D, Radda G K, Gadian D G, Rocker G, Esiri M, Falconer-Smith J 1981 Examination of a case of suspected McArdle's syndrome by ^{31}P nuclear magnetic resonance. New England Journal of Medicine 304:1338–1342
21. Holton J B 1990 Galactose disorders: an overview. Journal of Inherited Metabolic Disease 13:476–486
22. Ng W G, Xu Y K, Kaufman F R, Donnell G N 1989 Deficit of uridine diphosphate galactose in galactosaemia. Journal of Inherited Metabolic Disease 12:257–266
23. Green A, Holton J B, Honeyman M M, Leonard J V 1992, in press
24. Waggoner D D, Buist N R M, Donnell G N 1990 Long-term prognosis in galactosaemia: results of a survery of 350 cases. Journal of Inherited Metabolic Disease 13:802–818
25. Reichardt J K J, Packman S, Woo S L C 1991 Molecular characterization of two galactosaemia mutations: correlation of mutations with highly conserved domains in galactose-1-phosphate uridyl transferase. American Journal of Human Genetics 49: 860–867
26. Huttenlocher R R, Hillman R E, Hsia Y E 1970 Pseudotumour cerebri in galactosaemia. Journal of Pediatrics 76:902–905

27. Holton J B, Gillett M G, McFaul R, Young R 1981 Galactosaemia: a new severe variant due to uridine diphosphate galactose-4-epimerase deficiency. Archives of Disease in Childhood 56:885–887
28. Sardharwalla I B, Wraith J E, Bridge C et al 1987 A patient with a severe type of epimerase deficiency galactosaemia. Abstracts of the 25th Annual Symposium of the Society for the Study of Inborn Errors of Metabolism, SSIEM:91
29. Gillett M G 1985 Investigation of human uridine 5'-phosphate-4-epimerase. MSc thesis, University of Bath
30. Gitzelmann R 1969 Formation of galactose-1-phosphate from uridine diphosphate galactose in erythrocytes of patients with galactosaemia. Pediatric Research 3:279
31. Pourci M L, Mangeot M, Lemmonier A 1985 Origin of the galactose-1-phosphate present in erythrocytes and fibroblasts of treated galactosaemic patients. IRCS Medical Science 13:1232–1233
32. Cross K C, Acosta P B 1991 Fruits and vegetables are a source of galactose: implications in planning the diets of patients with galactosaemia. Journal of Inherited Metabolic Disease 14:253–258
33. Berry G T, Palmieri M J, Heales S et al 1992 Red blood cell uridine sugar nucleotide levels in patients with classic galactosaemia and other metabolic disorders. Metabolism 7:783–7
34. Winder A F 1982 Galactose intolerance and the risk of cataract. British Journal of Ophthalmology 66:438–441
35. Berry G T, Yandrasitz J R, Segal S 1981 Experimental galactose toxicity: effects on synaptosomal phosphatidylinositol metabolism. Journal of Neurochemistry 37:888–891
36. Starling J J, Kepler D O R 1977 Metabolism of 2-deoxy-D-galactose in liver induces phosphate and uridylate trapping. European Journal of Biochemistry 80:373–379
37. Dobbie J A, Holton J B, Clamp J R 1990 Defective galactosylation of proteins in cultured skin fibroblasts from galactosaemic patients. Annals of Clinical Biochemistry 27:274–275
38. Ormstein K S, McGuire E J, Berry G T 1992 Abnormal galactosylation of complex carbohydrates in cultured fibroblasts from patients with galactose-1-phosphate uridyl transferase deficiency. Pediatric Research 31:508–511
39. Green A, Holton J B, Roylance G, (in press)
40. Kaufman F R, Ng W G, Xu Y K et al 1989 Treatment of patients with classical galactosaemia with oral uridine. Pediatric Research 25:834
41. Gitzelmann R 1989 Disorders of galactose metabolism. In: Fernandes J, Saudubray G M, Tada K (eds) Inborn metabolic diseases: diagnosis and treatment. Springer-Verlag, Berlin, p 95–105
42. Beutler E, Baluda M 1966 A simple spot screening test for galactosaemia. Journal of Laboratory and Clinical Medicine 68:137–141
43. Monk A M, Mitchell A J H, Milligan D W A, Holton J B 1977 The diagnosis of classical galactosaemia. Archives of Diseases in Childhood 52:943–946
44. Kleijer W J, Janse H C, Macek M et al 1986 First trimester diagnosis of galactosaemia. Lancet 1:174
45. Holton J B, Allen J T, Gillett M 1989 Prenatal diagnosis of disorders of galactose metabolism. Journal of Inherited Metabolic Disease 12 Suppl 1:202–206
46. Paigen K, Pacholec F, Levy H L, 1982 A new method of screening for inherited disorders of galactose metabolism. Journal of Laboratory and Clinical Medicine 99:895–906
47. Kelly S 1979 Significance of the Duarte/classical galactosaemia genetic compound. Journal of Pediatrics 92:937
48. Shin Y S, Rimböck H, Endres W 1982 Fructose-1-phosphate aldolase activity in human fetal and adult tissues as well as leukocytes and cultured fibroblasts in hereditary fructose intolerance. Journal of Inherited Metabolic Disease 5 Suppl 1:45–46
49. Van den Berghe G 1991 Hereditary fructose intolerance. In: Schaub J, Van Hoof F, Vis H L (eds). Inborn errors of metabolism. Raven Press, New York, pp 181–192
50. Maggiori G, Borgna-Pignatti C 1982 Disseminated coagulopathy associated with hereditary fructose intolerance. American Journal of Diseases of Children 136:169–170
51. Gregori C, Schapira F, Kahn A et al 1982 Molecular studied of liver aldolase B in hereditary fructose intolerance using blotting and immunological techniques. Annals of Human Genetics 46:218–292
52. Cox T M, Ali M, Cross N C P 1991 Molecular genetics of hereditary fructose

intolerance. Proceedings of the 8th International Congress of Human Genetics. American Journal of Human Genetics 49 Suppl:184
53. Gitzelmann R, Steinmann B, Van den Berghe G 1989 Disorders of fructose metabolism. In: Scriver C R, Beaudet A L, Sly W S, Valle D (eds). The metabolic basis of inherited disease, 6th edn. McGraw – Hill, New York, p 412–417
54. Taunton O D, Greene H L, Stifel F B, 1978 Fructose-1,6-diphosphatase deficiency, hypoglycaemia and response to folate therapy in a mother and her daughter. Biochemical Medicine 19:260–264
55. Shin Y S, Reith M, Endres W, Haas P 1984 Sorbitol dehydrogenase deficiency in a family with congenital cataracts. Journal of Inherited Metabolic Disease 7 Suppl 2:151–152
56. Van Schaftingen E 1989 D-glycerate kinase deficiency as a cause of D-glyceric aciduria. FEBS Letters 243:127–131
57. Steinman B, Gitzelmann R 1981 The diagnosis of hereditary fructose intolerance. Helvetica Paediatrica Acta 36:297–316
58. Streb H, Posselt H G, Wolter K, Bender S W 1981 Aldolase activity of the small intestinal mucosa in malabsorption sites and in hereditary fructose intolerance. European Journal of Pediatrics 137:5–10
59. Baerlocher K, Gitzelmann R, Steinmann B 1980 Clinical and genetic studies in fructose metabolism. In: Burman D, Holton J B, Pennock C A (eds). Inherited disorders of carbohydrate metabolism. MTP Press, Lancaster, p 163–190
60. Gitzelmann R 1974 Enzymes of fructose and galactose metabolism. In: Curtius H Ch, Roth M (eds) Clinical biochemistry, principles and methods. De Gruyter, Berlin, p 1236–1251
61. Mock D M, Perman J A, Thaler M M, Morris R C 1983 Chronic fructose intolerance and infancy in children with hereditary fructose intolerance. A cause of growth retardation. New England Journal of Medicine 309:764–770
62. Pagliara A S, Karl I E, Keating J P et al 1972 Hepatic 1,6-diphosphatase deficiency. A cause of lactic acidosis and hypoglycaemia in infancy. Journal of Clinical Investigation 51:2115–2123

3. Amino acid disorders

R. J. Pollitt

The amino acids show great chemical diversity, the only common feature being the presence of a primary or secondary amino group and an acidic function. This is usually a carboxyl group but in some cases is an acidic sulphono or phosphono residue. Biochemically too this group is very heterogeneous. Amino acids are the primary components of proteins but some also act as intermediates in important metabolic cycles or function as neurotransmitters. Many of these functions are essential to life, even in utero, so that the defects that present as inherited metabolic disease are mainly confined to catabolic pathways. In keeping with their varied biochemistry, the clinical features associated with the amino acid disorders differ markedly. Only the disorders of the urea cycle share a common theme; the other groupings in this chapter reflect an attempt at biochemical order rather than a clinically useful classification.

DETECTION OF AMINO ACID DISORDERS

In contrast to the great biochemical and clinical heterogeneity of disorders of amino acid metabolism, their laboratory investigation follows a relatively simple common pattern. Nearly all can be detected by chromatographic examination of the urinary amino acids and in many cases the results of this investigation lead directly to the diagnosis. The ninhydrin reagent provides a sensitive and selective method of visualising and measuring amino acids and related compounds, and their chemical diversity facilitates chromatographic separation. The development of paper chromatography led to a rapid growth in knowledge of amino acid disorders during the late 1950s and the 1960s. Qualitative chromatography of amino acids is still the most widely performed investigation for symptomatic inherited metabolic disease, but the introduction of external quality assessment has shown that in inexperienced hands such chromatograms are frequently misinterpreted. Edwards et al[1] give a useful practical guide to problems likely to be encountered in routine investigation.

For urinary amino acids most laboratories rely on paper or thin-layer chromatographic methods[2,3] which, if critically applied, are highly satisfactory, though it is probably impracticable to design a routine procedure that will infallibly detect all known disorders. One-dimensional chromatography is rapid, and particularly valuable in the emergency investigation of the critically ill neonate for specific disorders such as maple syrup urine disease, argininosuccinic aciduria and citrullinaemia. However, its separation of the more polar amino acids is poor and its use in definitive investigations of patients with suspected metabolic disorders is to be deprecated. High-voltage electrophoresis at pH2 (Fig. 3.1) is the most useful one-dimensional system available. There are several two-dimensional thin-layer chromatography systems that give satisfactory results with urine without the need for any preliminary desalting.[3]

Disorders affecting amino acids with a high tubular reabsorbtion, partic-

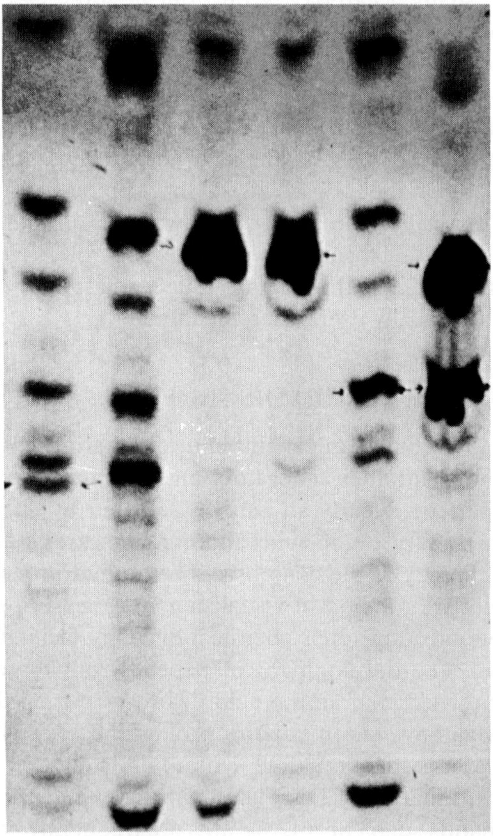

Fig. 3.1 Urinary amino acids separated on paper by high-voltage electrophoresis at pH2. Samples from left to right: phenylketonuria; normal subject, twice the usual volume applied; non-ketotic hyperglycinaemia with neonatal onset; non-ketotic hyperglycinaemia with late onset; homocystinuria due to cystathionine synthase deficiency; argininosuccinate lyase deficiency. The six most intense bands in the normal sample are, from top to bottom, histidine, glycine, alanine, serine, glutamine and taurine (close to the point of application).

ularly phenylalanine, tyrosine, methionine and the branched-chain amino acids, are more reliably diagnosed by the examination of plasma; in the immediate neonatal period and in mild or intermittent variants the plasma concentration of affected amino acids may be too low to produce any marked increase in urinary excretion. Moderate increases in the plasma concentration of these amino acids are, however, readily detectable by one-dimensional chromatography which is widely used in neonatal screening programmes.

Quantitative amino acid analysis is seldom required for the initial detection of a disorder but may be important in confirming the diagnosis and for monitoring any form of treatment. Some amino acids, e.g. phenylalanine, may be estimated by specific methods, but for most applications it is simpler and more satisfactory to use an automated amino acid analyser. High performance liquid chromatography with pre-column derivatisation offers a convenient and cheaper alternative to the dedicated amino acid analyser, but has limitations.

Recently, fast atom bombardment tandem mass spectrometry (Ch. 4), after conversion of amino acids to their butyl esters, has been developed to provide rapid (1 minute) semiquantitative analysis. This method cannot distinguish between isomers, however, and its general applicability has still to be fully assessed.

A detailed account of most of the methods just described, together with a comprehensive review of the chemistry of amino acids found in human body fluids in health and disease, is given in the monograph by Bremer et al.[3]

PHENYLKETONURIA, HYPERPHENYLALANINAEMIA AND RELATED CONDITIONS

Phenylalanine hydroxylase deficiency (McKusick 261600)

Phenylketonuria due to phenylalanine hydroxylase deficiency is the commonest of the amino acid disorders resulting in mental subnormality in most European populations. The disease was discovered by Følling in 1934 following the observation that the urine of two mentally deficient brothers, who had a peculiar musty odour, gave a green coloration with ferric chloride solution. For an interesting account of the history of phenylketonuria see Bickel.[4]

Biochemistry

In man phenylalanine is entirely of dietary origin. The major catabolic pathway is by the action of phenylalanine hydroxylase (phenylalanine mono-oxygenase, EC 1.14.16.1) to produce tyrosine (Fig. 3.2). In man this reaction is predominantly performed in liver. The status of phenylala-

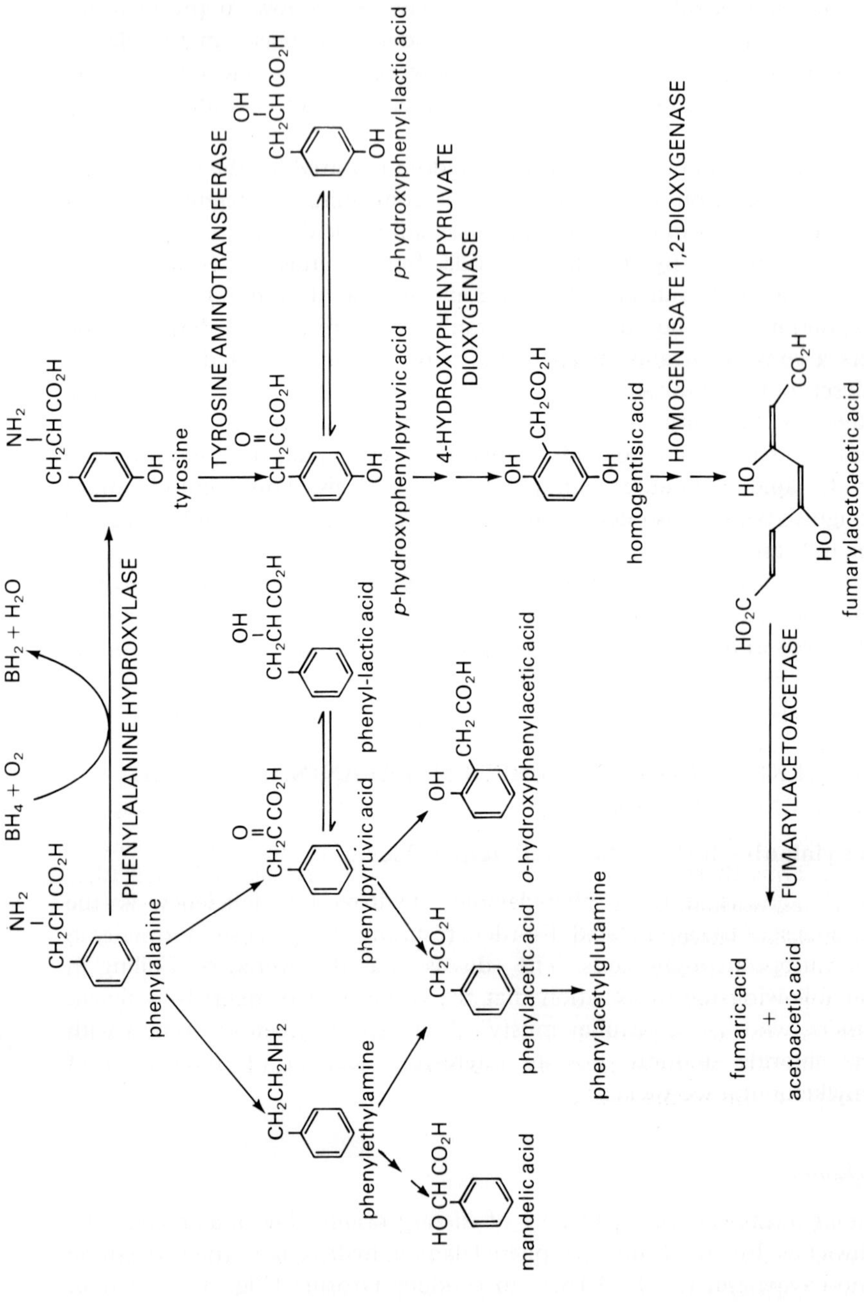

Fig. 3.2 Outline of phenylalanine metabolism showing the origin of the major abnormal metabolites found in phenylketonuria.

nine hydroxylase in kidney is uncertain and it cannot be detected in leucocytes, cultured fibroblasts or amniotic fluid cells. However, tyrosine hydroxylase (EC 1.14.16.2) shows some activity towards phenylalanine.

Tetrahydrobiopterin is necessary as a cofactor for phenylalanine hydroxylase, being oxidised, and then converted by pterin-4a-carbinolamine dehydratase to quinonoid dihydrobiopterin. The enzyme dihydropteridine reductase recycles the quinonoid dihydrobiopterin to tetrahydrobiopterin (Fig. 3.3).

In classical phenylketonuria there is a complete absence of phenylalanine hydroxylase activity, or at most very low residual activity. Affected individuals have near normal plasma phenylalanine concentrations at birth but these rise rapidly once feeding is established and usually reach 1.2–6.0 mmol/l within 2–3 weeks. Transamination leads to a series of overflow metabolites which appear in the urine: phenylpyruvic acid, phenyllactic acid, o-hydroxyphenylacetic acid, phenylacetic acid and phenylacetylglutamine. The last two metabolites may also arise following phenylalanine decarboxylation, as does mandelic acid, also excreted in excess. A host of minor metabolites have been reported. Phenylacetic acid is responsible for the characteristic smell of patients with untreated phenylketonuria. Phenylpyruvic acid gives a dark apple-green coloration with ferric chloride solution, as first observed by Følling. The increasing capacity for transamination with age is probably responsible for the lower plasma phenylalanine levels seen in older untreated patients compared to infants.

Patients with slight to moderate impairment of phenylalanine hydroxylation are often grouped together under the heading of hyperphenylalaninaemia, also referred to as mild, or atypical, phenylketonuria. Strict definition holds that there should be no phenylketonuria (i.e. no urinary excretion of phenylpyruvic acid) but in practise there are borderline patients who will occasionally excrete phenylpyruvic acid in readily detectable amounts, depending on dietary phenylalanine intake and other factors. Thus there is a complete gradation between classical phenylketonuria and normal. In some hyperphenylalaninaemic patients the phenylalanine decay curves following intravenous loads show that the residual phenylalanine hydroxylase is susceptible to substrate inhibition, suggesting an abnormal structure. A few reports have attributed hyperphenylalaninaemia in particular patients to defective phenylalanine transamination but, as levels of phenylalanine are regulated by the action of phenylalanine hydroxylase, this seems unlikely.

Diagnosis

In many countries with a high incidence, phenylketonuria is detected by neonatal screening for increased blood or plasma phenylalanine concentrations. The diagnosis is usually based on the increased phenylalanine in the absence of excess of any other plasma amino acid, tyrosine being normal

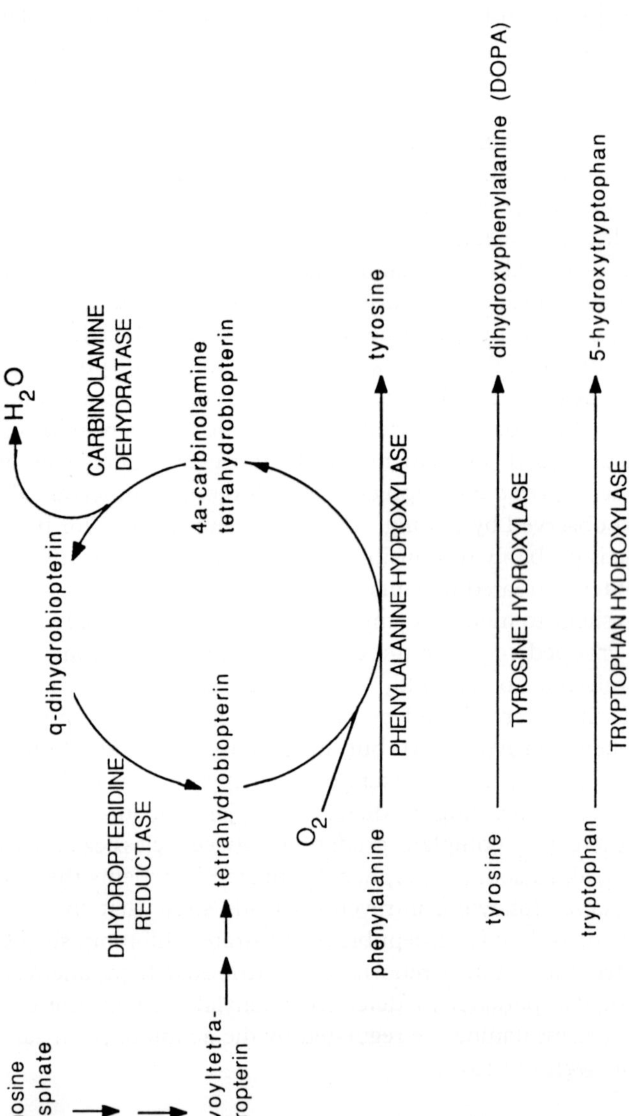

Fig. 3.3 Summary of tetrahydrobiopterin metabolism.

or somewhat reduced in concentration. With the prompt initiation of treatment it is unusual, in the neonatal period, for more than trace amounts of abnormal phenolic acids to be found in urine, but in older patients on an unrestricted diet these metabolites should be present. Enzyme studies (which involve liver biopsy) are unnecessary provided that the possibility of tetrahydrobiopterin deficiency (see below) is excluded by other methods.

The classification of patients with partial defects of phenylalanine hydroxylase is an unsolved problem. Not only is there a continuum from classical phenylketonuria to normality, but it is difficult to tell in the neonatal period whether a patient will need strict or only moderate restriction of dietary intake to control plasma phenylalanine levels later in childhood. Assay of hepatic phenylalanine hydroxylase, dietary challenges and phenylalanine load tests, with or without stable isotopic labelling, all show reasonable statistical correlations with dietary phenylalanine tolerance. However, such tests do not provide sufficiently reliable prognostic information in the individual patient to have a role in routine management. Attempts are being made to approach this problem through analysis of the quantitative effects of specific mutations on the expression and activity of the enzyme.[5]

Clinical features

Rapid exchange across the placenta keeps the phenylalanine levels essentially normal in the fetus with phenylalanine hydroxylase deficiency. After birth, however, the accumulation of phenylalanine and its metabolites inhibits mental development and progressively damages the brain. The baby with phenylketonuria usually appears normal for the first few months with no specific neurological signs, but by 6 months of age mental development is often obviously delayed. Untreated phenylketonuria usually leads to severe mental retardation with a high proportion of patients showing microcephaly and having seizures and other neurological abnormalities. Agitated and aggressive behaviour is common, often with autistic features. The hair and eye pigments are diluted, giving a tendency to blond hair and blue eyes. Eczema is found in about a quarter of the patients. A small proportion of untreated patients with the biochemical features of classical phenylketonuria are of normal intelligence. Others may escape with only mild mental retardation and perhaps one-sixth of the untreated cases are functioning 'normally' within the general community. The reason for this variability is unknown. Retrospective studies have suggested that patients with partial deficiency of phenylalanine hydroxylase, whose blood phenylalanine concentrations remain for the most part below 1.2 mmol/l (20 mg/dl), do not become markedly retarded.[6] Most paediatricians err on the side of safety and choose a lower limit, often 0.9 mmol/l but increasingly as low as 0.6 mmol/l, below which they do not treat.

The pathogenic mechanisms in phenylketonuria are still in dispute. Phenylalanine and its metabolites affect numerous areas of metabolism including the synthesis of indolamine and catecholamine neurotransmitters. The inhibitory effect of phenylalanine on the synthesis of cerebroside sulphatide seems likely to be responsible for the myelin deficiency seen in untreated phenylketonuria.[7] Given the individual variations in the threshold at which transamination becomes rapid, and the likelihood that phenylalanine itself plays a major role in pathogenesis, it is unsound to take the absence of urinary phenylpyruvic acid as a sign that dietary treatment is unnecessary.

Treatment

The aim of treatment is to prevent excessive phenylalanine accumulation by strict control of dietary protein intake coupled with the administration of a phenylalanine-free amino acid supplement to allow for the requirements of normal growth.[8] The original amino acid supplements were derived from acid-hydrolysed natural protein, the phenylalanine being removed by absorption on a charcoal column. Tyrosine is also retained by this column and tryptophan is destroyed during the hydrolysis, so that both must be added to the final product. Such preparations invariably have a most unpleasant taste and some of the earlier ones produced metabolic acidosis and anorexia. They have been superseded by mixtures of synthetic amino acids which are less distasteful. Such a diet requires careful attention to avoid vitamin and trace element deficiency and, as the patient grows older, to provide a degree of variety and to ensure palatability. Many special dietary products that help in these respects are now commercially available.

The blood phenylalanine concentration should be monitored regularly. Sufficient phenylalanine must be provided for the requirements of growth and tissue repair and it is usual to aim for a slight excess. The lower limit of acceptability for blood phenylalanine is usually set somewhere in the range of 0.1–0.2 mmol/l, normal being 0.06 ± 0.02 mmol/l. The upper limit is less generally agreed. Patients whose treatment started within the first few weeks of life and who have been well controlled have near-normal intelligence, but overall the treated group shows a deficit of 0.5 of the normal population standard deviation (corresponding to about 8 IQ points). Within the patient group lower IQ correlates with higher plasma phenylalanine concentrations at diagnosis, higher average phenylalanine exposures and later start to treatment.[9] Based on the data from the UK phenylketonuria register, Smith and colleagues tentatively suggest[9] maintaining non-fasting blood phenylalanine concentrations between 0.12 and 0.30 mmol/l for the first few years of life, though there are doubts as to the practicability of such tight control. There are still problems in interpreting existing data and some doubts as to whether there is a linear no-threshold effect of phenylalanine on intelligence or whether higher concentrations exert a disproportionate effect as suggested in the earlier literature.

Early practice was to completely abandon dietary treatment at around the age of 5 years when, it was argued, brain development would be substantially complete. This led in many cases to slow but very definite developmental regression and it is now realised that the period of vulnerability is much longer. There is clear evidence that exposure to excessive phenylalanine between 4 and 8 years of life leads to mental deterioration and strong indications that vulnerability persists, though to a lesser degree, into the early teens.[10] Coupled with this is increasing anxiety about the long-term outlook. Even with controlled relaxation of diet, allowing plasma phenylalanine to reach no higher than 1.2 mmol/l, some patients show deterioration in the EEG and there have been several reports of acute neurological deterioration in older patients on free diets[11], as well as reports of rather alarming magnetic resonance imaging abnormalities in brain, even in symptom-free individuals. For most children with phenylketonuria some degree of relaxation becomes unavoidable as they grow older and seems to be well tolerated but the current trend is towards 'diet for life', with phenylalanine concentrations maintained if possible below 0.9 mmol/l.

Genetics

Autosomal recessive inheritance has been demonstrated by showing a 1 in 4 incidence of phenylketonuria in sibs of index cases and an equal sex ratio. The heterozygotes have reduced capacity to hydroxylate phenylalanine and can as a group be distinguished by phenylalanine loading tests or by various measurements of plasma phenylalanine and tyrosine.[12] In individual cases, though, classification may be impossible because of overlap between the normal and heterozygote ranges and for family studies DNA methods are to be preferred. The incidence of phenylketonuria varies from country to country and even within regions of the United Kingdom. The overall average in the UK approximates to 10: 100 000. The highest incidence in the world seems to be in Turkey with 23 cases of classical phenylketonuria per 100 000.

The phenylalanine hydroxylase gene is located on chromosome 12 and is highly polymorphic.[13] The DNA sequence is 90 kb long and consists of 13 exons, resulting in mRNA of approximately 2.4 kb. Over 30 different mutations have so far been identified in association with phenylketonuria and over 50 haplotype patterns observed on restriction fragment length analysis. There is a high degree of linkage disequilibrium in Caucasian populations, with two haplotypes (numbered 2 and 3) very much over-represented in association with PKU alleles. Danish patients who are homozygous for haplotypes 2 or 3, or are mixed 2–3 heterozygotes tend to have classical PKU. Most of the mutations so far characterised in German and Danish patients are in exons 7 or 12, though a mutation in intron 12 accounts for 25% of the total.[5] Preliminary results from southern Europe indicate different haplotype distributions and it is likely that the final picture will be very complex.

First trimester prenatal diagnosis on the basis of restriction fragment length polymorphism is possible in most families but the apparently favourable outcome of early treatment has meant that in practice there has been rather little demand for this procedure.

Pregnancy in phenylketonuria

The fetus is adversely affected by high phenylalanine concentrations and, unless countermeasures are taken, babies born to phenylketonuric women show a very high incidence of microcephaly and mental retardation and an increased frequency of congenital heart defects and other abnormalities.[14] Such babies are said to suffer from maternal phenylketonuria. In the past this problem has been limited by the relatively small number of women with classical phenylketonuria who were of sufficient intelligence to participate in the general community, but it is increasing as more early-treated patients with good intellectual function reach sexual maturity. Very careful dietary control of phenylalanine levels prior to conception and throughout pregnancy will prevent fetal damage[15], though the degree of control required for complete protection may be very difficult to achieve. Patients with partial phenylalanine hydroxylase deficiency who were not considered to need treatment themselves in infancy may need dietary restriction during pregnancy. It has been belatedly recognised that systematic long-term follow-up of female patients with phenylketonuria, with very active counselling as the reproductive years approach, is essential if cases of fetal damage due to maternal phenylketonuria are to be prevented.

Tetrahydrobiopterin deficiencies

For each molecule of tyrosine synthesised by the action of phenylalanine hydroxylase a molecule of tetrahydrobiopterin is oxidised to 4a-carbinolamine-tetrahydrobiopterin. The latter is rapidly converted to quinonoid dihydrobiopterin by the enzyme pterin-4a-carbinolamine dehydratase. Normally the cycle is completed by the reduction of quinonoid dihydrobiopterin to tetrahydrobiopterin by dihydropteridine reductase (EC 1.6.99.7), a deficiency of which effectively prevents phenylalanine hydroxylation (Fig. 3.3). Patients with *dihydropteridine reductase deficiency* (McKusick 261630) may show typical biochemical features of classical phenylketonuria though they often have a fairly high tolerance to dietary phenylalanine. However tetrahydrobiopterin is also a cofactor for tyrosine hydroxylase and tryptophan hydroxylase, enzymes essential for the formation of the catecholamine neurotransmitters (dopamine, noradrenaline and adrenaline) and 5-hydroxytryptamine (serotonin) respectively. In dihydropteridine reductase deficiency depletion of these neurotransmitters often leads to progressive neurological deterioration with feeding difficulties, hypotonia, seizures and death. *Deficiency of pterin-4a-carbinolamine dehydratase* seems to be much milder, patients usually having normal levels of amine metabolites in CSF and only transient hyperphenylalaninaemia. This disorder results in the excretion of a range of 7-substituted pterins, 'primapterinuria'.

Defects on the pathway of de novo biopterin synthesis from guanosine triphosphate (McKusick 261640) can give rise to a clinical picture and secondary biochemical changes similar to those of dihydropteridine reductase deficiency. *Guanosine triphosphate cyclohydrolase* (EC 3.5.4.16) *deficiency* and *6-pyruvoyl-tetrahydropterin synthase deficiency* are now both well characterised.

These tetrahydrobiopterin deficiency disorders are sometimes referred to collectively as malignant or lethal hyperphenylalaninaemias but the clinical picture is very variable and some patients are only moderately affected, presenting late with mental retardation. Patients with dihydropteridine reductase deficiency may have only marginally increased blood phenylalanine concentrations, and it is uncertain how many escape detection during neonatal screening for phenylketonuria. In caucasian populations only 1–2% of cases of phenylketonuria/hyperphenylalaninaemia detected by neonatal blood-spot screening have tetrahydrobiopterin deficiency defects but some oriental countries experience a much greater proportion.

Detailed discussion of diagnosis is beyond the scope of this chapter and some aspects are still controversial. Dihydropteridine reductase is widely distributed in the body and may be assayed in fibroblasts, leucocytes or dried blood spots.[16] The *Crithidia fasiculata* assay for total blood biopterin, also applicable to dried blood spots[17], may be a useful screen for disorders of biopterin synthesis as is high performance liquid chromatography of urinary biopterins.[18] In most cases of tetrahydrobiopterin deficiency an oral dose of tetrahydrobiopterin produces a temporary reduction in blood phenylalanine concentrations. This could be a useful preliminary test but has given misleading results on occasions.

Treatment is by dietary phenylalanine restriction together with neurotransmitter replacement, using carefully controlled doses of L-dopa and L-5-hydroxytryptophan together with a peripheral decarboxylase inhibitor, and folinic acid to correct any secondary folate deficiency. The short-term effects are dramatic and many patients are now making good developmental progress. It remains to be seen how well such a regime can be supported on a long-term basis.

Dihydropteridine reductase deficiency can be diagnosed prenatally by enzyme assay on cultured amniotic fluid cells, and gene probes for restriction fragment polymorphism analysis are now available. Pterin analysis of amniotic fluid has also been successfully predictive in some tetrahydrobiopterin deficiency disorders.

Screening for phenylketonuria and other amino acid disorders

The demonstration in 1954 of the feasibility of dietary control of phenylketonuria created the need for a routine method for detecting babies with this condition before irreversible brain damage occurred. The first large-scale screening programmes[19] were based on the colour reaction of phenylpyruvic acid in the urine-soaked nappy with ferric chloride, usually in the form of the Phenistix® test stick. Because of the time taken for blood phenylalanine concentrations to increase after birth and for transamination to become established this test had to be performed at about 6 weeks of age and even so gave a false negative rate of about 10%.

With the development of the Guthrie bacterial inhibition assay (1960) it became possible to estimate the phenylalanine content of dried blood spots on a large scale and centralised screening using this assay became the method of choice. In the Guthrie method discs punched from the blood spot are applied to a nutrient agar gel containing spores of *Bacillus subtilis*. The medium also contains β-thienylalanine which inhibits the growth of the organism, this inhibition being overcome by phenylalanine. Thus after an overnight incubation each blood disc is surrounded by a zone of bacterial growth, the higher the phenylalanine content of the disc, the larger the growth zone. Use of this blood-based assay increased the sensitivity of detection of impaired phenylalanine hydroxylation and enabled screening to be carried out at an earlier age. In the UK it is recommended that the test be performed on or soon after the sixth day of life, providing that full protein feeding has been established for at least 48 h. Elsewhere, in the USA for example, the pattern of medical care may dictate that babies have to be tested much earlier. This reduces the sensitivity and selectivity of the screen but this may be partially overcome by replacing the microbiological assay by the more sensitive and accurate automated fluorometric method.

The introduction of blood testing for phenylketonuria produced almost universally about twice the number of patients anticipated, a common problem with screening programmes. A proportion of the excess could be ascribed to cases of classical phenylketonuria that would have been missed by the urine test, but most was due to the detection for the first time of patients with mild to moderate impairments of phenylalanine hydroxylase activity. These variants raised difficult problems in drawing the dividing line for non-treatment.

Whilst many screening programmes still use the original Guthrie method or an alternative specific fluorometric assay, others have taken advantage of the availability of blood samples to screen for additional amino acid disorders.[20] One-dimensional chromatography has proved popular, about one-third of the babies born in the UK being screened by chromatographic methods. Maple syrup urine disease, tyrosinaemia, some cases of homocystinuria, some of the urea cycle defects, and other rarer disorders may be detected in addition to phenylketonuria but, except in special populations, the additional yield of treatable disorders is rather low. Screening for congenital hypothyroidism is almost universal in Europe and the USA and dried blood spots are also used in some areas to screen for galactosaemia, congenital adrenal hyperplasia, biotinidase deficiency and other inherited metabolic disorders. Dried blood spots collected for neonatal screening are increasingly being used for anonymised mass surveillance of the HIV epidemic and remaining spots are often placed in long-term storage as a source of DNA for future genetic studies.

TYROSINAEMIAS

Four well-recognised inherited disorders of tyrosine metabolism produce tyrosinaemia. The best known, *tyrosinaemia Type I* (McKusick 276700), affects predominantly the liver and kidneys and has clinical features which may be confused with those of hereditary fructose intolerance and transferase-deficiency galactosaemia. The majority of cases are due to fumarylacetoacetase (EC 3.7.1.2) deficiency. This enzyme is on the tyrosine degradation pathway but follows homogentisic acid oxidase (Fig. 3.2). As a deficiency of the latter enzyme causes homogentisic aciduria but no tyrosinaemia, it follows that the amino acid abnormalities in tyrosinaemia Type I are secondary to liver damage. Indeed similar amino acid abnormalities are seen in advanced cases of galactosaemia and hereditary fructose intolerance. Tyrosinaemia Type I is therefore primarily a disorder of organic acid metabolism (Ch. 4).

A rare condition, *hawkinsinuria* (McKusick 140350), so far reported only from Australia, is due to a blockage in one of the steps in *p*-hydroxyphenylpyruvic acid oxidation and results in transient tyrosinaemia in infancy. Hawkinsin, 2-cystein-*S*-yl-1,4-dihydroxycyclohex-5-enylacetic acid, is detectable on amino acid chromatography and is a conjugate of a reactive intermediate in the oxidation sequence. This is a dominant condition suggesting that successive steps in the overall reaction occur with the substrate closely associated with a multienzyme complex.

Tyrosinaemia Type II (McKusick 276600) is associated with hyperkeratotic erosions of the palms and soles, corneal erosion and ulceration and variably with mild to moderate mental retardation. The dermatological features were described as the Richner–Hanhart syndrome before the biochemical nature of the disease became apparent. The biochemical features are a marked tyrosinaemia of 0.7–3.4 mmol/l, together with urinary excretion of excess of tyrosine and *p*-hydroxphenyllactic and *p*-hydroxyphenylpyruvic acids. The primary defect is in hepatic tyrosine aminotransferase (EC 2.6.1.5) which is responsible for the first step in tyrosine catabolism. This is a cytosolic enzyme. Mitochondrial aspartate aminotransferase will accept tyrosine as a substrate and this reaction, occurring in tissues which lack 4-hydroxyphenylpyruvate dioxygenase, accounts for the paradoxically high urinary output of *p*-hydroxy acids. A diet low in phenylalanine and tyrosine leads to rapid resolution of the dermatological problems and, presumably, if started early will remove the risk of mental retardation. Inheritance is autosomal recessive and the disease is particularly prevalent in populations of Italian origin.

Transient neonatal tyrosinaemia is particularly associated with prematurity and is ascribed to a temporary deficiency of *p*-hydroxyphenylpyruvate dioxygenase (EC 1.13.11.27) though there is no direct biochemical evidence for this. It cannot be easily distinguished from Type II tyrosinaemia except for the generally lower tyrosine levels. It is not usually treated but does appear to have a measurable deleterious effect on cognitive ability.[21] The incidence declined very markedly in the 1970s with the reduction in the protein level of artificial infant feeds and the trend to breast-feeding.

Other less well-defined disorders of tyrosine metabolism have been reported (reviewed, together with the disorders described above, by Goldsmith and Laberge[22]). Some cases apparently have a deficiency of *p*-hydroxyphenylpyruvate dioxygenase and are classed as *tyrosinaemia Type* III (McKusick 276710).

DISORDERS OF BRANCHED-CHAIN AMINO ACID CATABOLISM

The first two steps in catabolism are similar for the three branched-chain amino acids, leucine, isoleucine and valine (Fig. 3.4). In each case transamination yields the corresponding 2-oxo acid which then undergoes oxidative decarboxylation to yield the coenzyme A ester of a branched-chain carboxylic acid. This second step is mediated by the same enzyme for all three substrates.

Maple syrup urine disease (McKusick 248600)

In this disease there is deficient activity of the branched-chain oxo acid dehydrogenase (2-oxoisovalerate dehydrogenase (lipoamide), EC 1.2.4.4). Many of the clinical and biochemical features of maple syrup urine disease are due to accumulation of the branched-chain 2-oxo acids but the reversibility of branched-chain amino acid transamination under physiological conditions results in accumulation of the corresponding amino acids. Leucine is usually the most markedly elevated, in plasma sometimes reaching 5 mmol/l, giving rise to the alternative name of leucinosis. Corresponding isoleucine and valine levels are around 1 mmol/l. That valine accumulates to a smaller extent than might be expected is probably due to its very ready reduction to 2-hydroxyisovaleric acid. The 2-oxo acid arising from isoleucine retains a chiral centre at the 3-position and, in maple syrup urine disease, chemical racemisation followed by transamina-

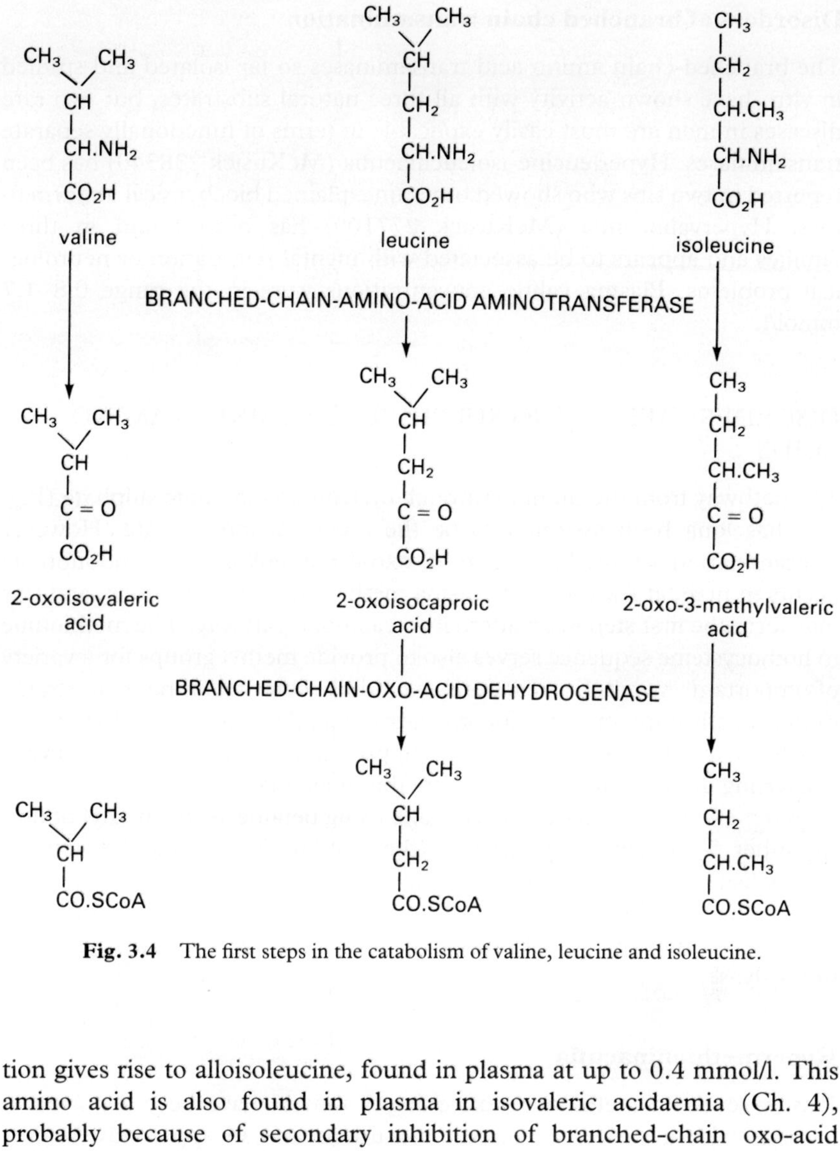

Fig. 3.4 The first steps in the catabolism of valine, leucine and isoleucine.

tion gives rise to alloisoleucine, found in plasma at up to 0.4 mmol/l. This amino acid is also found in plasma in isovaleric acidaemia (Ch. 4), probably because of secondary inhibition of branched-chain oxo-acid dehydrogenase by isovaleryl-CoA.

The classical form of maple syrup urine disease is associated with a virtual absence of branched-chain oxo acid dehydrogenase activity whilst milder and intermittent forms show significant residual activity. A thiamine responsive variant is known. Dihydrolipoyl-CoA dehydrogenase deficiency will also produce biochemical features of maple syrup urine disease and branched-chain amino acids are occasionally increased in some other organic acid disorders. For further details of maple syrup urine disease and these other conditions see Chapter 4.

Disorders of branched chain transamination

The branched-chain amino acid transaminases so far isolated and studied in vitro have shown activity with all three natural substrates, but two rare diseases in man are most easily explicable in terms of functionally separate transaminases. Hyperleucine-isoleucinaemia (McKusick 238340) has been reported in two sibs who showed other unexplained biochemical abnormalities. Hypervalinaemia (McKusick 277100) has been found in three families and appears to be associated with mental retardation or neurological problems. Plasma valine concentrations were in the range 0.8–1.7 mmol/l.

DISORDERS AFFECTING SULPHUR-CONTAINING AMINO ACIDS

The pathway from methionine through cysteine to inorganic sulphate (Fig. 3.5) has long been assumed to be the major catabolic route. However transamination of methionine to 2-oxo-4-methiolbutyrate undoubtedly occurs in man, at least at high plasma methionine concentrations, and this may form the first step in an alternative catabolic pathway. The methionine to homocysteine sequence serves also to provide methyl groups for a variety of important metabolic reactions including catecholamine neurotransmitter inactivation and creatine synthesis. The demand for methyl groups usually exceeds the methionine supply and a remethylation cycle, converting homocysteine back to methionine, makes up the deficiency. Two remethylation reactions occur, one using betaine as the methyl donor, the other 5-methyltetrahydrofolate (the 'methionine synthase' reaction). Catabolism of homocysteine is by conversion to cystathionine as the first step in the transfer of the –SH group to form cysteine. Cystathionine β-synthase, requires pyridoxal phosphate as cofactor, as also does cystathionine-γ-lyase.

Hypermethioninaemia

Plasma levels of methionine exceeding 1 mmol/l have been reported in patients with a variety of clinical conditions and in apparently healthy individuals too. Subjects with a simple deficiency of methionine *S*-adenosyltransferase (McKusick 250850) are generally asymptomatic but other forms of this heterogeneous condition are pathogenic. For a detailed review see Mudd et al.[23]

A mild degree of hypermethioninaemia is seen in cystathionine synthase deficiency (below). More severe hypermethioninaemia associated with other amino acid abnormalities is found as a secondary feature of severe liver damage in, for example, advanced cases of tyrosinaemia Type I and uridyl transferase deficiency galactosaemia.

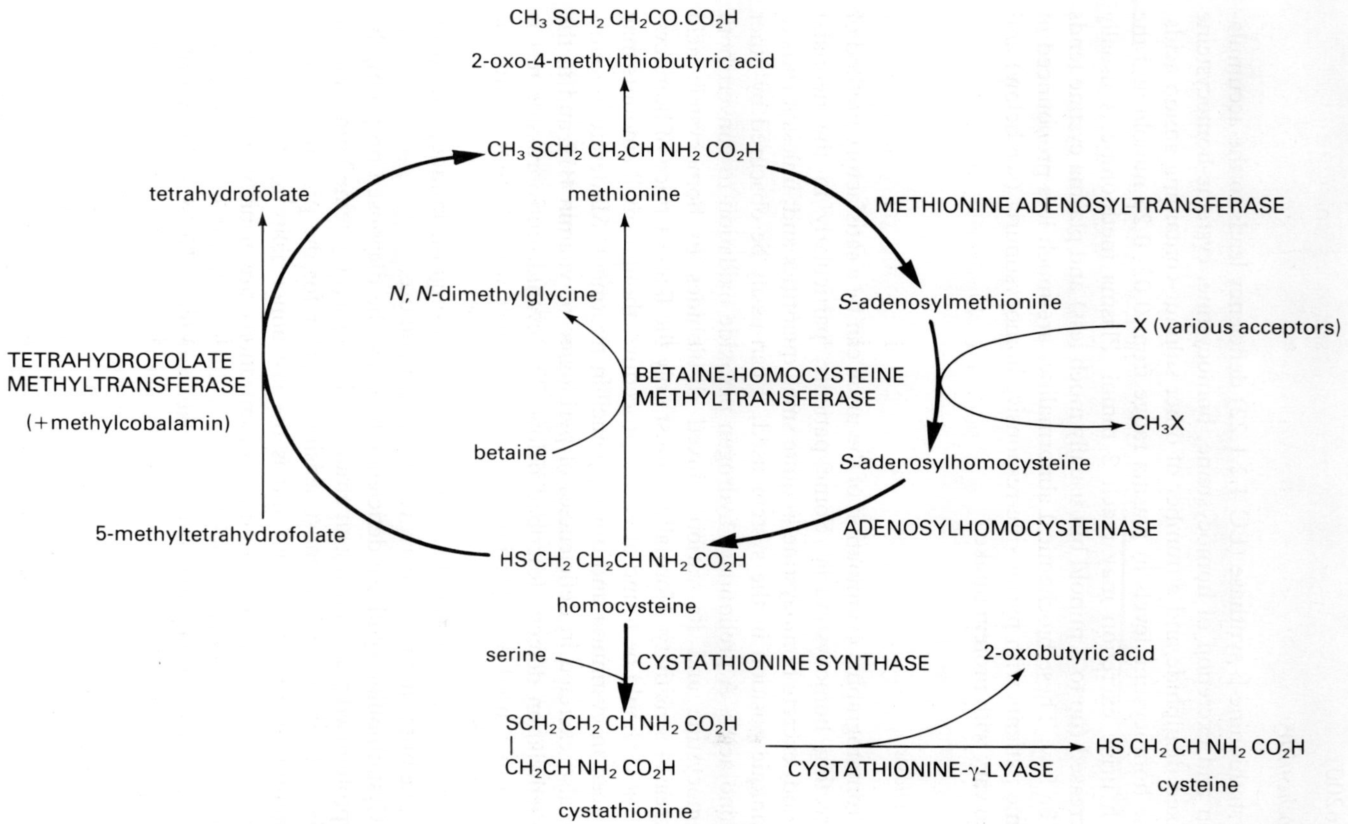

Fig. 3.5 The conversion of methionine to cysteine.

Homocystinuria: cystathionine synthase deficiency (McKusick 236200)

Biochemistry

Cystathionine-β-synthase (EC 4.2.1.22) deficiency leads to the accumulation and excretion of homocysteine, homocystine, cysteine-homocysteine mixed disulphide and a number of other sulphur-containing amino acids. The homocystine levels in plasma range from 0.02–0.25 mmol/l and the 24 h urine excretion may reach 2 mmol. Plasma methionine is usually increased (up to 2 mmol/l but usually much less) and plasma cystine tends to be low. These biochemical abnormalities are much less pronounced in some patients with pyridoxine-responsive homocystinuria (see below) and also vary with protein intake.

Diagnosis

Chromatographic examination of the urine can be a satisfactory method of detecting homocystinuria. Some patients, particularly in the neonatal period, excrete homocystine in quite small quantities and, unless it runs to a unique position in the system used, it can easily be obscured by other amino acids. A preliminary hydrogen peroxide oxidation to convert both homocystine and its various mixed disulphides to homocysteic acid increases sensitivity. Normally at most only the faintest trace of homocysteic acid should be found after this procedure, though small amounts may be seen in cystinuria and during penicillin treatment. Moderate amounts are also excreted in deficiencies of pyridoxine or vitamin B12 and in the remethylation defects described below. The cyanide–nitroprusside test is sometimes used as a preliminary screening test when homocystinuria is suspected but it is less sensitive than chromatography and may give false negative results. A variant of this test can distinguish homocystine from cystine but is not particularly reliable in general use.

Cystathionine synthase deficiency may also be diagnosed on promptly-deproteinised plasma using an amino acid analyser. Cysteine-homocysteine mixed disulphide is the most sensitive marker for the presence of small amounts of homocyst(e)ine and is the last abnormality to disappear on treatment. Plasma methionine concentrations are usually increased in cystathionine synthase deficiency which distinguishes this condition from the homocystinurias due to remethylation defects. However, some older untreated patients develop a partial defect in remethylation due to folate deficiency and may then show normal methionine levels. In these cases the diagnosis may be confirmed by the increase in plasma methionine following correction of the folate deficiency or by assay of cystathionine synthase. This enzyme is widely distributed amongst the tissues and can be assayed in cultured fibroblasts and in phytohaemagglutinin-stimulated lymphocytes as well as in liver biopsy. Occasionally unexpectedly high residual activity is found in a patient with an otherwise typical biochemical and clinical picture.

Neonatal screening for cystathionine synthase deficiency using chromatography or a bacterial inhibition test to detect hypermethioninaemia has proved unreliable, particularly for pyridoxine-responsive forms, as methionine is not always significantly increased at this time.

Clinical features

Patients with homocystinuria due to cystathionine synthase deficiency appear normal at birth but progressively develop a wide range of clinical abnormalities.[23,24] Dislocation of the lens is the most universal finding. In mild cases this may be the first clear sign of the disease though it may be preceded by myopia. In severe cases mental retardation is usually the first sign and there may be convulsions. Osteoporosis is common, often leading to spinal deformity. In later childhood excessive lengthening of the arms, legs and often fingers occurs giving a physical appearance similar to that of Marfan syndrome (Fig. 3.6). Knock knee often develops and the patient may walk like Charlie Chaplin. The clinical picture is further complicated by a marked tendency to arterial and venous thrombosis which may lead to a marked malar flush and livido reticularis. Thrombosis is a major cause of death.

Treatment

A marked biochemical response to high doses of pyridoxine (vitamin B_6) is seen in about half the patients. These responders have usually shown a milder clinical course prior to diagnosis and presumably have a structural variant of cystathionine synthase apoprotein that leads to defective binding of the pyridoxal phosphate cofactor. The dose required varies, some patients responding to as little as 2 mg of pyridoxine per 24 h others requiring 500 mg/24 h. It may be necessary to correct any coexisting folate deficiency if the full response to pyridoxine is to be achieved. Some authorities hold that such high doses should be continued for several weeks before a patient is definitely classified as non-responsive. Caution is required as very high doses of pyridoxine may produce sensory neuropathy in the normal adult. In general this has not been found to be a problem in patients with cystathionine synthase deficiency.

Patients who do not respond adequately to pyridoxine should be treated with a low-methionine high-cystine diet, following the same general principles as those used in the treatment of phenylketonuria, maple syrup urine disease, etc, and monitoring plasma methionine and homocystine levels. Plasma cystine tends to remain low despite dietary supplementation. As an adjunct to this treatment supplementary betaine or choline may be administered to promote the remethylation of homocysteine. The long-term

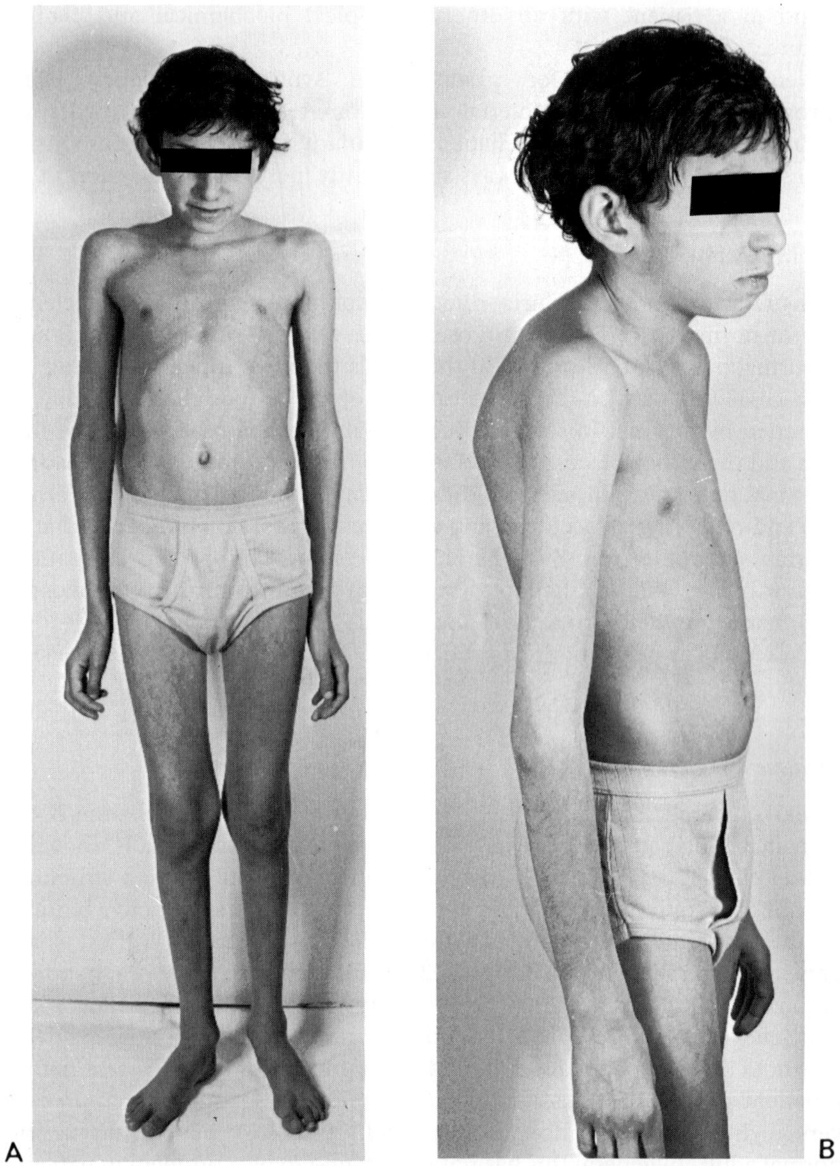

Fig. 3.6 A patient with untreated cystathionine synthase deficiency.

effects of treatment have not been evaluated in a sufficient number of early-diagnosed patients to draw firm conclusions, but it appears that in patients with the more complete deficiencies of cystathionine synthase activity, the degree of dietary control achieved has not always been sufficient to completely halt the progression of the disease.

Genetics

Cystathionine synthase deficiency is inherited as an autosomal recessive disorder. The disease has a worldwide distribution. The estimated incidence in Northern Ireland is 4:100 000 but elsewhere it appears to be much less common. Obligate heterozygotes have on average less than half the normal cystathionine synthase activity in liver, cultured fibroblasts and phytohaemagglutinin-stimulated lymphocytes, but individual results may be within the normal range. Carefully standardised methionine load tests with analysis of homocystine and other metabolites will also distinguish the majority of heterozygotes. Overlap of the normal and heterozygote ranges is to be expected in view of the heterogeneity of the biochemical disorder in clinically affected patients, many of whom presumably carry different mutations on the homologous chromosomes. Prenatal diagnosis is possible by enzyme assay on cultured amniotic fluid cells or cultured chorionic villus material.

Homocystinuria: remethylation defects

These conditions are less common than cystathionine synthase deficiency and are associated with impaired remethylation of homocysteine by 5-methyltetrahydrofolate. Two are well characterised, both showing moderate homocystinaemia, homocystinuria and sometimes cystathioninuria with normal or slightly low plasma methionine levels. Vascular changes similar to those in cystathionine synthase deficiency are seen.

Methylenetetrahydrofolate reductase deficiency (McKusick 236250)

In this disorder there is a reduced supply of 5-methyltetrahydrofolate for homocysteine remethylation. The clinical severity is variable and correlates with the decrease in methylenetetrahydrofolate reductase (EC 1.1.99.15) activity in cultured fibroblasts. The most severely affected cases die in early infancy with convulsions and other neurological symptoms. Less severe cases show mental retardation and spasticity and tend to die of thrombosis, presumably related to the homocystinuria. The late-onset form of the disease may present with a schizophrenia-like psychosis. Treatment with high doses of betaine, reinforced with folinic acid, pyridoxine and B_{12} seems to offer the best hope, though long-term experience is limited. Prenatal diagnosis is possible by enzyme assay on chorionic villus or cultured amniocytes.

Combined homocystinuria and methylmalonic aciduria

Methylmalonyl-CoA mutase (see Ch. 4) requires adenosylcobalamin as a cofactor; 5-methyltetrahydrofolate-homocysteine methyltransferase requires methylcobalamin. Two closely-related defects in cytosolic cobalamin metabolism, designated *cbl*C and *cbl*D (McKusick 277400 and 277410) on the basis of fibroblast complementation studies, and a defect in lysosomal cobalamin efflux (*cbl*F; McKusick 227380) result in a deficiency of both cofactors and hence in combined methylmalonic aciduria and homocystinuria. The clinical course is usually severe with failure to thrive, developmental delay, seizures and early death. Megaloblastic anaemia is often a feature. In some cases biochemical improvement has followed the administration of very large doses of hydroxocobalamin. Supplementary measures such as protein-restricted diet and betaine supplementation may be helpful.

Combined methylmalonic aciduria and homocystinuria may develop in severe nutritional B_{12} deficiency, defective B_{12} absorption and in some cases of severe transcobalamin II deficiency.

Other defects in methionine biosynthesis

Two disorders designated *cbl*E and *cbl*G are characterised by homocystinuria (without methylmalonic aciduria) and megaloblastic anaemia. Low levels of methylcobalamin are found in cultured cells and the methionine synthase reaction (tetrahydrofolate methyltransferase) under specific assay conditions is much reduced. It is unclear at present whether these diseases are primarily defects of B_{12} metabolism or are due to mutant methyltransferase with reduced cobalamin binding affinity. Treatment with hydroxocobalamin is sometimes effective.

Cystathioninuria (McKusick 219500)

This is a harmless biochemical abnormality and is due to a deficiency of cystathionine-γ-lyase, the enzyme that converts cystathionine to cysteine and 2-oxobutyrate. Cystathionine excretion varies with dietary methionine intake and may be as high as 12 mmol/24 h. In the majority of cases the cystathioninuria is reduced or abolished by large doses of pyridoxine. Diagnostic confusion may arise from bacterial contamination of cystathioninuric urine leading to the formation of homocystine. Cystathionine and homocystine may be excreted in modest quantities in pyridoxine deficiency.

Sulphite oxidase deficiency

Isolated deficiency of sulphite oxidase (EC 1.8.3.1, McKusick 272300) is extremely rare. *Combined deficiency of sulphite oxidase and xanthine oxidase* (McKusick 252150 and 252160) is slightly more common and is caused by deficiency of a specific pterin (molybdenum cofactor) necessary for the action of these two molybdenum-requiring enzymes. Though not strictly amino acid disorders, both forms may be detected by the urinary excretion of *S*-sulphocysteine (1–7 mmol/g creatinine) formed by the reaction of sulphite with cyst(e)ine. Plasma cystine is very low and urinary taurine is increased. Sulphite may be detected in completely fresh urine using the Merk SulfitTest® or similar strip but determination of the urinary thiosulphate to creatinine ratio is a better preliminary test.

Both disorders lead to severe neurological problems and early death. Dislocation of the ocular lens often occurs. Patients with the molybdenum cofactor defect may show characteristic slight abnormalities in the shape of the head. No treatment is available but sulphite oxidase can be measured in cultured amniotic fluid cells or chorionic villus biopsy and this enables prenatal diagnosis.

DISORDERS OF UREA SYNTHESIS

Any impediment in the synthesis of urea, the main nitrogenous excretion product in man, leads to accumulation of the ammonium ion which is toxic. Thus most of the urea cycle disorders[25] share a similar spectrum of clinical presentations and many of the treatment strategies are common to the entire group. In addition to disorders directly or indirectly affecting the activity of urea-synthesising enzymes, pathological impairment of the urea cycle occurs in two other disorders which seem to be primarily amino acid transport defects.

Deficiencies of urea cycle enzymes

Biochemistry

The synthesis of urea (Fig. 3.7) starts with the formation of carbamoyl phosphate from inorganic ammonia. A second nitrogen atom is introduced in the form of aspartate, derived from oxaloacetate by transamination. The complete reaction is essentially confined to liver but the three enzymes catalysing the sequence from citrulline to ornithine are present in a variety of tissues. There is normally a slow net outflow of citrulline from the liver and uptake of arginine and ornithine so that this part of the cycle is physiologically active in peripheral tissues. Metabolic defects occur in the synthesis of carbamoyl phosphate and at each of the enzymatic steps of the cycle proper. *Ornithine carbamoyltransferase (transcarbamylase) deficiency* (McKusick 311250) is sometimes called hyperammonaemia Type I with *carbamoyl phosphate synthase deficiency* (McKusick 237300) as Type II. This terminology is confusing and has no advantages. *Deficiencies of argininosuccinate synthase* (McKusick 215700), *argininosuccinate lyase* (McKusick 207900) and *arginase* (McKusick 207800) result in citrullinaemia, argininosuccinic aciduria and argininaemia, respectively and are often referred to under these names, though again there is sometimes scope for ambiguity.

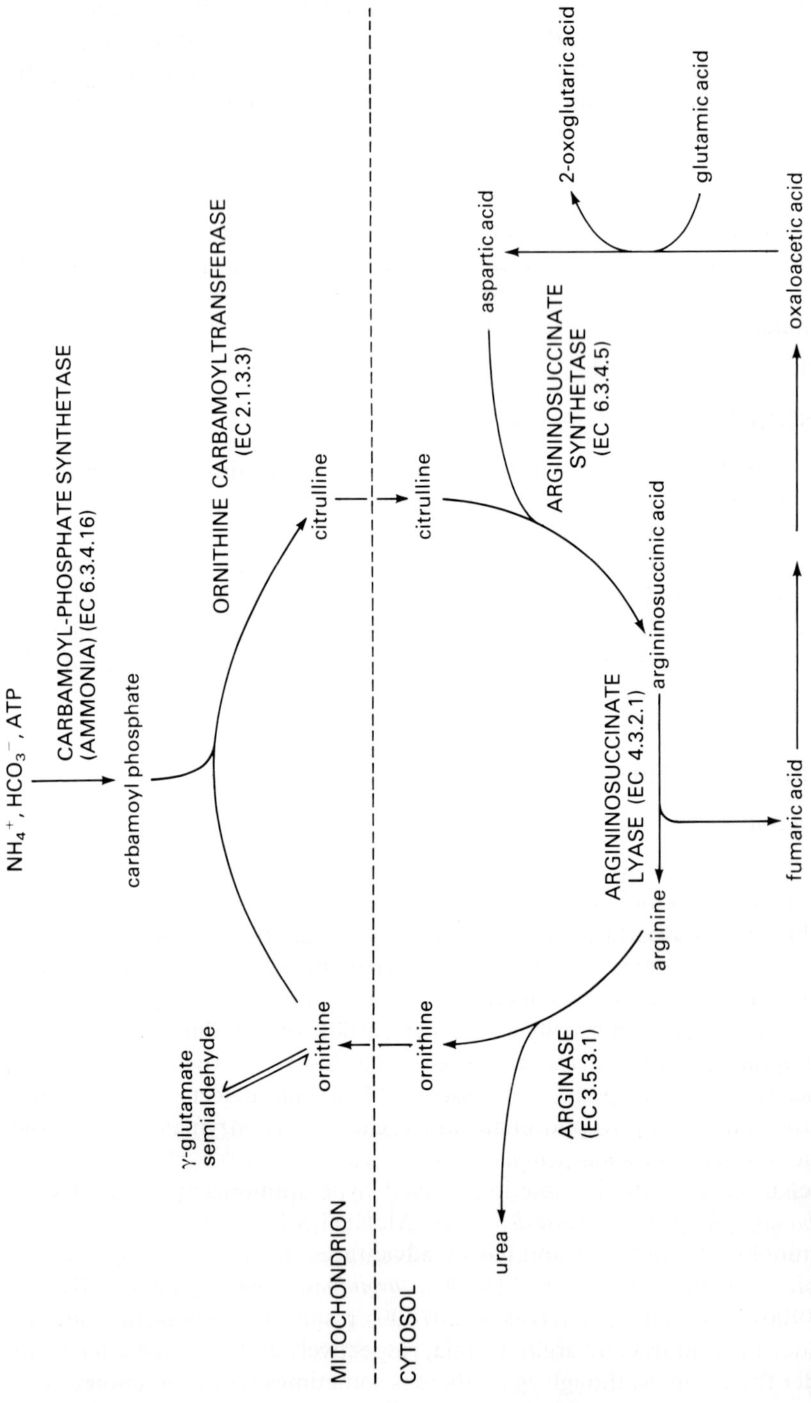

Fig. 3.7 The urea cycle.

The simplest biochemical picture is seen in carbamoyl phosphate synthase deficiency. Blood ammonia levels are much increased and glutamine, used to transport ammonia from the periphery to liver, is usually increased in plasma. Plasma glutamate is increased and 2-oxoglutarate decreased because of the effect of the excess ammonia on the glutamate dehydrogenase reaction. Plasma alanine is raised and there may be other non-specific changes in plasma amino acids. Blood urea is often low. Carbamoyl phosphate synthase requires *N*-acetylglutamate as an activator and in the few patients reported to have a *deficiency of N-acetylglutamate synthase* (McKusick 237310) the biochemical picture was similar to that of carbamoyl phosphate synthase deficiency.

In ornithine carbamoyltransferase deficiency additional biochemical features stem from the accumulation of carbamoyl phosphate, some of which passes into the cytosol and stimulates the synthesis of carbamoyl aspartate and thence pyrimidines. (Carbamoyl phosphate for pyrimidine biosynthesis is normally supplied by a cytosolic carbamoyl phosphate synthase that uses glutamine as a substrate.) Orotic acid, uracil, and uridine are excreted in excess in urine.

All these biochemical features – hyperammonaemia, increased glutamine, and pyrimidinuria – are seen, though often to a lesser degree, in the remaining three urea cycle enzyme defects in addition to the specific amino acid accumulations described below. Urinary pyrimidines are excreted in unexpectedly large amounts in arginase deficiency, possibly due to the combination of low mitochondrial ornithine levels with a stimulation of *N*-acetylglutamate synthase by arginine.

Clinical features

Hyperammonaemia is thought to be the main damaging factor in all the urea cycle defects other than arginase deficiency which is discussed separately below. The severity is very variable, each disorder having a form which proves rapidly fatal and milder forms usually with chronic presentations. Most patients who survive the first few days of life probably have residual enzyme activity.

The acute neonatal presentation is that of respiratory distress, poor feeding, vomiting, lethargy, hypotonia or spasticity, irritability and twitching, leading to convulsions, apnoea and death. Pulmonary and gastric haemorrhages occur particularly in deficiencies of carbamoyl phosphate synthase or ornithine carbamoyltransferase. In the chronic presentation with non-specific mental retardation there is often some history of episodic vomiting, lethargy, irritability or headache, often associated with high-protein meals, to indicate occasional ammonia intoxication, and there may have been seizures or even periods of coma. Some late-onset cases remain healthy until presenting in infancy or later childhood as an acute illness, often associated with an infection. Ornithine carbamoyltransferase deficiency, particularly, may cause sudden death in a previously asymptomatic child. In other cases there may be be an insidious neurological onset, sometimes with behavioural problems. An adult-onset form of citrullinaemia (Type II) is found in Japan; psychological disturbance is a marked feature.

Brittle hair with trichorrhexis nodosa is often seen in argininosuccinate lyase deficiency. It may reflect arginine deficiency and improves with age. Arginine depletion is a danger in the neonatal forms of all urea cycle defects except arginase deficiency.

In arginase deficiency there are usually only minor symptoms of irritability and mild developmental delay in infancy, but over the next few years progressive spasticity of the lower limbs, tremor, ataxia, choreoathetosis, seizures and severe mental retardation develop. These symptoms are presumed to be due mainly to direct toxic effects of arginine rather than to hyperammonaemia. Spasticity is also a feature in older patients with hyperammonaemic hyperornithinaemia with homocitrullinuria syndrome (see below).

Diagnosis

The urea cycle disorders have hyperammonaemia, intermittent in cases with subacute or late-onset presentations, as a common feature and plasma ammonia is often the first line of investigation. Care is needed with the technical aspects and also with interpretation.[26] Asymptomatic moderate hyperammonaemia occurs fairly frequently in neonates with birth weights under 2.5 kg; it is also common following perinatal asphyxia, and accompanies certain types of infection. Severe transient hyperammonaemia of the newborn is relatively rare and is usually found in premature infants of under 2 kg who develop respiratory distress in the first 24 h. It may be difficult to differentiate from a primary urea cycle defect on preliminary investigation, though clinical features provide a pointer.[27] Valproate therapy can cause mild hyperammonaemia and other drugs have from time to time been implicated. Hyperammonaemia also occurs in liver disease and is a particular feature of Reye's syndrome. Many of the organic acidaemias (Ch. 4) produce hyperammonaemia, probably by depleting hepatic intramitochondrial acetyl-CoA and thus preventing *N*-acetylglutamate synthesis. A careful examination for such disorders, particularly propionic acidaemia which is easy to miss, should be made in any child with hyperammonaemia and normal urinary orotic acid levels.

The presumptive diagnoses of carbamoyl phosphate synthase deficiency and ornithine carbamoyltransferase deficiency are usually made on the basis of hyperammonaemia in the absence of specific amino acid abnormalities. Plasma glutamine and glutamic acid are elevated, citrulline concentration usually abnormally low. An increased urinary orotic acid excretion separates ornithine carbamoyltransferase deficiency from carbamoyl phosphate synthase deficiency or *N*-acetylglutamate synthase deficiency. These last two can only be distinguished by enzyme assay in liver.

Deficiencies of argininosuccinate synthase, argininosuccinate lyase and arginase are easily recognisable by amino acid chromatography, even in the absence of hyperammonaemia. In argininosuccinate synthase deficiency plasma citrulline levels vary from 0.23 to over 4 mmol/l (normal 0.012–0.030 mmol/l) depending on protein intake, and urinary citrulline is grossly increased (3–15 mmol/24 h). Care is needed in patients with plasma citrulline at the lower end of the quoted range to distinguish between argininosuccinate synthase deficiency and the acute neonatal variant of pyruvate carboxylase deficiency (plasma citrulline approximately 0.2 mmol/l) described in Chapter 4.

A modest increase in plasma citrulline is also seen in argininosuccinate lyase deficiency but here the outstanding feature is the gross excretion of argininosuccinic acid and its anhydrides (combined output 5–30 mmol/24h), with lower levels (0.12–0.5 mmol/l) in plasma. Arginase deficiency leads to a 5–15-fold increase in plasma arginine. The urinary excretion is very variable and may be normal at times. When arginine is excreted in large amounts it is accompanied by lysine, cystine and traces of other amino acids, giving a pattern rather like that seen in cystine-lysinuria, due to defective renal tubular reabsorbtion. In all three disorders the specific amino acid abnormalities are accompanied by increased plasma and urinary glutamine levels and, particularly in the neonatal forms, by a number of less specific changes. Urinary pyrimidine excretion is increased.

The urea cycle enzymes can all be assayed in a single needle biopsy specimen of liver.[28] An alternative source of these enzymes is rectal mucosa but experience in its diagnostic use is limited. Other tissues, particularly cultured fibroblasts and lymphocytes, can be used to confirm argininosuccinate synthase and argininosuccinate lyase deficiency if required, though for argininosuccinate lyase deficiency several studies have shown discordant results between liver and other tissues. Erythrocytes are a ready source of arginase and show the defect in argininaemia.

Treatment

The hyperammonaemia of the severe neonatal forms must be corrected promptly if irreversible neurological damage is to be avoided. Haemodialysis is the best method currently available for rapid removal of ammonia. Haemofiltration is also effective. Intravenous arginine should be given in neonatal argininosuccinate lyase deficiency, because of the efficient urinary excretion of argininosuccinic acid, and is a useful adjunct in the other disorders. Amino nitrogen may also be trapped and excreted as hippuric acid and as phenylacetylglutamine, and the production of these compounds is increased by giving respectively sodium benzoate and sodium phenylacetate intravenously. Following this initial treatment, protein intake should be maintained at a minimum compatible with growth. Natural protein may be replaced by a mixture of essential amino acids but the practice of substituting 2-oxo acids for amino acids has been largely abandoned. Sodium benzoate and phenylacetic acid are given orally. Sodium phenylbutyrate is sometimes preferred to sodium phenylacetate as it has a less objectionable smell: it is converted to phenylacetic acid in vivo by β-oxidation.

Restriction of dietary protein intake is the mainstay of long-term treatment for the milder or late-onset forms of urea cycle disorder, but intercurrent attacks of hyperammonaemia need to be treated vigorously as above. Chronic oral administration of sodium benzoate and sodium phenylacetate or phenylbutyrate acid may be indicated. In argininosuccinate synthase and argininosuccinate lyase deficiencies substantial amounts of nitrogen are eliminated in the urine as citrulline and argininosuccinate respectively. The excretion of these metabolites may be yet further increased by augmenting the supply of the ornithine skeleton, and in all disorders except arginase deficiency supplementary arginine is beneficial. Detailed protocols for such treatments are to be found in the review by Brusilow and Horwich.[29]

In spite of very vigorous treatment, the neonatal onset forms of carbamoyl phosphate synthase deficiency and ornithine carbamoyltransferase deficiency carry a substantial immediate mortality rate and survivors show considerable handicap. Life-threatening hyperammonaemic crises are apt to recur unpredictably and the long-term outlook is poor. Patients with the milder varieties of these two disorders, and those with argininosuccinate synthase or argininosuccinate lyase deficiencies, have higher survival rates and may show normal development if promptly recognised and effectively treated. They too are susceptible to recurrent hyperammonaemic crises, particularly during infectious illness. Though arginase deficiency is seldom associated with severe illness in the neonatal period, the long-term outlook is problematical. Protein restriction would seem sensible but it is extremely difficult to effectively control the arginine accumulation.

Genetics

With the exception of ornithine carbamoyltransferase deficiency which is discussed in more detail below, the urea cycle disorders are inherited as autosomal recessive characters. Reduced levels of the appropriate enzyme have been demonstrated in various tissues of heterozygotes but the dependence of hepatic urea cycle enzyme activity on dietary protein intake must be remembered if this tissue is to be used for carrier detection. In practice carrier detection is of little importance as these defects are sufficiently rare for the risk to be very low of a carrier marrying (non-consanguineously) another carrier.

The main preventive measure is prenatal diagnosis but this is not always straightforward. Carbamoyl phosphate synthase deficiency can only be diagnosed directly by fetal liver biopsy but restriction fragment length polymorphism analysis is informative in some families and allows first trimester diagnosis on chorionic villus. Cultured amniotic fluid cells have detectable levels of argininosuccinate synthase, as measured directly or by the incorporation of ^{14}C from [*urideo_*^{14}C] citrulline into protein as arginine, but activity varies with the cell type. The slower-growing epithelial cells have low activity whereas the fibroblastoid amniotic fluid cells show high activity. This leads to a very broad normal range and may cause difficulties if the index case showed significant residual activity. The citrulline concentration in the amniotic fluid may provide a better guide or fetal liver biopsy may be performed. DNA-based diagnosis is hindered by the occurrence of a large number of pseudogenes. Argininosuccinate lyase may be determined in cultured amniotic fluid cells or chorionic villus biopsy, directly or by protein incorporation assay as for argininosuccinate synthase, or argininosuccinic acid may be determined in amniotic fluid as early as 12 weeks' gestation. Arginase deficiency can be detected in fetal erythrocytes obtained by fetoscopy and restriction fragment polymorphism analysis is informative in some families.

The gene for ornithine carbamoyltransferase is carried on the X-chromosome. Transmission from generation to generation is to be expected and in any one family the males will be more severely affected than the females. Where the male cases are mild or of late onset the female hemizygotes are usually clinically normal. Severe forms of ornithine carbamoyltransferase deficiency, usually lethal in the neonatal period in affected males, may also produce symptoms in the female hemizygotes. The severity of these symptoms is variable within a single family and reflects the degree to which Lyonization, the random inactivation of one X-chromosome in each somatic cell, has been unfavourable to the normal allele. A mosaic of normal and ornithine carbamoyltransferase-deficient cells can be demonstrated by enzyme histochemistry in the liver of affected females.

As in other X-linked metabolic diseases it may be difficult to assess carrier status in apparently healthy females as the proportion of cells carrying the mutant gene may be very low. Needle biopsy specimens of liver may show an essentially normal ornithine carbamoyltransferase activity. The urinary excretion of orotic acid following a protein load may be a better guide, and oral or intravenous alanine loads may be used to increase precision.

A more recent approach is to use allopurinol to inhibit the decarboxylation of orotidine-5-phosphate to uridine-5-phosphate. The consequent excretion of orotidine is much higher in carriers for ornithine carbamoyltransferase deficiency than in normal controls. However, even with this test a clear result cannot be expected in all instances. DNA-based studies may be useful but are uninformative in a fair proportion of cases. The situation is complicated by the frequent occurrence of de novo mutations, 'necessary' to maintain the frequency of the condition in the face of strong negative selection.

Ornithine carbamoyltransferase deficiency is probably the most common urea cycle defect and its X-linked mode of inheritance gives considerably greater scope for prevention by genetic counselling and prenatal diagnosis than the sporadically occurring disorders of enzymes coded on autosomal chromosomes. Prenatal diagnosis by enzyme assay on fetal liver biopsy (and possibly chorionic villus) should be possible in the male but will be unreliable if the fetus is female. DNA analysis, either for direct detection of the mutation or using linkage to restriction fragment length polymorphisms, can provide first trimester diagnosis in favourable families. Markedly impaired ammonia metabolism in the mother may damage the fetus irrespective of its genetic composition, further complicating family studies.

Hyperammonaemic hyperornithinaemia with homocitrullinuria (McKusick 238970)

The operation of the urea cycle within the hepatocyte requires the transport of ornithine into the mitochondria and citrulline out (Fig. 3.7). The mitochondrial ornithine tansporter is thought to be defective in a syndrome characterized by hyperammonaemia, hyperornithinaemia and homocitrullinuria (HHH). The hyperammonaemia probably arises through the impairment of the urea cycle by mitochondrial ornithine deficiency and is accompanied by a modest orotic aciduria. Ornithine catabolism also occurs within the mitochondria so that extramitochondrial ornithine concentration is increased. The homocitrulline seems to be synthesised directly from lysine and its output increases with the plasma lysine concentration and the load on the urea cycle. Clinically HHH presents as a relatively mild urea cycle disorder with typical symptoms of intermittent hyperammonaemia, though spasticity is a marked feature in some of the older patients (cf. argininaemia).

Diagnosis is based on the finding of all three cardinal biochemical features (HHH) but the first clues may be difficult to spot. The hyperammonaemia is intermittent, though it can exceed 1 mmol/l. The hyperornithinaemia is relatively modest, 0.4–0.9 mmol/l compared to a normal of below 0.12 mmol/l, and could be missed in the many chromatographic systems where lysine and ornithine run together. In some patients the ornithinaemia gives rise to an overflow amino aciduria but in others the urinary amino acids appear normal except for the presence of homocitrulline. This may occur at levels of up to 0.13 mol/mol creatinine but may be barely noticeable during clinical remission. The widespread use of sterilised cows' milk formulae in infant feeding militates against a chance finding of homocitrullinuria being taken seriously. Urea is present in high concentration in cows' milk and during the heat treatment this carbamylates the ε-amino groups of protein lysyl residues, the homocitrulline residues thus produced being liberated during digestion and excreted in the urine. In an ill infant an unequivocal diagnosis of HHH may be difficult to establish and confirmation may be obtained by demonstrating a reduced rate of incorporation of [^{14}C] ornithine (as proline and glutamate, see Fig. 3.8) into cell protein by phytohaemagglutinin-stimulated lymphocytes or cultured fibroblasts. This will not distinguish HHH from ornithine aminotransferase deficiency (see below) but this latter disorder is unlikely to be under consideration in the ill infant.

Treatment is primarily by protein restriction. Some patients respond to ornithine supplementation (oral ornithine or arginine hydrochlorides) with a reduction in hyperammonaemia. A normalisation of [^{14}C] ornithine incorporation into protein in response to increased ornithine concentration in the medium has been shown by fibroblasts from an ornithine-responsive patient, and this may provide a convenient way of assessing responsiveness in vivo. The association of hyperornithinaemia with gyrate atrophy of the choroid and retina (p. 99) should prompt caution in the long-term use of ornithine supplements. So far no patient with HHH has shown any indication of these ocular lesions.

Lysinuric protein intolerance (McKusick 222700)

Defective urea cycle operation in this disorder is evident from postprandial hyperammonaemia and increased orotic acid excretion. The disorder is ascribed to a functional deficiency of ornithine in the hepatic mitochondria but the exact mechanism is problematical.[30] Defective transport of dibasic amino acids at the basolateral membrane of the jejunal epithelium has been clearly demonstrated and is also present in the renal tubule and in cultured fibroblasts. Plasma concentrations of ornithine, arginine and lysine are subnormal but the citrulline concentration is elevated. Paradoxically the overall concentrations of these amino acids in liver are normal or increased. Diagnosis is based on the finding of a dibasic amino aciduria (usually without cystinuria) together with low plasma dibasic amino acid concentrations and hyperammonaemia.

The disease is particularly common in Finland (approximately 1.3: 100000 births) but is also found elsewhere. The symptoms include those of intermittent hyperammonaemia but lens opacities, hyperelastic skin, hyperextensible joints, and sparse, brittle hair are also commonly found. Treatment consists of a protein-restricted diet and supplementary citrulline.

ORNITHINE AMINOTRANSFERASE DEFICIENCY (McKusick 258870)

Ornithine synthesis and degradation (Fig. 3.8) are mediated by the same enzyme, ornithine-oxoacid aminotransferase (EC 2.6.1.13), which is present in the mitochondria of many cell types. Deficiency of this enzyme

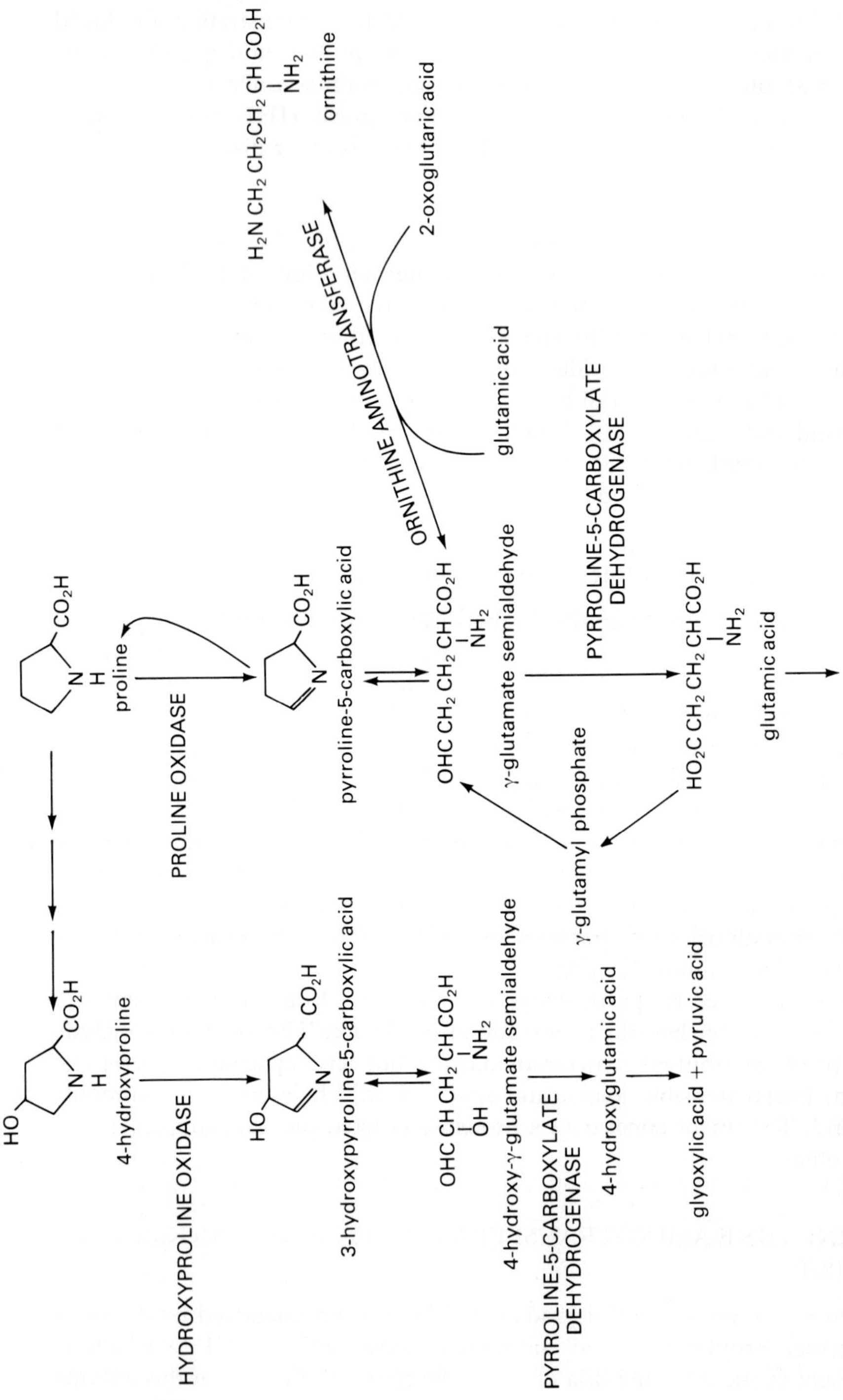

Fig. 3.8 The catabolism of ornithine, proline and hydroxyproline.

leads to hyperornithinaemia (0.4–1.4 mmol/l) with normal or low blood ammonia levels and no homocitrullinuria. A cystine-lysine-ornithinuria may be present.

The main clinical feature of ornithine aminotransferase deficiency is progressive loss of vision due to a characteristic degeneration (gyrate atrophy) of the choroid and retina. Symptoms usually become apparent in the first decade of life and progress to produce complete blindness at ages varying between 20 and 50 years. Histological changes are seen in liver mitochondria and in muscle but are asymptomatic.

Ornithine aminotransferase is a pyridoxal phosphate-requiring enzyme and a minority of patients respond biochemically to large doses of pyridoxine. Preliminary studies indicate a possible slowing of the rate of progression of chorioretinal degeneration but the slow and irregular course of the disease makes it impossible to evaluate treatments except over a very long period. For cases of pyridoxine-unresponsive ornithine aminotransferase deficiency, treatment aims at reducing plasma ornithine levels to near normal by severely restricting natural protein intake and supplementing with essential amino acids. This regime is difficult but has apparently had beneficial effects in some patients, with stabilisation of the visual defect. Ornithine cannot be synthesised in the absence of ornithine aminotransferase so that care is needed to avoid deficiency which rapidly leads to hyperammonaemia.

The absence of any clear idea of the pathophysiology of the chorioretinal degeneration has hindered attempts at alternative therapy. Based on the finding of low creatinine excretion, the administration of creatine (1.5 g/24 h orally) has also been tried and improves the histological appearance of muscle. Proline supplementation has been used to correct a hypothetical deficiency of proline in the retina, where both ornithine aminotransferase and pyrrolidone-5-carboxylate reductase are normally particularly active. Neither of these approaches can be recommended.

Ornithine aminotransferase deficiency is inherited as an autosomal recessive condition, can readily be detected in fibroblasts and presumably would be susceptible to prenatal diagnosis using cultured amniotic fluid cells or chorionic villus samples. The late age at diagnosis severely limits the potential of this approach.

NON-KETOTIC HYPERGLYCINAEMIA (McKusick 238300)

Hyperglycinaemia is a non-specific feature of several organic acidurias and in these cases is usually associated with intermittent ketosis (Ch. 4). Non-ketotic hyperglycinaemia[31] is a specific disorder of glycine catabolism due to a defect in the glycine cleavage system (Fig. 3.9). This system is present in liver, brain, and probably other organs but not in cultured fibroblasts. Four proteins are involved in the overall reaction: a pyridoxal phosphate-dependent glycine decarboxylase (P-protein), a lipoic acid containing

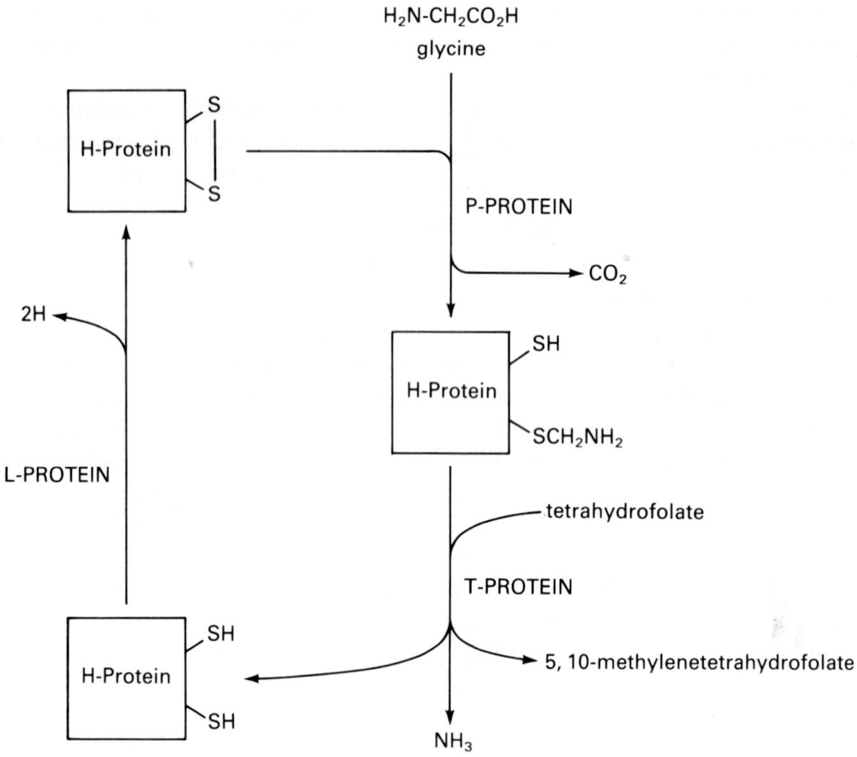

Fig. 3.9 The glycine cleavage system.

aminomethyl carrier protein (H-protein), a lipoamide dehydrogenase (L-protein) and a tetrahydrofolate-requiring methylene-group acceptor (T-protein). In the majority of cases of non-ketotic hyperglycinaemia the site of the defect has not been determined but those studied in detail have had deficiencies of either P-protein or T-protein.

In the most common form of non-ketotic hyperglycinaemia acute neurological problems may begin only a few hours after birth and generally in the first week of life. Somnolence, lethargy and lack of spontaneous movement progress to deep coma with apnoeic spells. Exaggerated reflexes may be present and there may be myoclonic seizures. The EEG shows a pattern of very low activity interspersed with occasional high-amplitude synchronous bursts. This abnormal pattern may be shown 30 min after birth in spite of apparent clinical normality at this stage. Milder forms of non-ketotic hyperglycinaemia may show non-specific mental retardation though some later-onset patients experience rapid neurological deterioration. As yet we cannot correlate the clinical variability with the biochemical heterogeneity.

Diagnosis. This is based on the finding of hyperglycinaemia and hyperglycinuria in the absence of an organic acid disorder. These abnormalities may be obvious but in a minority of cases the diagnosis must be actively sought as the plasma glycine levels may be only marginally increased and the glycinuria modest. If a diagnosis of non-ketotic hyperglycinaemia is suspected on clinical grounds, a quantitative amino acid analysis of plasma is mandatory. Spurious hyperglycinaemia can develop in infants fed on very low protein diets. Determination of CSF glycine will provide supporting evidence of non-ketotic hyperglycinaemia since, at least in the more severe forms of the disease, the CSF/plasma glycine ratio (0.2–0.33 compared with normal 0.02–0.03) as well as the absolute CSF glycine concentration (0.09–0.36 mmol/l, normal 0.004–0.010 mmol/l) are abnormally high. A transient neonatal form with the biochemical and clinical features of classical non-ketotic hyperglycinaemia but spontaneous normalisation has been described.

Glycine is an important inhibitory neurotransmitter in the central nervous system where the glycine cleavage system may well play a role in terminating its action. In patients with ketotic hyperglycinaemias (secondary to defects in organic acid metabolism) the CSF/plasma glycine ratio is similar to that in normal children, suggesting that in these disorders the liver is the main site of inhibition. Some such patients have experienced high plasma and CSF glycine concentrations for many years without neurological symptoms.

The glycine cleavage system is not expressed in cultured amniotic fluid cells. The glycine to serine ratio in amniotic fluid shows some discrimination between affected and unaffected fetuses but this is insufficient for the method to be reliable. Chorionic villus biopsy contains the glycine cleavage system and may be used for prenatal diagnosis[32] though a very large sample is required. Diagnosis by fetal liver biopsy is a theoretical possibility.

Treatment. Efforts aimed at reducing the overall glycine levels in the body by restricting supply or removal as conjugates have met with varied success. Of these, the administration of large doses of benzoate have been the most successful, as judged by reduction of CSF glycine concentration and of the frequency of seizures.[33] However, such manoeuvres have been uniformly unsuccessful in halting the overall course of the disease and allowing normal intellectual development. Supplementing the supply of various cofactors has been equally unsuccessful where it has been tried but there is no reason to suppose that cofactor responsive variants might not occur. In a few cases improvement in neurological function has been achieved by blocking glycine receptors with high doses of strychnine but results have mostly been disappointing. Diazepam in high dosage may have some benefit.

DEFECTS IN LYSINE DEGRADATION

The pathways for lysine catabolism are summarised in Figure 3.10. The major route is through saccharopine, 2-oxoadipic acid and glutaryl-CoA.

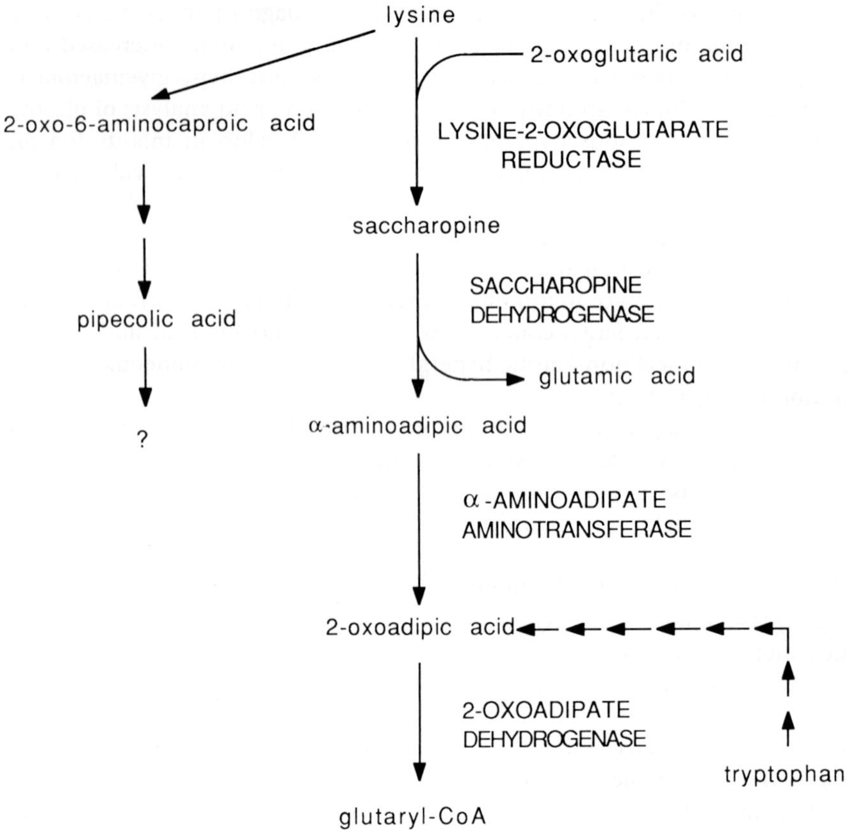

Fig. 3.10 Major pathways of lysine degradation.

Three inborn errors of metabolism are known to affect the early part of this pathway: hyperlysinaemia, saccharopinuria, and α-aminoadipic aciduria. In addition, pipecolic acid, an intermediate on a minor metabolic pathway of lysine, is excreted in excess in Zellweger disease and related peroxisomal disorders (see Ch. 6). Patients originally described as having pipecolataemia (McKusick 239400) fall within the Zellweger complementation group.

Hyperlysinaemia (McKusick 238700)

In this moderately rare condition plasma lysine concentrations range up to 1.5 mmol/l and large amounts of lysine but not of other dibasic amino acids or cystine are excreted in the urine. The lysine metabolites α-*N*-acetyl-lysine, ε-*N*-acetyl-lysine, homocitrulline and homoarginine are also excreted in excess. The basic defect is usually in lysine-2-oxoglutarate reductase, and in some patients an absence of saccharopine dehydrogenase has also been demonstrated. These two activities are combined in a single bifunctional enzyme. A variety of clinical symptoms have been described in association with hyperlysinaemia, mental retardation being prominent. However a limited prospective study[34] based on sibs of index cases and cases detected by neonatal screening suggests that the association of disease and hyperlysinaemia is in most cases fortuitous.

'Congenital lysine intolerance with periodic ammonia intoxication' (McKusick 238750) has been reported as a single case which is not easily explained in terms of current biochemical knowledge. Whilst there are theoretical reasons to predict that accumulation of lysine might interfere with the urea cycle, most cases of hyperlysinaemia show at most only marginally increased blood ammonia levels. Plasma lysine is sometimes increased in infants with ornithine carbamoyltransferase deficiency. Another disorder, with defective lysine transport into mitochondria (McKusick 238710), has been reported in two sibs.

Saccharopinuria (McKusick 268700)

A deficiency of saccharopine dehydrogenase has been reported in only a few patients. The other functional component of the complex, lysine-2-oxoglutarate reductase, is reduced in activity to a lesser extent. Saccharopine is excreted in large amounts (2 mmol/24 h) together with lysine, α-aminoadipic acid and, in one patient, citrulline. The clinical significance of this metabolic anomaly is unknown.

α-**Aminoadipic aciduria** (McKusick 204750)

Excessive excretion of 2-hydroxyadipic and 2-oxoadipic acids accompanies the α-aminoadipic aciduria in most, and possibly all, cases of this disorder. The output of these metabolites is very variable, all in the range 0.05–1.5 mmol/24 h. Plasma α-aminoadipic acid, below 5 μmol/l normally, is from 30 to 120 μmol/l. A deficiency of 2-oxoadipate dehydrogenase has been demonstrated in some cases but in another a defect in mitochondrial α-aminoadipate aminotransferase (EC 2.6.1.39) seemed more likely. The clinical presentations of the 20 or so cases so far reported have been very varied and could well be unrelated to the biochemical defect.

HISTIDINE METABOLISM

Histidinaemia (McKusick 235800)

The first step in the metabolism of histidine is the elimination of ammonia to form urocanic acid (Fig. 3.11). The enzyme histidine ammonia lyase (histidase, EC 4.3.1.3) is absent in histidinaemia. Histidine accumulates,

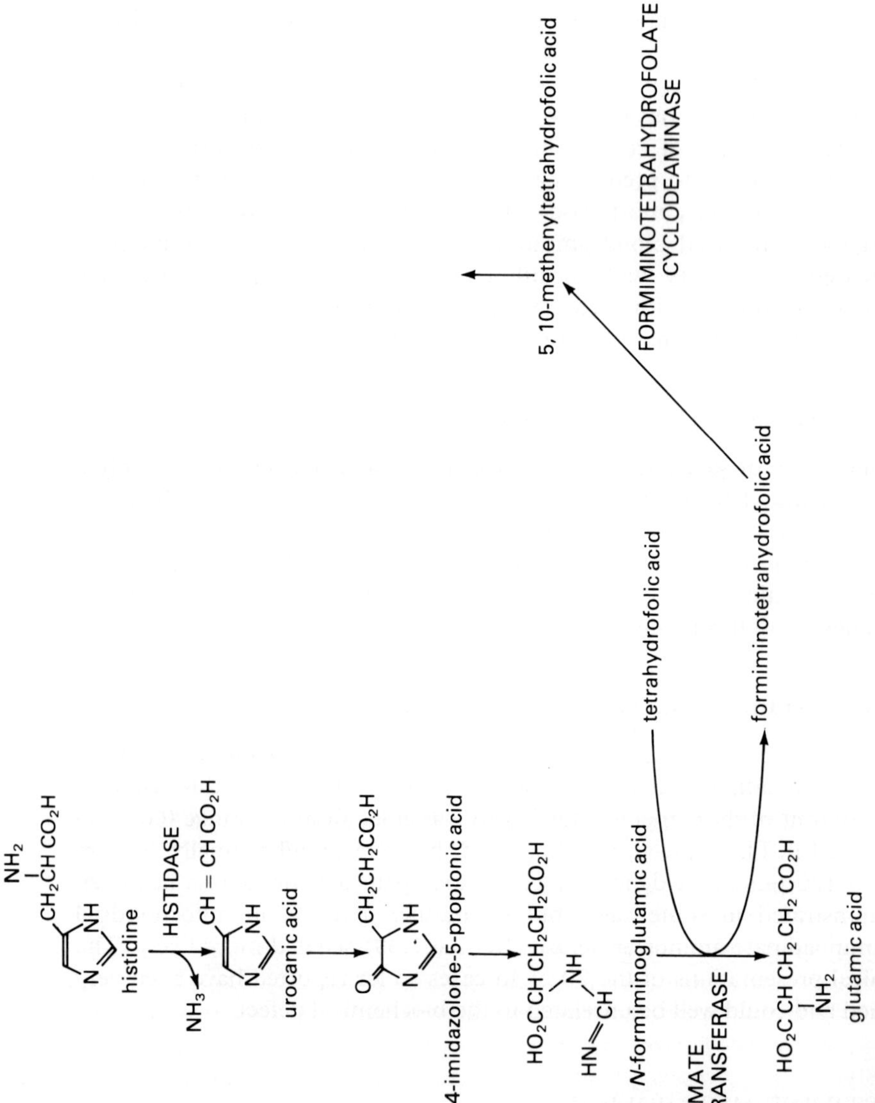

Fig. 3.11 Histidine catabolism.

plasma concentration 0.3–1.6 mmol/l (normal 0.05–0.2 mmol/l), and is excreted in excess in urine. Transamination leads to imidazolepyruvic acid, imidazolelactic acid and imidazoleacetic acid. With ferric chloride solution imidazolepyruvic acid gives a green coloration, similar to that given by phenylpyruvic acid only more transient, so that there is a danger of confusion with phenylketonuria. Histidine ammonia lyase can be measured in liver biopsy or in fresh skin, but not in cultured fibroblasts.

In caucasian populations histidinaemia occurs with a frequency approaching that of phenylketonuria and it is also common in Japan. For some years it was believed that histidinaemia caused mental retardation, generally less severe than that seen in phenylketonuria, and with a high proportion of patients with speech difficulties. However it has slowly become apparent that for the vast majority histidinaemia is a harmless biochemical anomaly, though the possibility remains that in a small number of individuals, at most 1%, histidinaemia has been a contributing factor to the development of some form of central nervous system dysfunction. This subject, and the difficulty of reconciling data from retrospective study of selected (diseased) populations with that derived from whole population screening, has been well reviewed by Scriver and colleagues[35–37]. Similar problems have arisen for other amino acid disorders and are particularly difficult to resolve for rare conditions.

Formiminoglutamic aciduria (McKusick 229100)

Further catabolism of urocanic acid produces formiminoglutamic acid (FIGLU, Fig. 3.11). The formyl group is then passed to tetrahydrofolate to form in turn 5-formiminotetrahydrofolate and 5,10-methenyltetrahydrofolate. These two reactions are performed by a single enzyme protein. There is some degree of confusion surrounding this disorder but patients described as having formiminoglutamic aciduria are postulated to fall into two groups.[38] A deficiency of glutamate formiminotransferase (EC 2.1.2.5) itself results in a massive excretion of FIGLU (up to 3.9 mmol/l). It has been associated with a relatively mild clinical presentation, mainly of psychomotor retardation and hypotonia, and there is a strong possibility that the condition is benign. The second type, reported from Japan, results in severe mental and physical retardation with cortical atrophy. There is a partial defect in formiminotransferase activity, coupled (it is hypothesised) with a severe defect in cyclodeaminase activity (EC 4.3.1.4). The excretion of FIGLU is less marked than in isolated formiminotransferase deficiency and may at times be normal. A histidine load test should be preformed if the diagnosis is doubtful. FIGLUuria may also occur in cobalamin disorders (*cbl*C, *cbl*D, *cb1*E and *cbl*G) and in B_{12} or folate deficiencies.

FIGLU does not normally react with ninhydrin though it may give a weak colour with some formulations and if the chromatogram is overheated. It also gives a peak on some automatic amino acid analysers.

DISORDERS OF PROLINE AND HYDROXYPROLINE METABOLISM

Proline is oxidised to pyrroline-5-carboxylic acid (which is in equilibrium with γ-glutamic semialdehyde) by proline oxidase, an enzyme that is tightly bound to the inner mitochondrial membrane (Fig. 3.8). γ-Glutamic semialdehyde can then be oxidised to glutamic acid by pyrroline-5-carboxylate dehydrogenase (EC 1.5.1.12) or can be converted to ornithine by ornithine aminotransferase. In *hyperprolinaemia Type 1* (McKusick 239500) proline oxidase activity is absent and proline accumulates in tissues (concentration in plasma 0.7–2.6 mmol/l) and is excreted in excess in the urine. In *hyperhydroxyprolinaemia* (McKusick 237000) there is a deficiency of the corresponding enzyme, hydroxyproline oxidase, leading to increased tissue levels of hydroxyproline and to increased urinary excretion. In *hyperprolinaemia Type II* (McKusick 239510) pyrroline-5-carboxylate dehydrogenase activity is deficient. This enzyme participates in the degradation of proline, hydroxyproline and ornithine but only proline accumulates, again giving hyperprolinaemia (up to 2.8 mmol/l in plasma) and prolinuria. The urine does however also contain both pyrroline-5-carboxylic acid (10–27 mmol/mol creatinine) and 3-hydroxypyrroline-5-carboxylic acid. Both types of hyperprolinaemia show increased urinary excretion of hydroxyproline and glycine due to partial saturation by proline of common renal transport sites. There is still some doubt as to whether Type II hyperprolinaemia is associated with neurological problems but the other two conditions are believed to be harmless.

Prolidase (proline dipeptidase, peptidase D, EC 3.4.13.9) cleaves proline or hydroxyproline from the C-terminus of peptides. *Prolidase deficiency* (McKusick 170100) results in the accumulation and excretion of a variety of proline- and hydroxyproline-containing peptides derived from the turnover of collagen and other proteins. Urinary bound proline and hydroxyproline are much increased. The diagnosis may be confirmed by assay of prolidase in erythrocytes, leucocytes or cultured fibroblasts, affected individuals generally showing less than 7% of normal activity.

Patients with this disorder show a wide range of symptoms, dermatitis and leg ulceration being the most common. Splenomegaly, mental retardation and bony deformities, particularly affecting the shape of the skull, are also frequently seen. There is no generally recognised treatment.

SPECIFIC DEFECTS OF RENAL TRANSPORT

There are many amino acid transport systems in the body. Of those concerned with transport within the cell, the systems of the mitochondrial inner membrane have been particularly well studied. They are in general highly specific, mediating the transport of a single metabolite or the counter-transport of a metabolically-related pair (see hyperammonaemic hyperornithinaemia with homocitrullinuria syndrome). Some information is available on transport across the lysosomal membrane (cystinosis). Transport across the outer cell membrane varies with cell type and function, and in epithelial cells from one face of the cell to another. Most of the systems studied in vitro will transport a range of amino acid substrates and most amino acids seem to be transported by more than one system. In vivo such transport systems are most conspicuous by their absence and the clearest examples are seen when the deficiency is expressed in the renal tubules.

Cystine-lysinuria (McKusick 220100)

The formation of cystine stones in bladder or kidney has been a recognised phenomenon for over 150 years, the name cystine being derived from the Greek *kystis* (bladder). Cystinuria was one of Garrod's original four inborn errors of metabolism. It is now recognised that the defect in cystinuria lies not in the metabolism of cystine but in its transport by the renal tubules since plasma cystine levels are normal or even low. In the most common form (cystine-lysinuria) the cystinuria is accompanied by excessive excretion of lysine, ornithine, and arginine which share with cystine a high affinity (low K_m) renal tubular transport system. This transport system is not expressed in cultured fibroblasts, but many cystinuric patients show intestinal malabsorption of cystine and the dibasic amino acids, indicating that the affected transport system is normally active at the brush border membrane. The unabsorbed dibasic amino acids are converted by bacterial action to putrescine, cadaverine and related products that may then appear in the urine. In those patients with a severe defect in the intestinal transport system some uptake of the affected amino acids occurs in the form of dipeptides which are hydrolysed intracellularly by the mucosal cell. By contrast, in lysinuric protein intolerance (p. 97) the intestinal defect in dibasic amino acid transport is at the basolateral membrane of the mucosal cell so that intestinal absorption as free amino acids or as dipeptides is equally affected; the lysinuria in this condition showing that a transport system of this type also exists in the kidney.

Isolated cystinuria (no excessive excretion of dibasic amino acids) is rarer than combined cystine-lysinuria and is thought to reflect a defect in a low-affinity transport system that is not shared with the dibasic amino acids. Hyper-dibasic aminoaciduria without cystinuria, which is very rare, is presumably due to a defect in the low affinity transport system specific for the dibasic amino acids. Thus it appears that in the kidney and probably many other organs there is a multiplicity of transport systems, the malfunction of any one of which can significantly affect the overall efficiency of amino acid transport in the organ concerned.

Diagnosis and classification

Diagnosis is based on the demonstration of grossly excessive urinary excretion of the appropriate amino acid(s) in the absence of any increase in their plasma concentration and, in the case of hyper-dibasic aminoaciduria, the absence of hyperammonaemia after a protein load. Amino acid excretion patterns superficially similar to those in cystine-lysinuria may be seen at times in hyperargininaemia and in hyperlysinaemia, the excessive load of the amino acid primarily affected hindering renal reabsorption of others sharing the same transporter.

The grossly excessive excretion of cystine in cystine-lysinuria and in isolated cystinuria may be detected by the cyanide-nitroprusside test. Though this is a convenient side-room test for the renal clinic, the use of solid sodium cyanide under these conditions is hazardous, and doubtful or false positive results are common. In the laboratory context this test is not worth performing if the specimen is to be examined for amino acids in any case. The other classical procedure, microscopy of urine sediment, has more to recommend it, in that the demonstration of the characteristic hexagonal crystals of cystine at least confirms that cystine is present in potentially stone-forming concentrations, but it should not be relied on to exclude the possibility of significant cystinuria.

The excretion of amino acids in homozygous cystine-lysinuria is rather variable, ranging from 0.2–0.3, 0.5–1.5, 0.2–0.9, and 0.1–0.7 mol/mol creatinine for cystine, lysine, arginine and ornithine respectively. The disorder is clearly heterogeneous. Some heterozygotes for cystine-lysinuria excrete cystine and lysine at about one-tenth the levels seen in the homozygous condition whilst others show no excessive excretion and this is used as a basis for classification. In Type I cystine-lysinuria the heterozygotes show no abnormality in urinary amino acid excretion and the homozygotes have a complete deficiency in intestinal absorption of cystine and dibasic amino acids. In Type II the heterozygotes show the amino aciduria but the homozygotes have some residual activity for the intestinal transport of cystine (but not lysine). Some authorities recognise a third type, similar to Type II but with a less severe intestinal transport defect.

Clinical expression and treatment

The only medical problems clearly associated with defects in the renal transport of cystine are those due to stone formation. Symptoms may first occur at any time from infancy to old age but onset is most common in the second and third decades of life. Renal colic, urinary obstruction, recurrent infection, and progressive loss of renal function develop as in urolithiasis from other causes.

Biochemical treatments aim at preventing saturation of the urine with cystine. Restriction of methionine intake, unless very drastic, probably has little effect on plasma cystine concentrations and hence on the filtered load. The simplest therapeutic measure is to maintain a high water intake so that the urine is always dilute. This requires particular attention at night, when the most concentrated urine is usually produced, and is not without its inconveniences. Alkalinisation of the urine by oral intake of sodium bicarbonate or citrate should help to decrease the possibility of the urine becoming saturated as the solubility of cystine increases rapidly at pH above 7.5. Small stones may even redissolve. If these simple measures fail, treatment with D-penicillamine, *N*-acetylpenicillamine or mercaptopropionylglycine, all of which form soluble mixed disulphides with cystine, may be effective but these drugs, particularly penicillamine, have severe side-effects in some patients. Without adequate treatment chronic renal failure can result and renal transplantation may be necessary. The transplanted kidney will not be affected by the transport defect elsewhere in the body and should remain disease-free.

Cystine-lysinuria can easily be detected in neonatal urine screening programmes. The incidence detected by such programmes has ranged from 6 to 50 per 100 000 which is much higher than that expected from the prevalence of cystine stones. Presumably many biochemically affected individuals never develop clinically significant stones so that the institution of alkalinisation and hydration therapy on a lifelong basis following such neonatal detection does not seem justified.

There have been several reports of an increased frequency of cystine-lysinuria in mentally retarded or psychiatrically disturbed populations but the reason for this is unclear.[39] It is also unclear whether isolated hyper-dibasic aminoaciduria has any clinical significance though there is a suggested association with severe mental retardation in the homozygous state. In assessing this and other possible associations between renal transport defects and disease it must be remembered that there is a multiplicity of transport systems within the body and present methods of characterising them are much less developed than methods for the investigation of enzyme defects. Given this heterogeneity, the possibility that in some cases the particular transport defect expressed in the kidney may have more serious effects elsewhere cannot be discounted, lysinuric protein intolerance being an example where this effect has been easy to demonstrate.

Iminoglycinuria (McKusick 242600)

The iminoacids, proline and hydroxyproline, share a renal tubular transport site with glycine. Deficient carrier activity at this site results in an hereditary iminoglycinuria. As in cystine-lysinuria, different types occur some of which also express the transport defect in the intestine. Heterozygotes may show isolated glycinuria. For a full discussion see Scriver.[40]

These abnormalities appear in general to have no clinical significance. Though the earliest cases were discovered in the course of investigation of patients with mental retardation or convulsions, the disorder has subsequently been found in healthy individuals. Babies discovered to have iminoglycinuria by newborn screening have remained healthy without treatment.

Transient iminoglycinuria due to immaturity of renal transport systems occurs frequently in the neonatal period. Iminoglycinuria also occurs through competition at the shared renal site(s) in hyperprolinaemia Types I and II and hyperhydroxyprolinaemia, but not in hyperglycinaemia.

Hartnup disease (McKusick 234500)

This is a combined renal and intestinal transport defect affecting predominantly the neutral amino acids, especially alanine, asparagine, glutamine, threonine, serine, the branched-chain amino acids, tryptophan, tyrosine, phenylalanine and histidine. These are present in the faeces and are excreted in excess in urine. Bacterial action on unabsorbed tryptophan in the gut gives rise to the rich variety of indoles that are excreted in urine in this condition. Plasma concentrations of the affected amino acids tend to be low.

The affected members of the Hartnup family, in whom the disease was originally discovered, showed symptoms only intermittently. The most striking problem was a pellagra-like rash, but there was also a cerebellar ataxia and psychological changes. These symptoms are relieved by oral nicotinamide and, though only a small proportion of tryptophan is converted to nicotinamide, are most likely to be due to nicotinamide deficiency secondary to the tryptophan malabsorption. The skin rash has been the most commonly reported symptom in subsequently diagnosed cases of Hartnup disease but expression seems to require some marginal degree of nutritional inadequacy. In newborn screening programmes in USA and in Australia, Hartnup 'disease' has been detected with a frequency of 5.6 and 4.3 per 100 000 births respectively. However, the clinical presentation is virtually unknown in these areas, which traditionally have a high meat consumption, and the condition is regarded as harmless. In this context it is interesting to note that tryptophanaemia (probably due to tryptophan pyrrolase deficiency) also appears to be asymptomatic.

DISORDERS OF METABOLISM OF β- AND γ-AMINO ACIDS

Abnormally high excretion of *R*(D, –)-β-aminoisobutyric acid (McKusick 210100) is a harmless genetic polymorphism resulting from low β-aminoisobutyrate-pyruvate aminotransferase activity. It occurs in about 5% of whites and in much higher proportions in some other races. This amino acid, an intermediate in thymine catabolism, is also excreted in larger amounts during periods of catabolism, and in cancer patients. High excretion of both *R* and *S*-β-aminoisobutyric acids, together with β–alanine occurs in *(methyl)malonic semialdehyde dehydrogenase deficiency*, a rare and apparently harmless biochemical anomaly. *Hyper-β-alaninaemia* (McKusick 237400) is associated with β-alaninuria, β-aminoisobutyric aciduria and γ-aminobutyric aciduria. Reported in a single family, it is a rapidly fatal neurological condition.

Carnosinase deficiency (McKusick 212200) and *homocarnosinosis* (McKusick 236130) may be identical disorders.[41] Urinary excretion of substantial quantities of carnosine continues even when meat is withdrawn from the diet. Increased concentrations of homocarnosine are found in CSF. It is doubtful if this condition produces disease.

The metabolism of γ-aminobutyric acid (GABA) within the central nervous system is abnormal in three conditions[42]: GABA-transaminase deficiency (McKusick 137150), succinic semialdehyde dehydrogenase deficiency (Ch. 4) and pyridoxine-dependent convulsions (McKusick 266100). GABA concentrations in CSF are increased in the first two of these conditions and decreased in the last, with no significant urinary amino acid findings.

OTHER DISORDERS

It has not been possible to cover all the known abnormalities of amino acid metabolism in man in this chapter. Of the better defined conditions, sarcosinaemia[43], β-mercaptolactate-cysteine disulphiduria and hydroxylysinuria are the most obvious omissions and the reader is referred to the larger monographs for information. In addition there are many individual reports in the literature which cannot be interpreted satisfactorily from the clinical or biochemical points of view and their elucidation must await the discovery of further similar cases. Certain disorders discussed in other chapters may also be detected through abnormalities of amino acid excretion. In addition to those examples already mentioned in passing, aspartylglycosaminuria may be detected by the excretion of asparaginyl-*N*-acetylglucosamine, hypophosphatasia by increased phosphoethanolamine excretion, some instances of generalised deficiency of acyl-CoA dehydrogenation by the associated sarcosinaemia and sarcosinuria, and some disorders of pyruvate metabolism by the associated hyperalaninaemia. Generalised amino aciduria may provide a clue to cystinosis and other causes of Fanconi syndrome, Wilson disease and galactosaemia.

ACKNOWLEDGEMENT

We would like to thank Dr B L Priestley for Figure 3.6.

REFERENCES

1. Edwards M A, Grant S, Green A 1988 A practical approach to the investigation of amino acid disorders. Annals of Clinical Biochemistry 25:129–141
2. Smith I, Seakins J W T (eds) 1976 Chromatographic and electrophoretic techniques. Vol 1, Paper and thin layer chromatography. Vol 2, Zone electrophoresis. Heinemann, London
3. Bremer H J, Duran M, Kamerling J P, Przyrembel H, Wadman S K 1981 Disturbances of amino acid metabolism: clinical chemistry and diagnosis. Urban and Schwarzenburg, Baltimore
4. Bickel H 1980 Phenylketonuria: Past, present and future, Journal of Inherited Metabolic Disease 3:123–132
5. Okano Y, Eisensmith R C, Guttler F et al 1991 Molecular basis of phenotypic heterogeneity in phenylketonuria. New England Journal of Medicine 324: 1232–1238
6. Waisbren S, Schnell R, Levy H L 1984 Intelligence and personality characteristics in adults with mild untreated atypical phenylketonuria and mild hyperphenylalaninemia. Journal of Pediatrics 105:955–958
7. Matuso K, Hommes F 1987 Regional distribution of the phenylalanine-sensitive ATP-sulphurylase in brain. Journal of Inherited Metabolic Disease 10:62–65
8. Francis D E M 1987 Diets for sick children, 3rd edn. Blackwell Scientific Publications, Oxford
9. Smith I, Beasley M G, Ades A E 1990 Intelligence and quality of dietary treatment in phenylketonuria. Archives of Disease in Childhood 65:472–478
10. Smith I, Beasley M G, Ades A E 1991 Effect on intelligence of relaxing the low phenylalanine diet in phenylketonuria. Archives of Disease in Childhood 66:311–316
11. Thompson A E, Smith I, Brenton D et al 1990 Neurological deterioration in young adults with phenylketonuria. Lancet 336:602–605
12. Guttler F, Hansen G 1977 Heterozygote detection in phenylketonuria. Clinical Genetics 11:137–146
13. Woo S L C 1989 Molecular basis and population genetics of phenylketonuria. Biochemistry (USA) 28:1–7
14. Lenke R R, Levy H L 1980 Maternal phenylketonuria and hyperphenylalaninemia. New England Journal of Medicine 303:1202–1208
15. Smith I, Glossop J, Beasley M 1990 Fetal damage due to maternal phenylketonuria: effects of dietary treatment and maternal phenylalanine concentration around the time of conception. Journal of Inherited Metabolic Disease 13:651–657
16. Surplice I M, Griffiths P D, Green A, Leeming R J 1990 Dihydropteridine reductase activity in dried blood spots: automation of an assay for a national screening service. Journal of Inherited Metabolic Disease 13:169–177
17. Leeming R J, Barford P A, Blair J A, Smith I 1984 Blood spots on Guthrie cards can be used for inherited tetrahydrobiopterin deficiency screening in hyperphenylalaninaemic infants. Archives of Disease in Childhood 59:59–61
18. Dhondt J L 1991 Strategy for the screening of tetrahydrobiopterin deficiency among hyperphenylalaninaemic patients: 15-years experience. Journal of Inherited Metabolic Disease 14:117–127
19. Medical Council Steering Committee for the MRC/DHSS Phenylketonuria Register 1981 Routine neonatal screening for phenylketonuria in the United Kingdom 1964–1978. British Medical Journal 282:1680–1684
20. Bickel H, Guthrie R, Hammersen G (eds) 1980 Neonatal screening for inborn errors of metabolism. Springer, Berlin
21. Rice D N, Houston I B, Lyon I C T, Macarthur B A, Mullins P R, Veale A M O, Guthrie R 1989 Transient neonatal tyrosinaemia. Journal of Inherited Metabolic Disease 12:13–22
22. Goldsmith L A, Laberge C 1989 Tyrosinemia and related disorders. In: Scriver C R, Beaudet A L, Sly W S, Valle D (eds) The metabolic basis of inherited disease. McGraw–Hill, New York, p 547–562
23. Mudd S H, Levy H L, Skovby F 1989 Disorders of transsulfuration. In: Scriver C R, Beaudet A L, Sly W S, Valle D (eds) The metabolic basis of inherited disease. McGraw–Hill, New York, p 693–734

24. Mudd S H, Skovby F, Levy H L et al 1985 The natural history of homocystinuria due to cystathionine-β-synthase deficiency. American Journal of Human Genetics 37:1–31
25. Urea Cycle Symposium 1981 Pediatrics 68:271–297, 446–472
26. Green A 1988 When and how should we measure plasma ammonia? Annals of Clinical Biochemistry 25:199–209
27. Hudak M, Jones M, Brusilow S 1985 Differentiation of transient hyperammonemia of the newborn and urea cycle enzyme defects by clinical presentation. Journal of Pediatrics 107:712–719
28. Nuzum C T, Snodgrass P J 1976 Multiple assays of the five urea-cycle enzymes in human liver homogenates. In: Grisolia S, Baguena R, Mayor F (eds) The urea cycle, Wiley, New York, p 325–349
29. Brusilow S W, Horwich A L 1989 Urea cycle enzymes. In: Scriver C R, Beaudet A L, Sly W S, Valle D (eds) The metabolic basis of inherited disease. McGraw–Hill, New York p 629–663
30. Simell O 1989 Lysinuric protein intolerance and other cationic aminoacidurias. In: Scriver C R, Beaudet A L, Sly W S, Valle D (eds) The metabolic basis of inherited disease. McGraw–Hill, New York, p 2497–2513
31. Carson N A J (ed) 1982 Selected reviews from the workshop on non-ketotic hyperglycinaemia. Journal of Inherited Metabolic Disease 5 Suppl 2:105–128
32. Hatasaka K, Tada K, Fueki N, Aikawa J 1990 Prenatal diagnosis of non-ketotic hyperglycinemia: enzymatic analysis of the glycine cleavage system in chorionic villi. Journal of Pediatrics 116:444–445
33. Wolff J A, Kulovich S, Yu A L, Qia C N, Nyhan W L 1989 The effectiveness of benzoate in the management of seizures in nonketotic hyperglycinemia. American Journal of Diseases of Children 140:596–602
34. Dancis J, Hutzler J, Ampola M G, Shih V E, van Gelderen H H, Kirby L T, Woody N C 1983 The prognosis of hyperlysinemia: An interim report. American Journal of Human Genetics 35:438–442
35. Scriver C R, Levy H L 1983 Histidinaemia. Part I: Reconciling retrospective and prospective findings. Journal of Inherited Metabolic Disease 6:51–53
36. Rosenmann A, Scriver C R, Clow C L, Levy H L 1983 Histidinaemia. Part II: Impact; a retrospective study. Journal of Inherited Metabolic Disease 6:54–57
37. Coulombe J T, Kammerer B L, Levy H L, Hirsch B Z, Scriver C R 1983 Histidinaemia. Part III: Impact; a prospective study. Journal of Inherited Metabolic Disease 6:58–61
38. Rowe P B 1983 Inherited disorders of folate metabolism. In Stanbury J B, Wyngaarden J B, Fredrickson D S, Goldstein J L, Brown M S (eds) The metabolic basis of inherited disease, 5th edn. McGraw – Hill, New York, p 498–521
39. Scriver C R, Whelan D T, Clow C L, Dallaire L 1970 Cystinuria: Increased prevalence in patients with mental disease. New England Journal of Medicine 283:783–786
40. Scriver C R 1989 Familial renal iminoglycinuria. In Scriver C R, Beaudet A L, Sly W S, Valle D (eds) The metabolic basis of inherited disease. McGraw–Hill, New York, p 2529–2538
41. Scriver C R, Perry T L 1989 Disorders of ω-amino acids in free and peptide-linked forms. In: Scriver C R, Beaudet A L, Sly W S, Valle D (eds) The metabolic basis of inherited disease. McGraw–Hill, New York, p 755–771
42. Jaeken J, Casaer P, Haegele K D, Schechter P J 1990 Normal and abnormal central nervous system GABA metabolism in childhood. Journal of Inherited Metabolic Disease 13:793–801
43. Levy H L, Coulombe J T, Benjamin R 1984 Massachusetts Metabolic Disease Screening Program. 3. Sarcosinemia. Pediatrics 74:509–513

4. Disorders of organic acid metabolism

R. A. Chalmers

INTRODUCTION

General concepts and definitions

Disorders of organic acid metabolism, more commonly referred to as organic acidurias or organic acidaemias, comprise a diverse group of diseases whose biochemistry encompasses several areas of intermediary metabolism. These include metabolic pathways associated with amino acid metabolism, particularly of L-leucine and other branched-chain amino acids; of L-lysine and of aromatic amino acids; pathways associated with fatty acid metabolism and ketogenesis, and also of pyruvate and carbohydrate metabolism including the tricarboxylic acid (TCA or Kreb's) cycle. Such disorders may occur in, or involve, many different organelles including the mitochondria, the cytosol, peroxisomes and microsomes, but only in one known instance, the lysosomes. These disorders share the common feature that they are characterised by the accumulation in body tissues and fluids, particularly urine, of organic acids and their esters and conjugates. Organic acids in this context are carboxylic acids that may contain a variety of other functional groups, for example hydroxyl, oxo (keto) and imino, and include conjugated organic acids, for example acylglycines and conjugates with other amino acids, including glutamate and aspartate, and glucuronides, but excludes the amino acids themselves. The characteristic features of such organic acids are high water solubility, acidity and ninhydrin-negativity. The range of biochemical and chemical properties is wide and not limited to that of relatively few compounds as in the case of physiological amino acids. Acyl moieties also conjugate with L-carnitine to form basic acylcarnitine esters, and this latter important group of metabolites is also considered here.

In addition to the common features of chemistry and biochemistry, these disorders of intermediary metabolism also share some common clinical characteristics, the patients frequently presenting with acute symptoms in early life with acidosis, ketosis, vomiting, convulsions and coma. The disorders are often lethal in the newborn and young children and survivors may be physically or mentally handicapped. Although the incidence of individual diseases may be low, collectively their overall incidence may be as high as 1:3000 liveborn infants. Thus, they present a significant clinical and biochemical challenge and, because of the nature of the disorders and their clinical manifestations, they place a disproportionate load on clinical paediatric services. Early and precise diagnosis is therefore essential since this, coupled with adequate early therapy, may result in greatly improved prognosis with normal subsequent physical and mental development. Other patients may present later in childhood with established failure to thrive, neurological deterioration or with sudden acute and profound attacks associated with infections and trauma. Careful investigation of such patients for metabolic disease is important.

As a result of their common clinical features, the organic acidurias cannot be diagnosed on purely clinical grounds. Organic acid analysis, particularly with gas chromatography and mass spectrometry, and other biochemical investigations are essential for their specific and unambiguous characterisation. Most of these disorders are of proven autosomal recessive inheritance, and good genetic counselling and prenatal diagnosis form an essential part of the overall care of the families in which an index case has been identified. This is discussed in more detail below in addition to specific examples related to individual diseases.

Diagnosis and screening for the organic acidurias

The primary populations at risk for the organic acidurias are newborns and infants, since most organic acidurias, including those that may be associated with neurological and physical handicap in later years, present with acute life-threatening illness in early life. It is these patients who need to be investigated in detail using the most comprehensive screening methods available. A suitable protocol for the investigation (or 'screening') of the neonate and child with suspected metabolic disease is shown in Figure 4.1. This is also applicable to those presenting in later childhood with failure to thrive, neurological problems or with acute symptoms indicative of a possible underlying metabolic disease. The latter patients include those presenting with Reye's syndrome-like attacks after a previously uneventful history, but with a possible metabolic basis, for example in fatty acid metabolism.

The initial clinical presentation giving suspicion of a metabolic disorder (Fig. 4.1) prompts the initiation of routine first-line tests and biochemistry designed to rapidly exclude traumatic, infective and acquired disorders, while also providing further indicators for possible metabolic disorders. Second-line biochemistry provides further indicators prior to the introduction of more specific and diagnostic investigations, including quantitative organic acid and amino acid analysis of blood and urine. Ideally, in positive cases, more than one sample should be analysed in order to exclude transient metabolic disorders, and careful interpretation of the results is necessary with due attention being given to the effects of diet and drugs employed at the time of sampling. Samples obtained during the initial

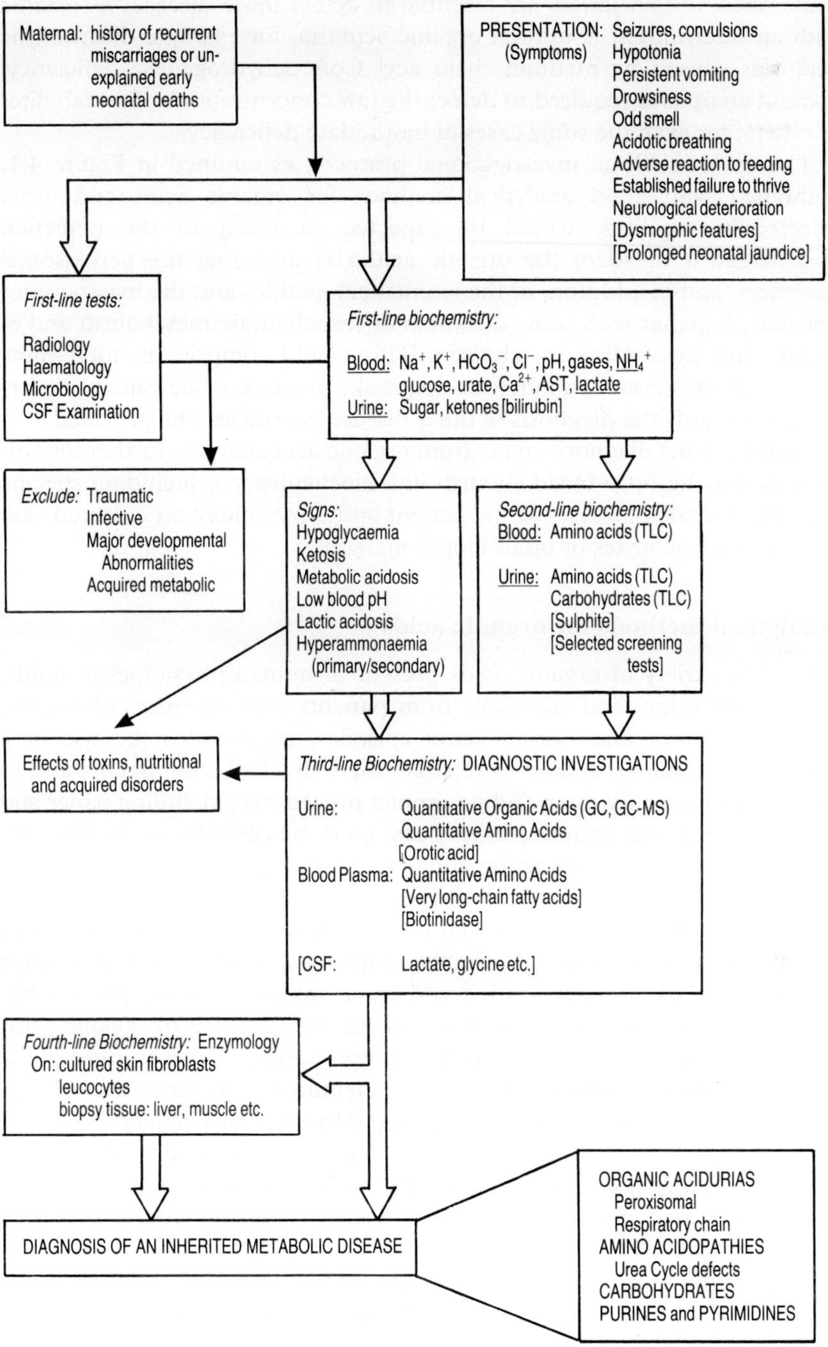

Fig. 4.1 Investigational protocol for the diagnosis of organic acidurias and other inherited metabolic diseases (© R A Chalmers).

acute phases of an illness are essential to detect those diseases associated with an intermittent abnormal organic aciduria, for example dicarboxylic acidurias caused by medium-chain acyl CoA dehydrogenase deficiency. Careful analysis is required to detect the low concentrations of metabolites in others, for example some cases of biotinidase deficiency.

The use of such an investigational protocol, as outlined in Figure 4.1, combined with good analytical methods for organic acids and other selected metabolites, would be expected to result in the detection and diagnosis of all of the organic acidurias including the peroxisomal disorders, and in addition, of the amino acidopathies and the hyperammonaemias, together with some disorders of carbohydrate metabolism and of purine and pyrimidine metabolism. This would comprise in total some two-thirds of the known inherited metabolic diseases, while valuable information towards the diagnosis of other diseases would also be provided.

Following the diagnosis made from organic acid analysis, further investigations may be introduced ('fourth-line biochemistry'), including specific loading or challenge tests of the patient and enzymology on cultured skin fibroblasts, leucocytes or other biopsy material.

Analytical methods for organic acids

The wide variety of organic acids present in human physiological fluids, particularly urine, and especially from patients with disorders of organic acid metabolism and during acute episodes, necessitates the use of a chromatographic procedure to separate the individual components and to identify and quantify them. While simpler procedures, including paper and thin-layer chromatography, have been used successfully in preliminary analyses, and liquid chromatography has been used by some workers for limited applications[1] and preliminary screening, in practical terms the use of gas chromatography is essential for the analysis of organic acids. The development of capillary gas chromatography, particularly with fused silica columns and chemically-bonded and cross-linked stationary phases, has allowed much qualitative, and most quantitative, analysis of organic acids to be achieved with use of gas chromatography alone. However, most of the known organic acidurias have been identified with the use of gas chromatography-mass spectrometry (GC-MS) and this remains essential for unambiguous identifications and diagnoses, detailed studies and quantification at low concentrations. Because of the current availability of small, dedicated and easily operated GC-MS instruments, most large clinical biochemistry departments can use this technique. More laboratories are now capable of diagnosing the organic acidurias, although the reliable use of GC-MS still needs the expertise of dedicated and experienced personnel.

Prior to gas chromatography and mass spectrometry organic acids must be extracted as a group from physiological fluids (using solvent or anion exchange extraction methods) and converted into volatile and thermally-stable derivatives (usually trimethylsilyl derivatives with keto acids stabilised as O-alkyloximes).

The derivatised organic acids are separated using programmed-temperature gas chromatography and quantified by reference to appropriate internal standards. Identifications may be made using retention data, usually expressed as methylene units, although absolute identifications necessitate the use of mass spectrometry. Full details of such procedures and the processes involved in the GC-MS of organic acids are given elsewhere.[1–3]. In addition to absolute identifications, GC-MS is also used for more specialised analyses for selected components by monitoring individual characteristic ions (SIM) for accurate quantification against appropriate internal standards. The latter is of particular value where low concentrations and very precise data are to be measured, for example in the prenatal diagnosis of the organic acidurias by direct chemical analysis of amniotic fluid (see below), and internal standards labelled with stable isotopes may also be employed in such analyses. Capillary gas–liquid chromatography also has application to specific problems, for example the separation and characterisation of enantiomers of hydroxyacids such as lactic acids and glyceric acids.

More recently proton nuclear magnetic resonance spectroscopy (^{1}H-NMR) has been applied successfully to the study of both organic acidurias and aminoacidopathies using unextracted biological fluids and may achieve greater application in the future[4, 5], but the very costly instrumentation and specialist interpretative skills required precludes the extension of this approach to all but the most specialised laboratories at present.

Urine is the most readily available physiological fluid for diagnostic and study purposes, particularly from an acutely ill baby or young infant, and is obtainable by essentially non-invasive methods. Urine has the further advantages that any organic acids that accumulate in blood plasma are also excreted into the urine, and many acids are found in measurable quantities only in urine. Thus, these disorders of organic acid metabolism are characterised more generally by an organic aciduria than by an organic acidaemia and urine has been the most extensively utilised and studied fluid.

Random, clean urine samples are sufficient for diagnostic purposes while for detailed patient monitoring and therapeutic studies timed (for example 6-hourly) collections are preferred. Complete 24-hour collections are extremely difficult to obtain especially from sick infants and neonates and are often of less value in detailed studies. The use of random and limited timed specimens necessitates the use of an endogenous metabolic internal standard with which to relate organic acid concentrations, in order to correct for widely differing urine flow rates and volumes. The most widely used standard is creatinine, the excretion of which is essentially related to mean muscle mass. While not the perfect standard, particularly in young metabolically unwell infants, it is generally accepted and used. Heparinised blood plasma is also used for specific studies, with methods scaled to deal with the small volumes available (100–200 μl).

Treatment and prognosis of the organic acidurias

Treatment

The large majority of patients with organic acidurias present with acute illness often associated with vomiting, metabolic acidosis, ketosis, hypoglycaemia and/or hyperammonaemia. Thus the immediate therapeutic measures undertaken, generally before a precise diagnosis has been made, are common to all or most organic acidurias, irrespective of the primary defect: they involve management of the acute episodes by supportive therapy, accompanied by detoxification measures to remove any accumulating metabolites and potentially toxic intermediates. Thus supportive measures introduced to any patient in acute metabolic decompensation include: assisted ventilation; control of acidosis with, for example, bicarbonate; restriction or cessation of protein intake, accompanied by oral or i.v. glucose to maintain calories and counter hypoglycaemia; and increased fluid (saline) intake to counter the frequently-associated dehydration and electrolyte loss. Such episodes are often precipitated by an intercurrent infection and this must also be sought for and treated actively where possible. Detoxification measures, especially in acute and unresponsive ketoacidosis, include exchange transfusions, peritoneal dialysis or forced diuresis.[6]

It is most important that such treatment is introduced immediately (but not delaying the collection and storage where necessary of samples for diagnosis) and not after a more specific diagnosis is made. These patients will often present to local or district hospitals and it is here that this immediate therapy must be instituted. Delay often means the eventual referral of the patient, often in a coma, to a more central paediatric hospital where adequate treatment may be applied too late to prevent irreversible neurological damage, giving rise to the poor prognosis often ascribed to many of the treatable organic acidurias.[6]

Once a more specific diagnosis has been established, perhaps by referral of the appropriate diagnostic specimens to a regional centre, more specific and individual therapeutic measures suited to particular disorders may be instituted. Such measures, directed towards the long-term management of the patient concerned, may involve environmental manipulation by reducing the load of substrate presented to the mutant or absent enzyme, including the use of dietary restriction; inhibition of substrate synthesis; substrate removal, and coenzyme supplementation at pharmacological levels (Table 4.1). Rarely, where the product of the missing or impaired enzyme reaction is an important intermediate, product replacement may also be attempted.

Table 4.1 Treatment of organic acidurias

1. Dietary and nutritional management	Protein restriction (1–1.5 g/kg per 24 h) Amino acid supplementation Hypercaloric diet Low fat if indicated; medium-chain triglycerides (MCT) in long-chain oxidation defects Frequent feeding, nocturnal/nasogastric if necessary; Corn starch supplements Mineral and vitamin supplements
2. Cofactor therapy (pharmacological doses)	Hydroxocobalamin D-Biotin Riboflavin Pyridoxine (thiamine; lipoate)
3. Substrate removal	Glycine (in isovaleric acidaemia) Antibiotics (metronidazole, amoxycillin) (in disorders of propionate metabolism) L-Carnitine
4. L-Carnitine	Acute management Long-term treatment (not in disorders of fatty acid metabolism or non-ketotic hypoglycaemias)

The most important general approach to the treatment of the organic acidurias is undoubtedly dietary manipulation. For disorders of amino acid catabolism this involves not only protein restriction, perhaps to 1–1.5 g/kg body weight per day, but also use of amino acid supplements, omitting those amino acid precursors associated with the particular disorder, to give an adequate amino acid and protein intake for normal growth and development and tailored to the specific requirements of the disease and the individual patient concerned. Additional supplements of selected amino acids have also been recommended (e.g. alanine, selected branched-chain amino acids) to promote growth. The use of hypercaloric diets, particularly during acute episodes, may be advantageous to prevent catabolism and frequent feeding, either orally or via nasogastric tube, including nocturnal feeding, may prove effective. Mineral and vitamin supplements are also required when partially artificial diets are employed, in order to avoid specific deficiencies, such as that of zinc, with the associated secondary clinical complications. Close collaboration between paediatrician, dietician and biochemist is essential in providing the optimal care and management of patients with organic acidurias.

In other organic acidurias, for example defects in β-oxidation of fatty acids and ketogenesis, with associated profound hypoglycaemic attacks and dicarboxylic aciduria, the use of low fat, high carbohydrate diets and of corn starch supplements is of value. In such disorders, the use of medium-chain triglycerides in the diet is to be avoided although, conversely, such supplements may be of value in the treatment of patients with defects in long-chain fatty acid β-oxidation. Patients with other organic acidurias may show secondary dicarboxylic aciduria, and appropriate measures need to be included in their management (see below).

The second most effective approach to treatment of the organic acidurias is the use of cofactors at pharmacological levels. This is based upon the primary defect being associated with a mutant enzyme, rather than a total absence, or on defects associated with the endogenous synthesis of the required cofactor. Some patients with methylmalonic aciduria may respond to vitamin B_{12} treatment, preferably using hydroxycobalamin, given in doses of 1 mg/24 h intramuscularly or 10 mg/24 h orally, resulting in considerable reduction in the excretion of methylmalonate by enhancement of residual enzyme activity. Similarly, D-biotin, in doses of 10 mg/24 h orally, abolishes the abnormal organic aciduria and prevents the clinical symptoms in patients with multicarboxylase deficiency caused by either holocarboxylase synthetase deficiency or secondary to biotinidase deficiency. Some patients with dicarboxylic aciduria, caused by medium-chain acyl CoA dehydrogenase deficiency, ethylmalonic-adipic aciduria, glutaric aciduria or multiple acyl CoA dehydrogenase deficiency, may respond well to riboflavin therapy. Finally, some patients with primary hyperoxaluria Type 1 (glycollic aciduria) with residual glyoxylate: alanine aminotransferase activity may respond to pharmacological doses of pyridoxine (vitamin B_6), reducing the urinary excretion of both oxalate and of glycollate and obviating the need for hepatic or renal transplantation.

Substrate removal is also an effective means of therapy in some organic acidurias. This may be by means of conjugation of accumulating substrate, for example in isovaleric acidaemia where isovaleryl CoA accumulates because of a specific dehydrogenase deficiency: isovaleryl groups are effectively conjugated with glycine via the action of glycine-N-acylase, and glycine therapy has proved valuable in the treatment of such patients, especially during acute episodes. Similarly L-carnitine conjugates with a number of acyl moieties including isovaleryl groups (see below) and is particularly effective for the treatment of patients with isovaleric acidaemia.[7] Substrate removal may also be effected by other means, such as the prevention, by use of antibiotics, of propionate production by colonic bacteria. For example the alternating use of metronidazole and amoxycillin in patients with methylmalonic aciduria and propionic acidaemia reduces the substrate load on the deficient enzyme systems and considerably reduces the accumulation and excretion of abnormal organic acids.[8,9]

Many organic acidurias are associated with the accumulation in tissues of acyl CoA esters, with consequent toxic effects due directly to the esters themselves and to metabolites produced by alternative pathways. Among the secondary effects of acyl CoA accumulation is the sequestration of available free coenzyme A, leading to severe inhibition of CoA-dependent metabolic processes including pyruvate oxidation, the tricarboxylic acid cycle and β-oxidation. This results in secondary lactic acidosis and dicarboxylic aciduria.

L-Carnitine (4-trimethylamino-3-hydroxybutyrate) is important in the modulation of availability of free CoA, and may exchange readily with acyl CoA esters to form acylcarnitine esters via the action of carnitine acyltransferases. This occurs in many of the organic acidurias, presumably as an attempt to detoxify acyl CoA esters accumulating in the mitochondria and increasing the removal of acyl moieties into the urine.[10] As a consequence, patients with many organic acidurias exhibit increased acylcarnitine excretion with resulting L-carnitine insufficiency or deficiency, and L-carnitine has been used in both the acute and long-term treatment of patients with these diseases. It has been of particular value in the treatment of patients with propionic acidaemia, methylmalonic aciduria and isovaleric acidaemia[7,11] and in the acute treatment of patients with medium-chain acyl CoA dehydrogenase deficiency and with 3-hydroxy-3-methylglutaric aciduria. However, in these latter disorders its use is perhaps contraindicated for maintenance therapy because of the enhanced transport of long-chain fatty acids into the mitochondria for β-oxidation, and hence increase of the substrate load. The efficacy of L-carnitine as a therapeutic measure in the organic acidurias is gaining acceptance because of proven clinical and biochemical effects, but its use requires careful assessment in each disorder concerned, and the individual patient's response to therapy also requires careful monitoring.

Prognosis

The increased efficacy of the combination of early diagnosis, adequate acute treatment and therapeutic advances based upon a better biochemical and clinical understanding of the conditions concerned, particularly with dietary, cofactor and L-carnitine therapy, has greatly improved the prognosis of patients with organic acidurias. Formerly, the large majority of patients with these diseases died during the early months or years of life; surviving patients showed severe neurological problems, poor development and a greatly reduced life expectancy, with a totally inadequate quality of life. Long-term survivors were almost certainly those with milder variants of the disorders concerned. Effective and early treatment has demonstrated that many patients with these disorders can show relatively normal growth and development, particularly if successful treatment and management is achieved during the early years of life. Medium-chain acyl CoA dehydrogenase deficiency and 3-hydroxy-3-methylglutaric aciduria can be considered treatable disorders, despite their associated acute and profound hypoglycaemic and Reye's syndrome-like attacks. The prognosis for patients with disorders such as isovaleric acidaemia and methylmalonic aciduria is also much improved. Other disorders may be considered curable, for example primary hyperoxaluria by hepatic transplantation.

As treatments improve other problems may become apparent however: for example in methylmalonic aciduria renal problems have now become generally evident in older patients. Also, in biotinidase deficiency where the response to biotin therapy is complete, there is now evidence that some permanent residual neurological damage may occur in patients treated late after an acute presentation.

It is also too early to be definitive about the longer-term outcome and survival of patients with some other disorders, particularly those with propionic acidaemia. Despite the survival of some patients into their second and third decades of life continued long-term assessment is still required.

Some disorders, for example multiple acyl CoA dehydrogenase deficiency caused by ETF and ETF dehydrogenase deficiency, are associated with severe and acute neonatal problems and with teratological and fetal developmental damage while others, for example glutaric aciduria Type 1, are associated with severe progressive and crippling neurological problems, and the prognosis of many such disorders remains extremely poor. In these latter disorders, as well as in many of the others for which the index patient presents a severe burden on the family concerned, prenatal diagnosis must remain an important consideration in overall care.

Prenatal diagnosis of the organic acidurias

The enzymatic bases for a considerable number of organic acidurias have now been identified and in many of these the enzyme activity, and hence its deficiency in affected cases, is demonstrable in cultured skin fibroblasts, cultured amniotic cells, and both directly and in culture in chorionic villi. Such disorders are therefore detectable in utero and prenatal diagnosis with termination of a pregnancy with an affected fetus is possible. Prenatal diagnosis is carried out with the prerequisite that the disorder has been previously diagnosed unambiguously in the index patient, and the mother is therefore 'at risk' for the disorder concerned.

Amniocentesis is generally performed at 14–16 weeks' gestation: cell cultures from the cells in the fluid may be established and the fluid itself may be analysed directly for accumulating metabolites excreted by the fetus. The procedure using cultured cells is obviously dependent upon obtaining a viable culture and sufficient cells for enzymology. Some 4 weeks are usually required from amniocentesis to final result. Thus repeat assays are generally not possible and relatively late terminations of affected fetuses are necessary.

More rapid and thus earlier diagnoses are obtainable by direct chemical analysis of the cell-free amniotic fluid supernatant and many organic acidurias have been diagnosed prenatally using this approach, with selected ion monitoring for specific metabolites using GC-MS[1,12] and, in some instances, the use of internal standards labelled with stable isotopes, although the latter are not usually essential (Table 4.2). Results are available within a few days of amniocentesis at 14–16 weeks' gestation and thus terminations are possible at around 15–17 weeks. The procedure is based upon the knowledge that the fetal bladder fills with urine from about 10 weeks' gestation onwards and this is excreted into the amniotic fluid thereby reflecting metabolic abnormalities in the fetus itself.

More recently this approach has been used earlier in pregnancy, with amniocentesis at around 10–11 weeks' gestation, based upon the permeability of the skin of the early fetus to blood metabolites. Amniotic fluid in the first trimester is essentially an ultrafiltrate of fetal blood plasma and thus reflects the metabolic state of the fetus. First trimester prenatal diagnoses by direct chemical analysis of amniotic fluid have been carried out for propionic acidaemia and methylmalonic aciduria and it is expected this list will grow rapidly. First trimester prenatal diagnosis is also carried out using chorionic villi obtained at 9–10 weeks' gestation either transcutaneously or transvaginally, with direct enzyme assays or, more rarely, DNA analysis. Enzymology results are often available on the day of biopsy or the day after. Cultures of chorionic villus cells may also be established and used for enzymology, but occasionally an enzyme activity expressed in direct biopsy material is not expressed in cultured villus cells.

Table 4.2 lists those organic acidurias for which prenatal diagnosis has been achieved, in the second trimester by using cultured cells or chemical analysis, and in the first trimester by direct enzyme assay, cultured cells or chemical analysis.

Table 4.2 Prenatal diagnosis of organic acidurias; + achieved; (+) possible;—not possible; ? unknown; GC-MS is direct gas chromatography and mass spectrometry of amniotic fluid

Disorder	Second trimester		First trimester	
	Enzymology on cultured amniocytes	GC-MS	GC-MS	Enzymology on chorionic villus tissue or cells
Methylmalonic aciduria	+	+	+	+
Propionic acidaemia	+	+	+	+
Branched-chain ketoaciduria	+	—	—	(+)
Isovaleric acidaemia	+	+	(+)	(+)
3-methylcrotonylglycinuria	(+)	(+)	(+)	(+)
Multicarboxylase deficiency				
Holocarboxylase synthetase	+	+	(+)	(+)
Biotinidase	(+)	—	—	(+)
Methylacetoacetyl CoA thiolase deficiency	(+)	(+)	?	(+)
2-oxoadipic aciduria	(+)	(+)	?	?
Glutaric aciduria	+	+	(+)	(+)
Medium-chain acyl CoA dehydrogenase deficiency	(+)	—	—	(+)
Long-chain acyl CoA dehydrogenase deficiency	(+)	—	—	(+)

Table 4.2 *contd*

Disorder	Second trimester		First trimester	
	Enzymology on cultured amniocytes	GC-MS	GC-MS	Enzymology on chorionic villus tissue or cells
Multiple acyl CoA dehydrogenase deficiency ('glutaric aciduria Type 2')	+	+	(+)	(+)
3-hydroxy-3-methylglutaric aciduria	+	+	+	+
Tyrosinaemia Type 1 (fumarylacetoacetase deficiency)	+	+	?	(+)
Pyruvate dehydrogenase deficiency, E1α deficiency (familial cases)	(+)	—	—	(+)
Pyruvate carboxylase deficiency	+	—	—	+
Fumaric aciduria	(+)	?	—	(+)
Primary hyperoxaluria Type 1*	—	—	—	—
D-Glyceric aciduria	(+)	(+)	?	?
4-hydroxybutyric aciduria	(+)	?	?	(+)
N-acetylaspartic aciduria (Canavan disease)	+	+	(+)	+

*possible on fetal liver tissue by direct enzymology

DISORDERS OF BRANCHED-CHAIN ORGANIC ACID METABOLISM

Introduction

The three neutral branched-chain amino acids are chemically similar and are all metabolised initially via a pyridoxal phosphate-dependent transamination with 2-oxoglutarate, and secondly by a thiamine pyrophosphate (TPP)-dependent oxidative decarboxylation (Fig. 4.2). Individual cytosolic transaminases occur, specific to 6-carbon and to 5-carbon amino acids, as indicated by the finding of isolated hypervalinaemia. The oxidative decarboxylation occurs via the action of a mitochondrial multienzyme complex, analogous to pyruvate dehydrogenase and 2-oxoglutarate dehydrogenase, associated with the inner mitochondrial membrane. The E3 enzyme (Fig. 4.3), dihydrolipoyl dehydrogenase (lipoamide dehydrogenase, EC 2.3.1.12), is common to all three dehydrogenase complexes and a deficiency of this latter enzyme produces a syndrome with features of congenital lactic acidosis, branched-chain ketoaciduria and 2-oxoglutaric aciduria. A deficiency of the specific branched-chain keto acid decarboxylase or the E2 enzyme leads to a severe disorder in which the metabolism of all three branched-chain amino acids is affected, branched-chain ketoaciduria or maple syrup urine disease (MSUD). Regulation of the enzyme complex may involve acyl CoA compounds and the activity in muscle, in which relatively large amounts of branched-chain amino acids are transaminated and oxidised, is stimulated by L-carnitine which may

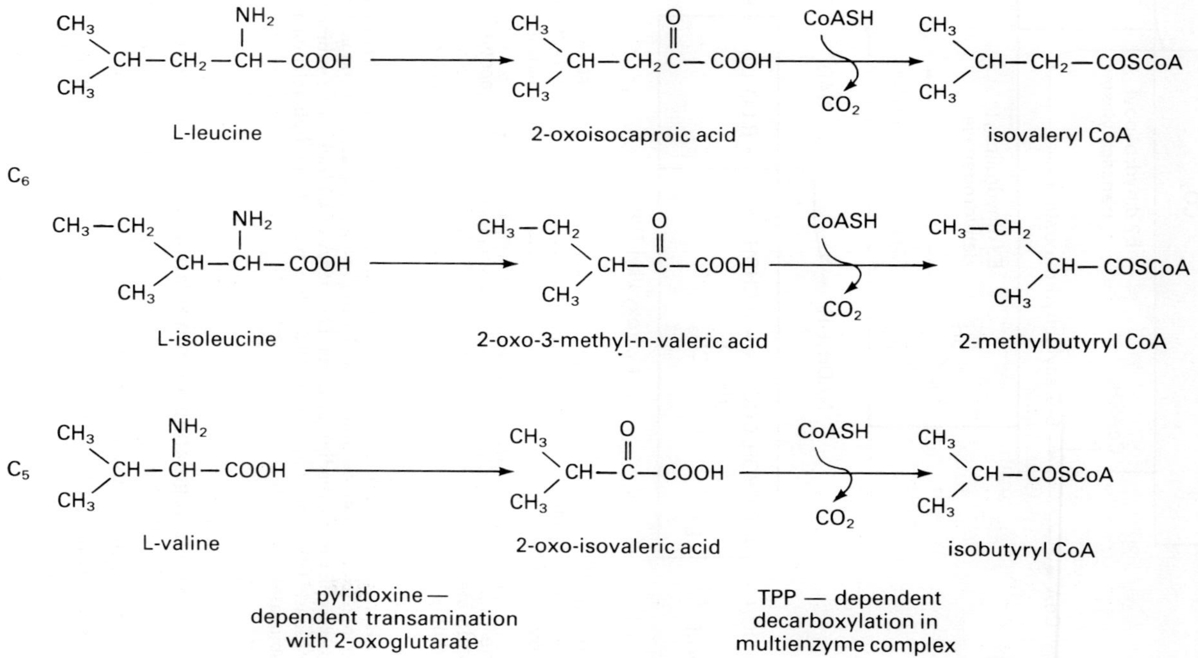

Fig. 4.2 Initial steps in the metabolism of branched-chain amino acids.

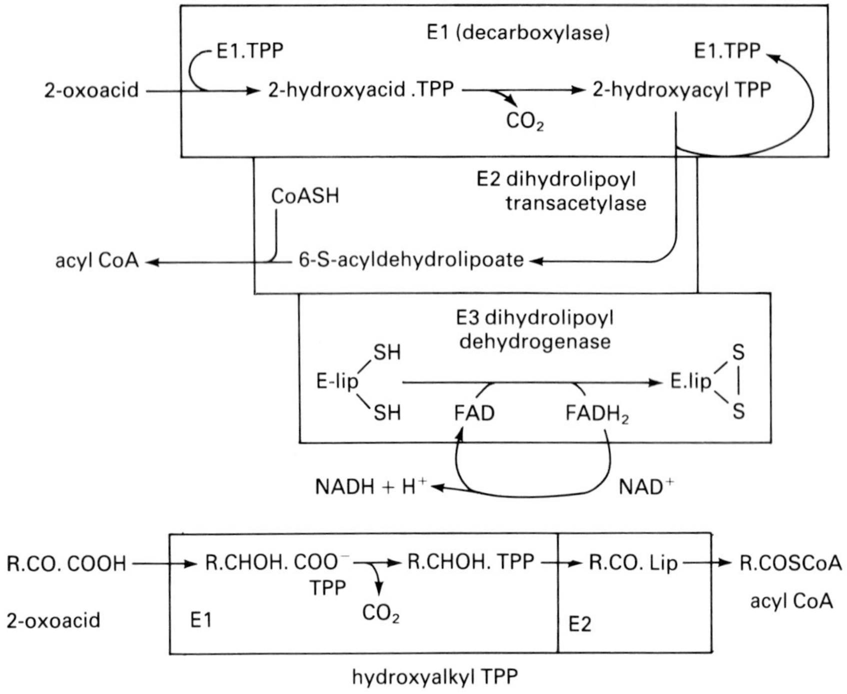

2-oxoisocaproate	isovaleryl CoA
2-oxo-3-methylvalerate	2-methylbutyryl CoA
2-oxoisovalerate	isobutyryl CoA
Pyruvate	acetyl CoA
2-oxoglutarate	succinyl CoA
2-oxoadipate	glutaryl CoA

Fig. 4.3 2-Oxoacid dehydrogenases and oxidative decarboxylation of 2-oxoacids. A defect in E1 leads to maple syrup urine disease (MSUD); in pyruvate decarboxylase, E1 to lactic acidosis; in 2-oxoglutarate decarboxylase, E1 to 2-oxoglutaric aciduria and in 2-oxoadipate decarboxylase, E1 to 2-oxoadipic aciduria. Deficiency of E3 leads to a combined dehydrogenase deficiency. The complexes are deactivated by phosphorylation and activated by phosphatases.

also thus exert a regulating or modulating effect on enzyme activity. In addition, like all the related dehydrogenase complexes, the enzyme complex is regulated by phosphorylation (deactivating) and dephosphorylation (activating) and is thus probably also under hormonal control.

Subsequent to this common 2-oxo acid decarboxylation, the degradative pathways of the three branched-chain amino acids are independent and distinctive. 2-oxoisocaproic acid (from L-leucine) is metabolised to isovaleryl CoA in the dehydrogenase step and subsequently to 3-methylcrotonyl CoA, 3-methylglutaconyl CoA, 3-hydroxy-3-methylglutaryl CoA and thence to acetyl CoA and acetoacetate, the latter being an obligate step in 'ketone body' formation. Patients with isolated defects in all stages of this pathway have been identified. The metabolism of 3-methylcrotonyl CoA (and of propionyl CoA and pyruvate) occurs via the action of D-biotin-dependent carboxylases. Defects in the synthesis (holocarboxylase synthetase) and recycling (biotinidase) of the biotin-containing holocarboxylases lead to further disorders related to multicarboxylase deficiency. In contrast to L-leucine metabolism, only one disorder associated with L-isoleucine catabolism, β-ketothiolase deficiency, or more correctly methylacetoacetyl CoA thiolase deficiency, has been identified, and only one associated with L-valine catabolism, namely 3-hydroxyisobutyryl CoA deacylase deficiency. These latter two branched-chain amino acids are of particular interest however, since they are both major precursors of propionyl CoA and methylmalonyl CoA, defects in the metabolism of which lead to the relatively common and severe propionic acidaemia and the methylmalonic acidurias respectively. These disorders are all described briefly in the following sections.

Branched-chain ketoaciduria: maple syrup urine disease, MSUD (McKusick 248600)

Branched-chain ketoaciduria is caused by deficient activity of branched-chain ketoacid decarboxylase (EC 1.2.4.4, E1 in Fig. 4.3) both in the E1α subunit and in the E1β subunit, affecting the metabolism of all three branched-chain oxo and amino acids. Defects have also been identified in the E2 enzyme of the dehydrogenase complex and detailed molecular analysis has demonstrated the complexities of phenotypic expression in the disorder.[13–15] In the classical presentation of the disease, little or no residual enzyme activity remains and branched-chain amino acids, keto acids and their hydroxy analogues accumulate in body fluids, with the keto acid of isoleucine, 2-oxo-3-methyl-n-valeric acid, apparently being responsible for the maple syrup smell apparent in the urine of some patients. Not all patients exhibit this sweet, caramel-like, odour, best observed in concentrated urine, but it does provide a useful additional indicator of the disease. Alloisoleucine may also accumulate in the disorder, caused by keto-enol tautomerism of 2-oxo-3-methylvalerate and reamination.

The classical form of the disease is inherited by an autosomal recessive mode with a usual incidence of 1:120 000 to 1:500 000 dependent upon the geographical area concerned, but with high incidences being recorded in Norway, Spain and inbred populations, such as the Mennonites of Pennsylvania, and a much lower incidence in England and Massachusetts. All racial types show cases of the disease. Variant forms have been recorded, including a late-presenting variant associated with acute intermittent attacks of ataxia, that may manifest as a result of an infection or other causes of stress; affected children are normal between attacks but there is the chance of permanent neurological damage from acute episodes. The possibility of compound heterozygosity in these patients has been suggested but it also appears likely that various levels of residual enzyme activity occur in patients with the same genotype (2–16%), leading to the wide spectrum of clinical and biochemical presentations observed. Other so-called variants are even more rare, with 'mild variant', 'valine-toxic' and apparently thiamine-responsive forms being recorded.[13,16]

Patients are apparently normal at birth with severe symptoms associated with ketoacidosis, poor feeding, vomiting and lethargy occurring within the first week of life. Muscular hypotonicity, abnormal movements and convulsions may also occur, death usually intervening within the first year of life following multiple intercurrent infections. Survivors generally suffer severe brain damage. Abnormal branched-chain amino acid and hydroxy and keto acid concentrations in blood and urine are apparent within the first week of life and the disorder may be readily diagnosed from both amino acid and organic acid analysis. CSF concentrations of these metabolites are also increased. Keto acids may be detected using 2, 4-dinitrophenylhydrazine (2, 4-DNP) or TLC but these and other organic acids are best determined using GC and MS of the TMS oxime, ethoxime or n-butyloxime derivatives. TMS-quinoxalinols are also useful for the determination of 2-oxoacids and ^{1}H-NMR allows simultaneous detection and measurement of both the branched-chain amino acids and the various keto and hydroxy acids. The renal clearance of the keto acids is very low (1–2 ml min^{-1} $1.73m^{-2}$) and hence there is a tendency to retain the keto acids in the blood, with excess hydroxyacids in the urine, with the retained keto acids probably exacerbating the severe symptoms still further. Lactic acidosis and ketoacidosis with associated organic aciduria may also occur, and branched-chain fatty acids are often elevated in the urine during ketoacidotic periods. Acylcarnitines are also elevated in the blood and urine and may be consistent with the accumulation of these branched-chain acyl moieties in the disease. The enzyme deficiency is expressed in leucocytes and cultured skin fibroblasts and may be demonstrated by measurement of the rate of oxidation of [1-^{14}C]-labelled branched-chain amino acids or keto acids to $^{14}CO_2$.

The severity of the disorder requires early diagnosis and vigorous treatment directed at removal of toxic metabolites and prevention of catabolism. Any delay in diagnosis or treatment may result in permanent neurological damage and early death. For effective treatment, diagnosis before about 10 days of age is imperative with initiation of intubation and intensive care for 3–5 days after diagnosis with monitoring of blood amino acids and urinary keto acids (using 2,4-DNP if necessary for rapid results). Intensive care may involve peritoneal dialysis for 1–3 days until blood leucine levels plateau (at around 1–1.5 mmol/L) and/or multiple or prolonged exchange transfusions.[6] Coma disappears within 6 days of treatment and abnormal movements and hypotonia also disappear within 2–3 weeks. Weight gain, associated with near normalisation of blood leucine levels and introduction of an anabolic state, occurs within 8 days.[6] This is assisted by a high calorie intake using intravenous glucose, with concomitant insulin administration, followed by gradual introduction of a diet low in branched-chain amino acids (40–60 mg/kg body weight per day) supplemented with artificial amino acid mixtures.[13] Most foods have relatively high contents of branched-chain amino acids and treatment with a restricted diet, while maintaining normal growth and development is difficult to maintain and requires close laboratory supervision.

With adequate therapy, the longer-term survival is good[13] but tolerance to dietary leucine and other branched-chain amino acids remains low throughout life except in the variant forms of the disease. In earlier cases, although maintenance of dietary therapy was believed to be adequate, ketoacidotic episodes associated with infections were recurrent and the long-term results of evaluation of psychomotor development were disappointing. Early diagnosis together with improved management and the availability of better commercial dietary preparations has improved outcome and prognosis considerably.[13] However, the severity of the disease and difficulties of management outside experienced centres means that prenatal diagnosis continues to be indicated in the overall care of affected families.

Disorders of the L-leucine pathway subsequent to isovaleryl CoA

After the transamination of L-leucine and the oxidative decarboxylation of its keto acid, 2-oxoisocaproic acid, to yield isovaleryl CoA, the further metabolism of the carbon skeleton of L-leucine follows a route that is quite distinct from that of the other branched-chain amino acids.

Isovaleryl CoA (Fig. 4.4) is metabolised by the specific FAD- and electron transfer flavoprotein (ETF)-dependent isovaleryl CoA dehydrogenase to 3-methylcrotonyl CoA, a defect in this dehydrogenase resulting in isovaleric acidaemia. Isovaleryl CoA dehydrogenase activity is also reduced in multiple acyl CoA dehydrogenase deficiency caused by defects in ETF and in ETF dehydrogenase, responsible for transfer of electrons from a variety of mitochondrial dehydrogenases into the respiratory chain.

3-Methylcrotonyl CoA is carboxylated by the specific D-biotin-dependent 3-methylcrotonyl CoA carboxylase to form 3-methylglutaconyl CoA. Deficient activity of the carboxylase apoenzyme causes isolated 3-methylcrotonylglycinuria with 3-hydroxyisovaleric aciduria. Secondary deficiency of this enzyme may also occur, firstly due to deficient activity of holocarboxylase synthetase, the enzyme responsible for attachment of the D-biotin to the apocarboxylase, and secondly, by deficient activity of biotinidase, responsible for release of free biotin from the lysyl residues (biocytin) arising from holocarboxylase turnover, and from intestinal absorption from the diet and gut bacterial turnover.

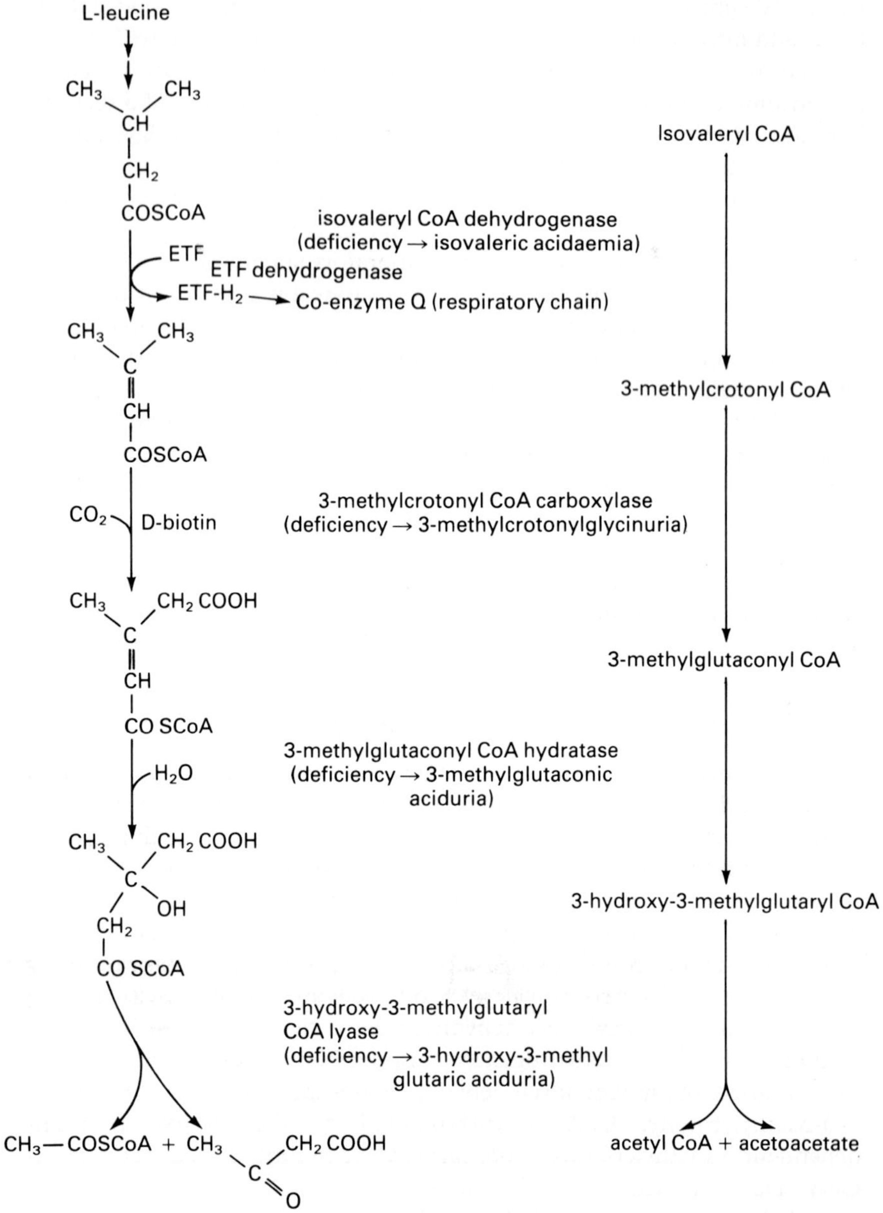

Fig. 4.4 Metabolism of isovaleryl CoA in the L-leucine metabolic pathway.

These disorders also affect other D-biotin-dependent carboxylase systems: holocarboxylase synthetase deficiency affects all three mitochondrial carboxylases (3-methylcrotonyl CoA carboxylase, propionyl CoA carboxylase and pyruvate carboxylase), and biotinidase deficiency affects the cytosolic acetyl CoA carboxylase in addition, to give rise to the multi-carboxylase deficiencies.

3-Methylglutaconyl CoA is metabolised by a hydratase to form 3-hydroxy-3-methylglutaryl CoA and possible deficiencies of this hydratase have also been described.

Finally, 3-hydroxy-3-methylglutaryl CoA is cleaved by a specific lyase to form acetoacetate and acetyl CoA. Deficient activity of the lyase results in 3-hydroxy-3-methylglutaric aciduria. The lyase deficiency is of interest since 3-hydroxy-3-methylglutaryl CoA is the obligate intermediate in the formation of ketone bodies, i.e. the synthesis of acetoacetate from acetoacetyl CoA, derived from butyryl CoA in the final stage of β-oxidation and of L-lysine metabolism. Patients with the lyase deficiency suffer from episodic acute and profound non-ketotic hypoglycaemia and this disorder is considered in detail with other disorders of this kind rather than as one of branched-chain amino acid catabolism.

Isovaleric acidaemia (McKusick 243500)

Isovaleric acidaemia is caused by deficient activity of the specific FAD- and ETF-dependent isovaleryl CoA dehydrogenase leading to intracellular accumulation of isovaleryl CoA, with the appearance of characteristic metabolites in body fluids and of a characteristic odour of sweaty feet or cheese during acute episodes. The disorder is characterised clinically by episodes of acidosis, vomiting, ataxia and tremors that may progress to lethargy and coma.[1,17] Many patients present acutely in the newborn period with severe metabolic acidosis and ketosis, lethargy and severe neurological symptoms including convulsions and coma. Death has occurred within a few weeks in about half of such cases, with overwhelming sepsis, leucopenia and pancytopenia contributing to the high mortality. Patients who survive this initial acute period show a subsequent course analogous to those presenting later in life. The differences in presentation are a reflection of the spectrum of disease associated with similar residual enzyme activity, environmental factors and the modifying effects of other related metabolic pathways in different individuals. This is supported by the occurrence of both neonatal and later-onset isovaleric acidaemia in the same sibships. Mild mental retardation may occur in surviving patients but prognosis with effective treatment, particularly during the first 1–2 years of life, is good.

More than 45 cases of isovaleric acidaemia are now recorded from 28 sibships with approximately equal numbers of males and females, consistent with an autosomal recessive mode of inheritance. The overall incidence of the disease has been estimated at less than 1:200 000. The enzyme deficiency is demonstrable in leucocytes and in cultured skin fibroblasts by reduced oxidation of [1-^{14}C]-isovalerate, reduced oxidation of [2-^{14}C]-leucine and reduced incorporation of [1-^{14}C]-isovalerate into protein.[7] Isovaleryl CoA dehydrogenase is a specific mitochondrial dehydrogenase with a tetrameric structure containing FAD, and direct assay of its activity by tritium release assays, using ^{3}H-isovaleryl CoA, to measure hydrogen elimination at the 2- and 3-carbons have confirmed the nature of the molecular defect in the disease. Molecular heterogeneity has been demonstrated by ^{35}S-methionine incorporation studies with five types of variant enzyme being identified. Complementation studies using cultured skin fibroblasts have shown a single complementation group, consistent with a single gene locus. The gene for isovaleric acidaemia is located on the long arm of chromosome 15 and at least five distinct variant alleles are known. Three mRNA species have been shown to hybridise to human isovaleryl CoA dehydrogenase cDNA in both normal and isovaleric acidaemia fibroblast lines from patients with different genotypes, suggesting the variants occur due to point mutations or small deletions.[18]

The accumulating isovaleryl CoA is metabolised to 3-hydroxyisovaleric acid and, via conjugation through the action of glycine-N-acylase, to isovalerylglycine, the latter being the most characteristic metabolite and always present in urine from affected patients. The characteristic odour is due to isovaleric acid itself, which only accumulates during acute episodes. Some patients excrete a number of other metabolites during acute ketoacidosis, including methylsuccinate, 4-hydroxyisovalerate, methylfumarate, 3-hydroxyisoheptanoate and other conjugates including isovalerylglutamate and isovalerylglucuronide.[7] The putative origins of some of these metabolites are indicated in Figure 4.5. During periods of remission, only isovalerylglycine is apparent, with concentrations in blood and urine increasing during metabolic decompensation (to more than 3 g/24 h in urine) and the detection of this metabolite is essential to the diagnosis. Typical chromatograms of urinary and blood metabolites have been published elsewhere[1,7] together with the mass spectra of characteristic metabolites. The proton NMR spectrum has also been published.[4]

The free isovaleric acid that accumulates in body fluids, including CSF, during acute ketoacidotic episodes shows an encephalopathic action in experimental animals and is probably the cause of the coma, in particular, and may be responsible for the mild neurological damage observed in some patients. Treatment of acute episodes in isovaleric acidaemia may require detoxification by peritoneal dialysis or exchange transfusions. Dietary management with a moderately reduced protein intake is also effective for longer-term care. The observation that glycine-N-acylase has a relatively high affinity for isovaleryl groups, leading to the increased excretion of isovalerylglycine in isovaleric acidaemia, prompted the use of supplemental glycine therapy in the disease. This may be of particular benefit during acute ketoacidotic episodes but may be of less benefit for long-term management in preventing further attacks.[19] Doses of 250 mg glycine/kg body weight per day have been used in acute episodes and up to 800 mg per day for chronic treatment, but some authorities have rejected its use in

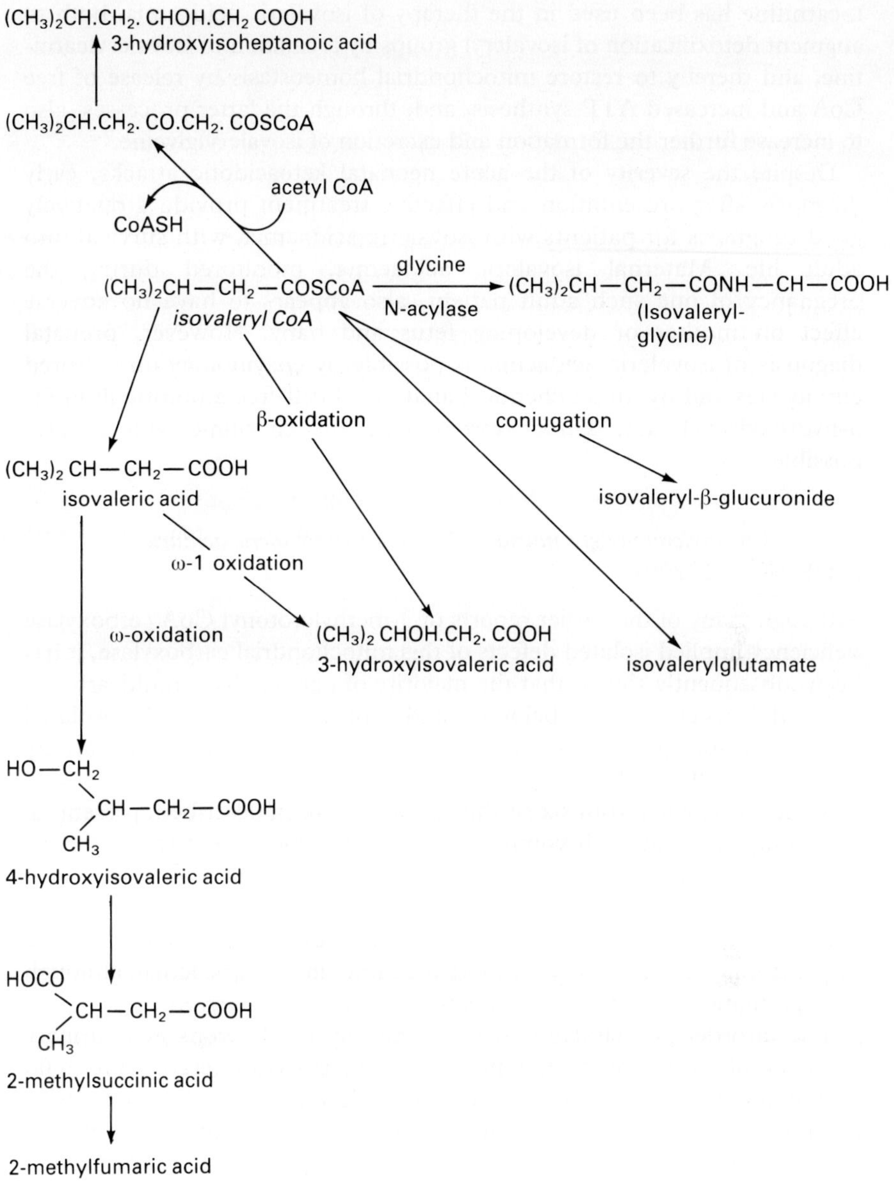

Fig. 4.5 Alternative pathways of isovaleryl CoA metabolism in isovaleric acidaemia.

less severely affected patients. Others have cautioned against the indiscriminate use of glycine therapy after observation of glycine-associated encephalopathy in one patient.[7] Patients with isovaleric acidaemia consistently show reduced free carnitine concentrations in plasma and greatly increased isovalerylcarnitine excretion into urine.[10] Supplemental

L-carnitine has been used in the therapy of isovaleric acidaemia, both to augment detoxification of isovaleryl groups by formation of isovalerylcarnitine, and thereby to restore mitochondrial homeostasis by release of free CoA and increased ATP synthesis, and, through the latter processes, also to increase further the formation and excretion of isovalerylglycine.[7]

Despite the severity of the acute neonatal ketoacidotic attacks, early diagnosis after presentation and effective treatment provide a relatively good prognosis for patients with isovaleric acidaemia, with survival into adult life. Maternal isovaleric acidaemia, monitored during the pregnancy of one such adult patient, also appears to have no adverse effect on mother or developing fetus and baby. However, prenatal diagnosis of isovaleric acidaemia is possible by enzymology on cultured amniocytes and by direct chemical analysis of cell-free amniotic fluid for 3-hydroxyisovalerate. Direct enzymology on chorionic villi is also possible.

Isolated 3-methylcrotonylglycinuria with 3-hydroxyisovaleric aciduria (McKusick 210200)

Although many of the earlier reports of 3-methylcrotonyl CoA carboxylase deficiency implied isolated defects of this mitochondrial carboxylase, it has been subsequently shown that the majority of patients have multicarboxylase deficiency (see below) and proven cases of isolated 3-methylcrotonylglycinuria appear rare, possibly because of the relatively mild clinical effects of this enzyme deficiency.

Some 11 patients from six sibships have now been described, presenting in infancy variously with vomiting, diarrhoea, hypotonia, and life-threatening hypoglycaemia, ketoacidosis, hyperammonaemia and coma, with micro- and macrovesicular fatty infiltration of the liver that may be secondary to the severe carnitine deficiency that is observed.[20,21] The disorder may be precipitated by mild infections and may be lethal, although asymptomatic affected siblings of patients have been observed.

The disorder is characterised biochemically by the consistent urinary excretion of greatly increased amounts of 3-hydroxyisovalerate (500–9000 mmol/mol creatinine) and 3-methyl-crotonylglycine (400–800 mmol/mol creatinine) in the absence of other metabolites associated with multicarboxylase deficiencies. Other characteristic metabolites may also be present including 3-methylcrotonylglutamate.[21] The enzyme deficiency is expressed in leucocytes and cultured skin fibroblasts where almost complete deficiency of 3-methylcrotonyl CoA carboxylase activity is observed in the presence of normal activities of other mitochondrial carboxylases and of biotinidase. The disorder appears to be inherited in an autosomal recessive mode. There is no response in vivo or in vitro to D-biotin therapy and treatment is by moderate protein restriction and essential L-carnitine supplementation.[20,21] The prognosis of treated patients appears good.

3-Methylglutaconic aciduria (McKusick 250950)

3-Methylglutaconic aciduria associated with proven 3-methylglutaconyl CoA hydratase deficiency has been reported only in two male siblings who presented with speech retardation as the only clinical symptom. Biochemically, the disorder is characterised by increased excretion of 3-methylglutaconic acid (500–1000 mmol/mol creatinine) and moderately increased 3-hydroxyisovaleric acid (150–250 mmol/mol creatinine), the excretion of which may be increased by a high protein diet and by L-leucine loading.[17] Two isomers of 3-methylglutaconate are found in urine in this condition and others in which this metabolite occurs, corresponding to the cis (*Z*) and trans (*E*) isomers. Very small but increased amounts of 3-methylglutarate may also occur but excretion of 3-hydroxy-3-methylglutarate is normal. The activity of 3-methylglutaconyl CoA hydratase is greatly reduced in cultured skin fibroblasts. However, the overall activity of the pathway, as measured by [1-^{14}C] isovalerate incorporation into protein, is only partially reduced, possibly indicating the presence of a bypass pathway. The mode of inheritance is unclear as is the requirement for treatment.

3-Methylglutaconic aciduria also occurs in other metabolic conditions as a secondary metabolite. In particular it has been reported in more than 17 patients presenting in infancy with abnormal neurological findings, including progressive developmental regression or neurological deterioration following normal early infancy, variously associated with dysmorphic features, multiple minor malformations, hypotonia, choreoathetosis with a slowly progressive encephalopathy and moderate dementia, spastic paraparesis and optic atrophy. Some patients show microcephaly and mental retardation. There is ketoacidosis, and organic acids in urine show only moderate increases in 3-methylglutaconic acid (generally 25–250 mmol/mol creatinine) and lesser amounts of 3-methylglutarate; 3-hydroxy-isovalerate and 3-hydroxy-3-methylglutarate levels are normal.

Oral loading with L-leucine inconsistently produces some increase in metabolite levels. The absence of increased excretion of 3-hydroxyisovalerate is not compatible with a defect in the metabolism of L-leucine at the proposed level, and this is supported by the finding of normal activity of 3-methylglutaconyl CoA hydratase in cultured fibroblasts. Some patients have been observed to always excrete increased amounts of tricarboxylic acid cycle metabolites and this, together with the marked lactic acidosis and ketosis that occurs[22,23], is suggestive of a defect or defects elsewhere than in L-leucine metabolism in this apparently heterogeneous group of patients.

3-Hydroxy-3-methylglutaric aciduria (McKusick 246450) is better classified as a disorder of ketogenesis than as a disorder of L-leucine metabolism, presenting primarily as non-ketotic hypoglycaemia, and is thus considered further below (p. 176).

Disorders of L-isoleucine metabolism

Following the decarboxylation of the 2-oxo-3-methyl-n-valerate formed from L-isoleucine, the product *S*-2-methylbutyryl CoA (Fig. 4.6) undergoes further catabolism to propionyl CoA. *S*-2-Methylbutyryl CoA is dehydrogenated by a specific FAD- and ETF-dependent 2-methyl-branched-chain acyl CoA dehydrogenase to form tiglyl CoA (2-methylcrotonyl CoA) which is then hydrated across the double bond to give 3-hydroxy-2-methylbutyryl CoA. The latter undergoes dehydrogenation to 2-methylacetoacetyl CoA which is then cleaved (thiolysed) to acetyl CoA and propionyl CoA, in an analogous manner to the metabolic steps in mitochondrial β-oxidation of fatty acids.

At least four 3-oxoacyl CoA thiolases occur in mammalian tissues, one in the cytosol that is specific for acetoacetyl CoA, one in the peroxisomes that has a broad chain length specificity and two in the mitochondria, one with a broad specificity, perhaps for longer chain acyl groups, and one specific for short-chain acetoacetyl CoA and methylacetoacetyl CoA. The peroxisomal enzyme functions in the β-oxidation of fatty acids whereas the cytosolic enzyme may be primarily involved in production of acetyl CoA from ketone bodies for steroid and lipid biosynthesis. The short-chain mitochondrial enzyme is activated by the potassium ion, K^+, unlike the other enzymes, and is primarily involved in energy production and catabolism. This is reflected in tissue distribution where the acetoacetyl CoA metabolising enzymes occur in brain, while liver shows all activities including the general catabolic mitochondrial enzyme. Deficient activity of K^+-activated short-chain methylacetoacetyl CoA thiolase leads to the metabolic condition described under various names including β-ketothiolase deficiency.

2-Methylacetoacetyl CoA thiolase deficiency (McKusick 203750)

This is characterised by early presentation with fever, vomiting and diarrhoea, with acidosis and ketosis during acute phases. Moderate hyperammonaemia may occur and frequent recurrent headaches have been an associated phenomenon. The disease is characterised biochemically by 3-hydroxy-2-methylbutyric aciduria and tiglylglycinuria, and 2-methylacetoacetic acid and butanone are also excreted during ketoacidosis. Hyperglycinaemia may also occur.

Since all three metabolites may also be excreted in increased amounts by patients with propionic acidaemia it is important to distinguish the two disorders on the basis of the other organic acids excreted by the latter patients. Similarly, patients with ketoacidosis in isolation or in association with other metabolic disorders may excrete increased amounts of 3-hydroxy-2-methylbutyrate and increased excretion of this metabolite alone is not diagnostic of 2-methylacetoacetyl CoA thiolase deficiency. Patients with 2-methylacetoacetyl CoA thiolase deficiency may have inter-

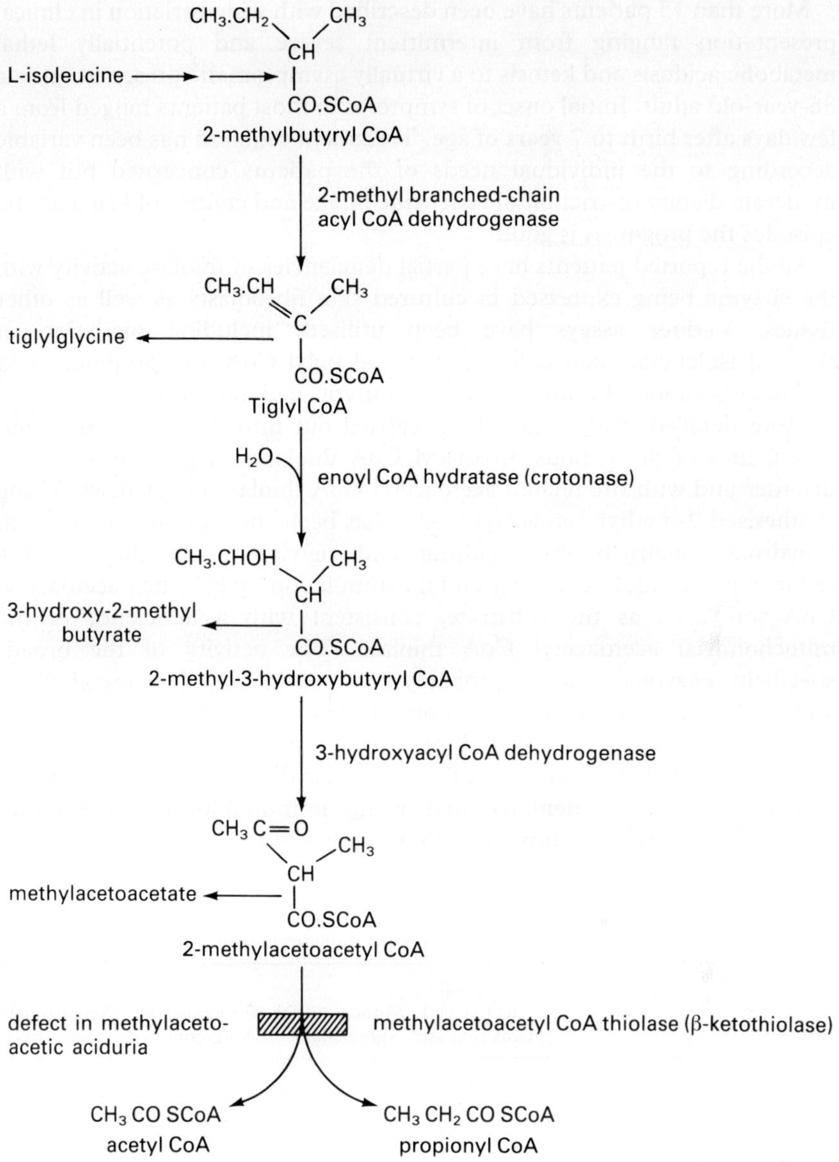

Fig. 4.6 Metabolism of 2-methylbutyryl CoA in the degradation of L-isoleucine, showing the defect in β-ketothiolase deficiency and metabolites accumulating in the disorder.

mittent or episodic variants with only moderate excretion of abnormal metabolites when clinically well and isolated tiglylglycinuria with small amounts of 3-hydroxy-2-methylbutyric aciduria is suggestive of the disorder. Oral loading with L-isoleucine (100 mg/kg body weight) with subsequent monitoring of tiglylglycine excretion is of diagnostic value.

More than 15 patients have been described with wide variation in clinical presentation ranging from intermittent severe and potentially lethal metabolic acidosis and ketosis to a virtually asymptomatic presentation in a 36-year-old adult. Initial onset of symptoms in most patients ranged from a few days after birth to 7 years of age. Treatment required has been variable according to the individual needs of the patients concerned but with moderate dietary restriction of isoleucine intake and control of ketoacidotic episodes the prognosis is good.

All the reported patients have partial deficiencies of thiolase activity with the enzyme being expressed in cultured skin fibroblasts as well as other tissues. Various assays have been utilised, including oxidation of [U-^{14}C] isoleucine, conversion of tritiated tiglyl CoA into propionic acid and incorporation of 2-methyl-[1-^{14}C]-butyric acid into protein.[17]

More detailed studies have been carried out into the relationship and specificities of the various 3-oxoacyl CoA thiolases in patients with this disorder and with the related acetoacetyl CoA thiolase deficiencies. Using synthesised 2-methylacetoacetyl CoA it has been shown that patients with 3-hydroxy-2-methylbutyric aciduria and tiglylglycinuria show greatly reduced β-ketothiolase activity and no stimulation by K^+ when acetoacetyl CoA was used as the substrate, consistent with a deficiency of the mitochondrial acetoacetyl CoA thiolase. The activity of the broad-specificity enzyme, which is probably involved in fatty acid metabolism, and of the cytosolic thiolase are normal. The specificities of the various 3-oxoacyl CoA thiolases (β-ketothiolases) are summarised in Table 4.3.

Considerable heterogeneity in the molecular defects responsible for the disorder have been demonstrated using immunoblotting and pulse-labelling methods[24], confirmed by PCR studies of the molecular defects at

Table 4.3 Substrate specificities of 3-oxoacyl CoA thiolases in man

Enzyme	Cytosolic acetoacetyl CoA thiolase[1]	Mitochondrial short-chain[2]	Mitochondrial long-chain[3]	Peroxisomal[4]
Acetoacetyl CoA	+	+	+	+
Acetoacetyl CoA, K^+ stimulated	—	+	—	—
2-Methylacetoacetyl CoA	—	+	—	—
3-Oxohexanoyl/3-oxo-octanoyl CoAs	—	—	+	+

1. The cytosolic acetoacetyl CoA-specific thiolase is primarily involved in sterol and lipid biosynthesis.
2. The mitochondrial short-chain thiolase is primarily involved in energy production and catabolism, is K^+ activated and metabolises both acetoacetyl CoA and methylacetoacetyl CoA.
3. The mitochondrial long-chain thiolase has a broader specificity and probably functions in thiolysis of oxoacyl CoA derivatives in fatty acid catabolism (see below).
4. The peroxisomal thiolase functions in the peroxisomal β-oxidation of fatty acids.

the DNA level that have shown various point mutations and transitions, some of which result in deletion of specific exons and truncated, and presumably unstable, enzyme proteins. Several patients are compound heterozygotes for different mutations.

The disorder is inherited in an autosomal recessive mode and, with the enzyme deficiency expressed in cultured skin fibroblasts and presumably in amniocytes, prenatal diagnosis is possible, although not yet reported. The relative ease of treatment once a diagnosis has been established, and the good prognosis, suggest prenatal diagnosis would not generally be required for this disorder.

Other thiolase disorders

Only two patients with *cytosolic acetoacetyl CoA thiolase deficiency* have been described, with differing clinical and biochemical presentations. One patient presented at 4 months of age with delayed motor development, ataxia, choreoathetosis, involuntary eye movements and hypotonia associated with raised lactate and pyruvate in blood.[25] Abnormally increased ketonaemia was induced following a ketogenic diet and severe neurological symptoms with epileptic fits developed despite treatment. Reduced activity of cytosolic acetoacetyl CoA thiolase was demonstrated in liver biopsy material in the presence of normal activity of several other enzymes studied. Studies on cultured skin fibroblasts confirmed the deficiency which was ascribed to altered kinetic properties of the enzyme.

The second patient was a severely mentally-retarded boy who presented from 7 months of age and who persistently excreted increased amounts of 3-hydroxybutyrate and acetoacetate.[26] Other organic acids were normal. Study of cultured skin fibroblasts showed reduced activity of 3-oxoacyl CoA thiolase when acetoacetyl CoA was used as substrate, with normal activity with methylacetoacetyl CoA and 3-oxohexanoyl CoA, suggesting a deficiency of cytosolic 3-oxoacyl CoA thiolase. Sterol synthesis rates from acetate were also reduced in the presence of normal fatty acid synthesis, consistent with this deficiency. Succinyl CoA:3-oxo acid CoA transferase activity (see below) was normal

Treatment, with reduced dietary fat intake, has been unsuccessful and, in view of the severe neurological symptoms associated with this condition and the expression of the defect in cultured skin fibroblasts, prenatal diagnosis should be considered in future pregnancies. The condition appears to be inherited in an autosomal recessive mode.

A single patient with *mitochondrial acetoacetyl CoA thiolase deficiency*[17] has also been described, with progressive neuropathy, growth retardation and ataxia associated with a persistent elevation of blood lactate, 3-hydroxybutyrate and acetoacetate. The activity of the K^+-activated mitochondrial acetoacetyl CoA thiolase in liver was reduced, whereas the activity of the cytosolic enzyme was normal. The activity of methylacetoacetyl CoA thiolase in cultured fibroblasts was also normal. The occurrence of only one peak for K^+-activated enzyme on chromatographic separation of the thiolases, compared to two in normal tissue, suggests the possibility of a deficiency of an organ-specific isozyme, although further study is required.

Other disorders of ketone body metabolism

Succinyl CoA: 3-oxoacid CoA transferase deficiency (McKusick 245050)

Tildon and Cornblath[27] described a baby who presented from the second day of life with tachypnoea and feeding difficulties associated with severe metabolic acidosis, ketonaemia, ketonuria and hyperuricaemia. Severe episodes continued to occur, with intolerance of dietary fat or protein, and the infant died at 197 days with sepsis, congestive heart failure and respiratory arrest. An apparently slightly milder case presented initially at 7 months of age and was managed with a high carbohydrate and low fat diet but died at 21 months with acute metabolic acidosis. Thiolase activities were normal but succinyl CoA-3-oxoacid CoA transferase activity was absent in brain, kidney and fibroblasts. This enzyme occurs exclusively in extrahepatic tissues and is responsible for conversion of acetoacetate to acetoacetyl CoA in these tissues for reutilisation via thiolysis to acetyl CoA. Thus severe neurological symptoms might be expected to occur in such disorders of ketone body utilisation and the disorder has several features in common with the thiolase deficiencies. Prognosis appears poor. The relative difficulty in distinguishing and diagnosing such patients with persistent ketoacidosis may mean that patients may remain undiagnosed.

Disorders of L-valine metabolism

After transamination of L-valine to 2-oxoisovaleric acid and oxidative decarboxylation of the latter to form isobutyryl CoA, the branched-chain acyl CoA ester is dehydrogenated to methacrylyl CoA, followed by hydration to 3-hydroxyisobutyryl CoA in a manner analogous to the metabolism of L-isoleucine (Fig. 4.7). The 3-hydroxyisobutyryl CoA is deacylated to the free acid which is then dehydrogenated to methylmalonyl semialdehyde with further metabolism to propionyl CoA. Only one disorder affecting this pathway has been described, namely 3-hydroxyisobutyryl CoA deacylase deficiency, although in multiple acyl CoA dehydrogenase deficiency the common deficiencies of ETF or ETF dehydrogenase affects all ETF-requiring dehydrogenase enzymes simultaneously, including isobutyryl CoA dehydrogenase (2-methyl-branched-chain acyl CoA dehydrogenase).

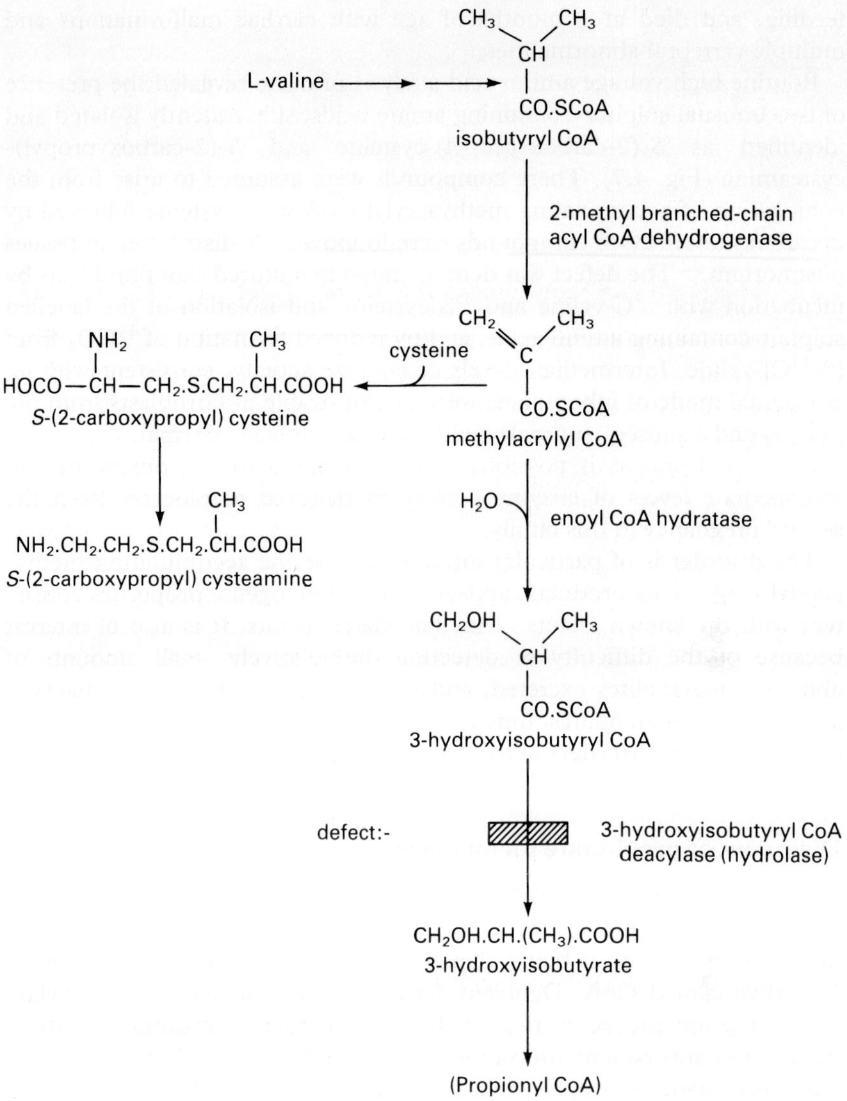

Fig. 4.7 Metabolism of isobutyryl CoA in the degradation of L-valine showing the defect in 3-hydroxyisobutyryl CoA deacylase deficiency and the metabolites that accumulate in this disorder.

3-Hydroxyisobutyryl CoA deacylase deficiency (McKusick 277080)

This has been described in only one infant, the first child of healthy first cousin Egyptian parents. The infant presented with multiple malformations, including dysmorphic facial features, and failure to thrive with poor feeding, and died at 3 months of age with cardiac malformations and multiple vertebral abnormalities.

Routine high voltage amino acid analysis of urine revealed the presence of two unusual sulphur-containing amino acids, subsequently isolated and identified as *S*-(2-carboxypropyl)-cysteine and *S*-(2-carboxypropyl)-cysteamine (Fig. 4.7). These compounds were assumed to arise from the conjugation of accumulating methyacrylyl CoA with cysteine followed by decarboxylation. Both compounds were found widely distributed in tissues postmortem.[28] The defect was demonstrated in cultured skin fibroblasts by incubation with ^{14}C-valine and ^{35}S-cysteine and isolation of the labelled sulphur-containing amino acids, and by reduced formation of $^{14}CO_2$ from [2-^{14}C]-valine. Intermediate levels of enzyme activity, consistent with an autosomal mode of inheritance, were demonstrable in fibroblasts from the parents and a subsequent male child who was clinically normal.

Prenatal diagnosis is possible, as demonstrated by the observation of intermediate levels of enzyme activity in cultured amniocytes from the second pregnancy in this family.

The disorder is of particular interest because the accumulating methyacrylyl CoA, or its products, appear to have teratogenic properties consistent with the known effects of methacrylates in rats. It is also of interest because of the difficulty of detecting the relatively small amounts of abnormal metabolites excreted, and the apparent absence of methacrylic acids or other metabolites, indicating potential difficulties in the diagnosis of this and other disorders of the L-valine (and L-isoleucine pathway).

Disorders of propionate metabolism

After the sequences of metabolic pathways described above, L-isoleucine and L-valine are metabolised to propionyl CoA which is subsequently metabolised, via the D-biotin-dependent propionyl CoA carboxylase, to *S*-methylmalonyl CoA. Deficient activity of propionyl CoA carboxylase leads to propionic acidaemia, with accumulation of propionyl CoA in tissues and subsequent utilisation of its alternative metabolic pathways. Other precursors of propionyl CoA include methionine, threonine, cholesterol and odd-carbon number fatty acids. Propionyl CoA and its alternative metabolites also accumulate when the further metabolism of methylmalonyl CoA is blocked (methylmalonic acidurias) and in multicarboxylase deficiency, and they cause many of the symptoms associated with these disorders (described below). Propionate is also produced normally by gut bacteria in substantial quantities[29]; it is then absorbed from the colon and utilised, via conversion into propionyl CoA and through the tricarboxylic acid cycle. Thus the intestine is an important source of propionate in these disorders and this is of relevance in the management of the patients concerned.

Propionic acidaemia (McKusick 232000 & 232050)

Propionic acidaemia is caused by deficient activity of propionyl CoA carboxylase. Propionyl CoA carboxylase is a mitochodrial enzyme, requiring D-biotin, ATP and magnesium ions for its activity. It is found in most tissues and cells studied, including fibroblasts and leucocytes, and occurs as a tetrameric protein containing four identical subunits of 128 000 daltons, made up of two non-identical subunits, α and β, of 72 000 and 56 000 daltons respectively. The gene for the α subunit has been localised to chromosome 13 and that for the β subunit to the long arm of chromosome 3. Four molecules of biotin are bound to each molecule of the apoenzyme, binding to the α subunit under the action of holocarboxylase synthetase, with D-biotinyladenylate being formed initially. This is then bound to the ε-lysyl group of the apoenzyme subunits to form the active holocarboxylase. Carboxylation occurs initially by formation of the carboxylated holocarboxylase with the biotin being carboxylated at the 1-N position, and then transfer of the carboxyl group from the biotin to the 2- or α-position of the propionyl CoA to form *S*-methylmalonyl CoA.

Clinical presentation. Patients with propionic acidaemia present with severe ketoacidosis, marked hypotonia, arreflexia, vomiting, hyperventilation, apnoea, lethargy and coma, usually in early infancy. Hypoglycaemia and hyperammonaemia with neutropenia, thrombocytopenia and pancytopenia may occur. Classically the disorder is associated with hyperglycinaemia (ketotic hyperglycinaemia)[30], although this is not observed in all cases. Patients may present acutely, in the newborn soon after initial protein feeding, or more chronically with recurrent episodes of ketosis, hyperammonaemia and hyperglycinaemia with periodic thrombocytopenia and neutropenia, often precipitated by intercurrent infections. Others may present with developmental retardation and essentially without ketosis.

While some of the acute cases respond to intensive intravenous glucose and bicarbonate therapy supplemented with peritoneal dialysis and other measures, the disorder is difficult to control and most patients die during such acute episodes with survivors frequently showing permanent neurological damage. Abnormal EEGs are recorded and CT scans show cerebral atrophy, confirmed on autopsy. These changes are probably secondary to hyperammonaemia, although on autopsy demyelination and spongy degeneration have been observed with lipids containing C_{15} and C_{17} straight-chain fatty acids accumulated both in brain and liver.

Early diagnosed and treated cases and the late-presenting cases often show no neurological abnormalities. The clinical spectrum observed is illustrative of the heterogeneity of the disease and the modification of the syndrome that can occur, dependent perhaps upon genetically determined molecular variations, resulting in differences in the ability of individual patients to metabolise accumulating compounds through alternative pathways. This is underlined by clinical heterogeneity within the same sibships.[30] Similarly, genetic complementation studies using cultured skin fibroblasts have demonstrated at least two major complementation groups in patients with propionic acidaemia (see below).

Biochemistry and diagnosis. Patients with propionic acidaemia consistently show increased excretion of methylcitric acids, generally associated with 3-hydroxypropionate and other metabolites of propionyl CoA. These include particularly, propionylglycine, 3-hydroxy-n-valerate and its precursor 3-oxo-n-valerate, formed by condensation of propionyl CoA with acetyl CoA. In addition, 2-methyl-3-oxo-n-valeric acid has also been found consistently, together with the corresponding hydroxy acid, being formed from the condensation of two molecules of propionyl CoA.[1] Methylmalonate excretion is normal or only very slightly increased. Accumulation of metabolites of isoleucine may also occur and tiglylglycine, 3-hydroxy-2-methylbutyrate and even 2-methylacetoacetate may be found in urine. 2-Methylbutyrylglycine may also be excreted following isoleucine loads. Methylcitric acid occurs in two isomeric forms, characterised as the 2*R*, 3*S*, and 2*S*, 3*S* isomers.[31] The two diastereoisomers are excreted in different ratios which are dependent upon the patient concerned and the metabolic and clinical condition at the time of study.[32] Long-chain ketones may also occur in urine, formed from the decarboxylation of 3-oxovaleric acids in a manner analogous to the formation of acetone from acetoacetate (3-oxo-n-butyrate). Similarly, the occurrence of 3-hydroxy-3-ethylglutarate in the urine of some patients suggests the substitution of 3-oxo-n valeryl CoA for acetoacetyl CoA in the hydroxymethylglutaryl CoA synthetase reaction, and may indicate that the free acid is formed via this route in a manner analogous to acetoacetate formation.

Propionyl CoA is the key intermediate in the formation of the majority of the abnormal metabolites observed and is also responsible for the accumulation of odd-carbon number fatty acids and abnormal triglycerides and lipids.[1] Secondary inhibition of other mitochondrial enzyme systems by propionyl CoA also occurs, for example inhibition of N-acetylglutamate synthesis probably underlying the hyperammonaemia observed, and it is also the cause of the secondary hypoglycaemia and hyperglycinaemia in patients with the disorder.[11] More direct evidence of the accumulation of propionyl CoA in propionic acidaemia has been presented by the observation of propionylcarnitine as the major acylcarnitine present in increased concentrations in urine, since propionylcarnitine can only be formed by transfer of the acyl moiety from propionyl CoA.[10] Administration of exogenous L-carnitine to patients with the disorder results in an increase in the excreted amounts of propionylcarnitine. Thus L-carnitine has value in the treatment of propionic acidaemia.

Genetics and prenatal diagnosis. Reference has been made above to genetic complementation studies on cultured skin fibroblasts from patients with propionic acidaemia that give evidence for at least two major complementation groups, designated *pccA* (McKusick 232000) and *pccBC* (McKusick 232050), the latter also being heterogeneous with the subgroups showing intragenic complementation. Studies of the biochemical properties of enzymes in cells from these patients showed differences in heat lability, potassium affinity and biotin-reactivation following avidin inactivation, suggesting that some patients have a structurally modified enzyme protein in which the ATP and carboxybiotin binding sites are affected. In addition, heterozygotes for the *pccA* group show classical gene dosage effects, with approximately half of normal activity of propionyl CoA carboxylase, whereas heterozygotes for the *pccBC* group(s) show normal activities. Studies using immunoprecipitation and gel electrophoresis have shown that fibroblasts from patients in the *pccA* group have primary deficiencies of the α subunit of propionyl CoA carboxylase due to absence of α subunit mRNA.[33] Both enzyme subunits are absent however due to the instability of the free β subunits. It is thus assumed that patients from the *pccBC* groups have deficiencies of the β subunit consistent with the different chromosomal location of the gene.

Propionic acidaemia is inherited in an autosomal recessive mode. The enzyme defect is expressed in cultured skin fibroblasts, amniocytes and chorionic villus tissue. The difficulty of treatment and relatively poor prognosis demands prenatal diagnosis of this condition, and this has been carried out on cultured amniocytes using both [1-^{14}C]-propionate incorporation into protein and by direct propionyl CoA carboxylase assay. Direct analysis of cell-free amniotic fluid supernatant for methylcitric acids has also been used successfully[12], both in the second trimester and, more recently, in the first trimester. First trimester prenatal diagnosis has also been made by direct propionyl CoA carboxylase assay on chorionic villi.

Treatment and prognosis. Treatment of propionic acidaemia, after management of acute ketoacidotic and hyperammonaemic episodes, depends upon dietary manipulation, with minimal natural protein intake (around 1–1.5 g/kg body weight per day) supplemented with amino acid mixtures, omitting isoleucine and valine in particular, and with carbohydrate and fat to supply the other calorie requirements. Dietary requirements need to be tailored to suit individual patients and close monitoring of urinary ketones and organic acids is of value, particularly during the initial establishment of the diet. Monitoring of growth and development is important and it has been suggested that supplemental L-alanine (100 mg/kg per 24 h) may be valuable to promote growth in these patients. Increased fluid intake is also important to avoid the recurrent episodes of dehydration and the use of nasogastric feeding or intravenous treatment may be necessary. Although reports of biotin responsiveness in propionic acidaemia are variable, residual enzyme activity (probably of other carboxylases) may be enhanced by oral biotin (10–50 mg/24 h) and this is always worth investigation. L-Carnitine has been shown to increase the urinary excretion of propionyl groups by patients with propionic acidaemia[10], with secondary biochemical effects suggesting increased availability of free coenzyme A and improvements in energy metabolism, although with little direct effect upon other propionyl metabolites. Administration of L-carnitine (100–400mg/kg body weight per 24 h orally or up to 50 mg/kg per 24 h intravenously) appears to be of value both for regular therapy and especially for the management of acute episodes. Detoxification and supportive measures, introduced earlier in this chapter, are also essential during acute episodes as are mineral and vitamin supplements during regular therapy. Recently, use of antibiotics, particularly metronidazole, has been shown to markedly reduce metabolite excretion in patients both with methylmalonic acidurias and with propionic acidaemia[8,9], by prevention of propionate production by colonic bacteria. The use of antibiotic therapy represents a major advance in the treatment of these disorders.

The prognosis of patients with propionic acidaemia remains generally poor by comparison with the majority of other disorders of branched-chain amino acid metabolism, although advances in therapy offer some improvements. However, detailed information on reasonably large numbers of patients remains limited and a fuller survey of the outcome of such patients is important. Early accurate diagnosis, combined with effective acute treatment to prevent irreversible neurological damage and effective maintenance therapy with rapid response to acute episodes, is improving the prognosis of patients with propionic acidaemia and some patients have now lived into their second and third decades of life.

The methylmalonic acidurias (McKusick 251000, 251100, 251110, 277400 & 277410)

Carboxylation of propionyl CoA leads to the formation of *S*-methylmalonyl CoA which is itself metabolised, firstly by racemisation to *R*-methylmalonyl CoA and thence, via the action of a specific vitamin B_{12}-dependent mutase, to succinyl CoA for entry into the tricarboxylic acid cycle (Fig. 4.8). Methylmalonyl CoA racemase acts by removing the α-hydrogen on *S*-methylmalonyl CoA; the mutase enzyme acts by transfer of the CoA carboxyl group and requires 5'-deoxyadenosylcobalamin as cofactor. Although a single report of racemase deficiency has appeared, subsequent investigation of cultured fibroblasts from the patient concerned demonstrated a deficiency of methylmalonyl CoA apomutase and thus all patients described with methylmalonic aciduria (more than 100) have deficiencies affecting the apomutase or of the synthesis or attachment of the essential cobalamin cofactor.

The mutase exists as a dimer in which both subunits have a molecular mass of 70 000 daltons; each subunit binds 5'-deoxyadenosylcobalamin (AdoCbl), and both show catalytic activity. The gene for the mutase enzyme subunit is located on chromosome 6 (p12–21.2).

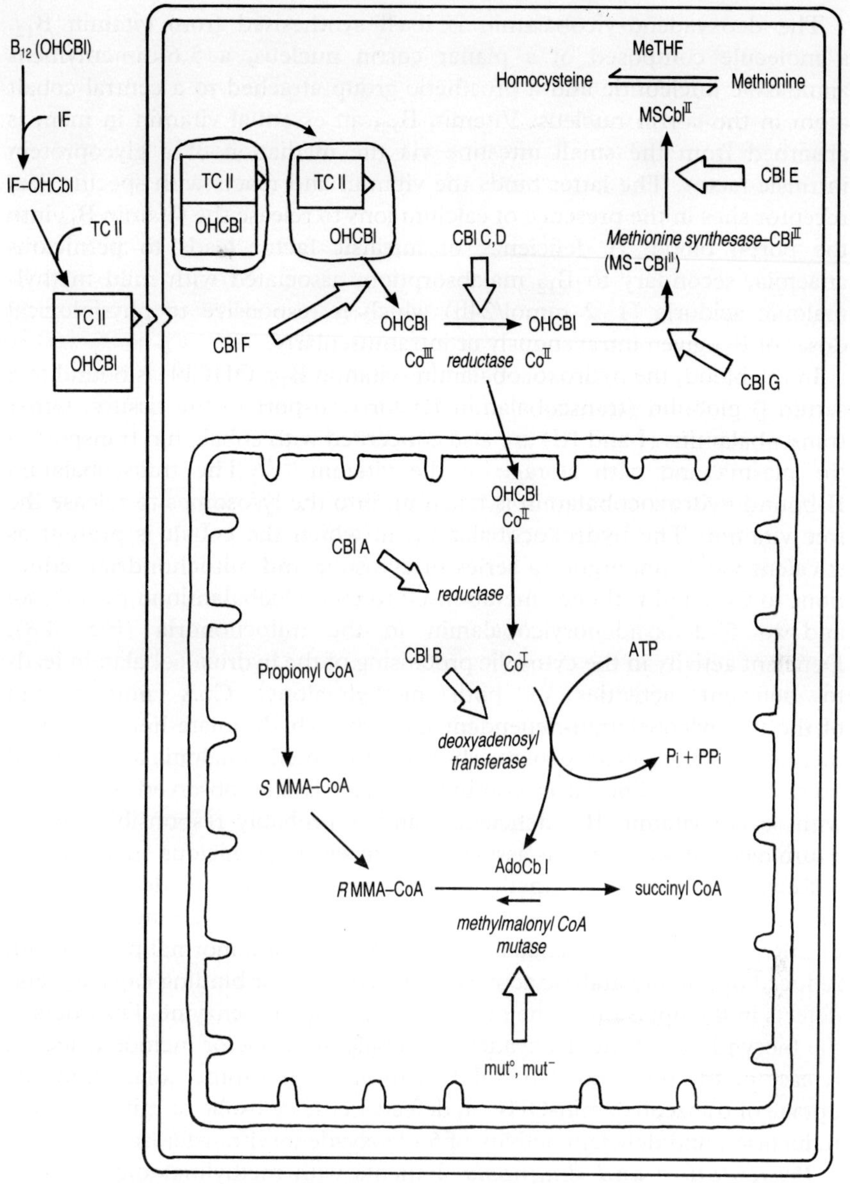

Fig. 4.8 Schematic representation of the absorption, transport and cellular metabolism of hydroxocobalamin (vitamin B_{12}, OHCbl) and metabolism of propionyl CoA, methylmalonyl CoA (MMA-CoA), and the methylmalonic acidurias. Defects in the mutase (mut°, mut⁻), deoxyadenosyltransferase (Cbl B) and mitochondrial CobIIalamin reductase (Cbl A) all lead to methylmalonic aciduria with subgroups designated by the complementation groups given. Defects in the lysosomal release of hydroxocobalamin (Cbl F) and in the cytosolic processing of hydroxocobalamin (Cbl C and Cbl D) lead to combined methylmalonic aciduria and homocystinuria. (Defects in the synthesis and attachment of methylcobalamin, causing isolated homocystinuria are designated Cbl E and Cbl G see e.g. reference 39.) TC II–transcobalmin II, IF–intrinsic factor, AdoCbl–deoxyadenosylcobalmin, MeTHF–methyltetrahydrofolate. (See text for further detail.)

The deoxyadenosylcobalamin is itself synthesised from vitamin B_{12}, a molecule composed of a planar corrin nucleus, a 5,6-dimethylbenzimidazole nucleotide and a prosthetic group attached to a central cobalt atom in the corrin nucleus. Vitamin B_{12}, an essential vitamin in man, is absorbed from the small intestine via the mediation of a glycoprotein intrinsic factor. The latter binds the vitamin and reacts with specific ileal receptor sites in the presence of calcium ions to release the vitamin B_{12} into the portal blood. A deficiency of intrinsic factor leads to pernicious anaemia, secondary to B_{12} malabsorption, associated with mild methylmalonic aciduria (1–2 mmol/24h) which is responsive to physiological doses of B_{12} given intravenously or intramuscularly.

In the blood, the hydroxocobalamin (vitamin B_{12}, OHCbl) is bound to a serum β globulin (transcobalamin II) for transport to the tissues. Other transcobalamins (I and III) are also concerned with cobalamin transport in the plasma and with storage of the vitamin.[34,35] The transcobalamin II-bound hydroxocobalamin is taken up into the lysosomes to release the free vitamin. The hydroxocobalamin, in which the cobalt is present as trivalent Co^{III}, undergoes a series of cytosolic and mitochondrial reductions to Co^{I}, and is thence metabolised to methylcobalamin in the cytosol and to 5'-deoxyadenosylcobalamin in the mitochondria (Fig. 4.8). Deficient activity in the cytosolic processing of the hydroxocobalamin leads to deficient activities of both methylmalonyl CoA mutase and of the methylcobalamin-dependent methyltetrahydrofolate-homocysteine: methyltransferase, with patients showing both methylmalonic aciduria and homocystinuria. The latter combined defect is also observed in patients with severe vitamin B_{12} deficiency, and is probably responsible for the neurological manifestations associated with severe pernicious anaemia.

Recognised causes of methylmalonic aciduria include defects in the biosynthesis of methylmalonyl CoA mutase itself, with varying expression of mRNA leading to absence of enzyme protein, or abnormal protein with reduced or absent catalytic activity; reduced cofactor binding capacity, and defects in the uptake into the mitochondria of the proenzyme. Disorders in the biosynthesis of the deoxyadenosylcobalamin cofactor include defective release of the precursor Co^{III}OHCbl from the lysosome, after endocytic uptake of transcobalamin-OHCbl; defects in the cytosolic or mitochondrial reductases, and deficient activity of 5'-deoxyadenosyltransferase.

Presentation and diagnosis. Patients with methylmalonic acidurias generally present with an acute illness within the first month of life, with low blood pH, failure to thrive, hypotonia, ketoacidosis and frequently with hyperglycinaemia, hyperuricaemia, hypoglycaemia and hyperammonaemia. There is often associated vomiting, dehydration, and lethargy, leading to coma and death if untreated. Neutropenia, thrombocytopenia and recurrent acute episodes associated with minor infections are common. Acute extrapyramidal disease with bilateral destruction of the globi pallidi has been reported in several patients after acute metabolic decompensation, and this must contribute to continuing neurological dysfunction.

The patients show a greatly increased urinary excretion of methylmalonic acid accompanied by increased excretion of methylcitric acids, 3-hydroxypropionic acid and other metabolites of propionyl CoA. Methylmalonate concentrations in urine may be very great, being around 10–30 mol/mol creatinine or 2–50 mmol/24 h, and increased concentrations are also observed in blood plasma (0.2–3.0 mmol/l) and in cerebrospinal fluid. Propionic acid may also accumulate in blood plasma, particularly during acute episodes. A number of reported cases were responsive to pharmacological doses of B_{12} (usually given as cyanocobalamin or hydroxocobalamin, 1 mg/24 h intramuscularly) with concomitant major reduction of methylmalonate concentrations and of propionyl metabolites. Withdrawal of therapy restored the metabolite concentrations to pretreatment levels, this being the true evaluation of vitamin responsiveness in this and other metabolic disorders, although difficult to achieve with vitamin B_{12} because of the storage of this vitamin.

Patients with combined methylmalonic aciduria and homocystinuria show lower concentrations of methylmalonate in blood and urine, and propionyl metabolites are present at generally low levels, if at all. However, these patients are severely affected clinically, with moderate to severe mental retardation associated with lethargy, seizures, megaloblastic anaemia and cerebellar dysfunction, but without ketosis. Some patients show a later onset with intellectual deterioration, lethargy and dementia but without anaemia although the bone marrow shows megaloblastic changes. Abnormalities of the brain are seen postmortem, similar to those in the subacute combined degeneration of pernicious anaemia. Accumulation of abnormal brain lipids containing odd-carbon number and methyl-branched fatty acids have also been reported. These patients do not appear to respond to vitamin B_{12} (cyanocobalamin) therapy although in vitro responsiveness to methylcobalamin suggests the need for more specific cofactor therapy.

Patients with combined methylmalonic aciduria show greatly increased concentration ratios of acylcarnitine to free carnitine in urine and blood. Here the predominant acylcarnitine is propionylcarnitine, providing direct evidence for the accumulation of propionyl CoA and for secondary carnitine insufficiency in this disorder. The implications of these observations regarding therapeutic manoeuvres are discussed further below.

It is obviously of importance to exclude vitamin B_{12} deficiency in the diagnosis of methylmalonic aciduria: mild asymptomatic methylmalonic aciduria may be observed during neonatal screening programmes. Transient neonatal acidosis associated with methylmalonic aciduria and B_{12} deficiency has also been recorded, and severe megaloblastic anaemia with combined methylmalonic aciduria and homocystinuria has been reported in the breast-fed infant of a strictly vegetarian mother. Rapid responses to single dose B_{12} therapy are recorded in these cases, with complete abolition of the metabolic abnormalities and no recurrence, given adequate dietary intake.

Treatment and prognosis. The treatment of patients with methylmalonic acidurias is similar to that of patients with propionic acidaemia, with reduced dietary protein intake of isoleucine, valine, threonine and methionine, and supplementation with other essential amino acids, including leucine and alanine.

Some patients respond well to vitamin B_{12} treatment (1 mg/24 h i.m. initially, with 10 mg/24 h orally being suitable for maintenance therapy in many patients). This should always be initiated early on in the evaluation of the patient with methylmalonic aciduria. True responsiveness should ideally be established, either by temporary withdrawal of the vitamin (for several weeks if necessary) or by L-leucine loading tests. Some cases have been reported to be unresponsive to cyanocobalamin, and hydroxocobalamin may be preferred for treatment as the natural form of the vitamin. It appears that 5'-deoxyadenosylcobalamin offers no advantages for therapy and evidence suggests that this form of the cofactor is hydrolysed back to hydroxycobalamin on administration.[36] True vitamin-responsive patients generally require only minimal dietary restriction.

In unresponsive cases increased carbohydrate is important, with frequent feeding and use of nasogastric feeding as necessary, to overcome the severe anorexia associated with these forms of methylmalonic aciduria. Regular monitoring and rapid response to acute episodes is essential but failure to thrive and to grow are continuing problems in methylmalonic aciduria, with developmental retardation being a consistent feature of the disorder. Osteoporosis may occur and hyperuricaemia with impairment of renal function is often evident and requires appropriate treatment. Chronic and progressive renal failure associated with renal tubular dysfunction develops in cobalamin-unresponsive patients, despite treatment.[37,38] This appears unique to methylmalonic aciduria and thus is probably caused by accumulation of methylmalonyl CoA or its metabolites.

Patients show favourable biochemical and clinical responses to administration of L-carnitine, both under basal metabolic conditions and during severe acute metabolic decompensation, when reduced organic acid excretion is associated with increased propionylcarnitine excretion. L-Carnitine has a proven place in the treatment of these patients.

Propionate produced by colonic bacteria also forms an important precursor to methylmalonate and other metabolites in this disorder, and the use of antibiotic therapy[8,9], particularly alternate metronidazole and amoxycillin (Bain et al, unpublished), has proved very effective in greatly reducing the abnormal organic aciduria and improving clinical progress and prognosis. The possible beneficial effects of significant lowering of the renal load of methylmalonate on renal function remains to be evaluated.

The prognosis of patients with methylmalonic acidurias is variable but is improving as developments in therapy, for example L-carnitine and antibiotics occur. However, the continuing difficulty of long-term management of patients with vitamin-unresponsive methylmalonic acidurias and the severity of acute episodes, with associated neurological damage and developmental retardation, make a poor prognosis for many patients. The prognosis of the true B_{12}-responsive patient is good and such patients generally show normal growth and development under minimal dietary restriction. Treatment appears necessary for life however, with clinical deterioration associated with withdrawal of vitamin B_{12} therapy.

Genetics, enzymology and prenatal diagnosis. Seven classes of methylmalonic aciduria have been defined on the basis of fibroblast enzyme and complementation studies. About one-half to three-quarters of all patients with methylmalonic aciduria have mutase apoenzyme defects (McKusick 251000), subdivided into mut°, that show no increase in enzyme activity when cells are cultured in the presence of saturating concentrations of cofactor, and mut^{-} in which a structurally altered apoenzyme apparently exists with reduced cofactor affinity. Mut° patients show variable expression of mRNA, associated with no detectable enzyme protein (CRM –ve), unstable protein (CRM +ve, 3–40% of normal) and defective import of proenzyme into mitochondria. Mut^{-} patients show between 20 and 100% of cross-reacting material in cultured cells.

The remainder of the patients have cobalamin cofactor uptake, release or synthetic defects, classified on the basis of complementation and enzymological studies into Cbl A, B, C, D and F groups: Cbl A variants (McKusick 251100) have defects in the mitochondrial cobalamin reductase (Fig. 4.8); Cbl B variants (McKusick 251110) have deoxyadenosyltransferase deficiency; Cbl C (McKusick 277400) and Cbl D (McKusick 277410) have defects in the cytosolic processing and reduction of hydroxocobalamin and are associated with combined methylmalonic aciduria and homocystinuria, and Cbl F variants have a defect in the lysosomal release of hydroxocobalamin after uptake into the cells,[1,34,35,39] (Table 4.4). Other cobalamin cofactor synthetic defects (Cbl E and Cbl G; McKusick 236270 and 250940 respectively) affect only the production or utilisation of methylcobalamin, associated with isolated homocystinuria and not with methylmalonic aciduria.[35,40]

Each variant of methylmalonic aciduria appears to be inherited in an autosomal recessive mode with an overall incidence of around 1 in 50 000 live births and occurrence in most ethnic groups. The enzyme defects are expressed in cultured skin fibroblasts and amniocytes and are relatively simple to detect by measurement of [1-^{14}C] propionate incorporation into protein (acid-insoluble material) in cultured fibroblasts in subconfluent culture. However direct measurement of methylmalonyl CoA mutase with and without added cofactor is necessary for more detailed study and classification of patients.[36]

Prenatal diagnosis is usually carried out using the propionate-incorpora-

Table 4.4 Methylmalonic aciduria complementation groups. 'Cells' refers to cultured skin fibroblasts; +, normal; -, markedly deficient or undetectable; ±, partially deficient; total, enzyme activity in presence of saturating cofactor concentrations; holo, without added cofactor

	Cobalamin disorders				Apomutase disorders	
	Cbl A	Cbl B	Cbl C/D	Cbl F	Mut°	Mut⁻
Enzyme activities in cell extracts						
Holomutase	—	—	—	—	—	—
Total mutase	+	+	+	+	—	±
Holomethyltransferase	+	+	—	—	+	+
Total methyltransferase	+	+	±	±	+	+
Adenosyltransferase	+	—	+	+	+	+
Cobalamin metabolism in intact cells						
AdoCbl synthesis	—	—	—	—	+	+
MeCbl synthesis	+	+	—	—	+	+
Substrate fixation in intact cells						
[1-^{14}C] propionate	—	—	—	—	—	—
[^{14}C-Me] methyltetrahydrofolate	+	+	—	—	+	+

tion assay since relatively few cells are required and it is rapid to perform. Prenatal diagnosis is also performed by direct measurement of methylmalonate and methylcitrates in amniotic fluid supernatant by quantitative selected ion monitoring, with use of chemically-related internal standards, for example methylsuccinate and homocitrate respectively, or using stable isotope dilution analysis. This approach has recently been applied successfully to first trimester prenatal diagnosis. First trimester diagnosis is also possible using either propionate incorporation assays or direct mutase assays on chorionic villi.

Multicarboxylase deficiencies (McKusick 253260 & 253270)

Introduction

As stated earlier, the three mitochondrial carboxylase enzymes, 3-methylcrotonyl CoA carboxylase, propionyl CoA carboxylase and pyruvate carboxylase, and the cytosolic acetyl CoA carboxylase are all dependent upon D-biotin for their activity; D-biotin being attached to the apoenzymes to form the active holoenzymes by the action of a fifth enzyme, holocarboxylase synthetase.[1,41] A deficiency of the latter enzyme in the mitochondria results in deficient activity of all four carboxylases, with clinical symptoms and biochemical findings associated with the deficiencies of the individual enzymes.[42]

Following the turnover and degradation of the holocarboxylases, the biotin-containing residue biocytin, composed simply of biotin attached to the ε-lysyl residue of the enzyme, is degraded further to release free

D-biotin for reutilisation, through the action of a further enzyme biotinidase (Fig. 4.9). D-Biotin is also made available from intestinal bacteria as an important source in man, but this is also presented in the form of biocytin or other biotinyl peptides, as is that from many dietary sources. Thus although free D-biotin is also available from the diet, a lack of biotinidase results in a deficiency of D-biotin with the activities of both the mitochondrial and cytosolic carboxylases being affected and consequent severe clinical and biochemical manifestations. Similar features are also observed in patients with severe dietary biotin deficiency and the multicarboxylase deficiencies, both inherited and acquired, are important metabolic disorders of children.

Since they are readily treatable with oral D-biotin but may be fatal or associated with marked neurological sequelae if left untreated, their early diagnosis is most important. Holocarboxylase synthetase-deficient patients present early and acutely with severe acidosis whereas biotinidase-deficient patients present later in infancy with neurological, skin and other abnormalities. The long-term prognosis may be different between the two disorders and differential diagnosis remains important. A further complication is

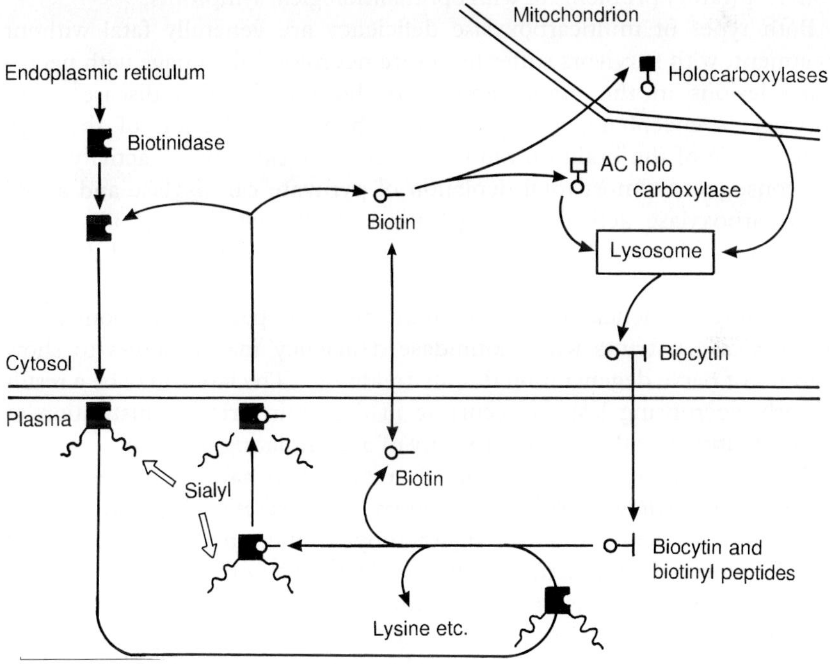

Fig. 4.9 Mitochondrial and cytosolic carboxylases and the recycling and metabolism of biotin via biotinidase. Biotinidase is sialylated on leaving the cell and functions to cleave biocytin and other biotinyl peptides and transport biotin into the cell. The mitochondrial holocarboxylases are propionyl CoA carboxylase, 3-methylcrotonyl CoA carboxylase and pyruvate carboxylase. AC represents cytosolic acetyl CoA carboxylase.

introduced by the relatively minor abnormal or absent organic aciduria in some patients with biotinidase deficiency and careful clinical and biochemical evaluation is essential.

Presentation and diagnosis

The majority of patients with holocarboxylase synthetase deficiency (*early-onset multicarboxylase deficiency,* McKusick 253270) present in the neonatal period with vomiting, ketoacidosis, hyperammonaemia, lactic acidosis, convulsions and profound hypotonia, leading to coma and death in most cases if untreated. Patients presenting later also show features associated with dietary biotin deficiency, including alopecia and an erythematomous rash similar to those seen in patients with biotinidase deficiency. Infants with biotinidase deficiency (*late-onset or juvenile multicarboxylase deficiency, McKusick 253260*) show these features, again associated with hypotonia, metabolic acidosis and with seizures, breathing difficulties, developmental delay, ataxia, kerato-conjunctivitis, optic nerve atrophy and severe deafness. Not all of these symptoms may be present however and patients are recorded who presented primarily with progressive neurological deterioration, respiratory problems or with ophthalmological symptoms.

Both types of multicarboxylase deficiency are generally fatal without treatment, with survivors suffering severe neurological damage with necrotising lesions in the brain, similar to those in Leigh's disease[43] and Wernicke's encephalopathy. This is probably a reflection of the high dependence of the brain on biotin recycling for carboxylase activity, with the consequent almost total depletion of pyruvate carboxylase and acetyl CoA carboxylase activities being critical in the aetiology of the severe neurological damage.[44] However, both types of patient respond dramatically to treatment with D-biotin (10 mg/24 h, orally). Some holocarboxylase synthetase-deficient patients may be only partially responsive to D-biotin and patients with biotinidase deficiency may progress to show features of nerve degeneration despite treatment. The latter may be a result of early necrotising lesions occurring in the brain prior to institution of biotin treatment rather than to toxicity of accumulating biocytin.

The first patient who was originally reported to have biotin-responsive 3-methylcrotonylglycinuria was shown to excrete, in addition to 3-hydroxy-isovalerate and 3-methylcrotonylglycine, increased amounts of 3-hydroxypropionate, methylcitrates and lactate[42,1], providing the basis for the subsequent demonstration of multicarboxylase deficiency caused by holocarboxylase synthetase deficiency.[45] All untreated patients with holocarboxylase synthetase deficiency have this characteristic overt organic aciduria (illustrated most clearly by Chalmers[2]) but patients with biotinidase deficiency may show only a moderate and intermittent abnormal organic aciduria with low but increased levels of some metabolites, for example lactate and 3-hydroxy-isovalerate, but very low levels of

Table 4.5 Typical ranges of urinary organic acids in multicarboxylase deficiencies (Expressed as mmol/mol creatinine)

Metabolite	Biotinidase deficiency	Holocarboxylase deficiency
3-Hydroxyisovalerate	220 –680	1500 –14000
3-Methylcrotonylglycine	11 – 79	226 –3600
3-Hydroxypropionate	nil –113	560 –6300
Methylcitrates	22 – 30	110 – 900

other characteristic metabolites such as methylcitrates and 3-methylcrotonylglycine (Table 4.5). Biotinidase-deficient patients have low levels of biotin in blood and urine and commonly excrete increased amounts of biocytin. Biotinidase deficiency is much more difficult to diagnose on the basis of the organic aciduria and careful, quantitative analytical methods are required. In some cases the diagnosis is dependent on demonstration of low or absent activity of biotinidase, and enzymology may become essential in the evaluation of patients with unexplained neurological deterioration. Treatment with D-biotin rapidly abolishes the abnormal organic aciduria in most patients with multicarboxylase deficiency, and hence diagnostic samples must be obtained prior to commencement of any vitamin therapy.

Biotinidase deficiency can be demonstrated in plasma, serum, leucocytes and cultured skin fibroblasts and is most simply determined using blood plasma. Carboxylase enzyme activities in cultured skin fibroblasts are reduced when the cells are cultured in biotin-deficient medium, but normal when biotin-containing media (i.e. with fetal calf serum) are used. This distinguishes biotinidase-deficient patients from those with holocarboxylase synthetase deficiency where marked deficiency of all three mitochondrial carboxylases occurs, responding in vitro only to supplemental biotin concentrations in excess of 1 µmol/l. Direct assay of holocarboxylase synthetase is more complex, requiring an apocarboxylase as substrate, and generally patients with a deficiency of this enzyme are diagnosed on the basis of their organic aciduria and multiple carboxylase deficiencies.

Treatment, genetics and prognosis

As stated above, treatment of both conditions is simple, with supplemental D-biotin, 10–50 mg/24 h orally. Response, both clinical and biochemical, is dramatic and rapid but regular maintenance therapy with D-biotin is required, since abnormal signs return within a few days of cessation of therapy. Pretreatment, plasma and urine biotin concentrations are normal in patients with holocarboxylase synthetase deficiency, but reduced in biotinidase-deficient patients. A minority of patients with severe holocarboxylase synthetase deficiency show only a moderate response to biotin and it could be expected that a total deficiency of this enzyme would be incompatible with life.

Prognosis for treated holocarboxylase synthetase-deficient patients is very good with the first reported patient being into his third decade, still on biotin therapy. Screening programmes for biotinidase deficiency (see below) have revealed patients with partial enzyme deficiencies. The majority of such patients have no clinical or biochemical abnormalities, but biotin therapy has been advocated for such patients to avoid possible neurological damage.[46]

Cultured fibroblasts from patients with holocarboxylase synthetase deficiency complement those from patients with propionic acidaemias and have been designated the *bio* complementation group. As would be expected, cells from this group also complement those from patients with biotinidase deficiency. However, little is known of the molecular basis for the disorders. Holocarboxylase synthetase deficiency is rare, several of the papers in the literature relating to studies on the same patients. However, newborn screening programmes have shown the incidence of profound biotinidase deficiency to be between 1:85 000 and 1:145 000 live-born infants and that of the partial deficiency to be around 1:130 000, with an overall frequency of about 1:60 000.[47] The frequency of heterozygotes has been estimated at 1 in 123.

Both conditions are inherited in an autosomal recessive mode. Prenatal diagnosis is possible for the severe forms of holocarboxylase synthetase deficiency by both enzymology on cultured amniocytes and chorionic villus tissue, and by direct analysis of amniotic fluid for 3-hydroxyisovalerate and methylcitrates. Prenatal diagnosis of biotinidase deficiency is possible both in the first and second trimesters by direct enzymology. Generally however, the ease of treatment and good prognosis of the majority of patients with these conditions make prenatal diagnosis unnecessary.

DISORDERS OF L-LYSINE (AND L-TRYPTOPHAN) METABOLISM

Introduction

In mammals L-lysine is primarily metabolised via saccharopine and thence to 2-aminoadipic acid (Fig. 4.10). 2-Aminoadipic acid is transaminated to 2-ketoadipic acid, which is also an intermediate in the catabolism of L-tryptophan and of hydroxylysine. 2-Oxoadipic acid or 2-ketoadipic acid is dehydrogenated (decarboxylated) via a reaction similar to pyruvate and 2-oxoglutarate dehydrogenation (see Fig. 4.3) to form glutaryl CoA. The glutaryl CoA formed is dehydrogenated in the mitochondria via an FAD-linked enzyme to glutaconyl CoA, followed by decarboxylation on the same enzyme protein to crotonyl CoA, and thence by β-oxidation to finally yield

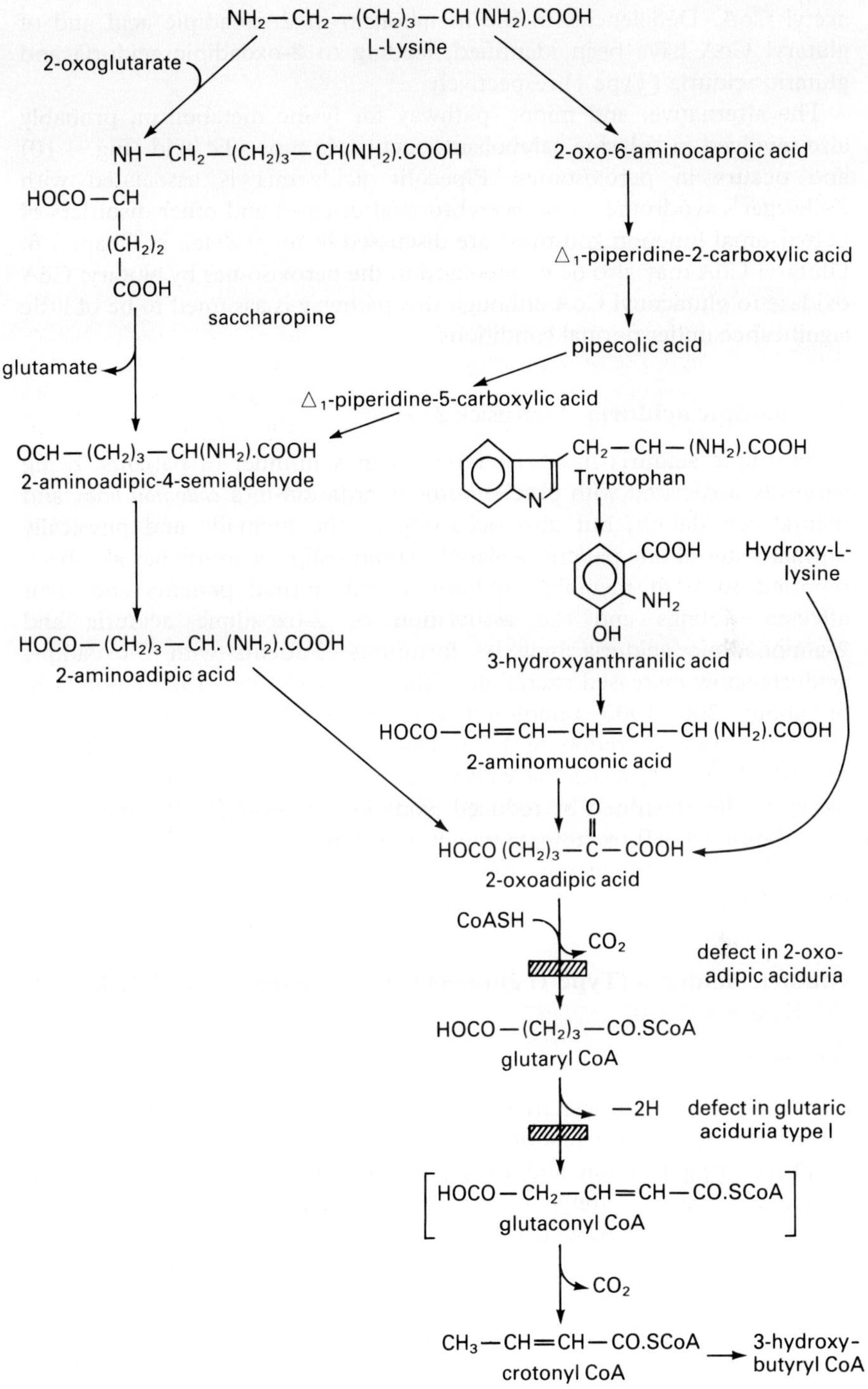

Fig. 4.10 Catabolism of L-lysine and L-tryptophan with positions of defects in 2-oxoadipic aciduria and glutaric aciduria Type 1.

acetyl CoA. Deficiencies in the metabolism of 2-oxoadipic acid and of glutaryl CoA have been identified, leading to 2-oxoadipic aciduria and glutaric aciduria (Type 1) respectively.

The alternative, and minor, pathway for lysine metabolism, probably also involved in D-lysine catabolism, occurs via pipecolic acid (Fig. 4.10) and occurs in peroxisomes. Pipecolic acidaemia is associated with Zellweger's syndrome (hepatocerebrorenal disease) and other disorders of peroxisomal function and these are discussed in more detail in Chapter 6. Glutaryl CoA may also be metabolised in the peroxisomes by glutaryl CoA oxidase to glutaconyl CoA although this pathway is assumed to be of little significance under normal conditions.

2-Oxoadipic aciduria (McKusick 245130)

2-Oxoadipic aciduria has been reported in a number of patients, being variously associated with psychomotor retardation in a *collodion baby* and mental retardation, but also occurring in the mentally and physically normal sister of one patient. Isolated 2-aminoadipic aciduria has also been reported in both mentally subnormal and normal patients and their affected siblings and the association of 2-oxoadipic aciduria and 2-aminoadipic aciduria may be fortuitous. Patients with 2-oxoadipic aciduria show increased excretion of the keto acid (500–1500 μmol/24 h, or about 200–1000 mmol/mol creatinine) and of 2-hydroxyadipic acid. Increased excretion of 1,2-butene dicarboxylic acid, glutaric acid and 3-hydroxybutyric acid have also been observed. The enzyme deficiency has been demonstrated by reduced oxidation of D,L-2-[1-^{14}C] aminoadipate and of 2-[^{14}C] oxoadipate in cultured skin fibroblasts. The disorder is probably inherited in an autosomal recessive mode, and prenatal diagnosis should be possible if required.

Glutaric aciduria (Type 1; glutaryl CoA dehydrogenase deficiency) (McKusick 231670)

Introduction

Following the dehydrogenation of 2-oxoadipic acid to form glutaryl CoA (Fig. 4.10), the latter is first dehydrogenated to form glutaconyl CoA in an FAD-requiring reaction and then decarboxylated on the same enzyme protein to give crotonyl CoA. The crotonyl CoA is hydrated to 3-hydroxybutyryl CoA, which is then metabolised to acetoacetyl CoA and thence to acetyl CoA. Deficient activity of the glutaryl CoA dehydrogenase enzyme that catalyses both stages of glutaryl CoA metabolism leads to glutaric aciduria. This disorder has been designated in the literature as glutaric aciduria 'Type 1' because glutaric aciduria also occurs in multiple acyl CoA dehydrogenase deficiency (MACDD; see below), formerly designated as 'glutaric aciduria Type 2'.

Presentation, diagnosis and biochemistry

Patients with glutaric aciduria are characterised by severe progressive neurological deterioration, generalised dystonic cerebral palsy and choreoathetosis. Macrocephaly is generally present. Convulsions and ketoacidotic episodes may occur with death resulting, associated with some similarities to Reye's syndrome. The patients appear to be of normal intelligence although this may be difficult to assess because of the severely dysarthric speech and severe impairment of motor function that leads to almost total helplessness. CT brain scans have shown localised frontotemporal atrophy associated in some cases with ventricular enlargement, white matter hypodensity and diffuse cortical atrophy.[48] Some patients have shown degeneration of the globi palladi (cf. methylmalonic aciduria above) and spongy degeneration of cortical white matter.[49] MRI scans have shown bilateral temporal lobe atrophy and hyperlucency of the caudate nucleus, and there is evidence for loss of γ-aminobutyric acid (GABA)-containing neurones and gliosis in the basal ganglia and substantia nigra. Macrocephaly, and abnormalities in CT and MRI scans, may precede onset of acute symptoms and provide an indicator for biochemical investigation.

The disorder is generally associated with greatly increased excretion of glutaric acid (to more than 20 000 mmol/mol creatinine) and of 3-hydroxyglutaric acid (to more than 500 mmol/mol creatinine) and increased concentrations of glutaconic acid have been observed during acute episodes. Glutarylglycine excretion may also be increased. Excretion of 2-oxoglutarate is always increased and there may be a moderate associated increase in 2-hydroxyglutaric acid excretion. Since only the latter is increased in MACDD ('glutaric aciduria Type 2') and 3-hydroxyglutarate is unique to glutaric aciduria Type 1 it is important to distinguish between the two hydroxyglutaric acids in the diagnosis of this condition. Glutarylcarnitine excretion is also increased and carnitine deficiency may develop. Some patients with similar clinical symptomatology have been reported to have minimal or absent abnormal organic aciduria and demonstrable glutaryl CoA dehydrogenase deficiency in cultured cells. However, the abnormal organic aciduria may be abolished when a low lysine diet is employed, and the clinical and dietary status of the reported cases is too unclear for adequate evaluation of these reports. Patients have also been reported with major organic aciduria but without clinical manifestations in the same sibships as clinically-affected individuals[48]: it is apparent that some major metabolic perturbation occurs as the precipitating factor in the production of severe brain lesions and overt clinical manifestations.

The disorder is caused by deficient activity of mitochondrial FAD-dependent glutaryl CoA dehydrogenase, specifically in the dehydrogenation rather than the decarboxylation reaction[50], with the abnormal metabolites occurring via alternative metabolism of the accumulating glutaryl CoA and glutarate. The enzyme defect has been demonstrated in cultured skin fibroblasts, leucocytes and other tissues, using assays based upon decarboxylation of [1,5-^{14}C] glutaryl CoA and [1,5-^{14}C] glutaric acid; tritium release from [2,3,4-^{3}H] glutaryl CoA; oxidation of [6-^{14}C] lysine, which is decarboxylated specifically at the glutaryl CoA dehydrogenase step, and by an ETF-based dehydrogenase assay with glutaryl CoA as substrate.

Treatment and prognosis

Treatment with a diet low in lysine and, in some cases in tryptophan, has been of value in reducing the excretion of glutaric acid and other metabolites. Similarly, treatment with riboflavin, the precursor to the FAD cofactor for the enzyme, will also reduce glutarate in some patients with residual enzyme activity.[51] In most cases dietary management is by low protein, low lysine diet, which essentially abolishes the abnormal organic aciduria. However, after presentation with severe neurological symptoms, little clinical benefit appears to result. Following suggestions that the neurological damage may be due to defective function of the basal ganglia, caused by inhibition of GABA synthesis by glutarate and its metabolites, some patients have been treated with the GABA analogue lioresil (Baclofen) (4-amino-4-(4-chlorophenyl)-butyric acid), with some improvement in clinical function.[51] More recently, use of γ-vinyl-GABA (vigabatrin), an irreversible inhibitor of GABA transaminase, has also been tried with better success.[52]

However, the disorder is extremely severe and possibly progressive following the initial neurological damage, and the prognosis is generally very poor except in early detected and treated cases and the rare patient with high residual enzyme activity who responds to high doses of riboflavin and dietary restriction. Biochemical riboflavin-responsiveness has also been reported in a single patient with peroxisomal glutaryl CoA oxidase deficiency who excreted moderately increased amounts of glutarate only (to around 500 mmol/mol creatinine). The significance of the metabolic block to the patient's symptoms, that were dissimilar to those in patients with glutaryl CoA dehydrogenase deficiency, was unclear.

Genetics and prenatal diagnosis

The disorder is inherited in an autosomal recessive mode and prenatal diagnosis is possible, both by direct enzymology and by measurement of glutarate in amniotic fluid. The enzyme activity is expressed in chorionic villi and first trimester diagnosis is also possible. cDNA clones encoding human glutaryl CoA dehydrogenase have been isolated and sequenced but identification of mutations causing glutaryl CoA dehydrogenase deficiency has not been reported.

DICARBOXYLIC ACIDURIAS AND NON-KETOTIC HYPOGLYCAEMIAS: DISORDERS OF FATTY ACID METABOLISM AND KETOGENESIS

Introduction

The β-oxidation of fatty acids has been a relatively neglected area of intermediary metabolism but the identification of inherited disorders of key enzymes in the pathway, initially in the acyl CoA dehydrogenases, has stimulated much interest in this area. The β-oxidation of fatty acids provides the major part of the energy requirements of liver and muscle, particularly during fasting and catabolism. The brain does not directly β-oxidise fatty acids but utilises the ketone bodies produced by other tissues.

In the β-oxidative process, long-chain fatty acids are taken up by the cell, activated by conversion into their corresponding acyl CoA esters, via the action of acyl CoA synthetases, and transported for β-oxidation into the mitochondria by an L-carnitine-mediated process involving two carnitine palmitoyltransferases (CPT) and a specific carnitine-acylcarnitine translocase[53] (Fig. 4.11). L-Carnitine facilitates the process by allowing transfer of the acyl moieties without loss of the high energy bond introduced on synthesis of the acyl CoA esters.

Once within the mitochondria and converted back to their acyl CoA esters, the long-chain fatty acids enter the β-oxidation spiral (Fig. 4.11). The acyl CoA esters are first dehydrogenated to *trans*-2-enoyl CoA esters, and these are hydrated to L-3-hydroxyacyl CoA esters that are then dehydrogenated to the corresponding 3-ketoacyl CoA esters. Finally the latter are cleaved to yield acetyl CoA and an acyl CoA ester that is chain-shortened by two carbons from the initial substrate. The whole process is repeated down to butyryl CoA (C_4) which is finally β-oxidised to yield acetoacetyl CoA. Odd-carbon number fatty acids are oxidised by the same process to finally yield propionyl CoA, which is then metabolised as described above.

Unsaturated (*cis*) fatty acids are also metabolised by β-oxidation until the unsaturated bond is reached: at this stage enoyl CoA isomerase and 2,4-dienoyl CoA reductase act to transfer the double bond to the 2 position and to reduce double bonds in the 2 position.[53]

In muscle tissues the acetyl CoA produced is oxidised to CO_2 via the tricarboxylic acid cycle. In liver it is primarily converted into ketone bodies via obligatory conversion into 3-hydroxy-3-methylglutaryl (HMG) CoA followed by cleavage of the HMG CoA by HMG CoA lyase to yield acetoacetate and acetyl CoA (Fig. 4.11).

Enzymes differing in their carbon chain length specificities occur at almost every stage in the β-oxidation pathway and many inherited disorders have been characterised since about 1983, particularly medium-chain acyl CoA dehydrogenase deficiency.

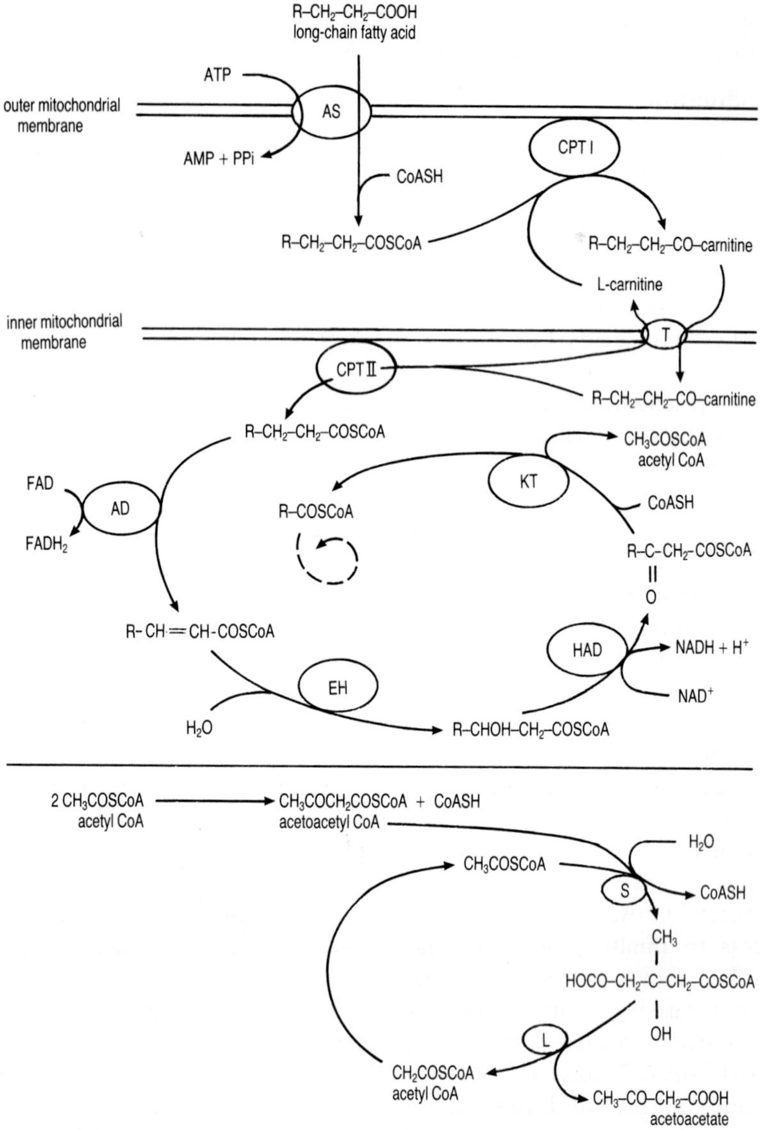

Fig. 4.11 Mitochondrial long-chain fatty acid β-oxidation and ketone body formation. Showing the activation of the fatty acid through the acyl CoA synthetase (AS), formation of acylcarnitine via carnitine palmitoyl transferase I (CPT I) for specific translocation (T) through the inner mitochondrial membrane and reconversion back to acyl CoA ester via carnitine palmitoyl transferase II (CPT II). The β-oxidative spiral includes the action of the acyl CoA dehydrogenases (AD), enoyl CoA hydratase (EH), 3-hydroxyacyl CoA dehydrogenases (HAD) and ketothiolases (KT). Acetyl CoA (and acetoacetyl CoA) is converted into ketone bodies (the so-called 'McGarry–Foster cycle') via the obligatory action of 3-hydroxy-3-methylglutaryl CoA synthetase (S) and 3-hydroxy-3-methylglutaryl CoA lyase (L). (See text for further details.)

Abnormalities in mitochondrial β-oxidation, particularly deficient activity of the fatty acyl CoA dehydrogenases, leads to accumulation of the intermediate acyl CoA esters and their metabolism elsewhere in the cell. Long-chain fatty acids accumulate and are ω-oxidised on the microsomes through the action of a cytochrome P_{450}-linked mixed function oxygenase to produce dicarboxylic acids; ω-1 oxidation occurs by a similar process to produce ω-1 hydroxymonocarboxylic acids. Defects in the β-oxidative pathway are thus generally associated with an abnormal dicarboxylic aciduria although this may be intermittent, depending upon the fatty acyl load presented to the mutant enzyme system. These disorders are commonly associated with profound hypoglycaemia and failure to adequately synthesise ketone bodies (non-ketotic hypoglycaemia). A similar clinical presentation is also associated with 3-hydroxy-3-methylglutaryl CoA lyase deficiency (3-hydroxy-3-methylglutaric aciduria) in the catabolic pathway of L-leucine, but the major functional and symptom-producing defect is in ketone body synthesis, and the disorder has been included in this section rather than under L-leucine metabolism.

Long-chain dicarboxylic acids produced on the microsomes are activated there to the corresponding diacyl-mono-CoA esters. These long-chain dicarboxyl moieties are chain-shortened in the peroxisomes, probably normally to C_{14}, and the chain-shortened dicarboxyl moieties are then transported, probably as their acylcarnitine esters, to the mitochondria for further β-oxidation. Thus, defects in the β-oxidation pathway at the medium-chain level also result in accumulation of medium-chain length dicarboxyl CoA esters and excretion of characteristic metabolites into the urine. Very long-chain fatty acids ($>C_{22}$) are also metabolised initially in peroxisomes via the action of acyl CoA oxidases, and defects in this processing prior to further β-oxidation in the mitochondria, or lack of other peroxisomal functions, may result in a mild dicarboxylic aciduria. Peroxisomal disorders are described more generally and specifically in Chapter 6, although selected disorders associated with abnormal organic aciduria are included where appropriate in this chapter.

Disorders of mitochondrial acyl CoA dehydrogenases

Glutaryl CoA dehydrogenase, described briefly above, is one of at least six mitochondrial FAD-dependent acyl CoA dehydrogenases. These include those involved in β-oxidation of fatty acyl CoA esters and those involved in branched-chain amino acid metabolism, also discussed earlier (isovaleryl CoA dehydrogenase and 2-methylbutyryl CoA dehydrogenase). Other FAD-dependent mitochondrial dehydrogenases include sarcosine dehydrogenase and dimethylglycine dehydrogenase, both specifically associated with the metabolism of choline and betaine. The FAD cofactor associated with the dehydrogenases is reduced and passes its electrons to a common electron transfer flavoprotein (ETF), which in turn passes them to coenzyme Q in the electron transport chain via the action of ETF dehydrogenase (Fig. 4.12). A defect in either ETF or ETF dehydrogenase will affect simultaneously all associated dehydrogenase systems to produce a multiple (acyl CoA) dehydrogenase deficiency (MACDD) in which other ETF-dependent dehydrogenases are also affected.

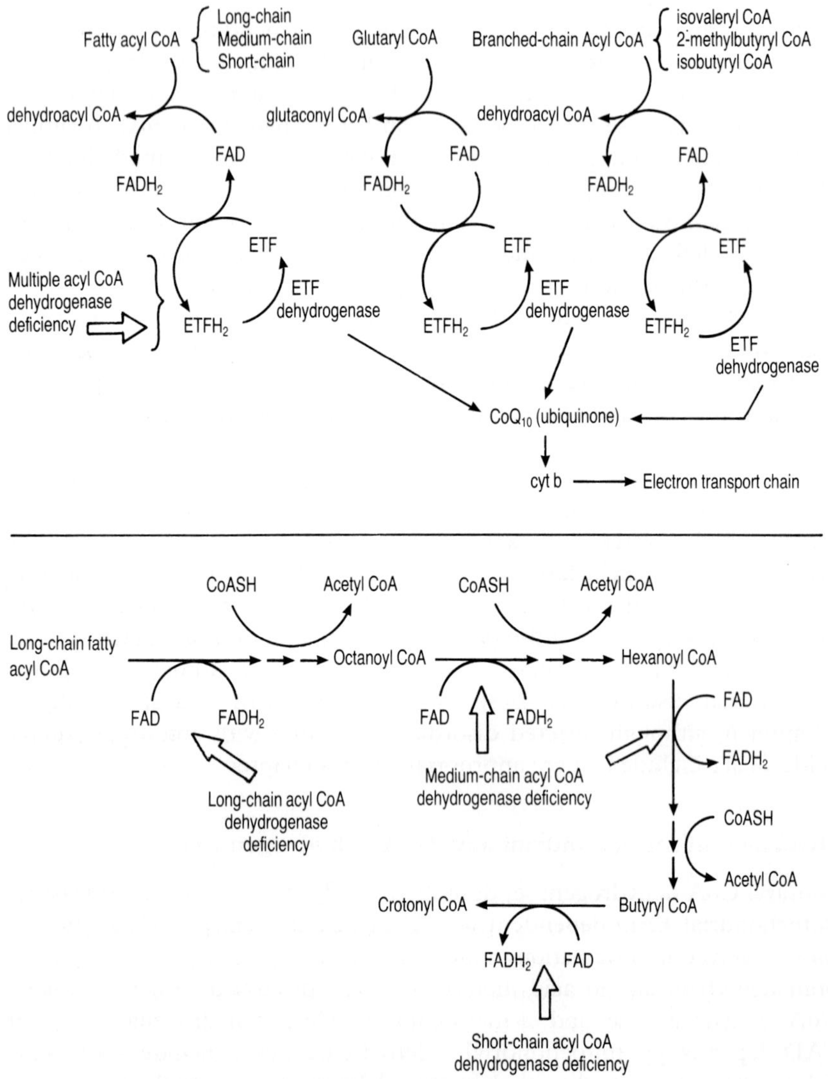

Fig. 4.12 Mitochondrial FAD and ETF-dependent acyl CoA dehydrogenases and disorders of fatty acid β-oxidation. Deficiency of ETF (electron-transfer flavoprotein) or of ETF dehydrogenase will result in deficiencies of all dependent dehydrogenases including sarcosine, dimethylglycine and 2-hydroxyglutarate dehydrogenases (not shown here).

Accumulating acyl CoA esters in patients with these dehydrogenase deficiencies are also converted into their corresponding acylcarnitine esters both for transport out of the mitochondria and within the cell, and as a detoxification process for subsequent excretion into the urine. Systemic carnitine deficiency caused by a specific inherited transport defect in muscle and kidney (and fibroblasts) but not liver also occurs, associated with hypoglycaemia, progressive hypertrophic cardiomyopathy and skeletal muscle weakness[54] (and see McKusick 212140): no abnormalities of organic acid metabolism are evident in such patients and the disorder is not considered further here.

Medium-chain acyl CoA dehydrogenase (MCAD) deficiency (McKusick 201450)

Presentation. Patients with medium-chain acyl CoA dehydrogenase (MCAD) deficiency may present acutely with acidosis, hyperammonaemia, profound non-ketotic hypoglycaemia, encephalopathy, hepatomegaly and pathologically with severe microvesicular fatty infiltration of the liver. Features may thus closely resemble those of Reye's syndrome and differential diagnosis is most important. The age of initial presentation varies widely, with some patients presenting acutely in early infancy with all the features described above, while others present in later childhood or even as adults, primarily with hypoglycaemic episodes or muscular weakness, although the clinical history often reveals milder episodes preceding the more acute presentation. The disorder is probably the underlying cause of some cases of Reye's syndrome and has been implicated as underlying some cases of sudden infant death syndrome (SIDS). However, recent prospective studies of SIDS have shown no cases of MCAD deficiency (or of other disorders of organic acid metabolism)[55], and it may be concluded that while patients with such disorders may die suddenly in infancy, these disorders very rarely present as true cases of sudden infant death syndrome.

Biochemistry. Patients excrete large amounts of dicarboxylic acids (C_6 $-C_{10}$) and unsaturated dicarboxylic acids during acute episodes, in which suberic acid (C_8) and its conjugates predominate. Suberylglycine (derived from the block in medium-chain dicarboxylic acid β-oxidation) is excreted as a most characteristic and diagnostic metabolite. Other metabolites include (ω-1)-oxidised fatty acids, particularly 5-hydroxyhexanoic acid and 7-hydroxyoctanoic acid, octanoylglucuronide and dicarboxylate glucuronide species, hexanoylglycine and phenylpropionylglycine[11,56]. Phenylpropionate is derived from gut bacterial metabolism of phenylalanine and normally β-oxidised to benzoate through the mitochondrial fatty acid β-oxidation pathway: MCAD deficiency leads to accumulation of this intermediate and conjugation with glycine to yield the latter characteristic metabolite.

However, suberylglycine is the most characteristic and consistent acylglycine excreted, the levels observed always greatly exceeding those of other acylglycines. C_8–C_{10} fatty acids also accumulate in blood plasma and *cis*-dec-4-enoic acid has been shown to be particularly characteristic of the disorder.[57] This arises from the metabolism of unsaturated fatty acids, for example linoleic acid, which is metabolised by β-oxidation and the action of enoyl CoA isomerase to 4-*cis*-decenoyl CoA: this is normally dehydrogenated to 2-*trans*, 4-*cis*-decadienoyl CoA by MCAD[52] but this does not occur in MCAD deficiency.

The enzyme deficiency leads to accumulation of medium-chain acyl CoA esters which are then converted into their corresponding acylcarnitine esters. These accumulate in the blood and are excreted into the urine: the disorder is thus characterised also by increased excretion of esterified carnitine into the urine, primarily as octanoylcarnitine with smaller amounts of hexanoylcarnitine, and free carnitine concentrations may be low. Octenoylcarnitine and decenoylcarnitine are also excreted into the urine, indicating the specificity of MCAD for acyl CoA esters of chain lengths C_6–unsaturated C_{10}.

Experience has shown that patients originally described in the literature with suberylglycinuria, dicarboxylic aciduria, and systemic carnitine deficiency with non-ketotic responses to fasting, all probably had MCAD deficiency, although more recently specific systemic carnitine deficiency has been described, caused by a defect in the membrane transport of L-carnitine. Although described as a non-ketotic disorder, some patients, with higher residual MCAD activity, do show a moderate but inadequate ketonuria in conjunction with the dicarboxylic aciduria, and the ketogenic response to fat intake may be increased by administration of riboflavin.

Diagnosis. This may not be easy since patients generally show no dicarboxylic aciduria when clinically well and careful assessment of patients with recurrent hypoglycaemia and suspected MCAD deficiency is essential. Asymptomatic patients usually excrete detectable amounts of octanoylcarnitine (increased on L-carnitine administration, 100 mg/kg) and suberylglycine, and careful analysis can usually differentiate the patient with MCAD deficiency. Prolonged fasting and particularly the use of medium-chain triglyceride loading must be strictly avoided since this can precipitate acute and lethal attacks. Instead, loading with phenylpropionic acid (20mg/kg) or with moderate amounts of long-chain fats (equivalent to less than the normal daily fat intake *for the individual patient*) or 1–1.5 g/kg, with analysis of urine for phenylpropionylglycine or dicarboxylic acids, suberylglycine and octanoylcarnitine should be employed. These tests represent more physiological assessments of the ability of the patient to metabolise fatty acids. Medium-chain triglycerides (MCT) and MCT-containing infant formulas may in themselves provoke a dicarboxylic aciduria, even in normal subjects: sebacic (C_{10}) acid predominates in the dicarboxylic aciduria and although octanoylcarnitine concentrations may increase, these are very low and no excretion of significant concentrations of suberylglycine occurs. While plasma medium-chain fatty acids also increase on MCT administration, the plasma concentrations of dec-4-enoic acid do not increase, indicating the particular diagnostic value of this metabolite.

Accumulating evidence suggests that MCAD is relatively common (see below) with more than 100 known cases, although many cases probably remain undiagnosed. There is a spectrum of clinical presentations dependent upon the level of residual fatty acid oxidising ability and individual genotypic variations.

Acute management of patients with MCAD deficiency is directed towards rapid correction of the profound and potentially lethal hypoglycaemia; L-carnitine may also be of value in acute episodes by promoting excretion of accumulating medium-chain acyl moieties as acylcarnitines. Therapy with L-carnitine is however probably contraindicated for maintenance because under more basal conditions it will promote long-chain fatty acid uptake into mitochondria and thereby possibly exacerbate accumulation of medium-chain intermediates with adverse clinical consequences. Regular maintenance is relatively simple with avoidance of fasting, particularly when extended periods of exercise are possible, and use of a diet with moderate restriction of fat intake (often naturally assumed by patients with MCAD deficiency) and increased carbohydrate with, particularly, a carbohydrate-containing drink or snack before bedtime. In some instances, the use of corn starch may be of value as a bedtime drink.

Since acute episodes may be induced by mild infections and after immunisations, care must be taken during such events to monitor the patient and maintain blood glucose levels. Similar caveats apply during any prolonged surgical procedure and with appropriate measures, no adverse effects have been noted. Prognosis of the correctly diagnosed and treated patient appears excellent and prenatal diagnosis, although possible, should be unnecessary.

Enzymology and genetics. The enzyme deficiency is expressed in cultured skin fibroblasts and other tissues and is demonstrable by measurement of [1-^{14}C] octanoate oxidation in intact fibroblasts, preferably growing in monolayer for good assay reproducibility, in comparison (as a ratio) to normal oxidation of butyrate (C_4) and oleate (C_{18}) or palmitate (C_{16}). Most patients show varying levels of residual oxidative capacity in cultured fibroblasts, from 15–45% of normal activities. However, direct measurement of enzyme activity in disrupted cells using assays based upon ETF as natural cofactor show very low activities, and it is clear that residual oxidative capacity and survival of the patients is dependent upon overlapping enzyme specificities and, more importantly, on the availability of alternative pathways for medium-chain fatty acid oxidation, for example in the peroxisomes, under the abnormal circumstances pertaining in these patients.

Medium-chain acyl CoA dehydrogenase is a homotetramer, with a subunit molecular mass of approximately 44 kDa. Each subunit contains one molecule of FAD. The monomeric subunits are nuclear-encoded and translated from mRNA to a precursor protein with an arginine-rich leader sequence of about 4 kDa to direct uptake into the mitochondria. Cultured skin fibroblasts from several patients with MCAD deficiency have been shown to synthesise normal amounts of subunit protein of normal molecular size, suggesting the majority of patients had a point mutation affecting catalytic activity.[56,58]

The cDNA encoding human MCAD has been cloned and the gene assigned to the short arm of chromosome 1. The mRNA has been sequenced, and studies in a number of laboratories, using both the PCR reaction with NcoI restriction endonuclease and site-specific oligonucleotide hybridization, have shown that the molecular defect in more than 88% of MCAD patients is a common point mutation at position 985 relative to the adenine at the start codon, in exon 11 of the gene. This results in an A to G conversion causing a lysine to glutamate conversion at position 304 in the mature enzyme.[59–61] This finding is unusual in a metabolic condition, in comparison for example with the extensive molecular heterogeneity found in isovaleric acidaemia and methylmalonic aciduria, and suggests a founder effect.

Other rare molecular defects have been identified and are summarised in Table 4.6.[62]

Genotypically, more than 80% of patients are homozygous for the $A \rightarrow G_{985}$, with the remainder being compound heterozygotes for this mutation and one of the rarer mutations (Table 4.6) and fewer than 3% being compound heterozygotes for these rare mutations only.

The lysine at position 304 in the mature enzyme is not involved in

Table 4.6 Molecular defects and genotypes in medium-chain acyl CoA dehydrogenase deficiency (based on data from Coates & Tanaka[62])

Molecular defects (n = 344)		
$A \xrightarrow{985} G$	306	(88.9%)
13 bp tandem repeat insertion +999	3	
4 bp deletion 1100–1103 (AGTT)	2	
$G \xrightarrow{799} A$	2	
$C \xrightarrow{157} T$	1	
$G \xrightarrow{447} A$	1	
$T \xrightarrow{730} C$	1	
$T \xrightarrow{1124} C$	1	
Unidentified	27	(7.8%)
Genotypes (n = 172)		
$A \xrightarrow{985} G$	138	(80.2%)
G/non G	30	
non G/ non G	4	

substrate or cofactor binding, occurring in the H-helix of the monomer structure, the alteration from the basic lysine to the acidic glutamate appearing to affect the assembly of the mature tetrameric structure.[62] This has been confirmed by studies on the incorporation of mutant enzyme into isolated mitochondria, when little detectable uptake occurs, consistent with such a defect in the quaternary structure of the enzyme.

Also of interest is the finding of numerous mRNA splicing defects in this condition: a common polymorphism in the normal sequence appears to increase splicing defects in the normal enzyme but this, in combination with the common point mutation in MCAD-deficient patients, increases the incidence of splicing defects.[60] Thus the point mutation appears also to affect the tertiary structure of the pre-mRNA resulting in the defects observed.

MCAD deficiency has a high frequency in, and appears exclusive to, caucasian populations of Anglo-Saxon origin, supporting the concept of a founder effect, with estimated frequencies being between 1:6500 to 1:20 000 in these populations. Preliminary newborn screening using both PCR/NcoI, oligonucleotide hybridization and FAB-MS of dried blood spots collected for PKU screening have revealed carrier frequencies of 1:40 to 1:100 in these populations.[62] Based on similar studies, the frequency of the condition in Japan, Finland and Italy appears to be negligible.

Screening applied to samples from SIDS babies (see above), in three independent studies in Anglo-Saxon populations, have shown the frequency of the $A \rightarrow G_{985}$ mutation to be less than the background in the populations concerned, confirming that MCAD deficiency does not contribute to the incidence of SIDS.

Long-chain acyl CoA dehydrogenase (LCAD) deficiency (McKusick 201460)

Some 14 patients with proven long-chain acyl CoA dehydrogenase (LCAD) deficiency have been described.[62] Typical features include early presentation in the first few months of life with hypoglycaemia without ketosis, a low plasma free carnitine and increased acylcarnitine (mainly acetylcarnitine) excretion. Long-chain acylcarnitines are elevated in plasma. Patients are hypotonic with lethargy, persistent vomiting, cardiomegaly and skeletal muscle weakness; pathologically there is macro- and microvesicular fatty infiltration of liver, heart and other tissues. However not all these features may be present. Several of the early-presenting patients have died during severe episodes. Other patients may be neurologically damaged; two patients have been microcephalic, both severely retarded, and a third patient died.

Conversely in older children with proven LCAD deficiency the presentation is of fasting-induced intermittent hypoglycaemia, lethargy and coma, muscle pain and possible myoglobinuria. A dicarboxylic aciduria and acidaemia with C_{12} and C_{14} dicarboxylic acids is present in those patients in whom it has been studied, but without suberylglycinuria or phenylpropionylglycinuria.

The enzyme deficiency is expressed in liver, leucocytes and cultured skin fibroblasts where oxidation of palmitate is greatly reduced in the presence of normal oxidation of octanoate and butyrate. Direct measurement of acyl CoA dehydrogenases shows a major deficiency of long-chain acyl CoA dehydrogenase in the presence of normal medium-chain and short-chain enzymes.[63] The gene encoding human LCAD has been cloned and assigned to chromosome 2 (q34 – q35).

Treatment with a high carbohydrate, low fat diet, with medium-chain triglyceride supplementation has been used with avoidance of fasting and, although development continued to be slow, cardiac hypertrophy and hepatomegaly resolved. Therapy with L-carnitine has also been used, but as with MCAD deficiency it may be expected to exacerbate the symptoms by increasing uptake of long-chain fatty acids into mitochondria, together with stimulation of β-oxidation. It is apparent that, given the early presentation and severe clinical and neurological consequences of acute episodes in some patients, the prognosis for many patients is poor, especially when diagnosis is delayed. The disorder appears to be inherited in an autosomal recessive mode and prenatal diagnosis on cultured amniocytes and on chorionic villi should be possible.

Short-chain acyl CoA dehydrogenase deficiency (McKusick 201470)

Relatively few patients with proven short-chain acyl CoA dehydrogenase deficiency have been described, three infants presenting variously in the first days of life with vomiting, poor feeding, acidosis, hypoglycaemia, lethargy and hypotonia, and hyperpnoea. One infant died despite supportive therapy, one survived and has since developed normally without further episodes, while the third has shown developmental delay with progressive muscle weakness and hypotonia, hepatomegaly and microcephaly. All three infants showed increased excretion of lactate, ethylmalonate and methylsuccinate with some adipate, and had a generalised amino aciduria. Free carnitine concentrations in plasma were low and acylcarnitines elevated.

Ethylmalonic acid is formed as its CoA ester by carboxylation of butyryl CoA, catalysed by propionyl CoA carboxylase. The presence of this metabolite and associated compounds in urine is believed to indicate a defect in short-chain acyl CoA dehydrogenase (SCAD) or possibly in electron transport affecting especially this enzyme system. Studies in cultured skin fibroblasts have shown reduced activity of this enzyme measured with ETF as electron acceptor. Because of apparently overlapping specificities with MCAD, considerable activity is still observed, but when assayed in the presence of antiMCAD antibody, very low residual activity of short-chain acyl CoA dehydrogenase is observed.[56] A myopathic form of butyryl CoA dehydrogenase deficiency has also been described in two adults in which the enzyme defect is expressed only in muscle.

Short-chain acyl CoA dehydrogenase is, like the other acyl CoA dehydrogenases, a homotetramer with subunits of 41 kDa, each containing one molecule of FAD. The human gene has been sequenced and assigned to chromosome 12 (q22–qter).

Ethylmalonic-adipic aciduria. Several other infants have also been described with ethylmalonic-adipic aciduria (under McKusick 231690) who have presented with potentially lethal severe hypoketotic, hypoglycaemic, acidotic attacks. Analysis of urine for organic acids showed increased concentrations of ethylmalonate, adipate and hexanoylglycine. Butyric acid and butyrylglycine concentrations were also increased and carnitine concentrations greatly reduced. During periods of remission the abnormal organic aciduria may be minimal or absent. Some cases appeared to be clinically responsive to riboflavin treatment (200 mg/24 h) but others showed no response. Early treatment with a low fat, high carbohydrate diet suggests a good prognosis for patients with this disorder. Oxidation of [1-^{14}C]butyrate is reduced in comparison to control values and residual activities ranging from 14 to 45% have been recorded. Oxidation of lysine and leucine were reduced in one patient suggesting again a defect associated with a common electron transport process. Ethylmalonic-adipic aciduria also occurs as a persistent feature in patients with riboflavin-responsive multiple acyl CoA dehydrogenase deficiency (MACDD) (see below) and it is possible that these patients represent part of the spectrum of this disorder.

Multiple acyl CoA dehydrogenase deficiency (MACDD) (McKusick 231680)

Patients with the most severe form of multiple acyl CoA dehydrogenase deficiency present in the neonatal period with severe hypoketotic hypoglycaemia, metabolic acidosis, hepatomegaly, hypotonia, hyperammonaemia, convulsions and neurological symptoms, with death within the first months of life. Dysmorphic features are often observed with large head, depressed nasal bridge and other features, and pathologically there is severe microvesicular fatty infiltration of the liver, heart and other organs and grossly enlarged polycystic kidneys.[64,65] In a less severe but still neonatal presentation, dysmorphic features and polycystic kidneys are not observed but these cases are also associated with similarly severe clinical features. Other patients have presented later in infancy and childhood, but acute episodes may occur with cardiomyopathy and death in some cases. The mildest cases have presented in adult life and maternal MACDD[66] may cause adverse effects in the fetus and newborn, although this is not invariable.

It is evident that these patients represent a spectrum of disease manifestations associated with a common cause or causes modified by residual enzyme activities and by the variable genetic phenotypes of individuals.

The disorder is readily distinguished from other disorders of fatty acid metabolism, and from isolated glutaryl CoA dehydrogenase deficiency, by the characteristic organic aciduria: glutaric acid is prominent but there are also major increases in 3-hydroxyisovaleric acid, isovalerylglycine, ethylmalonic acid, 2-hydroxyglutarate and C_8-C_{10} dicarboxylic acids and associated metabolites. Other glycine conjugates may also be observed including hexanoylglycine, isobutyrylglycine and 2-methylbutyrylglycine, but the amounts of suberylglycine are insignificant. Short-chain fatty acids may be elevated during acute attacks, providing the basis for the *sweaty feet* or *cheesy* odour associated with these episodes. Amino acids, particularly lysine, may also be elevated and there is a prominent sarcosinaemia and sarcosinuria together with dimethylglycinuria in patients without dysmorphic features or polycystic kidneys.

The spectrum of biochemical abnormalities observed in this organic aciduria is indicative of the inhibition, or loss of activity, of a variety of acyl CoA dehydrogenases including those involved in fatty acid β-oxidation at all levels, glutaryl CoA dehydrogenase, and those involved in branched-chain amino acid metabolism (isovaleryl CoA dehydrogenase, 2-methylbutyryl CoA dehydrogenase and isobutyryl CoA dehydrogenase). Other mitochondrial FAD-dependent dehydrogenases are also affected, including sarcosine dehydrogenase, dimethylglycine dehydrogenase and 2-hydroxyglutarate dehydrogenase. The common feature of these enzyme systems is their dependence upon FAD for electron transfer and subsequently upon ETF and ETF dehydrogenase for electron transfer into the electron transport chain (Fig. 4.12). Some patients have been shown to respond to riboflavin therapy and FAD synthesis from riboflavin has been shown to be normal in tissues from at least one patient.

Electron transfer flavoprotein (ETF) is an αβ dimer containing one flavin which becomes reduced to its semiquinone on electron transfer from the dehydrogenases. The α subunit (α-ETF), to which the FAD is believed to be bound, is about 32 kDa and the β subunit (β-ETF), which may interact directly with the dehydrogenases, is 27 kDa. ETF dehydrogenase (ETF: ubiquinone oxidoreductase) is a 67 kDa protein in the inner mitochondrial membrane and contains one flavin and one Fe_4S_4 iron–sulphur cluster per monomer. The sequence of electron transfer probably involves firstly reduction of the flavin and the iron–sulphur complex, followed by electron transfer to the ubiquinone (coenzyme Q_{10}). Studies, using electron paramagnetic resonance (epr) spectroscopy and direct assays of ETF and of ETF dehydrogenase, have shown that in some patients with the severe neonatal form of the disease, associated with dysmorphic features and polycystic kidneys, the defect is in ETF dehydrogenase. The gene for ETF dehydrogenase has been cloned and two different point mutations identified in two patients.[62] Defects in the α-ETF subunit have been identified in some patients with the severe forms of MACDD[67], whereas a defect in β-ETF has been identified in some patients with the late-onset form of the disease.[62] This is perhaps in accord with the presumed functions of the two subunits. The gene for α-ETF has been assigned to chromosome 15 (q23–q25) and that for β-ETF has been assigned to chromosome 19.

The disorder may be diagnosed, in addition to the characteristic abnormal organic aciduria, by enzymology on cultured skin fibroblasts and other tissues, in which the oxidation of fatty acid substrates, oxidation of [6-^{14}C]-L-lysine and incorporation of isovalerate and other substrates into protein are all greatly reduced. More direct dehydrogenase assays may also be used but more detailed studies on the electron transfer processes have usually required other biopsy material, for example, liver.

No successful treatment of the severe neonatal patients has been reported, although milder cases may respond to moderate reduction of protein and fat intake with increased carbohydrate, and particularly addition of riboflavin. Treatment with riboflavin is also of value in maternal cases.[66] Supplementation with L-carnitine to counter the adverse effects of the chronic carnitine deficiency have also been of benefit.[68] The severity of the neonatal forms, with evidence of intrauterine damage to the fetus with polycystic kidneys and dysmorphic features being evident at around 19 weeks' gestation,[69] makes prenatal diagnosis most important.

All the disorders appear to be inherited in autosomal recessive modes, with both males and females being affected in the same sibships and the forms of the disease remaining true within sibships. The disorder appears not uncommon. Prenatal diagnosis has been made by direct analysis of cell-free amniotic fluid in which glutarate and 2-hydroxyglutarate concentrations are elevated, and by enzymology on cultured amniocytes.[69] Dicarboxylic acids are not consistently elevated in amniotic fluid and use of these acids for prenatal diagnosis is unreliable.

Other disorders of mitochondrial fatty acid β-oxidation

3-Hydroxyacyl CoA dehydrogenase deficiency

At least two chain-length-specific 3-hydroxyacyl CoA dehydrogenases occur in mammalian tissues, one specific for short-chain substrates and one that metabolises medium-chain and long-chain substrates. A number of patients have recently been identified, presenting with Reye's syndrome-like disorders and hepatic dysfunction, who excrete, in addition to a dicarboxylic aciduria that extends from C_6 to C_{10}, increased amounts of 3-hydroxydicarboylic acids of chain lengths from C_6 to C_{12}. Acylglycines are not detectable.[70] 3-Hydroxy-monocarboxylic acids are elevated in plasma. At least some of these patients have a primary defect in fatty acid oxidation as demonstrated by reduced oxidation of [16-^{14}C] palmitic acid and tritiated water release from [9,10-^{3}H] myristic acid.[70] However similar organic aciduria has been observed in other patients, presenting with Reye's-syndrome-like attacks, who showed no evidence for a permanent metabolic disorder on subsequent investigation.[62,71] A few patients, presenting in a similar manner but with recurrent episodes of hypoglycaemia, hypotonia and coma, associated with myopathy, cardiomyopathy and carnitine deficiency, have been shown to have a deficiency of membrane-bound long-chain 3-hydroxyacyl CoA dehydrogenase.[62,72] The occurrence of patients with proven 3-hydroxyacyl-CoA dehydrogenase deficiency, including one who had a much milder presentation and course[73] and those without identifiable enzyme disorders but with apparently closely similar abnormal organic aciduria, is indicative of the complexity of the definition and diagnosis of disorders in this area.

In addition to the disorders that have been characterised and are described in the sections above, a considerable number of patients are identified with features indicating an underlying disorder of fatty acid metabolism but in whom no specific enzyme deficiency can be demonstrated. The complexity of mitochondrial and peroxisomal β-oxidation in man and of the alternative pathways for fatty acid metabolism with currently unexplored enzymes is certain to yield further inherited disorders in this area of intermediary metabolism.

Disorders of peroxisomal fatty acid metabolism

These peroxisomal disorders are described in detail in Chapter 6, p 243.

Refsum's disease (McKusick 266500) or phytanic acid storage disease is a disorder characterised by peripheral neuropathy, cerebellar ataxia and retinitis pigmentosa. The disorder occurs in older children and adults; is of autosomal recessive inheritance, and is caused by accumulation of phytanic acid (3,7,11,15-tetramethylhexadecanoic acid) in tissues and blood. This acid is derived exclusively from dietary sources containing free phytol and phytanic acid (e.g. dairy products and ruminant meats). Phytanic acid is degraded normally in man by an exclusive α-oxidation pathway that is now believed to occur in the peroxisomes and involves an initial α-hydroxylation followed by decarboxylation to form pristanic acid. This latter C_{19} fatty acid is then metabolised via normal β-oxidation to yield propionyl CoA, acetyl CoA and isobutyryl CoA. The disorder is caused by deficient activity of phytanic acid α-hydroxylase and is expressed in cultured skin fibroblasts. Treatment is by a diet low in phytol and phytanic acid and this may be combined with plasmapheresis. For full success treatment must be instituted prior to the occurrence of permanent neurological damage.

3-Hydroxy-3-methylglutaric aciduria (McKusick 246450)

3-Hydroxy-3-methylglutaric aciduria (HMG aciduria) is caused by deficient activity of 3-hydroxy-3-methylglutaryl CoA lyase, a key enzyme in

L-leucine catabolism and also in the formation of acetoacetate, and hence 'ketone bodies', from acetoacetyl CoA and acetyl CoA (Fig. 4.13). A deficiency of this enzyme is characterised clinically by profound hypoglycaemic attacks, which may be of very sudden onset, with minimal or absent ketosis, and associated with cyanosis, vomiting and apnoea, leading rapidly

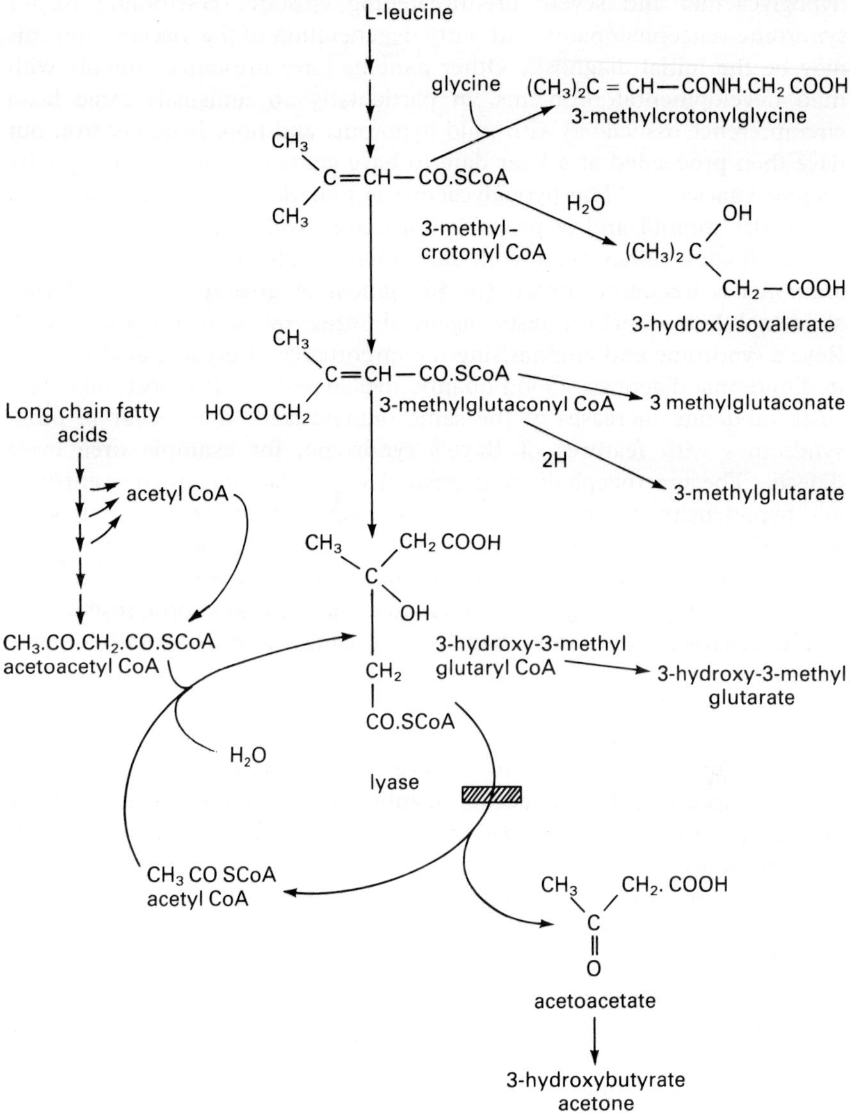

Fig. 4.13 Metabolism of 3-hydroxy-3-methylglutaryl CoA showing its dual position, in the catabolism of L-leucine and as the obligate intermediate in the formation of acetoacetate from acetoacetyl CoA (see also Fig. 4.11). The origins of the metabolites accumulating in 3-hydroxy-3-methylglutaryl CoA lyase deficiency are also shown.

to coma and life-threatening illness. The symptoms observed may be ascribed primarily to the inability to form ketone bodies, rather than to the associated defect in L-leucine catabolism, and the disorder is best classified as a non-ketotic hypoglycaemia or disorder of ketogenesis.

More than 40 patients have been described with this disorder, most patients presenting for the first time with acidosis, profound non-ketotic hypoglycaemia and severe life-threatening episodes resembling Reye's syndrome (encephalopathy with fatty degeneration of the viscera) and this may be the initial diagnosis. Other patients have presented initially with mild developmental problems, in particularly an unusually large head circumference associated with mild hypotonia and poor head control, but have then proceeded at a later date to have acute and profound hypoglycaemic attacks.[74,75] The hypoglycaemia is remarkable with glucose levels below 0.1 mmol/l and is probably associated with the inability to form ketone bodies rather than with inhibition of gluconeogenesis.[75] Blood ammonia is frequently raised (to 500 μmol/l or greater) associated with abnormal liver function tests, again showing marked similarities with Reye's syndrome and emphasising the importance of organic acid analysis in differential diagnosis. Good quantitative analysis is also most important since moderate increases of the same organic acids may occur in other syndromes with features of Reye's syndrome, for example urea cycle defects. The macrocephaly is associated with dilatation of the ventricles and hypodensity of white matter, and permanent brain damage may occur although this may be prevented by rapid and effective treatment. The acute acidotic attacks may prove lethal[76] but in the majority of other cases effective acute therapy during attacks leads to a relatively good prognosis.

The characteristic and diagnostic organic aciduria (and organic acidaemia) includes greatly increased concentrations of 3-hydroxy-3-methylglutaric acid (to above 11 mol/mol creatinine) with associated increases in 3-hydroxyisovaleric acid (to above 2 mol/mol creatinine), 3-methylglutaconic acid (to above 6 mol/mol creatinine) and 3-methylglutaric acid (to above 1 mol/mol creatinine). During acute episodes, and in the immediate period leading to an attack, 3-methylcrotonylglycine is also excreted (Fig. 4.13) into the urine, and the patients display the very characteristic and distinctive odour of tomcats' urine (probably caused by 3-methylcrotonic acid). Inhibition of fatty acid β-oxidation may also occur and a prominent dicarboxylic aciduria with saturated and unsaturated acids and 5-hydroxyhexanoic aciduria may result. In common with patients with other conditions in which acyl CoA esters accumulate, patients with 3-hydroxy-3-methylglutaric aciduria show increased acylcarnitine excretion into urine with evidence for carnitine insufficiency. Acylcarnitines excreted by these patients have been shown to include 3-methylglutarylcarnitine and 3-hydroxyisovaleryl-carnitine, giving direct evidence for the role of L-carnitine in the transport and metabolism of diacyl and hydroxyacyl moieties.[77]

Acute management must be swift and positive and is directed at the rapid correction of the profound hypoglycaemia, reduction of the acidosis with concomitant fluid replacement and, in cases of severe hyperammonaemia, with exchange transfusions and peritoneal dialysis. Intravenous L-carnitine has also proved very effective in conjunction with i.v. glucose therapy in increasing the response to therapy and in reversal of the profound coma associated with this disorder (see below). Longer-term management has been directed towards reduction in L-leucine intake, by moderate protein restriction[74,75] together with a reduced fat intake, and towards careful regulation of blood glucose, especially in early life. The latter is accomplished by frequent feeding including nocturnal feeding if required (with corn starch if necessary) to avoid overnight hypoglycaemia, supplemented as needed with high glucose drinks. However, studies on the contribution of protein catabolism to metabolic decompensation in the disorder[78] have indicated the significance of fat metabolism in such episodes and emphasised the importance of dietary fat restriction.

The prognosis of well-treated cases appears excellent although there is always the risk of sudden acute and potentially lethal hypoglycaemic and acidotic attacks with devastating clinical and residual neurological effects.[75,76] Careful consideration needs to be given to immunisation in these patients, severe and potentially lethal reactions having occurred in at least two cases.[74] If immunisation is given this should be carried out in hospital with close and appropriate monitoring. Similarly, avoidance of prolonged fasting is important and this also must be considered if anaesthetics are to be administered.

During acute episodes, L-carnitine has been used effectively to assist in the detoxification and removal of accumulating acyl moieties. The concomitant restoration of mitochondrial homeostasis is shown by recovery of normal β-oxidation and abolition of dicarboxylic aciduria (above). However maintenance therapy with L-carnitine may be contraindicated because of the unwanted stimulation of fatty acid β-oxidation and hence increased attempts to form ketone bodies.

3-Hydroxy-3-methylglutaric aciduria is inherited in an autosomal recessive mode and the HMG lyase activity is demonstrable in leucocytes and cultured skin fibroblasts with intermediate levels of activity being recorded in the cells of heterozygotes. Genetic complementation studies have shown a single complementation group consistent with the monomeric enzyme, but detailed molecular studies have not been reported.

Prenatal diagnosis may be requested by parents of patients with the disease because of the severity of hypoglycaemic attacks, possibility of neurological damage and the uncertainties of long-term survival, although current experience suggests the chance of this is good. Prenatal diagnosis has been carried out in the first trimester by direct enzymology in chorionic villi and during the second trimester by enzymology on cultured amniocytes, using both direct lyase assays or measurement of [1-^{14}C]- isovalerate incorporation into protein, and by direct GC-MS analysis of organic acids in cell-free amniotic fluid supernatant.

HEREDITARY TYROSINAEMIAS AND RELATED ORGANIC ACIDURIAS

Introduction

L-Tyrosine is a 'non-essential' amino acid derived both from the diet and from the metabolism (4-hydroxylation) of L-phenylalanine. It is metabolised in the cytosol by pyridoxine-dependent tyrosine aminotransferase, which has a specific requirement for 2-oxoglutarate as coreactant, to form 4-hydroxyphenylpyruvate. The latter is then metabolised to homogentisic acid (3,6-dihydroxyphenylacetic acid) in an unusual reaction involving side-chain transfer catalysed by 4-hydroxyphenylpyruvate dioxygenase. Homogentisic acid accumulates in alkaptonuria (*homogentisic aciduria*, McKusick 203500), due to a deficiency of homogentisate oxidase, and is the cause of the ochronosis observed. This enzyme normally cleaves the aromatic ring to give maleylacetoacetate which is isomerised to fumarylacetoacetate, the latter being cleaved by fumarylacetoacetase to form fumarate and acetoacetate (Fig. 4.14). The fumarate is converted into malate by the action of cytosolic fumarase for transport into the mitochondria and further metabolism in the tricarboxylic acid cycle.

Several disorders occur in which plasma tyrosine concentrations are increased and in which a tyrosyluria, urinary excretion of the metabolites of tyrosine, 4-hydroxyphenylpyruvate, 4-hydroxyphenyllactate and 4-hydroxyphenylacetate, occurs. Deficiency of fumarylacetoacetase has been shown to be the cause of 'tyrosinaemia Type 1' and tyrosine aminotransferase deficiency results in tyrosinaemia Type 2 (Richner – Hanhart syndrome). The apparently rare deficiency of 4-hydroxyphenylpyruvate dioxygenase has been designated tyrosinaemia Type 3. These are described below in order of the appearance of the relevant enzymes in the metabolic pathway.

Other causes of overt tyrosyluria include transient *neonatal tyrosinaemia* that is particularly common in premature infants and is probably caused by delayed maturation of hepatic enzymes. The tyrosyluria is often responsive to a single dose of ascorbate (vitamin C), the required cofactor for the 4-hydroxyphenylpyruvate dioxygenase.

Tyrosinaemia has also been noted in patients with and without acidosis who excreted an unusual sulphur-containing metabolite into their urine (2-L-cysteinyl-1,4-dihydroxycyclohexanylacetic acid, 'Hawkinsin'), and also *cis* and *trans* 4-hydroxycyclohexylacetic acid. This disorder

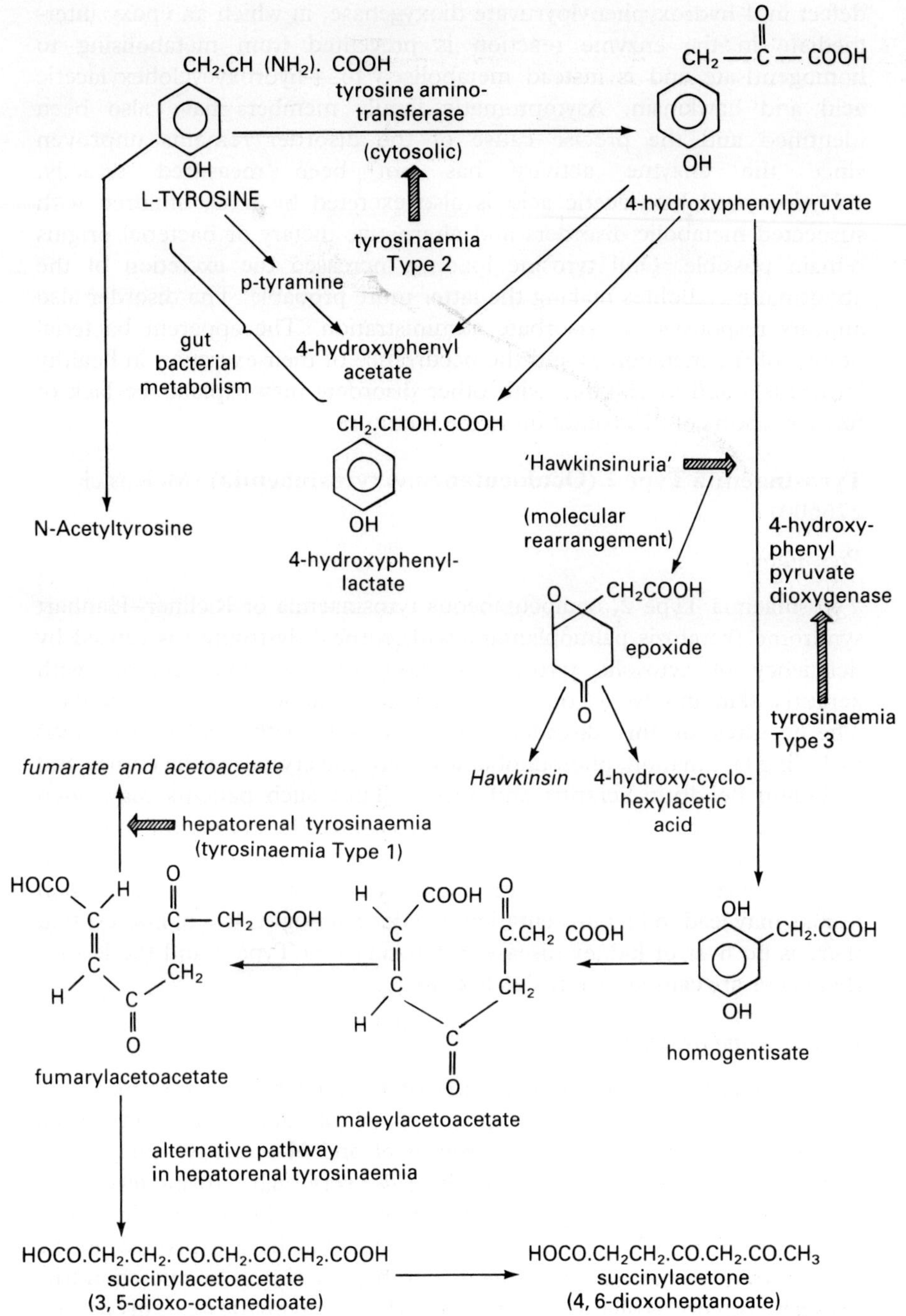

Fig. 4.14 Metabolism of L-tyrosine and site of defects in the hereditary tyrosinaemias with origins of the metabolites observed.

(*'Hawkinsinuria'*, McKusick 140350) has been supposed to be caused by a defect in 4-hydroxyphenylpyruvate dioxygenase, in which an epoxy intermediate in the enzyme reaction is prevented from metabolising to homogentisate and is instead metabolised to 4-hydroxycyclohexylacetic acid and hawkinsin. Asymptomatic family members have also been identified and the precise cause of the disorder remains unproven since the enzyme activity has not been measured directly. 4-Hydroxycyclohexylacetic acid is also excreted by other children with suspected metabolic disorders and alternative dietary or bacterial origins remain possible. Oral tyrosine loading increased the excretion of the abnormal metabolites making the latter more probable. The disorder also appears responsive to ascorbate administration. The apparent bacterial origins of the metabolites and the occurrence of their excretion in healthy individuals and in children with other disorders may explain the lack of further reports of this condition in the literature.

Tyrosinaemia Type 2 (Oculocutaneous tyrosinaemia) (McKusick 276600)

Presentation

Tyrosinaemia Type 2, oculocutaneous tyrosinaemia or Richner–Hanhart syndrome (keratosis palmoplantaris with corneal dystrophy) is caused by deficiency of cytosolic tyrosine aminotransferase, and presents with keratitis, skin and eye lesions, with mental retardation in some patients.[79] The features of this disorder are remarkable with ocular symptoms including lacrimation, photophobia with tyrosine crystals in the cornea and including dendritic keratitis and ulcers. Thus such patients may often present initially to an ophthalmologist and, since the eye lesions in particular are often evident at an early age, it is important to determine blood tyrosine levels in any patient with unexplained keratitis. Similarly the skin lesions may lead to first presentation to a dermatologist. It is of interest that there is no liver or kidney disease in tyrosinaemia Type 2 and the lesions that occur are caused by tyrosine toxicity.

Diagnosis and treatment

The diagnosis is made on the basis of elevated plasma tyrosine (1–3 mmol/l) and of urinary tyrosine. Tyrosyluria also occurs in which 4-hydroxyphenylacetate is quite prominent and N-acetyl-tyrosine is also excreted in large amounts, as a result of the very high tyrosine levels and probably reduced hepatic formation of other tyrosine metabolites. The formation of the other metabolites of tyrosine has been explained on the basis of transamination of tyrosine in extrahepatic tissues by mitochondrial aspartate aminotransferase to give 4-hydroxyphenylpyruvate. This cannot be metabolised further in these tissues but is reduced to 4-hydroxyphenyllactate and decarboxylated to 4-hydroxyphenylacetate in the liver. The latter metabolite is probably further increased by bacterial metabolism of L-tyrosine secreted into the small intestine where it is converted into 4-tyramine and subsequently oxidised.

Treatment is by protein restriction or, where necessary, by a diet low in phenylalanine and tyrosine, to bring plasma tyrosine concentrations towards 1 mmol/l. Early therapy may prevent possible neurological damage and in all cases dietary treatment will relieve the other symptoms, although residual corneal scarring may occur. Symptoms may recur on relaxation of treatment. Prognosis on such a diet is good and several adult female patients have had normal children.

Genetics

The disorder is inherited in an autosomal recessive mode. Many reported cases are of Mediterranean origin, particularly Italian, but cases are reported in many other ethnic groups. Human tyrosine aminotransferase is a phosphoprotein that shows three fractions on isoelectric focusing and appears to be subject to hormonal control. The gene for tyrosine aminotransferase has been mapped to chromosome 16 (q22–q24).

Tyrosinaemia Type 3 (4-hydroxyphenylpyruvate dioxygenase deficiency) (McKusick 276710)

This has been described in only two patients, one a 17-month-old Egyptian girl with drowsiness and ataxia associated with tyrosinaemia and tyrosyluria. A liver biopsy showed undetectable activity of 4-hydroxyphenylpyruvate dioxygenase in the presence of a normal activity of tyrosine aminotransferase.[80] The second child was Japanese and presented at 21 days with seizures and mild brain atrophy on CAT scan. He died at 3 months after accidental asphyxia. Liver 4-hydroxyphenylpyruvate dioxygenase activity was 5% of control values whereas tyrosine aminotransferase and fumarylacetoacetase activities were normal.[81]

Tyrosinaemia Type 1 (Hepatorenal tyrosinaemia) (McKusick 276700)

Presentation and diagnosis

Patients with tyrosinaemia Type 1 or hepatorenal tyrosinaemia usually present acutely in early infancy with failure to thrive, vomiting, diarrhoea and hepatomegaly with early death occurring due to hepatic failure. Patients show hypertyrosinaemia and hypermethioninaemia, the latter often manifesting before the tyrosinaemia, and a 'cabbage-like' odour may be present. Death from liver failure occurs within the first year of life in untreated patients. Patients with a more chronic form of the disease may occur within the same sibships as those with the acute presentation, and are characterised by liver disease, renal tubular dysfunction and a Fanconi syndrome associated with hypophosphataemia and rickets. Hepatic cirrhosis, hepatoma and renal failure may develop chronically[82] and patients usually die within the first decade of life if untreated. Episodes of acute severe peripheral neuropathy may occur associated with hypotonia, vomiting, seizures, self-mutilation and respiratory insufficiency[83], with similarities to neurological attacks in acute intermittent porphyria and perhaps associated with inhibition of δ-aminolaevulinic dehydratase.

There is a profound tyrosyluria in which, however, excretion of 4-hydroxyphenylacetate is not particularly prominent. Excretion of N-acetyltyrosine may also occur when plasma tyrosine levels are particularly elevated. Hypoglycaemia, unresponsive to glucagon, is common and there may be a more generalised aminoacidaemia in which cystathione, proline and hydroxyproline are prominent. Increased excretion of catecholamines, δ-aminolaevulinic acid and sugars (glucose, fructose and galactose) may occur. The last of these features is particularly evident in patients presenting more chronically. Diagnosis may be confirmed by demonstration of succinylacetone (4,6-dioxo-heptanoic acid) and succinylacetoacetate (3,5-dioxo-octanedioic acid) in urine (see below), generally with use of special analytical methods, utilising GC-MS, because of the relatively low levels observed.

Biochemistry and pathogenesis

Tyrosinaemia Type 1 is caused by deficient activity of cytosolic fumarylacetoacetase (fumarylacetoacetate hydrolase). Fumarylacetoacetate and its metabolic precursor maleylacetoacetate (Fig. 4.14) are believed to accumulate, with the latter acting as a potent sulphydryl group inhibitor. A variety of other enzyme systems are thereby inhibited, including δ-aminolaevulinic acid dehydratase, causing the renal tubular and hepatic dysfunction and the multiple biochemical and clinical abnormalities observed. Succinylacetoacetate and succinylacetone also accumulate from metabolism of the unstable fumarylacetoacetate (Fig. 4.14) and are excreted into the urine to give the characteristic organic aciduria in addition to the tyrosyluria. Fumarylacetoacetase deficiency is demonstrable in skin fibroblasts and lymphocytes and this, together with succinylacetone excretion in urine has been taken as diagnostic of tyrosinaemia Type 1. Liver tissue from patients with a variety of liver diseases may show reduced enzyme activities and this tissue is not suitable for diagnosis.[82] Because of the existence of a pseudodeficiency gene (see below), demonstration of the enzyme deficiency alone without other findings is not diagnostic.

Treatment and prognosis

Patients with hepatorenal tyrosinaemia are difficult to treat effectively although use of diets low in phenylalanine and tyrosine have been of apparent benefit. Treatment needs to be started as early in life as possible and results in improvement of renal tubular dysfunction, although varied effects on hepatic dysfunction have been reported. Succinylacetone excretion, as well as the tyrosyluria, may be completely abolished by strict adherence to dietary restriction. Administration of compounds containing sulphydryl groups may possibly be of benefit but effective treatment relies upon liver transplantation. Patients receiving liver transplants may still excrete succinylacetone, ascribed to fumarylacetoacetase deficiency in extrahepatic tissues, and hepatic transplantation should perhaps be coupled with dietary restriction to reduce the continued excretion of succinylacetone and accumulation of its toxic metabolic precursors. Liver transplantation should also be considered early to avoid development of hepatocellular carcinoma and other clinical problems associated with chronic tyrosinaemia Type 1.[84]

Genetics

The disorder is inherited in an autosomal recessive mode with an overall incidence, from neonatal well-baby screening programmes, of around 1 per 100 000 live births. There is a high incidence of the disease in the French-Canadian population of Quebec, with a frequency of 1 in 700 occurring in some interbred communities, with a known founder effect. Fumarylacetoacetase is a homodimer with subunits of 43kDa. Immunoblotting studies have shown no cross-reacting material in fibroblasts from patients with the acute form of the disease with varying amounts in patients with the chronic presentation. Pulse-labelling studies have shown that cells from both patient types produce immunoreactive material that was more unstable in cells from patients with the acute form, although this is not a consistent finding.[85] The gene has been mapped to chromosome 15 (q23–q25).

Lymphocytes of some control subjects show low fumarylacetoacetase activities associated with low δ-aminolaevulinic acid dehydratase activities but without tyrosinaemia or tyrosyluria in the subjects concerned: family studies have revealed an autosomal dominant trait which could act as a pseudodeficiency gene, making heterozygote detection for the disorder outside known families with a proven index case very difficult.

Prenatal diagnosis remains of importance in the management of the families concerned and has been made on the basis of the measurement of succinylacetone concentrations in amniotic fluid supernatant using GC-MS, and also from the measurement of fumarylacetoacetase activity in cultured amniocytes and chorionic villus tissue.

DISORDERS OF PYRUVATE METABOLISM, THE TRICARBOXYLIC ACID CYCLE AND THE RESPIRATORY CHAIN

Introduction

Pyruvate has a central role in intermediary metabolism, being utilised in both lipogenesis and gluconeogenesis and in energy production via oxidation. It is metabolised by oxidative decarboxylation via the thiamine pyrophosphate, lipoate and coenzyme A-dependent pyruvate dehydrogenase (PDH) complex to form acetyl CoA (Fig. 4.15), which becomes available for citrate synthesis and fatty acid biosynthesis or which may be oxidised through the tricarboxylic acid cycle and the respiratory chain. Pyruvate is also utilised for gluconeogenesis via conversion to oxaloacetate through the action of biotin-dependent pyruvate carboxylase, and thence to phosphoenolpyruvate via GTP-dependent phosphoenolpyruvate carboxykinase (PEPCK). Pyruvate dehydrogenase activity is regulated via the action of an activating phosphatase and an inactivating kinase, and the ratios of acetyl CoA to free CoA and of NADH to NAD^+. Pyruvate carboxylase activity and pyruvate initiated gluconeogenesis is regulated by the mitochondrial malate translocase, necessary for oxaloacetate transport via conversion to malate.

Pyruvate is also converted by transamination to and from alanine and is reduced by lactate dehydrogenase to L-lactate, the latter being the end-product of the glycolytic pathway that is essential for ATP generation in several tissues. Lactate produced by anaerobic glycolysis in other tissues such as brain and muscle may be reutilised by the liver by conversion back to pyruvate (the Cori cycle), the latter again catalysed by lactate dehydrogenase.[86] In the fed state, a large proportion of ingested glucose is utilised in the brain, particularly in infants and during fasting, and glucose produced by the liver is also primarily utilised in the brain.[86] Normal activity of the pathways shown in Figure 4.15 is thus essential for brain function and maintenance of glucose output during fasting.

Lactate concentrations in body fluids (normally 1–2 mmol/l in blood) depend upon the pyruvate concentrations and upon the relative amounts of reduced and oxidised cytosolic NAD:

$$\left[\frac{[\text{lactate}]\,[\text{NAD}^+]}{[\text{pyruvate}]\,[\text{NADH}]\,[\text{H}^+]} = K \right]$$

Thus when the ratio NAD/NADH is constant, changes in lactate concentration depend upon the pyruvate concentration and rate of pyruvate formation. Conversely, lowering of the NAD/NADH ratio will also lead to a rise in lactate concentration.

Lactate concentrations do not alter significantly under normal conditions, including mild infections, but rise appreciably during exercise (and, for example, fitting and convulsions) due to production from muscle.

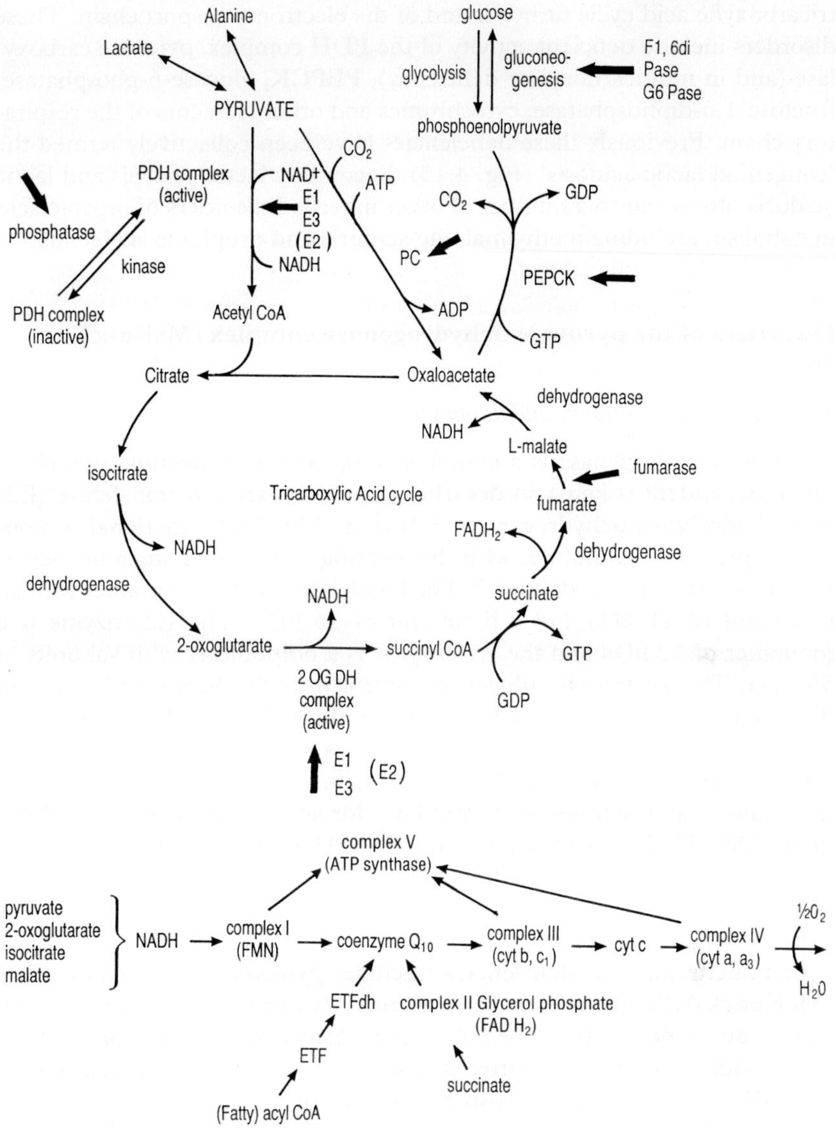

Fig. 4.15 Pyruvate metabolism, gluconeogenesis, the tricarboxylic acid cycle and the respiratory chain, arrows showing identified inherited enzyme deficiencies. PDH–pyruvate dehydrogenase complex, PC pyruvate carboxylase, PEPCK–phosphoenolpyruvate carboxykinase, 2 OG DH–2-oxoglutarate dehydrogenase, cyt–cytochromes. See text for further detail.

Major increases occur in a variety of conditions including hypoxia and circulatory failure. Lactic acid is also the predominant and characteristic metabolite observed when the systems outlined in Figure 4.15 fail or are deficient, as in disorders of pyruvate metabolism, of gluconeogenesis, of tricarboxylic acid cycle turnover and of the electron transport chain. These disorders include deficient activity of the PDH complex, pyruvate carboxylase (and in multicarboxylase deficiency), PEPCK, glucose-6-phosphatase, fructose-1,6-diphosphatase, cytochromes and other elements of the respiratory chain. Previously these deficiencies have been collectively termed the 'congenital lactic acidosis' (Fig. 4.15). Secondary lactic acidosis and lactic aciduria also occur in a number of other inherited disorders of organic acid metabolism including methylmalonic aciduria and propionic acidaemia.[1]

Disorders of the pyruvate dehydrogenase complex (McKusick 208800)

Biochemistry, presentation and diagnosis

Pyruvate dehydrogenase is a complex composed of a thiamine pyrophosphate dependent α-ketoacid decarboxylase (E1), an acyl transferase (E2) and dihydrolipoyl dehydrogenase (E3) (Fig. 4.3). Each functional component is present in multiples, with the working complex having a molecular mass of several million daltons.[86] The E1 enzyme is a $\alpha_2\beta_2$ tetramer with an α subunit of 41 kDa and a β subunit of 36 kDa. The E2 enzyme is a monomer of 52 kDa and the E3 enzyme is a homodimer with subunits of 55 kDa. The enzyme is subject to control through phosphorylation and dephosphorylation of the E1α subunits by the actions of PDH kinase and PDH phosphatase respectively. The kinase is a heterodimer and phosphorylates 3 serine residues in the E1α protein; the phosphatase is again a heterodimer and requires Mg^{2+} and Ca^{2+} for activity. Increased mitochondrial NADH/NAD^+ and acetyl CoA/CoASH ratios stimulate the kinase and reduce the activity of the complex. The complex also includes a 'protein X' of unknown function that may be related to the E2 enzyme and contains lipoate.

Identified enzyme deficiencies include *pyruvate decarboxylase (E1)* (McKusick 312170), affecting a large majority of patients (over 90%) with PDH deficiencies (see below), and *lipoamide dehydrogenase (E3)* (McKusick 246900). The latter is associated with combined deficiencies of PDH, 2-oxoglutarate dehydrogenase and of branched-chain keto acid dehydrogenase, all three enzyme complexes sharing the same E3 enzyme[87] (Fig. 4.3).

Patients deficient in lipoamide dehydrogenase present within the first few months of life with delayed physical and mental development and death in the first years of life from overwhelming acidosis. These patients show a combination of elevated urinary lactate, pyruvate, 2-oxoglutarate and 2-hydroxybutyrate, with moderate elevation of branched-chain keto and hydroxy acids[88] and a moderate increase in plasma branched-chain amino acids.

Few reports have appeared consistent with a deficiency of the E2 enzyme, *dihydrolipoyl transacetylase*, but identification of this deficiency and of the *X-protein* in patients with lactic acidemia has recently been made.[89] One case has been reported of apparent combined deficiencies of the E1 enzymes of both the PDH and 2-oxoglutarate dehydrogenase, apparently caused by altered binding of thiamine pyrophosphate. Patients with defects in the activation of the PDH complex, caused by deficient activity of *PDH phosphate phosphatase*, have also been recorded, presenting with overwhelming acidosis and features of Leigh's disease.[86]

The clinical presentation of patients with *pyruvate decarboxylase (E1) deficiency* may be divided into three groups: those presenting acutely in neonatal and early infantile life with severe acidosis and a rapidly progressive fatal illness; those presenting in later infancy and childhood with delayed motor and neurological development, ataxia and features of Leigh's encephalomyelopathy with survival into early childhood; and those with subacute or chronic neurodegenerative disease, often with survival into adult life. The last of these patients may not show systemic lactic acidosis, and more chronic presentation in late childhood may show no overt metabolic abnormalities ('cerebral' lactic acidosis).[90] Patients presenting acutely in infancy are characterised by an organic aciduria in which concentrations of both lactate and pyruvate are greatly increased with a normal L/P ratio, reduced citrate excretion and increased 2-oxoglutarate excretion.[88] Of particular importance is an elevation of CSF lactate (and pyruvate) in *all* presentations of the condition: CSF lactate (and ideally pyruvate) should form part of the diagnostic investigation (Fig. 4.1) of any patient with lactic acidosis or with chronic neurodegenerative disease of unknown cause, with or without elevated blood lactates.

The enzyme deficiency is expressed in cultured skin fibroblasts with the level of residual enzyme activity ranging from 2% of normal activity in fibroblasts in the severely affected neonatal cases, to above 40% in the less severely affected cases. A strict correlation of the degree of enzyme deficiency and the lactate concentrations in body fluids does not occur, although there is a general trend of blood lactates of more than 20 mmol/l in the neonatal cases to 3–5 mmol/l in others. Patients presenting in infancy may show characteristic dysmorphic features with a narrowed head and wide nasal bridge with associated microcephaly. Agenesis of the corpus callosum, with absent medullary pyramids and abnormal inferior olives, has been observed in some cases and cystic lesions affecting the brain stems and basal ganglia, cerebral atrophy and generalised hypomyelination in others. There may be evidence of abnormal fetal development and possibly defective embryogenesis.

Genetics

Equal numbers of males and females are affected with pyruvate decarboxylase (E1) deficiency and from this it was assumed that the disorder was inherited in an autosomal recessive manner. However, E1α cDNA clones have been recently isolated and characterised and the gene for the subunit has been mapped to the X chromosome (p22.1).[91] (The genes for the E1β subunit and E3 enzyme have been mapped to chromosomes 3 and 7 respectively.[86]) Numerous different mutations of the E1α gene have been identified including small deletions, point mutations, and insertion-duplications.[92–94] Some of these affect the serine phosphorylation sites in the protein leading to inactivation and most appear to be sporadic new mutations, the parents being completely normal.

The X-chromosome location of the gene provides an explanation of the heterogeneity observed in pyruvate decarboxylase (E1α) deficiency, with males generally being severely affected, and some males and most females showing a variety of presentations due to X-inactivation affecting different tissues to varying degrees. Complete absence of the subunit in male patients would be expected to be lethal in utero.

Finally it is of particular interest that a different gene for the E1α subunit exists on chromosome 4, being expressed in testis only at spermatogenesis to produce this essential component of the PDH complex in spermatozoa. The gene on chromosome 4 is continuous ('intronless') but shows considerable homology with the X-chromosome gene.

Treatment and prognosis

Attempts at treatment, including the use of high fat, low carbohydrate diets, lipoic acid, thiamine, biotin and citrate have been universally unsuccessful, although lipoate-responsive lactic acidaemia has been observed.[95] The prognosis is generally poor and prenatal diagnosis can be considered in familial cases.

Disorders of gluconeogenesis

These disorders include *fructose-1,6,-bisphosphatase deficiency* (McKusick 229700; see p. 55), characterised by fasting hypoglycaemia with hepatomegaly and by increased urinary concentrations of lactate, 2-oxoglutarate and glyceraldehyde-3-phosphate. Similar clinical features characterise the *Type 1 glycogenoses* (*see* p. 26) in which greatly increased urinary concentrations of lactate and 2-oxoglutarate have been recorded. *Phosphoenolpyruvate carboxykinase (PEPCK) deficiency* (McKusick 261650) has only been reported in a few patients who were characterised by non-ketotic hypoglycaemia, hypotonia and moderate lactic acidosis, with fatty deposits in liver and other tissues. The PEPCK enzyme occurs in both cytosol and mitochondria, and in one series of patients the defect appeared localised to the cytosolic enzyme while in another the mitochondrial form was clearly deficient.[86] Hepatomegaly and hypertriglyceridaemia with hypercholesterolaemia may occur in the latter patients.

Pyruvate carboxylase deficiency (McKusick 266150)

Pyruvate carboxylase is a biotin-dependent enzyme occurring as a homotetramer in the mitochondria. Each 125 kDa subunit contains one molecule of biotin. The enzyme exerts a key regulatory role in gluconeogenesis in liver and kidney, and enzyme activity is controlled by acetyl CoA as allosteric activator. In other tissues pyruvate carboxylase is important for the maintenance of 4-carbon intermediates in the tricarboxylic acid cycle and appears important for normal brain development (see multicarboxylase deficiencies above). Isolated pyruvate carboxylase deficiency has been described in more than 20 patients who were generally characterised by acidosis, hypotonia, seizures and retarded development. Fasting hypoglycaemia is rarely recorded and the age of presentation and symptoms observed are very variable, as is the degree of enzyme deficiency in individual patients.

The patients may be divided into two groups, one associated with early infantile presentation and longer-term survival (for several years of life), but with gross retardation and with an organic aciduria in which lactate concentrations greatly exceed those of pyruvate. Citrate excretion is normal but increased excretion of fumarate, malate and 2-oxoglutarate occurs.[88,96] The second group is associated with neonatal presentation with hepatomegaly, ketosis, hyperammonaemia and citrullinaemia, and death within 3 months of birth.[86] The former patients have been shown to have enzyme protein present (cross-reacting material positive or CRM+) but with greatly reduced activity, whereas the latter group are CRM–, with no residual enzyme activity present. Four of these patients have been shown to lack mRNA for pyruvate carboxylase. The CRM—patients are unable to synthesise oxaloacetate from pyruvate at all, and utilise aspartate, glutamine and glutamate. This results in reduced availability of aspartate, affecting the urea cycle and the equilibrium of cytosolic and mitochondrial redox states, resulting in the hyperammonaemia, citrullinaemia and ketosis observed. Hepatomegaly, with lipid droplet accumulation, is frequently observed[86], and defective myelin formation is observed in the brain in conjunction with other neuronal changes.

Treatment of patients has included dietary supplementation with L-glutamine and aspartate to increase availability of oxaloacetate, and thiamine has also been used. Unlike the response observed in patients with multicarboxylase deficiency, D-biotin has no effect in the absence of much residual enzyme activity.

Both groups of pyruvate carboxylase-deficient patients show apparent autosomal recessive inheritance and cases have been reported in several ethnic groups. The enzyme deficiency is demonstrable in cultured skin fibroblasts as well as other tissues and prenatal diagnosis has been carried out in both the second and first trimesters, the latter by direct enzymology on chorionic villi.

Fumaric aciduria (McKusick 136850)

Fumarase (fumarate hydratase) occurs in cytosol and mitochondria in isoenzymic forms in all tissues except brain, where only the mitochondrial form has been identified. Numerous electrophoretic species have been identified, both isoenzymes being determined by the same autosomal gene locus on the long arm of chromosome 1. Both isoenzymes are tetrameric with mature subunits of 45 kDa. Evidence suggests that a single fumarase mRNA produces two distinct proteins, which differ slightly in amino acid sequence, and one of which has a leader sequence that directs uptake into the mitochondria. Fumarase exerts key roles in both the mitochondrial tricarboxylic acid cycle and in metabolism of large amounts of fumarate produced in the cytosol by the urea cycle as well as the cytosolic production from the purine nucleotide pathway and from tyrosine catabolism.

Five patients with proven fumarase deficiency have been described, presenting in the first months of life with failure to thrive, developmental delay, hypotonia, seizures, cerebral atrophy and mental retardation. Dysmorphic facial features may also be evident. Pathologically, patients show agenesis of the corpus callosum and microcephaly. Most patients have died within the first year of life.[97–100] Two adult siblings with severe mental retardation have also been described but enzymology was not performed. Infantile patients show an abnormal organic aciduria in which fumarate is greatly elevated (between 400 and 4000 mmol/mol creatinine) with associated increases in 2-oxoglutarate and succinate, although the latter may be normal.[99] Malate may also be elevated on some occasions. There are no abnormalities in other organic acids, in amino acids or in urea cycle metabolites. Almost complete deficiency of both mitochondrial and cytosolic isoenzymes occur in all tissues examined although in the one surviving case some residual mitochondrial activity remained.[98] Clinically, fumarase deficiency affects primarily the brain in which the enzyme is expressed only in mitochondria, and has thus been characterised as a mitochondrial encephalopathy. A human cDNA clone for liver fumarase has been identified and studies on the molecular basis of the disorder are in progress. The prognosis is very poor and prenatal exclusion has been carried out by enzymology on cultured amniocytes and on chorionic villus tissue.

Disorders of the respiratory chain

These are described in detail in Chapter 7.

DISORDERS OF OXALATE, GLYOXYLATE AND GLYCERATE METABOLISM

The metabolism of glyoxylate, oxalate and glycerate is interconnected through glycine and serine and by the occurrence of two forms of primary hyperoxaluria, associated with glycollic aciduria and with L-glyceric aciduria. Glyoxylate may be produced from glycine by the action of peroxisomal D-amino acid oxidase and by various transamination reactions. The major route of metabolism of the peroxisomally-generated glyoxylate is transamination to glycine by the action of peroxisomal alanine: glyoxylate aminotransferase in liver and kidney (Fig. 4.16). Lesser amounts of glyoxylate are also metabolised by cytosolic and mitochondrial glutamate:glyoxylate aminotransferase and cytosolic glyoxylate reductase (to produce glycollate). Glyoxylate may also be metabolised via mitochondrial glyoxylate:2-oxoglutarate carboligase, an enzyme closely associated with 2-oxoglutarate dehydrogenase. The activity of this enzyme is normal in

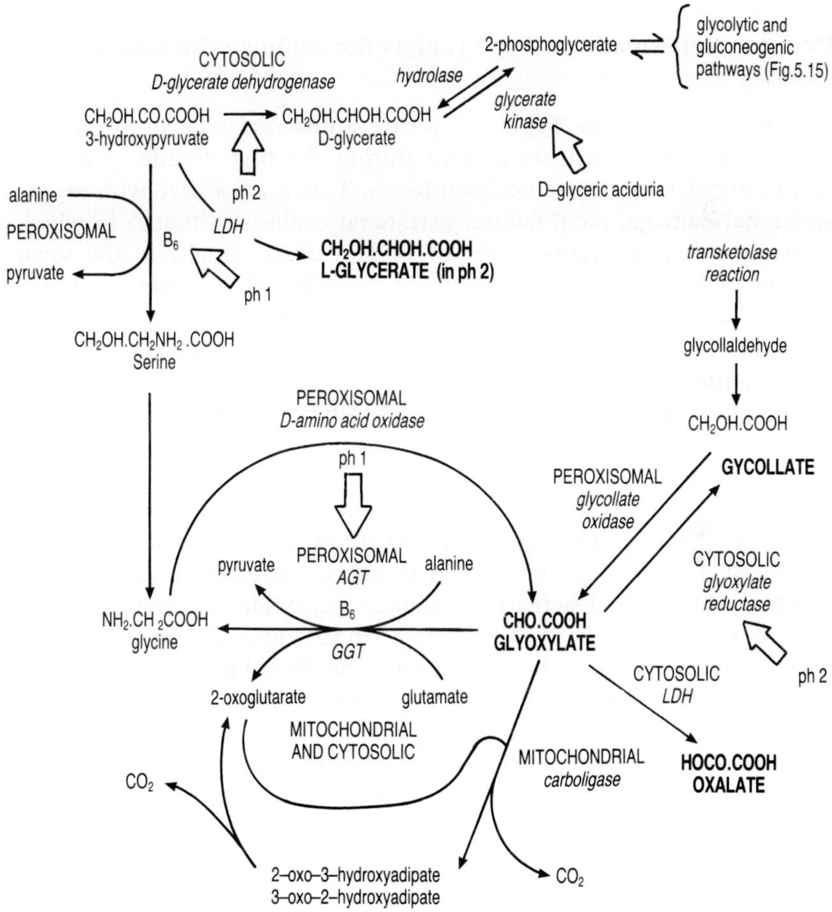

Fig. 4.16 Metabolism of glyoxylate, glycerate and oxalate, showing the positions of the defects in primary hyperoxaluria (ph) Type 1 (glycollic aciduria), Type 2 (L-glyceric aciduria) and in D-glyceric aciduria.

primary hyperoxaluria Type 1 but for many years it was believed that deficient activity of a cytosolic carboligase was the underlying cause.[101] Cytosolic carboligase was in fact an artefact from damaged mitochondria. Glycine is also interconverted into serine which is further metabolised to hydroxypyruvate and thence to D-glycerate via the action of D-glycerate dehydrogenase. D-Glycerate may also be produced from D-glyceraldehyde and is metabolised to 2-phosphoglycerate in the glycolytic and gluconeogenic pathways. Disorders of glyoxylate metabolism result in increased oxidation of glyoxylate to oxalate, giving rise to hyperoxaluria and oxalosis. Defective D-glycerate dehydrogenase activity results in L-glyceric aciduria and hyperoxaluria and isolated D-glyceric aciduria also occurs (Fig. 4.16).

Primary hyperoxaluria Type 1: glycollic aciduria (McKusick 259900)

Primary hyperoxaluria Type 1 is a rare autosomal recessively inherited disorder in which patients present during the first decade of life with recurrent calcium oxalate nephrolithiasis. This is associated with progressive renal damage, renal failure, extrarenal oxalosis in tissues in which a high calcium flux occurs, heart block and death usually in the second decade of life. There is considerable variation in presentation ranging from a severe neonatal presentation with rapidly progressive oxalosis, renal failure and death, to a relatively mild form with less severe clinical manifestations.

Primary hyperoxaluria Type 1 is caused by deficient activity of peroxisomal alanine:glyoxylate aminotransferase (AGT).[102] The accumulating glyoxylate is oxidised via the action of lactate dehydrogenase to oxalate and reduced to glycollate by glyoxylate reductase. Alanine: glyoxylate aminotransferase, which has been shown to be identical with serine:pyruvate aminotransferase, occurs exclusively in the peroxisomes in human liver. A spectrum of residual activity of hepatic peroxisomal alanine:glyoxylate aminotransferase has been demonstrated in patients with primary hyperoxaluria Type 1, corresponding to the range of clinical presentation. In most patients with residual activity and CRM+ material present, activity is confined to peroxisomes, but two patients have also been identified in which AGT is absent from the peroxisomes but occurs abnormally in the mitochondria due to an intracellular signalling defect.[103] Location of the enzyme in the mitochondria prevents the AGT from fulfilling its normal metabolic function and results in clinical and biochemical manifestations of primary hyperoxaluria Type 1.

Several patients with primary hyperoxaluria Type 1 respond to pharmacological doses of pyridoxine (vitamin B_6), presumably due to activation of residual AGT or of alternative transaminases and these patients show a much more favourable prognosis, with reduced oxalate (and glycollate) excretion. Very high doses of pyridoxine may be of value even in the severe neonatal cases where there is no detectable residual AGT activity. Other methods of treatment have been directed towards increasing the solubility of the urinary oxalate, with increased fluid intake and magnesium oxide. Renal transplantation is universally unsuccessful. The most effective treatment for patients with pyridoxine-resistant hyperoxaluria is enzyme replacement therapy through liver transplantation. Hepatic transplantation is followed by an immediate reduction of urinary glycollate to normal levels, followed by a slower fall of urinary oxalate to normal as extrarenal stores of oxalate are solubilised.[101]

Primary hyperoxaluria Type 2: L-glyceric aciduria (McKusick 260000)

Several patients have been identified as having hyperoxaluria Type 2, which is caused by deficient activity of cytosolic D-glycerate dehydrogenase (Fig. 4.16). The enzyme deficiency results in the accumulation of 3-hydroxypyruvate with subsequent reduction of this intermediate, by lactate dehydrogenase, to L-glycerate. Glyoxylate reductase is identical with D-glycerate dehydrogenase,[104] and absence of the former enzyme activity results in accumulation of glyoxylate in the cytosol, with subsequent oxidation to oxalate. Thus the single enzyme deficiency results in the characteristic organic aciduria observed. Survival of these patients appears much better than those with Type 1 primary hyperoxaluria with patients surviving well into their fourth and fifth decades, despite excretion of amounts of urinary oxalate similar to those seen in patients with glycollic aciduria. This suggests that other factors may reduce extensive calcium oxalate deposition and retard both urinary stone formation and extrarenal oxalosis: it is possible that the large amount of L-glycerate excreted by these patients sequesters much of the available calcium as soluble calcium glycerate, reducing the formation of calcium oxalate.[101]

D-Glyceric aciduria (McKusick 220120)

Five patients with D-glyceric aciduria have been described, presenting with severe hypotonia, choreoathetosis and fits or with severe metabolic acidosis and retardation. Greatly increased concentrations of D-glyceric acid were found in urine in the absence of other abnormal organic aciduria.[105] The very rare disorder is probably caused by deficient activity of D-glycerate kinase.[106] The disorder is probably of autosomal recessive inheritance. (See also Chapter 2, p. 56)

DISORDERS OF GLUTAMIC ACID AND GAMMA-AMINO BUTYRIC ACID (GABA) METABOLISM

5-Oxo-L-prolinuria (Pyroglutamic aciduria) (McKusick 266130)

5-Oxo-L-prolinuria was first reported in a 19-year-old mentally subnormal man with cerebellar ataxia who excreted 24–35 g of pyroglutamic acid (5-oxoproline) per day, with increased concentrations in blood and cerebrospinal fluid. Several patients have now been described with the consistent features of a chronic metabolic acidosis of neonatal presentation and progressive haemolytic anaemia, with untreated patients showing psychomotor retardation and others dying within the first year of life with pronounced cerebellar damage. Pyroglutamic acid occurs as an intermediate in the γ-glutamyl pathway (Fig. 4.17), and in this disorder it accumulates as a result of a generalised deficiency of glutathione synthetase[107], due in part to increased synthesis of, and in part to loss of feedback inhibition of, γ-glutamyl synthetase. Increased pyroglutamate excretion may also occur as a secondary phenomenon in other organic acidurias associated with hyperammonaemia and from dietary sources[1]: diagnosis is dependent upon erythrocyte glutathione and glutathione synthetase determinations to avoid ambiguity. Treatment involves correction of the acidosis with bicarbonate and citrate. The disorder is of autosomal recessive inheritance.

Glutathione synthetase deficiency without pyroglutamic aciduria may occur in patients with haemolytic anaemia with an isolated enzyme deficiency in erythrocytes. Pyroglutamic aciduria without haemolytic anaemia or neurological abnormalities has been reported in two brothers with enterocolitis, calcium oxalate renal stones and 5-oxoprolinase deficiency in fibroblasts and leucocytes. However, 5-oxoprolinase deficiency has been observed in an asymptomatic adult[107] and the relationship of the enzyme deficiency to clinical symptoms remains unclear.

4-Hydroxybutyric aciduria (Succinic semialdehyde dehydrogenase deficiency) (McKusick 271980)

4-Hydroxybutyric aciduria has been reported in several patients with marked hypotonia, non-progressive ataxia, ocular dyspraxia and mental retardation, or with severe developmental delay.[108,109] Succinic semialdehyde excretion was also increased and study of lymphocytes showed the primary defect to be in succinic semialdehyde dehydrogenase, a key enzyme in 4-aminobutyric acid (GABA) metabolism. Other metabolites related to 4-hydroxybutyrate, including 3,4-dihydroxybutyrate (2-deoxytetronic acid), and glycollate are frequently elevated. A persistent dicarboxylic aciduria has been recorded in some patients. Blood glycine levels may also be increased.

Most attempts at treatment have been essentially unsuccessful but improvement in the cerebellar symptoms occurred over several years. More

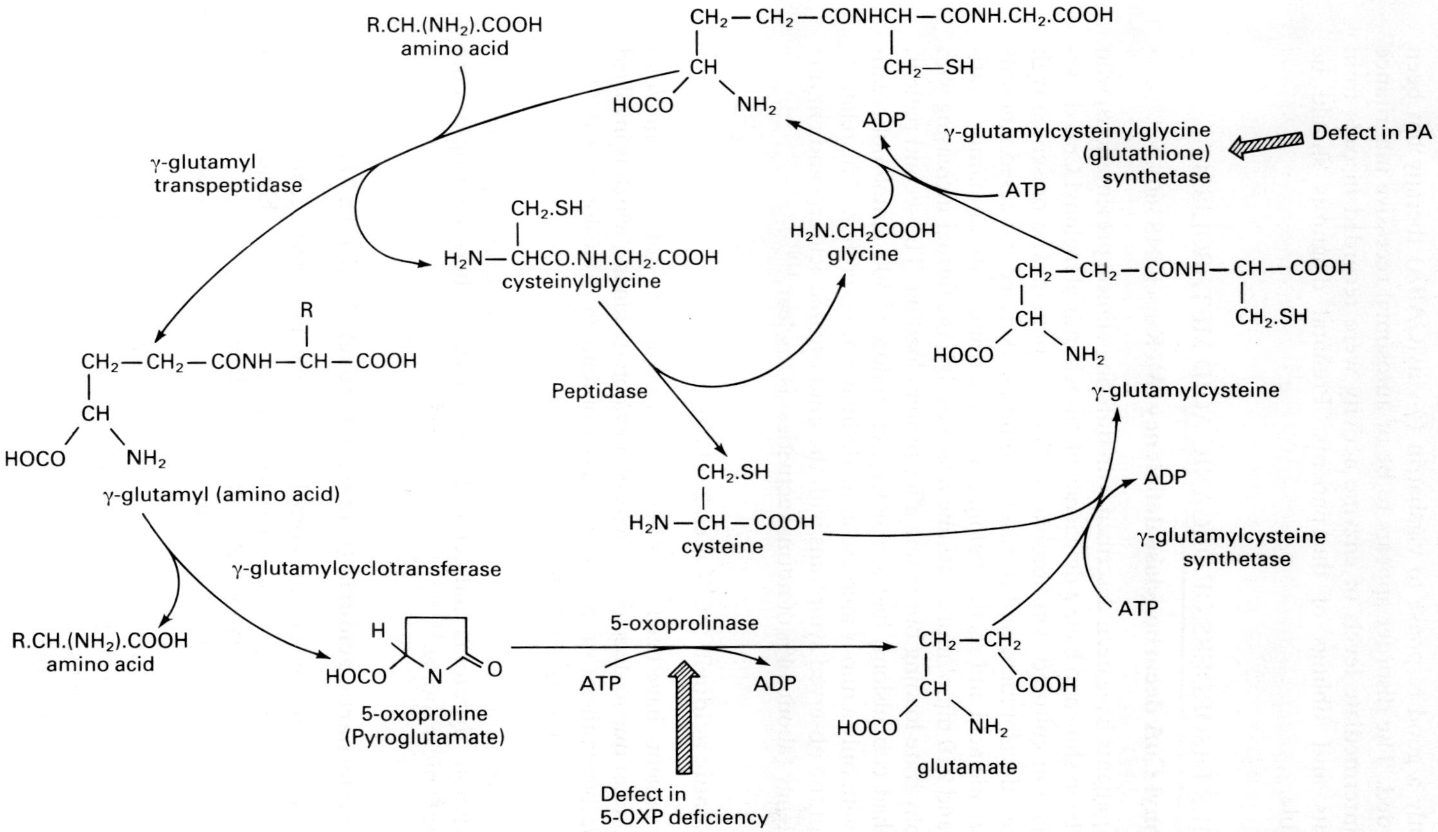

Fig. 4.17 The γ-glutamyl cycle, pyroglutamate and glutamate metabolism showing the positions of the defects in 5-oxoprolinuria (pyroglutamic aciduria) (PA) and 5-oxoprolidase deficiency (50XP).

recently a good response to vigabatrin (γ-vinylGABA) therapy has been recorded. The disorder appears to be of autosomal recessive inheritance and intermediate levels of enzyme activity were recorded in cells from parents and siblings of the patients. Prenatal diagnosis should be possible.

OTHER DISORDERS OF ORGANIC ACID METABOLISM

Malonyl CoA decarboxylase deficiency (McKusick 248360)

Two patients have been described with differing clinical presentations, who have been shown to have a deficiency of mitochondrial malonyl CoA decarboxylase in cultured skin fibroblasts. The first patient who presented with delayed development and persistent vomiting excreted increased amounts of malonic acid and methylmalonate into the urine (240 mmol/mol creatinine and 210 mmol/mol creatinine respectively), the former increasing with carbohydrate loading but falling after protein loading. The second patient, who had convulsions, had a malonate excretion of 308 mmol/mol creatinine with only a minor increase in methylmalonate excretion. The relationship of the observed symptoms with the mild organic aciduria and enzyme deficiency (about 14% of normal activities) is unclear.[110]

Mevalonic aciduria (McKusick 251170)

Four patients have been described with mevalonic aciduria (1–2 mol/mol creatinine) due to deficient activity of mevalonate kinase, which is involved in the biosynthesis of cholesterol and isoprenoids. Mevalonic acid (3,5-dihydroxy-3-methylvaleric acid) is formed from 3-hydroxy-3-methylglutaryl CoA by the action of 3-hydroxy-3-methylglutaryl CoA reductase. Patients present with a variety of symptoms, including severe psychomotor retardation, hypotonia and cerebellar ataxia with others showing a more severe clinical course.[111]

N-acetylaspartic aciduria (Canavan disease) (McKusick 271900)

Canavan disease is an autosomal recessively inherited leukodystrophy associated with hypotonia, spasticity, megalencephaly, blindness and severe mental retardation. Recently this disorder has been shown, in studies on more than 20 patients, to be characterised biochemically by N-acetylaspartic aciduria (500–4000 mmol/mol creatinine), caused by deficiency of aspartoacylase.[112,113] N-acetylaspartate concentrations are also elevated in blood plasma, CSF and brain. Pathologically, the disorder is characterised by spongy degeneration of the brain with hypodensity of white matter and demyelination. The enzyme deficiency is expressed in cultured skin fibroblasts, and prenatal diagnosis has been carried out using cultured amniocytes, chorionic villus material and by measurement of N-acetylaspartate in amniotic fluid.

REFERENCES

1. Chalmers R A, Lawson A M 1982 Organic acids in man. Analytical chemistry, biochemistry and diagnosis of the organic acidurias. Chapman and Hall, London
2. Chalmers R A 1989 Organic acids. In: Lawson A M (ed) Mass spectrometry. Walter de Gruyter, Berlin, ch 6, p 352–403
3. Sweetman L 1991 Organic acid analysis. In: Hommes F A (ed) Techniques in diagnostic human biochemical genetics. Wiley-Liss, New York, ch 11, p 143–176
4. Iles R A, Hind A J, Chalmers R A 1985 Use of proton nuclear magnetic resonance spectroscopy in detection and study of organic acidurias. Clinical Chemistry 31: 1795–1801
5. Davies S E C D, Iles R A, Stacey T E, de Sousa C, Chalmers R A 1991 Carnitine therapy and metabolism in the disorders of propionyl-CoA metabolism studied using ^{1}H-NMR spectroscopy. Clinica Chimica Acta 204:263–278
6. Saudubray J-M, Ogier H, Charpentier C et al 1984 Neonatal management of organic acidurias. Clinical update. Journal of Inherited Metabolic Disease 7 (Suppl 1):2–9
7. De Sousa C, Chalmers R A, Stacey T E, Tracey B M, Weaver C M, Bradley D 1986 The response to L-carnitine and glycine therapy in isovaleric acidaemia. European Journal of Pediatrics 144:451–456
8. Bain M D, Jones M, Boriello S P, Reed P J, Tracey B M, Chalmers R A, Stacey T E 1988 Contribution of gut bacterial metabolism to human metabolic disease. Lancet 1: 1078–1079
9. Thompson G N, Chalmers R A, Walter J H et al 1990 The use of metronidazole in management of methylmalonic and propionic acidaemias. European Journal of Paediatrics 149:792–796
10. Chalmers R A, Roe C R, Stacey T E, Hoppel C L 1984 Urinary excretion of L-carnitine and acyl-carnitines by patients with disorders of organic acid metabolism: evidence for secondary insufficiency of L-carnitine. Pediatric Research 18:1325–1328
11. Chalmers R A 1989 Current research in the organic acidurias. Journal of Inherited Metabolic Disease 12:225–239
12. Sweetman L 1984 Prenatal diagnosis of the organic acidurias. Journal of Inherited Metabolic Disease 7 (Suppl 1):18–22
13. Danner D J, Elsas L J 1989 In: Scriver C R, Beaudet A L, Sly W S, Valle D (eds) The metabolic basis of inherited disease, 6th edn. McGraw–Hill, New York, ch 22, p 671–692
14. Fisher C W, Chuang J L, Griffin T A, Lau K S, Cox R P, Chuang D T 1989 Molecular phenotypes in cultured maple syrup urine disease cells. Complete E1α cDNA sequence and mRNA and subunit contents of the human branched chain α-keto acid dehydrogenase complex. Journal of Biological Chemistry 264:3448–3453
15. Nobukini Y, Mitsubichi H, Endo F, Akaboshi I, Asaka J, Matsuda I 1990 Maple syrup urine disease. Complete primary structure of the E1β subunit of human branched chain α-ketoacid dehydrogenase complex deduced from the nucleotide sequence and a gene analysis of patients with this disease. Journal of Clinical Investigation 86:242–247
16. Nyhan W L 1984 Maple syrup urine disease. In: Nyhan W L (ed) Abnormalities in amino acid metabolism in clinical medicine. Appleton-Century-Crofts, Norwalk, Connecticut, ch 2, p 21–35
17. Sweetman L 1989 In: Scriver C R, Beaudet A L, Sly W S, Valle D (eds) The metabolic basis of inherited disease, 6th, edn. McGraw–Hill, New York, 28, p 791–819
18. Matsubara Y, Ito, Glassberg R, Satyabhama S, Ikeda Y, Tanaka K 1990 Nucleotide sequence of messenger RNA encoding human isovaleryl-coenzyme A dehydrogenase and its expression in isovaleric acidaemia fibroblasts. Journal of Clinical Investigation 85:1058–1064
19. Krieger I, Tanaka K 1976 Therapeutic effects of glycine in isovaleric acidaemia. Pediatric Research 10:25–29

20. Tsai M Y, Johnson D D, Sweetman L, Berry S A 1989 Two siblings with biotin resistant 3-methylcrotonyl-coenzyme A carboxylase deficiency. Journal of Pediatrics 115:110–113
21. Rolland M O, Divry P, Zabot M T, Guibaud P, Gomez S, Lachaux A, Loras I 1991 Isolated 3-methylcrotonyl-CoA carboxylase deficiency in a 16-month-old child. Journal of Inherited Metabolic Disease 14: 838–839
22. Haan E A, Scholem R D, Pitt J J, Wraith J E, Brown G K 1987 Episodes of severe metabolic acidosis in a patient with 3-methylglutaconic aciduria. European Journal of Pediatrics 146:484–488
23. Elpeleg O N, Meiron D, Barash V, Hurwitz Y, Tal I, Amir N 1990 3-methylglutaconic aciduria with persistent metabolic acidosis and 'uncoupling episodes'. Journal of Inherited Metabolic Disease 13:235–236
24. Nagasawa H, Yamaguchi S, Orii T, Schutgens R B H, Sweetman L, Hashimoto T 1989 Heterogeneity of defects in mitochondrial acetoacetyl-CoA thiolase biosynthesis in fibroblasts from four patients with 3-ketothiolase deficiency. Pediatric Research 26:145–149
25. De Groot C J, Luit-de Haan G, Hulstaert C E, Hommes F A 1977 A patient with severe neurological symptoms and acetoacetyl-CoA thiolase deficiency. Pediatric Research 11:1112–1116
26. Bennett M J, Hosking G P, Smith M F, Gray R G F, Middleton B 1984 Biochemical Investigations on a patient with a defect in cytosolic acetoacetyl-CoA thiolase, associated with mental retardation. Journal of Inherited Metabolic Disease 7:125–128
27. Tildon J T, Cornblath M 1972 Succinyl-CoA: 3-ketoacid CoA-transferase deficiency. A cause for ketoacidosis in infancy. Journal of Clinical Investigation 51:493–495
28. Brown G K, Hunt S M, Schlolem R et al 1982 β-Hydroxy-isobutyryl coenzyme A deacylase deficiency: A defect in valine metabolism associated with physical malformations. Pediatrics 70:532–538
29. Thompson G N, Walter J H, Bresson J-L et al 1990 Sources of propionate in inborn errors of propionated metabolism. Metabolism 39:1133–1137
30. Wolf B, Hsia Y E, Sweetman L, Gravel R, Harris D J, Nyhan W L 1981 Propionic acidaemia: A clinical update. Journal of Pediatrics 99:835–846
31. Brandänge S, Josephson S, Måhlen A, Mörch L 1984 Characterisation of the citrate synthetase reaction with propionyl CoA. Acta Chemica Scandinavica B38:695–700
32. Davies S E C, Chalmers R A, Iles R A 1987 Influences on the stereochemistry of citrate-synthase-catalysed methylcitrate formation. Biochemical Society Transactions 15:841–842
33. Lamhonwah A-M, Gravel R A 1987 Propionic acidemia: Absence of alpha-chain mRNA in fibroblasts from patients of the *pccA* complementation group. American Journal of Human Genetics 41:1124–1131
34. Rosenberg L E, Fenton W A 1989 In: Scriver C R, Beaudet A L, Sly W S, Valle D (eds) The metabolic basis of inherited disease, 6th edn. McGraw–Hill, New York, ch 29, p 821–844
35. Fenton W A, Rosenberg L E 1989 In: Scriver C R, Beaudet A L, Sly W S, Valle D (eds) The metabolic basis of inherited disease, 6th edn, McGraw–Hill, New York, ch 82, p 2065–2082
36. Chalmers R A, Bain M D, Mistry J, Tracey B M, Weaver C 1991 Enzymological studies on patients with methylmalonic aciduria: Basis for a clinical trial of deoxyadenosyl cobalamin in a hydroxocobalamin-unresponsive patient. Pediatric Research 30:560–563
37. Molteni K H, Oberley T D, Wolff J A, Friedman A L 1991 Progressive renal insufficiency in methylmalonic acidemia. Pediatric Nephrology 5:323–326
38. D'Angio C T, Dillon M J, Leonard J V 1991 Renal tubular dysfunction in methylmalonic acidaemia. European Journal of Pediatrics 150:259–263
39. Shih V E, Axel S M, Tewksbury J C, Watkins D, Cooper B A, Rosenblatt D S 1989 Defective lysosomal release of vitamin B_{12} (cblF): A hereditary cobalamin metabolic disorder associated with sudden death. American Journal of Medical Genetics 33:555–563
40. Watkins D, Rosenblatt D S 1989 Functional methionine synthase deficiency (cblE and cbIG): Clinical and biochemical heterogeneity. American Journal of Medical Genetics 34:427–434
41. Wolf B, Heard G S 1989 In: Scriver C R, Beaudet A L, Sly W S, Valle D (eds) The

metabolic basis of inherited disease, 6th edn. McGraw–Hill, New York, Ch 83, p 2083–2103
42. Chalmers R A, Lawson A M, Watts R W E 1974 Studies on the urinary acidic metabolites excreted by patients with β-methylcrotonylglycinuria, propionic acidaemia and methylmalonic acidaemia, using gas-liquid chromatography and mass spectrometry. Clinica Chimica Acta 52:43–51
43. Baumgartner E R, Suormala T M, Wick H et al. 1989 Biotinidase deficiency: A cause of subacute necrotizing encephalomyelopathy (Leigh syndrome). Report of a case with lethal outcome. Pediatric Research 26:260–266
44. Hanovar M, Janota I, Neville B G R, Chalmers R A 1992 Neuropathology of biotinidase deficiency. Acta Neuropathologica 84:461–464
45. Burri B J, Sweetman L, Nyhan W L 1981 Mutant holocarboxylase synthetase. Evidence for the enzyme defect in early infantile biotin-responsive multiple carboxylase deficiency. Journal of Clinical Investigation 68:1491–1495
46. Suormala T M, Baumgartner E R, Wick H, Scheibenreiter S, Schweitzer S 1990 Comparison of patients with complete and partial biotinidase deficiency: Biochemical studies. Journal of Inherited Metabolic Disease 13:76–92
47. Wolf B 1991 Worldwide survey of neonatal screening for biotinidase deficiency. Journal of Inherited Metabolic Disease 14:923–927
48. Amir N, Elpeleg O N, Shalev R S, Christensen E 1989 Glutaric aciduria type 1: Enzymatic and neurologic investigations of two kindreds. Journal of Pediatrics 114:983–989
49. Goodman S I, Frerman F E 1989 In: Scriver C R, Beaudet A L, Sly W S, Valle D (eds) The metabolic basis of inherited disease, 6th edn. McGraw–Hill, New York, ch 30, p 845–853
50. Hyman D B, Tanaka K 1984 Specific glutaryl-CoA dehydrogenating activity is deficient in cultured fibroblasts from glutaric aciduria patients. Journal of Clinical Investigation 73:778–784
51. Brandt N J, Gregersen N, Christensen E, Grøn I H, Rasmussen K 1979 Treatment of glutaryl CoA dehydrogenase deficiency (Glutaric aciduria) – Experience with diet, riboflavin and GABA analogues. Journal of Pediatrics 94:669–673
52. Francois B, Jaeken J, Gillis P 1990 Vigabatrin in the treatment of glutaric aciduria type I. Journal of Inherited Metabolic Disease 13:352–354
53. Schulz H 1990 Mitochondrial β-oxidation. In: Tanaka K, Coates P M (eds) Fatty acid oxidation. Clinical, biochemical and molecular aspects. Alan R Liss, New York, p 23–26
54. Stanley C A, Treem W R, Hale D E, Coates P M 1990 A genetic defect in carnitine transport causing primary carnitine deficiency. In: Tanaka K, Coates P M (eds) Fatty acid oxidation. Clinical, biochemical and molecular aspects. Alan R Liss, New York, p 457–464
55. Holton J B, Allen J T, Green C A, Partington S, Gilbert R E, Berry P J 1991 Inherited metabolic disease in the sudden infant death syndrome. Archives of Disease in Childhood 66:1315–1317
56. Roe C R, Coates P M 1989 In: Scriver C R, Beaudet A L, Sly W S, Valle D (eds) The metabolic basis of inherited disease, 6th edn. McGraw – Hill, New York, ch 33, p 889–914
57. Duran M, Bruinvis L, Ketting D, de Klerk J B C, Wadman S K 1988 *Cis*-4-decenoic acid in plasma: a characteristic metabolite in medium-chain acyl-CoA dehydrogenase deficiency. Clinical Chemistry 34:548–551
58. Ikeda Y, Hale D E, Keese S M, Coates P M, Tanaka K 1986 Biosynthesis of variant medium chain acyl-CoA dehydrogenase in cultured fibroblasts from patients with medium chain acyl-CoA dehydrogenase deficiency. Pediatric Research 20:843–847
59. Yokota I, Indo Y, Coates P M, Tanaka K 1990 Molecular basis of medium chain acyl-coenzyme A dehydrogenase deficiency. An A to G transition at position 985 that causes a lysine-304 to glutamate substitution in the mature protein is the single prevalent mutation. Journal of Clinical Investigation 86:1000–1003
60. Kelly D P, Whelan A J, Ogden M L et al 1990 Molecular characterization of inherited medium-chain acyl-CoA dehydrogenase deficiency. Proceedings of the National Academy of Sciences USA 87:9236–9240
61. Gregersen N, Andresen B S, Bross P et al 1991 Characterization of a disease-causing

Lys329 to Glu mutation in 16 patients with medium-chain acyl-CoA dehydrogenase deficiency. Journal of Inherited Metabolic Disease 14:314–316
62. Coates P M, Tanaka K and various authors 1992 In: Proceedings of the Second International Symposium on Fatty Acid Oxidation: Clinical, biochemical and molecular aspects, Philadelphia, November 3–6, 1991, Wiley–Liss, New York, in press
63. Hale D E, Stanley C A, Coates P M 1990 The long-chain acyl CoA dehydrogenase deficiency In: Tanaka K, Coates P M (eds) Fatty acid oxidation. Clinical, biochemical and molecular aspects. Alan R Liss, New York, p 303–311
64. Lehnert W, Wendel U, Lindenmaier, Böhm N 1982 Multiple acyl-CoA dehydrogenation deficiency (Glutaric aciduria type II), congenital polycystic kidneys, and symmetric warty dysplasia of the cerebral cortex in two brothers I: Clinical, metabolical, and biochemical findings. European Journal of Pediatrics 139:56–59
65. Böhm N, Uy J, Kiessling M, Lehnert W 1982 Multiple acyl-CoA dehydrogenation deficiency (Glutaric aciduria type II), congenital polycystic kidneys, and symmetric warty dysplasia of the cerebral cortex in two newborn brothers II: Morphology and pathogenesis. European Journal of Pediatrics 139:60–65
66. Harpey J-P, Charpentier C, Goodman S I, Darbois Y, Lefèbre G, Sebbah J 1983 Multiple acyl-CoA dehydrogenase deficiency occurring in pregnancy and caused by a defect in riboflavin metabolism in the mother. Journal of Pediatrics 103:394–398
67. Finocchiaro G, Ikeda Y, Ito M, Tanaka K 1990 Biosynthesis, molecular cloning and sequencing of electron transfer flavoprotein. In: Tanaka K, Coates P M (eds) Fatty acid oxidation. Clinical, biochemical and molecular aspects. Alan R Liss, New York, p 637–652
68. Mandel H, Africk D, Blitzer M, Shapira E 1988 The importance of recognizing secondary carnitine deficiency in organic acidaemias: Case report in glutaric acidaemia type II. Journal of Inherited Metabolic Disease 11:397–402
69. Chalmers R A, Tracey B M, King G S et al 1985 The prenatal diagnosis of glutaric aciduria type II, using quantitative GC-MS. Journal of Inherited Metabolic Disease 8 Suppl 2:145–146
70. Pollitt R J 1990 Clinical and biochemical presentations in 20 cases of hydroxydicarboxylic aciduria. In: Tanaka K, Coates P M (eds) Fatty acid oxidation. Clinical, biochemical and molecular aspects. Alan R Liss, New York, p 495–502
71. Tracey B M, Cheng K N, Rosankiewiczs J, Stacey T E, Chalmers R A 1988 Urinary C6–C12 dicarboxylic acylcarnitines in Reye's syndrome. Clinica Chimica Acta 175:79–88
72. Rocchiccioli R, Wanders R J A, Aubourg P et al 1990 Deficiency of long-chain 3-hydroxyacyl-CoA dehydrogenase: A cause of lethal myopathy and cardiomyopathy in early childhood. Pediatric Research 28:657–662
73. Przyrembel H, Jakobs C, Ijlst L, de Klerk J B C, Wanders R J A 1991 Long-chain 3-hydroxyacyl-CoA dehydrogenase deficiency. Journal of Inherited Metabolic Disease 14:674–680
74. Stacey T E, de Sousa C, Tracey B M et al 1985 Dizygotic twins with 3-hydroxy-3-methylglutaric aciduria; unusual presentation, family studies and dietary management. European Journal of Pediatrics 144:177–181
75. Gibson K M, Breuer J, Nyhan W L 1988 3-Hydroxy-3-methyl glutaryl-coenzyme A lyase deficiency: review of 18 reported patients. European Journal of Pediatrics 148:180–186
76. Ozand P T, Al Aqeel A, Gascon G, Thomas E, Gleispach H 1991 3-Hydroxy-3-methylglutaryl-coenzyme A (HMG-CoA) lyase deficiency in Saudi Arabia. Journal of Inherited Metabolic Disease 14:174–188
77. Chalmers R A, Tracey B M, Stacey T E, Cheng K N, Madigan M J, Lawson A M 1986 The use of fast atom bombardment mass spectrometry to identify and study urinary acylcarnitines in disorders of organic acid metabolism. Biochemical Society Transactions 14:967–969
78. Thompson G N, Chalmers R A, Halliday D 1990 The contribution of protein catabolism to metabolic decompensation in 3-hydroxy-3-methylglutaric aciduria. European Journal of Pediatrics 149:346–350
79. Goldsmith L A, Kang E, Beinfang D C, Jimbow K, Gerald P, Baden H P 1973 Tyrosinemia with planter and palmar keratosis and keratitis. Journal of Pediatrics 83:798–805

80. Giardini O, Cantani A, Kennaway N G, D'Eufemia P 1983 Chronic typosinemia associated with 4-hydroxyphenylpyruvate dioxygenase deficiency with acute intermittent ataxia and without visceral and bone involvement. Pediatric Research 17:25–29
81. Endo, F, Kitano A, Uehara I et al 1983 4-hydroxyphenyl pyruvic acid oxidase deficiency with normal fumaryl acetoacetase: a new variant form of hereditary hypertyrosinemia. Pediatric Research 17:92–96
82. Kvittingen E A 1991 Tyrosinaemia type I – an update. Journal of Inherited Metabolic Disease 14:554–562
83. Mitchell G, Larochelle J, Lambert M et al 1990 Neurologic crises in hereditary tyrosinemia. New England Journal of Medicine 322:432–437
84. Flye M W, Riely C A, Hainline B E et al 1990 The effects of early treatment of hereditary tyrosinaemia type I in infancy by orthotopic liver transplantation. Transplantation 49:916–921
85. Kvittingen E A, Rootwelt H, van Dam T, van Faassen H, Berger R 1992 Hereditary tyrosinaemia type I: Lack of correlation between clinical findings and amount of immunoreactive fumarylacetoacetase protein. Pediatric Research 31:43–46
86. Robinson B H 1989 Lactic acidemia. In: Scriver C R, Beaudet A L, Sly W S, Valle D (eds) The metabolic basis of inherited disease, 6th edn, McGraw–Hill, New York, ch 32, p 869–888
87. Munnich A, Saudubray J-M, Taylor J et al 1982 Congenital lactic acidosis, α-ketoglutaric aciduria and variant form of maple syrup urine disease due to a single enzyme defect: Dihydrolipoyl dehydrogenase deficiency. Acta Paediatrica Scandinavica 71:167–171
88. Chalmers R A 1984 Organic acids in urine of patients with congenital lactic acidoses: An aid to differential diagnosis. Journal of Inherited Metabolic Disease 7 Suppl 1:79–89
89. Robinson B H, MacKay N, Petrova-Benedict R, Ozalp I, Coskun T, Stacpoole P W 1990 Defects in the E2 lipoyl transacetylase and the X-lipoyl-containing component of the pyruvate dehydrogenase complex in patients with lactic acidemia. Journal of Clinical Investigation 85:1821–1824
90. Brown G K, Haan E A, Kirby D M et al 1988 'Cerebral' lactic acidosis: defects in pyruvate metabolism with profound brain damage and minimal systemic acidosis. European Journal of Pediatrics 147:10–14
91. Robinson B H, Chun K, MacKay N, Otulakowski G, Petrova-Benedict R, Willard H 1989 Isolated and combined deficiencies of the α-keto dehydrogenase complexes. Annals of the New York Academy of Sciences 573:337–346
92. Hansen L L, Brown G K, Kirby D M, Dahl H-H M 1991 Characterization of the mutations in three patients with pyruvate dehydrogenase E1α deficiency. Journal of Inherited Metabolic Disease 14:140–151
93. De Meirleir L J, Lissens W, Vamos E, Liebaers I 1991 Pyruvate dehydrogenase deficiency due to a mutation of the E1α subunit. Journal of Inherited Metabolic Disease 14:301–304
94. Endo H, Miyabayashi S, Tada K, Narisawa K 1991 A four-nucleotide insertion at the E1α gene in a patient with pyruvate dehydrogenase deficiency. Journal of Inherited Metabolic Disease 14:793–799
95. Byrd D J, Krohn H-P, Winkler L et al 1989 Neonatal pyruvate dehydrogenase deficiency with lipoate responsive lactic acidaemia and hyperammonaemia. European Journal of Pediatrics 148:543–547
96. Van Biervliet J P G M, Bruinvis L et al 1977 Report of a patient with severe, chronic lactic acidaemia and pyruvate carboxylase deficiency. Developmental Medicine and Child Neurology 19:392–401
97. Zinn A B, Kerr D S, Hoppel C L 1986 Fumarase deficiency: a new cause of mitochondrial encephalomyopathy. New England Journal of Medicine 315:469–475
98. Petrova-Benedict R, Robinson B H, Stacey T E, Mistry J, Chalmers R A 1987 Deficient fumarase activity in an infant with fumaricacidemia and its distribution between the different forms of the enzyme seen on isoelectric focusing. American Journal of Human Genetics 40:257–266
99. Walker V, Mills G A, Hall M A, Millward-Sadler G H, English N R, Chalmers R A 1989 A fourth case of fumarase deficiency. Journal of Inherited Metabolic Disease 12:331–332

100. Gellera C, Uziel G, Rimoldi M et al 1990 Fumarase deficiency is an autosomal recessive encephalopathy affecting both the mitochondrial and cytosolic enzymes. Neurology 40:495–499
101. Chalmers R A, Purkiss P 1991 Oxalic acid in plasma and urine. In: Hommes F A (ed) Techniques in diagnostic human biochemical genetics. Wiley-Liss, New York, ch 23, p 359–376
102. Danpure C J, Jennings P R, Watts R W E 1987 Enzymological diagnosis of primary hyperoxaluria type 1 by measurement of hepatic alanine:glyoxylate aminotransferase activity. Lancet 1:289–291
103. Danpure C J, Cooper P J, Wise P J, Jennings P R 1989 An enzyme trafficking defect in two patients with primary hyperoxaluria type 1: Peroxisomal alanine/glyoxylate aminotransferase rerouted to mitochondria. Journal of Cell Biology 108:1345–1352
104. Mistry J, Danpure C J, Chalmers R A 1988 Hepatic D-glycerate dehydrogenase and glyoxylate reductase deficiency in primary hyperoxaluria type 2. Biochemical Society Transactions 16:626–627
105. Fontaine M, Porchet N, Largilliere C et al 1989 Biochemical contribution to diagnosis and study of a new case of D-glyceric acidemia/aciduria. Clinical Chemistry 35:2148–2151
106. Van Schaftingen E 1989 D-Glycerate kinase deficiency as a cause of D-glyceric aciduria. FEBS Letters 243:127–131
107. Meister A, Larsson A 1989 Glutathione synthase deficiency and other disorders of the γ-glutamyl cycle. In: Scriver C R, Beaudet A L, Sly W S, Valle D (eds) The metabolic basis of inherited disease, 6th edn, McGraw–Hill, New York, ch 31, p 855–868
108. Onkenhout W, Maaswinkel-Mooij P D, Poorthuis B J H M 1989 4-hydroxybutyric aciduria: further clinical heterogeneity in a new case. European Journal of Pediatrics 149:194–196
109. Gibson K I, Goodman S I, Frerman F E, Glasgow A M 1989 Succinic semialdehyde dehydrogenase deficiency associated with combined 4-hydroxybutyric and dicarboxylic acidurias: Potential for clinical misdiagnosis based on urinary organic acid profiling. Journal of Pediatrics 114:607–610
110. Brown G K, Scholem R D, Bankier A, Danks D M 1984 Malonyl coenzyme A decarboxylase deficiency. Journal of Inherited Metabolic Disease 7:21–26
111. Gibson K M, Hoffmann G, Nyhan W L et al 1989 Mevalonate kinase deficiency in a child with cerebellar ataxia, hypotonia and mevalonic aciduria. European Journal of Pediatrics 148:250–252
112. Matalon R, Michals K, Sebesta D, Deanching M, Gashkoff P, Casanova J 1988 Aspartoacylase deficiency and N-acetylaspartic aciduria in patients with Canavan disease. American Journal of Medical Genetics 29:463–471
113. Matalon R, Kaul R, Casanova J et al 1989 Aspartoacylase deficiency: The enzyme defect in Canavan disease. Journal of Inherited Metabolic Disease 12 Suppl 2:329–331

5. Lysosomal storage disorders

C. A. Pennock

INTRODUCTION

Lysosomes are intracellular cytoplasmic particles containing many acid hydrolases able to digest a wide range of macromolecules.[1] These enzymes are retained within a tripartite impermeable membrane in most primary lysosomes (those which are not actively digesting macromolecular material). These primary lysosomes are formed from endocytic vesicles which become true lysosomes when enzymes are incorporated. There is considerable evidence now that the enzymes are transferred to the lysosomes and taken up by adsorptive pinocytosis and some of these hydrolases are identified by the presence of mannose-6-phosphate which is attached to the enzyme and acts as a recognition marker.[2] A disease entity is known in which there is failure of this uptake, resulting in abnormal catabolism of several different types of macromolecule due to multiple hydrolase deficiency. The condition is known as inclusion cell (I-cell) disease and will be discussed later. Lysosomes which have taken up their enzymes and macromolecules are usually called secondary lysosomes.

The material digested by lysosomes is either exogenous material taken up by endocytosis or is endogenous material separated from other intracellular materials by autophagy. Sometimes lysosomal hydrolases are excreted by exocytosis to degrade extracellular molecules. It has long been known that lysosomes degrade chondromucoprotein and the proteoglycans of cartilage in this way. The wide range of hydrolases in normal lysosomes provides great opportunity for genetic abnormality which can lead to the accumulation or storage of macromolecules which have not been appropriately digested on account of an inadequate or absent enzyme.[3]

There are many ways in which a lysosomal storage disease may occur. The commonest of these is failure of a gene to produce adequate levels of an active enzyme, or the production of an enzyme showing only partial activity due to altered kinetics. Other possibilities include failure to incorporate the enzyme into the lysosome because of failure of lysosomal transport. This might arise because the enzyme recognition marker has not been synthesised or has not been exposed by a specific enzymatic process as well as owing to a primary defect in the receptor protein. It is also possible for an enzyme to undergo premature proteolysis before adequate lysosomal uptake can occur. Alternatively, there may be a mutation of the primary enzyme which, while not affecting its potential activity, affects that portion of the molecule which identifies it as an enzyme destined for lysosomal uptake and thus a substrate for the phosphorylating enzyme. An example of the latter has already been noted as a rare form of GM_2 gangliosidosis (Tay Sachs disease). Lysosomal storage disorders may also arise from defects in specific transporters located in the lysosomal membrane, resulting in failure of egress of metabolites produced within the lysosome (cystinosis, sialic acid storage disease).

Observation and investigation of the lysosomal storage disorders has, in a relatively short space of time, taken us through almost all of the phases in our understanding of inherited metabolic disease as outlined by O'Brien.[4] Careful clinical delineation and classification has been followed by absolute identity of the mode of inheritance and, in some instances, discovery of information about the chromosome on which the abnormal gene is located. Chemical analysis of accumulated or excreted metabolites has suggested the possible metabolic block which has been confirmed sometimes in a most elegant fashion using complementation studies in tissue culture. The actual enzyme involved in most of these disorders has been identified and in many cases its physical characteristics have been described. Such has been the progress in our understanding of this group of disorders that we are now able to offer sound genetic advice, carrier detection and prenatal diagnosis of the affected fetus in most of these rare, but sadly progressive, afflictions of the human body and mind.

All that is not to say that much remains to be done. Classification of these disorders (discussed later) in many ways remains cumbersome, not least because some enzyme defects may result in accumulation of more than one type of macromolecule. The latter also leads to problems of differential diagnosis based on clinical presentation which is made worse by the considerable genetic heterogeneity of phenotypic expression seen throughout the lysosomal storage diseases. O'Brien's concept of one gene–one enzyme– many substrates model for metabolic disorders is amply illustrated.[4]

Their rarity means that most physicians will not have seen enough of them to be able to suggest a possible clinical diagnosis with ease, and the chemist will be confronted with a multitude of problems of methodology which precludes a wide-ranging screening approach to assist the clinician. Prenatal diagnosis and termination of affected pregnancies is not necessarily an ethically acceptable approach to either treatment or abnormal gene eradication, and errors of diagnosis can still be made with ease by the unwary or inexperienced. Current attempts at treatment are fraught with difficulty, either because the diagnosis has been made too late to reverse some of the handicap or because possible treatment regimes are potentially lethal in their own right. In spite of enthusiasm for treatment by bone marrow transplantation[5,6] these disorders will remain largely untreatable until methods have been devised in animal models to target DNA specific to the enzyme deficiency into haematopoeitic stem cells.[7]

DEFECTS IN THE LYSOSOMAL STORAGE DISEASES

The majority of the currently known lysosomal storage diseases have now been shown to arise from defects in enzymes which are sugar hydrolases responsible for degradation of complex carbohydrate sequences attached to glycoproteins, glycosaminoglycans and glycolipids.

Glycoproteins, as the term implies, are proteins with carbohydrates attached. Strictly speaking, the glycosaminoglycans involved in lysosomal disorders are also glycoproteins in the sense that they are carbohydrate polymers usually attached to protein and usually called proteoglycans. The old term mucopolysaccharide is only retained in the description of the disease affecting such polymers – mucopolysaccharidoses. The term glycolipid, replacing older terms which include mucolipid, designates molecules with carbohydrate attached to a lipid moiety such as ceramide. Thus all of these compounds have one thing in common – a carbohydrate portion attached to protein or lipid – and they may be classified under the general term of glycoconjugates.

There has been a dramatic increase in our knowledge of complex carbohydrate (glycoconjugate) synthesis and catabolism[8] and it is inevitable that many other inheritable disorders affecting metabolism of these macromolecules will be described in the years ahead. Of the many possible glycoconjugate structures already known, some relatively common examples are illustrated in the following classification.

Glycolipids

Galactosyl or glucosyl linkage to ceramide is common to the sphingolipids, globosides, gangliosides and lipid sulphates, all of which may be regarded as glycolipids. Degradation of these substances ultimately results in release of individual sugars and ceramide along the lines shown in the simplistic overview in Figure 5.1 which also identifies the site of the defect for lysosomal glycolipid disorders described later in this chapter.

The lipid moiety is a long-chain amino-alcohol base to which one of a variety of carboxylic acids of variable chain length (C_{16}–C_{26}) is attached via an amide bond. The trivial name of ceramide has been used for structures of this type in Figure 5.1 but represents a gross oversimplification. Other glycoceramides and cholesteryl esters involved in lipid metabolism may be involved in lysosomal storage disease.

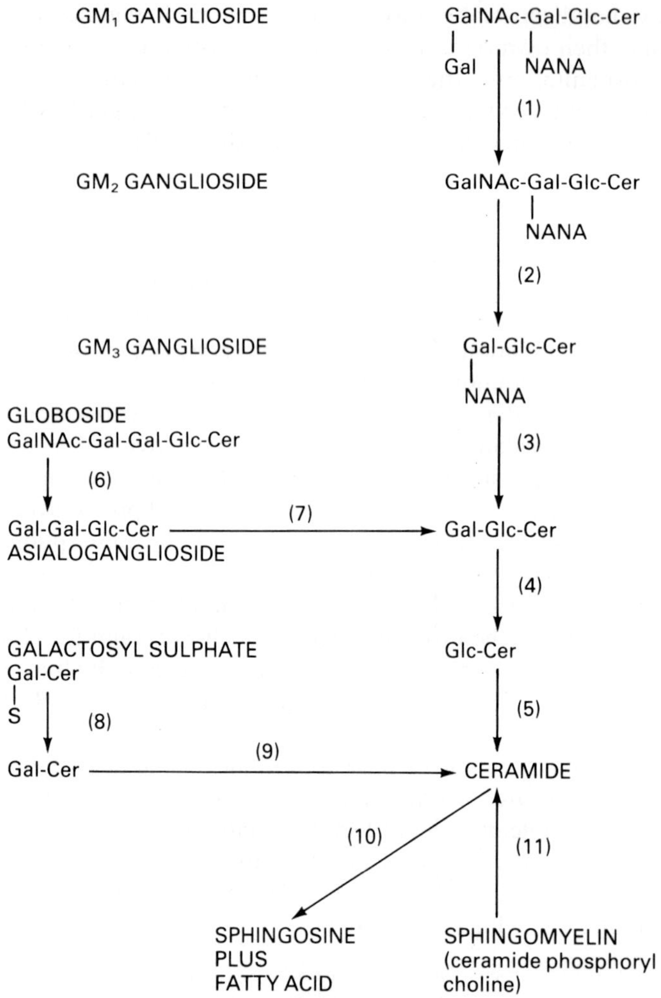

Fig. 5.1 Simplified view of the interrelationships of ceramide glycoconjugates and lysosomal storage disease. Gal – galactose, Glc – glucose, GalNac – N-acetylgalactosamine, NANA – N-acetylneuraminic acid, Cer – ceramide, S – sulphate. Numbers in parentheses identify the sites of defects giving rise to lysosomal glycolipid disorders, see Table 5.3.

Glycosaminoglycans

Glycosaminoglycans (GAG, or mucopolysaccharides) are the major polymers of the ground substance of connective tissue and are high molecular weight polymers of repeating dimers of an amino sugar usually linked to a hexuronic acid.[9] The amino sugar is usually glucosamine or galactosamine both of which are usually acetylated or sulphated at the amino group and both of which may be sulphated at either carbon-4 or -6 of the hexose ring. The hexuronic acid is either glucuronic acid or its C5 epimer, iduronic acid. These may also be sulphated at their carboxyl group in the most complex of these compounds or, more rarely, O-sulphated at C2. GAG molecules, with the exception of hyaluronic acid, are usually linked in a comb-like structure to a protein core through a short neutral carbohydrate region (usually galactosyl-galactosyl-xylose) linked to serine or threonine. Keratan sulphate is unusual in having galactose instead of a hexuronic acid and it may also contain small amounts of fucose and mannose. The principal features of these structures are summarised in Table 5.1. Heparan and dermatan sulphate figure prominently as accumulated molecules in the group of disorders called mucopolysaccharidoses while keratan sulphate accumulates in only one of these conditions although it may also be found in some other lysosomal disorders.

Glycoproteins

The sugar fraction of glycoproteins may represent anything from 1 to 85% of a molecule with N-acetyl-D-glucosamine, D-galactose, N-acetyl-D-galactosamine, D-mannose, L-fucose and sialic acid as the principal sugars present.[8] N-acetyl glucosamine linked to the amide nitrogen of asparagine is the most common linkage of carbohydrate to protein in serum glycoproteins. N-acetyl-galactosamine is linked to the hydroxyl group of serine or threonine in proteoglycans, blood group substances and mucins and galactose is linked to hydroxylysine in collagen.

Lysosomal degradation of glycoprotein occurs in three stages, with the protein core being digested by proteases to leave a glycopeptide from which the oligosaccharide is released by the action of N-aspartyl-β-glucosaminidase, before further degradation into the constituent sugars by exoglycosidases which sequentially remove single monosaccharides from the non-reducing end of the chain. These lysosomal enzymes are synthesised in the form of proenzymes which are phosphorylated before transfer to the lysosome by which they are taken up by specific receptors in the lysosomal membrane, which recognises mannose-6-phosphate as the enzyme marker. Some enzymes may be produced in a high molecular weight form which undergoes partial proteolytic digestion after incorporation into the lysosome thus releasing its active form.

Three principal groups of carbohydrate structure are found in glycoproteins[8]:

1. High mannose structures

```
                           M-M-M         Asn = asparagine
                           |          GlcNAc = N-Acetyl
e.g. Asn-GlcNAc-GlcNAc — M                     glucosamine
                           |
                           M-M-M           M = mannose
                           |
                           M-M
```

Table 5.1 Structure and nomenclature of glycosaminoglycans (GAG), formerly called acid mucopolysaccharides (MPS). GlcA – glucuronic acid, IdA – iduronic acid, Gal – galactose, GlcNS – N-sulphated glucosamine, GlcN – glucosamine, GlcNAc – N-acetylglucosamine, GalNac – N-acetylgalactosamine

Current nomenclature	Previous nomenclature	Abbreviation	Hexuronic acid	Hexosamine	Sulphate link	Sulphate
Hyaluronic acid	Hyaluronic acid	HA	GlcA	GlcNAc	O	C–6 GlcNAc
Chondroitin-4-sulphate	Chondroitin sulphate A	C4S	GlcA	GalNAc	O	C–4 GalNAc
Chondroitin-6-sulphate	Chondroitin sulphate C	C6S	GlcA	GalNAc	O	C–6 GalNAc
Dermatan sulphate	Chondroitin sulphate B	DS	IdA and GlcA	GalNAc	O	C–4 GalNAc
Keratan sulphate	Keratosulphate	KS	None; Gal instead	GlcNAc	O	C–6 GlcNAc
Heparin Heparan sulphate	Heparin Heparitin sulphate	Hep } HS }	IdA and GlcA	GlcNAc GlcNS	O and N	C–2 IdA C–6 GlcNAc N–S GlcN

The above structure, often referred to as M9, has been isolated from Chinese hamster ovary. Variants with 5–9 mannose residues are widespread and the majority of the lysosomal enzymes are also glycoproteins of the high mannose type in which some of the mannose residues are phosphorylated to create a recognition marker which enables them to be targeted to the lysosome.

2. Intermediate structures

```
    F                  M-GlcNAc         F = fucose
    |                  |              Gal = galactose

Asn-GlcNAc-GlcNAc — M
                       |
                       M-GlcNAc-Gal
```

These are found in human immunoglobulin IgG. Note that several lysosomal enzymes are required for degradation, namely a galactosidase, glucosaminidase, mannosidase, fucosidase and aspartylglucosaminidase. The outer ends of the chain may also be sialylated and a sialidase will be required for degradation. All of these enzymes have been implicated in lysosomal storage disease and a hypothetical model of such a glycoprotein is shown in Figure 5.2 to illustrate these possible disorders.

3. Complex structures: in these the intermediate structure, or variants of it are identifiable in which the carbohydrate chain is complex, usually mannose-free and linked to the protein core through N-acetylgalactosamine α-linked to serine or threonine. Many anomalous sequences have also been identified which are not consistent with our current knowledge of complex carbohydrate synthesis. Others are specific to certain types of macromolecule such as the Ser-Xyl-Gal-Gal-GlcNAc linkage sequence found in proteoglycans, and the hydroxyproline-galactose portions of collagen.

In addition to these, mucin sequences are identifiable in which the carbohydrate chain is complex, usually mannose-free and linked to the protein core through N-acetylgalactosamine α-linked to serine or threonine rather than N-linked. Less is known about degradative pathways of these O-linked chains than about the N-linked glycoproteins referred to above.

CLASSIFICATION OF LYSOSOMAL DISEASE

Classification of the lysosomal storage disorders is somewhat confused. Some attempts have been made to overcome these problems[10] but we are still left with a strange mixture of titles sometimes eponymous, sometimes based on the enzyme that is absent and sometimes, as in the case of mucopolysaccharidoses, numerical. None of these approaches is perfect

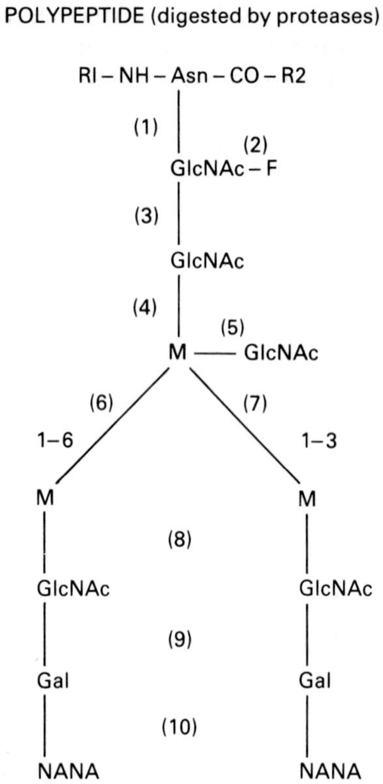

Fig. 5.2 Hypothetical degradation of a complex glycoprotein. Asn – asparagine, GlcNAc – N-acetylglucosamine, F – fucose, M – mannose Gal – galactose, NANA – N acetylneuraminic acid. Lysosomal storage diseases are known which affect each of the sugar hydrolases shown: (1) β-aspartylglucosaminidase; (2) α-1–6 fucosidase; (3) β-1–4 endohexosaminidase; (4) β-1–4 mannosidase; (5) β-1–4 hexosaminidase; (6) α-1–6 mannosidase: (7) α-1–3 mannosidase; (8) β-1–2 hexosaminidase; (9) β-1–4 galactosidase; (10) α-2–6 neuraminidase (sialidase).

and the difficulties are compounded by the heterogeneity of the phenotypic expression of what appears to be the same enzyme defect. Such heterogeneity may even occur within the same family. Disorders of β-galactosidase activity, for example, range from an infantile generalised ganglioside storage disorder, with late infantile and adult forms of milder presentation, through to a bone dysplasia of the Morquio type. Deficiencies of β-galactosidase may thus be classified as gangliosidoses, oligosaccharidoses, or mucopolysaccharidoses dependent on the major stored or excreted metabolite.[11] In the following account lysosomal disorders are assigned to groups which seems most appropriate in the light of our current knowledge but which will change as our understanding evolves. Only the more common conditions in each group are discussed in detail and description of the rare conditions such as I-cell disease is only made where it introduces new concepts or aids our understanding of the more common problems.

Glycogenosis II has been singled out as it does not fit into the above classification. Cystinosis and sialic acid storage disease are part of a heterogeneous group of lysosomal transport defects. The term mucolipidosis has not been used since a mucolipid is not a defined chemical compound and in many of these disorders storage of mucopolysaccharide or lipid does not occur. Some have been classified as oligosaccharidoses as proposed by Leroy in 1982.[11] The same argument has been applied to the so called glycoproteinoses[12] where the defect affects the carbohydrate portion rather than the protein moiety, resulting in oligosaccharide accumulation and excretion. These have also been grouped under oligosaccharidoses. The currently known lysosomal disorders are summarised in Table 5.2.

GENETICS

All of the lysosomal storage disorders are inherited in an autosomal recessive fashion with the exception of Hunter syndrome and Fabry disease which are X-linked disorders.[13] The majority are rare with less than 50 patients having been described in the current medical literature. Some have a predilection for certain ethnic groups. Glycolipid disorders are relatively common among Aschkenazic Jews of whom about 4% are carriers for Tay Sachs disease, 1% carriers for Niemann–Pick disease (Type A) and 0.04% for Gaucher disease. The majority of patients with aspartylglucosaminuria have been found in Finland, although the incidence is still rare. In some conditions, such as Maroteaux–Lamy syndrome, the incidence is unknown while in others failure of biochemical recognition and diagnosis may produce a falsely low apparent incidence. Incorrect diagnosis is especially a problem in Morquio disease which may be readily confused with a wide range of other hereditary bone dysplasias, especially in adults where urinary excretion of keratan sulphate, a glycosaminoglycan which accumulates and is excreted in younger patients with the disease, may be undetectable.

The most likely conditions to be seen in Europe and North America have a pan-ethnic distribution and a birth incidence of 1:100 000 or less and include Hurler and Sanfilippo syndrome and the metachromatic leukodystrophies. The commonest of these, Sanfilippo syndrome, may be especially difficult to diagnose[14] since affected individuals may appear to be physically normal, the skeletal defects of the disease may be minimal and progression of the mental handicap may be slow. Families may have had more than one affected child before a diagnosis is made and it may be too late to give genetic advice.

Consistent with the possession of half the normal gene dose, the other half being the abnormal gene, the majority of heterozygous or hemizygous

Table 5.2 Lysosomal storage disorders

Disorder	Synonym or eponym	McKusick number[13]	Enzyme defect	Principal storage material	Comments
Glycogenosis I	Pompe disease	232300	α 1–4 Glucosidase (acid maltase)	Glycogen α 1-4 linked oligosaccharides	Infantile childhood and adult forms exist
Gaucher disease					
Type I	Non-cerebral juvenile Gaucher	230800	Glucocerebrosidase	Glucosylceramide	Lipid-laden Gaucher cells are found in bone marrow.
Type II	Infantile cerebral	230900			
Type III	Juvenile or adult Gaucher	231000			
Sphingomyelin lipidosis	Niemann–Pick disease. (Types A,B,C)	257200 257220	Sphingomyelinase	Sphingomyelin	Typical lipid-laden foam cells are found in the marrow
Sphingomyelin lipidosis	Niemann-Pick disease (Nova Scotia NP) (Type D)	257250	Not known	Sphingomyelin	
Galactosyl-ceramide lipidosis	Krabbe disease, globoid cell leuko dystrophy	245200	Galactocerebroside-β-galactosidase	Galactocerebroside and its derivatives	
α-Galactosidase deficiency	Fabry disease Angiokeratoma corporis diffusum	301500	α-Galactosidase	Globosides	Sex-linked inheritance
GM_1 gangliosidosis					
Type I	Generalized	230500	β-Galactosidase	GM_1 gangliosides *keratan sulphate *galactosyl-oligosaccharides	See also MPS IV B
Type II	Juvenile				
Type III	Adult				
GM_2 gangliosidosis					
Type I	Tay Sachs	272800	β-D-N acetyl hexosaminidase A	GM_2 ganglioside	
Type II	Sandhoff disease	268800	β-D-N acetyl hexosaminidase A and B	GM_2 ganglioside	

Table 5.2 Lysosomal storage disorders (*contd*)

Disorder	Synonym or eponym	McKusick number[13]	Enzyme defect	Principal storage material	Comments
Type III	Juvenile Tay Sachs	230700	β-D-N acetyl hexosaminidase	GM_2 ganglioside	
Type IV	Adult (chronic)	272800	β-D-N acetyl	GM_2 ganglioside	
Type V	Activator-deficient Tay Sachs	272750	Hexosaminidase activator peptide	GM_2 ganglioside	
Metachromatic leukodystrophy	Sulphatidosis MLD		Arylsulphatase A	*Sulphatides	
Late infantile		250100			
Juvenile		250100			
Adult		250100			
Multiple sulphatase deficiency	MLD juvenile Austin type	272200	Multiple sulphatase	Sulphatides, *glycosaminoglycans	Excrete abnormal urinary GAG
Wolman disease		278000	Acid lipase	Cholesteryl esters	
Cholesteryl ester storage disease			Acid lipase	Cholesteryl esters	
Ceramidase deficiency	Farber lipogranulomatosis	228000	Ceramidase	Ceramide	
Mucopolysaccharidosis					
MPS I H	Hurler	252800	α-L-Iduronidase	*Heparan and *dermatan sulphates	
MPS I S	Scheie	252800	α-L-Iduronidase		
MPS I H/S	Hurler/Scheie compound		α-L-Iduronidase		
MPS II	Hunter syndrome (mild and severe forms)	309900	Iduronate-2-sulphate sulphatase	*Heparan and *dermatan sulphates	

Table 5.2 Lysosomal storage disorders (*contd*)

Disorder	Synonym or eponym	McKusick number[13]	Enzyme defect	Principal storage material	Comments
MPS III A	Sanfilippo disease	252900	Heparan-N-sulphamidase	*Heparan sulphate	
B		252920	N-acetyl-α-D-glucosaminidase	*Heparan sulphate	
C		252930	Acetyl CoA: α–glucosaminide transferase	*Heparan sulphate	
D		252940	N-acetyl-α-D-glucosamine-6-sulphate sulphatase	*Heparan sulphate	
MPS IV A	Morquio disease	253000	N-acetyl galactosamine-6-sulphate sulphatase	*Keratan sulphate	
IV B	Morquio disease	253010	β-Galactosidase	*Keratan sulphate	
MPS V	Scheie disease	—	—	—	Redesignated MPS IS
MPS VI	Maroteaux–Lamy disease (mild and severe forms)	253200	N-acetyl-galactosamine-4-sulphate sulphatase	*Dermatan sulphate	
MPS VII	Sly disease	253220	β-Glucuronidase	Not clearly defined	May excrete excess GAG
Sialidosis	Mucolipidosis I (MLI) normosomatic type or	256550	Sialidase (neuraminidase)	*Sialyloligosaccharides	
	cherry red spot, myoclonus syndrome and dysmorphic type	252400			This was the original MLI
Galactosialidosis	Golberg syndrome	256540	Protective protein deficiency, galactosidase, sialidase both appear deficient	Sialyloligosaccharides	

Table 5.2 Lysosomal storage disorders (*contd*)

Disorder	Synonym or eponym	McKusick number[13]	Enzyme defect	Principal storage material	Comments
α-Mannosidosis		248500	α-Mannosidase	*Mannose-rich oligosaccharides	
β-Mannosidosis		248510	β-Mannosidase		
Fucosidosis		230000	Fucosidase	*Fucosyl oligosaccharides	A genetic variant with low plasma fucosidase exists, McKusick 229950
Aspartylglucosaminuria		208400	Aspartamido-β-N-acetyl glucosamine amidohydrolase	*Aspartylglucosamine asparagines	
I-cell disease	Mucolipidosis II (ML II)	252500	UDP-N-acetyl glucosamine glycoprotein phosphotransferase	*GAG especially heparan sulphate *Oligosaccharides Glycolipids	
Pseudo-Hurler polydystrophy	ML III	252600			Partial enzyme defect in ML III
Cystinosis		219750	Transport defect	Free cystine	Nephropathic and benign forms exist with much heterogeneity
Sialic acid	Salla disease	268740	Transport defect	Free sialic acid and glucuronic acid	

*Detectable in urine

carriers of these conditions exhibit half the enzyme activity in selected tissues especially peripheral blood leucocytes, cultured skin fibroblasts and even blood serum. This feature has been used to detect carriers in high risk populations such as Aschkenazic Jews in whom Tay Sachs disease is so common.

LYSOSOMAL STORAGE DISEASES

Glycogenosis II (Pompe)

This condition has a special place in the study of lysosomal storage disorders[15] being the first disease to be recognised as such by Hers who demonstrated that the stored material was enclosed in membrane-bound vesicles. The other glycogenoses (see Ch. 2) are due to defects in cytoplasmic enzymes. Although cytoplasmic glycogen accumulation can be demonstrated in Pompe disease it is readily dispersed by giving glucagon or adrenaline to stimulate the normal glycogenolytic pathway. Furthermore, the enzyme now known to be deficient, acid maltase ($\alpha 1-4$ glucosidase) sediments in normal cells in the lysosomal cell fraction unlike the enzymes involved in the other glycogenoses.

This disease also illustrates the genetic heterogeneity so common in the lysosomal disorders with infantile, early childhood and adult forms. The relevant cDNA has been isolated and at least four different mutations may produce the disease. In the adult form, glycogen does not accumulate probably due to a small amount of residual enzyme activity. Pompe disease may also be regarded as an oligosaccharidosis in that oligosaccharides with frequent $\alpha 1-4$ linkages appear in the urine.

Heterozygote detection is difficult because a renal $\alpha 1-4$ glucosidase isoenzyme is present in serum as well as a neutral maltase which may interfere with assays on cellular microsomes. Diagnosis of the condition may be difficult for precisely the same reason and it is important to use two different types of assay or to remove the renal isoenzyme by isoelectric focusing. Alternatively, it is possible to use glycogen as the substrate in the presence of antibodies to the interfering enzyme in the assay. Since the renal isoenzyme appears in urine it is not possible to make a prenatal diagnosis on the direct examination of amniotic fluid and diagnosis requires culture of amniotic cells or chorionic villio.

Although at least three different presentations of this condition exist they do not usually occur within the same family, unlike the pleomorphic presentation sometimes seen in GM_1 gangliosidosis (see p. 222). The infantile form of Pompe disease presents sometime between birth and 6 months of age with severe hypotonia and muscle weakness associated with cardiac hypertrophy and culminating in early death, usually within the first year of life, from cardiorespiratory failure. Unlike the other glycogenoses, the liver is not enlarged (except later on due to cardiac congestion) and abnormalities of glucose homeostasis and lactate metabolism are not found, although the author has seen one patient with episodes of profound unexplained hypoglycaemia. The tongue is often enlarged and this is associated with feeding difficulties. This clinical feature, with hypotonia, may occur in hypothyroidism, a diagnosis which can be easily excluded by measurement of serum thyroxine.

The later infantile and early childhood form of the disease is mainly associated with muscle weakness and a relatively slower progression without cardiac abnormalities, and may be similar in presentation to the muscular dystrophies. Death in this group of patients is usually due to respiratory failure sometime before adulthood. The adult form of the disease usually presents over the age of 30 but careful questioning reveals that patients have had muscular weakness for many years associated with a respiratory problem prior to their presentation. There is progression of these two clinical features throughout adult life and the diagnosis is probably frequently missed since the condition mimics so many other chronic myopathies with little evidence of cardiac disease. The diagnosis may be established in all of these conditions by the demonstration of increased glycogen in muscle tissue and a deficiency of acid maltase in leucocytes, bearing in mind the possible influence of other isoenzymes.

Glycolipidoses (see Table 5.3)

Gaucher disease

This is the most common of the glycolipidoses and, like Tay Sachs disease, is prominent among Aschkenazic Jews with an incidence of 1: 2500 (Type I) with another two clinical types (II and III) seen in non-Jewish populations. Type I is a chronic non-neuropathic disease principally seen in

Table 5.3 Enzymes and associated deficiency disorders. Numbers in parentheses identify the sites of defects as shown in Figure 5.1

Enzyme	Deficiency disorder
β-Galactosidase (1)	GM_1 gangliosidosis
Hexosaminidase (2)	GM_2 gangliosidosis
Neuraminidase (3)	GM_3 gangliosidosis*
β Galactosidase (4)	?
Glucocerebrosidase (5)	Gaucher
N-acetylgalactosamidase (6)	?
α-Galactosidase (7)	Fabry
Arylsulphatase A (8)	Metachromatic leukodystrophy
Galactocerebrosidase (9)	Krabbe
Ceramidase (10)	Farber
Sphingomyelinase (11)	Niemann–Pick

*GM_3 accumulates in sialic acid storage disease although glycoproteins and sialyl oligosaccharides are the chief stored substances

adults, although the clinical story probably starts in childhood. Patients present with splenomegaly, thrombocytopenia, leukopenia and anaemia. The liver also becomes involved and increased serum liver enzymes are associated with developing hepatomegaly. Aseptic necrosis of the femoral heads and areas of diminished bone density in both ends of the long bones are seen radiologically and are often associated with intermittent episodes of severe bone pain and hyperpyrexia. The most severely affected patients have lung disease with cor pulmonale, pulmonary hypertension and frequent episodes of bronchopneumonia. The condition is slowly progressive. In Type II the presentation is very early, in the first few months of life, with hepatosplenomegaly and neurological complications typified by affected cranial nerves, poor feeding and misdirection of food due to abnormal function of the pharyngeal musculature. Progressive spasticity develops and death occurs within a couple of years of birth. Type III is a milder condition with some of the features of both of the other types.

Hepatomegaly and neurological changes are also seen in Niemann–Pick disease, GM_1 gangliosidosis and Wolmans disease but in Niemann–Pick disease the child is usually hypotonic and has cherry red maculae. Infants with GM_1 gangliosidosis often show coarse facial features and radiological changes more akin to those seen in the mucopolysaccharidoses while patients with the very rare Wolmans disease have calcified adrenals detectable radiologically.

In all three types of Gaucher disease, large lipid-laden foam cells derived from splenic histiocytes are to be found throughout the reticuloendothelial system. Identification of the so-called Gaucher cells in marrow is virtually diagnostic even though foam cells are seen in other lipidoses. Gaucher cells are strongly positive for acid phosphatase activity (the activity of tartrate labile/formol stable acid phosphatase is also markedly increased in serum) and have rod-like inclusions in the cytoplasm, thought to be due to glycolipid aggregating with protein to form tubular inclusion bodies.

The glycolipids accumulating have been shown to be glucosylceramide (glucocerebroside), but the view that most of the clinical features result from physical damage due to accumulation is difficult to reconcile with the fact that clinical severity does not correlate with the number of Gaucher cells or the density of inclusions and this problem remains to be resolved. Acitivity of several lysosomal acid hydrolases is increased but in all three types there is a deficiency of lysosomal glucocerebrosidase which cleaves glucose from glucosylceramide. It seems likely that uptake of glucosylceramide by macrophage lysosomes results in release of other enzymes and macrophage products which damage nearby tissues and account for the progressive destructive nature of the disorder. The major source of the glucosylceramide appears to be the turnover of the erythrocytes, leucocytes and platelets as well as the small contribution made by the slower turnover of other cell membranes.

The presence of several other β-glucosidases in peripheral blood leucocytes has, in the past, precluded the use of an artificial methylumbelliferyl glucopyranoside substrate for enzyme assay for confirmation of the diagnosis. Radioactively–labelled glucocerebroside has been the substrate of choice, although recent use of detergents or sodium taurocholate has improved specificity of the assay using less expensive artificial substrate. The labelled substrate is preferred for heterozygote detection, although identification may still be unreliable, and is essential for prenatal diagnosis.

The gene has been mapped to chromosome 1q21 and it has been cloned and sequenced. Several point mutations have been described associated with the disease[16] and some studies have shown that more than 25% of the abnormal alleles are identifiable. Mutational analysis may be an option for prenatal diagnosis in some families and population screening may become feasible in some ethnic groups with a very high incidence of the disease. Glucocerebrosidase also requires an activator protein, saposine C, the gene for which is on chromosome 10.

Treatment by splenectomy relieves the haematological problems but may accelerate progression of the disease, although this is still in debate. Attempts to treat by injection of enzyme with an added mannose recognition signal for lysosomal uptake (see I-cell disease) has met with some success and the enzyme is currently available as 'Ceredase'. More recent attempts to effect gene transfer with a suitable viral vector have been successful in cell culture and may offer a suitable future treatment.[16]

Sphingomyelin-lipidoses (Niemann – Pick disease)

There are several types of Niemann – Pick disease, formerly designated A, B, C, D and E, in which sphingomyelin may accumulate in the brain and viscera, and in which sphingomyelinase activity may or may not be deficient. An improved classification[17] but still one likely to require future amendment, divides the Niemann – Pick group of diseases into Type I, with sphingomyelin deficiency and accumulation of sphingomyelin and cholesterol, and Type II disease with less marked accumulation and often enzyme activity which is normal in tissues although reduced in fibroblasts. Both types may be indistinguishable clinically, presenting with hepatosplenomegaly, feeding difficulties and cachexia in the first few months of life. Rapid neurological degeneration occurs and a cherry red spot can be observed within the macula in some patients. The skin takes on a brownish hue and death occurs within 6 years.

Subacute(S) and chronic(C) forms of both types exist which are more slowly progressive. Type I S patients have little evidence of neurological involvement whereas Type II S patients may have psychomotor retardation and seizures. Type I C presents with unexplained hepatomegaly in adulthood and Type II C with neurological problems without hepatomegaly.

Diagnosis of Niemann – Pick disease Type I is based on the demonstration of typical large lipid-laden foam cells in the marrow (which are quite different from those seen in Gaucher disease when examined by electronmicroscopy) and is confirmed by demonstration of diminished sphingomyelinase activity in peripheral leucocytes, using a chromogenic analogue of sphingomyelin which is water-soluble. Identification of heterozygotes and prenatal detection of an affected fetus are feasible for Type I but not reliable in the other types of Niemann–Pick disease.

Adequate laboratory tests for detection of Type II have yet to be defined but refined techniques to demonstrate partial deficiency of sphingomyelinase in tissue culture appear to be possible, although characterisation of the gene is more likely to provide suitable tests. No treatment exists for either type.

Galactosylceramide lipidosis (Krabbe disease)

Krabbe disease, also known as globoid cell leukodystrophy, is an exceedingly rare inherited defect in galactocerebroside β-galactosidase activity, leading to a generalised accumulation of galactoceramide and its derivatives. Interestingly, early accumulation inhibits myelin formation so that there is no overall increase of galactocerebroside in brain. The condition is untreatable and is usually fatal in the first few months of life with very rapid neurological degeneration and flaccid paralysis associated with blindness and deafness.

α-Galactosidase deficiency (Fabry disease)

Fabry disease is a very rare disorder inherited in an X-linked manner in which glycosphingolipids of the globoside type accumulate due to deficiency of α-galactosidase. Deposition is generalised and associated with widespread pain and parathesiae (often accompanied by severe pyrexia), corneal opacities, and the development of angiokeratomata in skin and mucous membranes throughout childhood. Death is usually due to renal failure.

Carrier females are also known to exhibit the full clinical picture usually seen in hemizygous males. Restriction fragment length polymorphisms (RFLPs) have been found which offer reliable detection of carrier females. Time of presentation in both sexes is very variable and treatment has been directed largely at the relief of severe pain although some success has been obtained by replacement of the defective enzyme, α-galactosidase. Only quite a low percentage of normal activity has to be replaced to normalise metabolism (about 5%). Fetal liver transplantation has also been tried with limited success. End-stage renal disease may be relieved by renal transplantation or dialysis.

GM_1 gangliosidosis

Many different subtypes of this disorder may be seen ranging from a rapidly fatal infantile form with severe neurological degeneration and dysostosis multiplex to an adult form with chronic neurological disease.[18] Another type resembles mucopolysaccharidosis IV (Morquio disease) with which it is usually classified since ganglioside metabolism does not seem to be impaired, at least in nervous tissue. The infantile form usually presents as a hypotonic inactive infant with gargoyle-like facies and dysostosis multiplex. A cherry red macular spot is seen in over half of the patients, hepatosplenomegaly and corneal opacities rapidly develop and the condition may be mistaken for an early Hurler syndrome, I-cell disease or pseudo–Hurler polydystrophy. The milder juvenile type presents later, often with seizures, and the facial features are usually normal, although progressive neurological degeneration occurs at an exponential pace. The late adult form usually presents with cerebellar dysarthria starting as a young adult and associated with a progressive spastic ataxia.

In all patients the disorder is due to a greater or lesser diminution of the activity of lysosomal β-galactosidase which cleaves galactose from GM_1 ganglioside, keratan sulphate and many galactose-containing oligosaccharides. The enzyme exists as either a monomer, dimer or polymer and its pleiotrophic effects have been explained by the one gene–one enzyme–many substrates model of O'Brien.[4] Residual activity of the enzyme to a selected substrate influences the type and relative amount of substrate which accumulates. This would explain how the biochemical defect in Morquio B is almost confined to a block in keratan sulphate catabolism. Some patients with β-galactosidase defects may be K_m mutants and may be difficult to diagnose if reliance is placed on enzyme assay of a single point, single substrate concentration type usually used to diagnose lysosomal enzyme defects.

GM_1 gangliosidosis may present with very similar features to Hurler syndrome or other mucopolysaccharidoses but the latter may be distinguished by a distinctive pattern of urinary mucopolysaccharide (glycosaminoglycan) excretion. A cherry red macula is also seen in children with Tay Sachs disease but they do not have hepatomegaly.

GM_2 gangliosidosis (Tay Sachs and Sandhoff diseases)

GM_2 gangliosidosis or Tay Sachs disease figures prominently in any general text on lyosomal disorders. It has a high incidence amongst Ashkenazic Jewish populations (about 1:30 are heterozygous carriers compared with about one-tenth of this incidence in non-Jews), and was one of the first lipidoses to be described and studied as a result of Tay's description of the macular cherry red spot, which is almost pathognomonic for this and a few very closely related conditions of abnormal sphingolipid metabolism. As in the case of many lysosomal disorders, GM_2 gangliosidosis has infantile, juvenile and adult forms with considerable phenotypic variability. Clinical presentation is usually that of a hypotonic infant with an exaggerated startle response to noise. The muscle weakness is slowly progressive. Although crawling may be achieved, these infants never walk and pursue a rapid downhill path of motor and mental deterioration from the end of their first year, usually associated with marked feeding problems, blindness, deafness and convulsions, and finally ending in a state of decerebrate cortical rigidity by the age of 2–3 years.

Sandhoff disease is virtually identical, clinically. A later-onset juvenile form of GM_2 gangliosidosis is often mistakenly diagnosed as Batten's disease or Spielmeyer–Vogt disease in which retinitis pigmentosa is an important differentiating feature. A late-onset slowly progressive adult form also exists.

All of these conditions are due to deficient activity of β-D-N acetyl hexosaminidase, essential for degradation of GM_2 gangliosides. Two lysosomal forms of this enzyme exist, hexosaminidase A, which is heat-labile, and heat-stable hexosaminidase B. Deficiency of A is complete in Tay Sachs disease, at least when pure GM_2 ganglioside is used as substrate, and partial in the juvenile and adult forms, while both enzymes are affected in Sandhoff disease. The B enzyme is not involved in GM_2 ganglioside catabolism but is important in degradation of oligosaccharides so that Sandhoff disease is sometimes classified as an oligosaccharidosis. Infantile, juvenile and adult forms of that condition also exist. The situation has been complicated by the discovery of an activating polypeptide for hexosaminidase activity, synthesis of which is also genetically determined and absence of which may cause a similar disorder.

The mean hexosaminidase A activity (measured as a ratio of heat-labile activity to heat-stable activity) in serum of heterozygous carriers is about half that found in homozygous normal individuals and follows a Gaussian distribution curve which overlaps the lower end of the reference range for non-carriers. Where the results in the overlap area are inconclusive, designation of genetic status can be confirmed using leucocytes. These tests are now widely used in mass population screening in communities at risk for Tay Sachs disease thus enabling sound genetic advice and prenatal diagnosis to be offered to couples who are both carriers. Such programmes have reduced the incidence of Tay Sachs disease in North America to about one-third of what it used to be and the programmes have provided a prototype for the detection of other genetic diseases in high risk populations. Such programmes have proven value in medical audit, having cost less than one-fifth of the care for affected individuals born if the screening programme had not been initiated.

Sulphatidoses

Metachromatic leukodystrophy

Metachromatic leukodystrophy (MLD) encompasses a group of at least six disorders affecting myelin metabolism, with similar clinical presentation associated with increased urinary galactosyl sulphate (cerebroside sulphate) excretion and tissue accumulation of cerebroside sulphatide due to defective action of cerebroside sulphatase (arylsulphatase A).[19] The most common variant, a late infantile form, presents at about 18 months to 2 years of age with delayed neuromuscular development, hypotonia, a progressive loss of speech and onset of ataxia ultimately ending with spastic quadriparesis within about 5 years. This is rapidly followed by a downhill course leading to death at about the age of 7 years. Optic atrophy is also a prominent feature also seen in a later onset juvenile form which shows slower progression. An adult form may be difficult to diagnose clinically and presents with dementia and psychosis associated with ataxia which may also progress very slowly to spastic quadriparesis. This diagnosis is probably quite often missed

A congenital form of the disease is thought to exist but this is based on limited information on two infants presenting with apnoea and cyanosis, seizures with muscular weakness and death in the first few weeks of life. The biochemical lesion in this condition has not been confirmed but in the other types described above there is deficient activity of arylsulphatase A with accumulation of metachromatic material in neuronal tissues, which has been identified as cerebroside sulphate and is associated with progressive demyelination. There is also a markedly raised protein concentration in cerebrospinal fluid.

Arylsulphatase A is a heat-labile component of cerebroside sulphatase which is associated with a heat-stable activator of the enzyme, deficiency of which can also lead to a rare form of metachromatic leukodystrophy. These patients show arylsulphatase A activity in the heterozygous range in cultured fibroblasts but the activity can be enhanced to normal levels by the addition of the heat-stable protein activator. These patients present clinically with the features of juvenile MLD.

Another condition presents with all the features of late infantile MLD plus abnormal coarse facies, hepatosplenomegaly, dysostosis multiplex, ichthyosis and deafness. Not only do these patients excrete metachromatic cerebroside sulphate but they also have excess glycosaminoglycan excretion of a similar pattern to I-cell disease, with heparan sulphate, dermatan sulphate and possibly keratan sulphate present. Metachromatic granules are seen in leucocytes which also distinguishes this from other forms of MLD. This fascinating condition results from a single gene mutation which affects several sulphatases and is thus usually designated multiple sulphatase deficiency. The disorder thus represents a complex presentation of the features of MLD (aryl sulphatase A deficiency), Maroteaux–Lamy disease (MPS IV, arylsulphatase B deficiency), X-linked ichthyosis (aryl sulphatase deficiency), Hunter disease (MPS II, iduronate-2-sulphate sulphatase deficiency), Sanfilippo A disease (MPS III A, heparan-N-sulphamidase deficiency), Morquio disease (MPS IV, N-acetyl-galactosamine-6-sulphate sulphatase deficiency) and DiFerrante disease (MPS VIII, N-acetyl-glucosamine-6-sulphate sulphatase deficiency).

Diagnosis of MLD sometimes requires histological confirmation or identification of urinary metachromatic granular deposits, since although arylsulphate A activity is easily measured with p-nitrocatechol sulphate as substrate, individuals with protein activated deficiency may have residual enzyme activity and metachromatic granules present in their urine. Furthermore, some members of the population may have a pseudo-deficiency gene but sulphatiduria does not occur. The enzyme is less stable in urine and plasma than in leucocytes. The enzyme assay can be made more specific by separating the various arylsulphatases before assay or by using the natural cerebroside substrate. Heterozygote detection is possible, but the presence of the low activity pseudo-deficiency allele for arylsulphatase activity among some otherwise normal members of the population may produce low results suggestive of MLD if the artificial substrate is used. Prenatal diagnosis is feasible and potential treatment now exists in the form of bone marrow transplantation if only one could be assured that the enzyme could be targeted to the oligodendroglial cells across the 'blood–brain barrier'.

Other lipid storage disorders

Acid lipase deficiency

Hydrolysis of the cholesteryl esters derived from low density lipoprotein requires active lipase which is deficient in the two related disorders, Wolman's disease and cholesteryl ester storage disease. Wolman's disease is usually fatal in the first year of life with progressive failure to thrive, hepatosplenomegaly and adrenal calcification. The condition is untreatable but prenatal diagnosis has been achieved and heterozygotes can be detected. Cholesteryl ester storage disease which has a slower, more benign course, may be confused clinically with Type I glycogenosis (see also p. 26).

Ceramidase deficiency (Farber's lipogranulomatosis)

Farber's lipogranulomatosis is a very rare lipid disorder resulting from a deficiency of lysosomal acid ceramidase thus leading to the accumulation of ceramide. The latter leads to painful deformity of the joints, multiple subcutaneous nodules especially in pressure-bearing areas and a hoarse voice due to laryngeal and lung involvement. This clinical triad is unique to Farber's disease. Death is usually early and there is no treatment.

Mucopolysaccharidoses

Mucopolysaccharidosis IH (Hurler syndrome)

This condition is the classic mucopolysaccharide storage disorder described by Hurler in which there is a distinctive bone dysplasia (dysostosis multiplex) associated with severe mental retardation.[13]

Patients with this condition usually present in infancy and early childhood with progressive deterioration of mental and physical ability associated with distinctive facial features. The head is large and bulging with a marked increase in the anteroposterior diameter due to premature closure of the sagittal sutures, thus producing a scaphocephalic skull. These patients have coarse features and thick hair with marked hypertelorism, flattening of the bridge of the nose making it saddle-shaped, wide nostrils, thick patulous lips, an enlarged protruding tongue and open mouth which, with their coarse facial skin and hair, gives them a distinctive appearance. Narrowing of the nasopharynx and the enlarged tongue lead to a snuffling respiration associated with chronic rhinitis.

There is progressive clouding of the cornea during the early months of life associated with retinal degeneration. The neck is short so that the head appears to rest directly on the thorax. The abdomen is protuberant and inguinal and umbilical herniae are common. The liver and spleen are both grossly enlarged from about 6 months of age. Progressive kyphosis and gibbus formation of the lumbar region of the spine give these patients a cat-like position. The hands are broad and stubby, flexion contractures of the elbows and hands develop progressively (claw-hand deformity), and the fifth finger is usually bent radially. Bilateral dislocation of the hip is common.

Growth is rapid during the first year of life but falls below the third percentile later. Neurological development may appear normal at first but eventually there is a delay in sitting and walking, and toilet training is rarely achieved. The progressive thickening of the skull due to hyperostosis is ultimately associated with a conductive deafness. Hydrocephalus is a prominent feature which may require treatment. These children reach a learning plateau before the age of 2 years, and death from respiratory or cardiac failure usually occurs before the age of 10 years. Respiratory infections are frequent.

The radiological features are distinctive with thickening of the calvarium, microcephaly and a J-shaped sella turcica. The ribs are spatulate and the chest is wide. The vertebrae are immature and there is usually anterior beaking of T12 and L1. The ilia are flared, the femoral epiphyses are dysplastic and there is marked shortening of the shafts of the long bones with irregular diaphyses. Short bones show metaphyseal widening and dysplastic epiphyses. The terminal phalanges are particularly hypoplastic, and the metacarpals broad and tapering proximally.

The biochemical defect is due to deficient activity of α-L-iduronidase, a lysosomal enzyme which is required for the degradation of heparan sulphate and dermatan sulphate. Those two glycosaminoglycans accumulate in the tissues within the lysosomes and can be seen as metachromatic granules in peripheral blood lymphocytes. Heparan and dermatan sulphate are excreted in the urine with dermatan sulphate in excess. There also appears to be a partial deficiency of β-galactosidase activity which may be due to the inhibition of the enzyme by accumulated glycosaminoglycans.

Mucopolysaccharidosis IS (Scheie syndrome)

This condition was first described as a variant of Hurler syndrome with which it has many features in common. Patients have coarse facial features with a large tongue and broad mouth associated with a square mandible. Very marked clouding of the cornea occurs, maximal at the periphery, and may be associated with retinitis pigmentosa and glaucoma later in life. Inguinal herniae are common and the liver may be enlarged. There are marked joint contractures which are usually more severe than seen in Hurler syndrome with a particularly severe claw-hand deformity.

In common with other mucopolysaccharidoses these patients have excessive body hair. Their stature is usually normal although their bone age is retarded. Their neurological development is normal except that they may develop carpal tunnel syndrome. Scheie syndrome shows a later progression than that seen in Type IH, and intellect is normal. Spinal changes are minimal and there are only mild changes in the femur and long bones.

The condition is allelic with Hurler syndrome, and the biochemical abnormality is identical in that α-L-iduronidase activity is defective, and the patients excrete excessive amounts of dermatan sulphate and heparan sulphate.

An intermediate condition between Type IH and Type IS has also been described which has all the features of Hurler syndrome but milder radiological features associated with severe joint contractures and later progression of the disease.

Mucopolysaccharidosis II (Hunter syndrome)

This condition is less severe than Hurler syndrome and there appear to be two allelic types based on the severity and survival, a juvenile and a late form. These patients have plethoric facies with many of the features of Hurler syndrome. There is no corneal clouding except in older patients, and this is usually only revealed by slit lamp examination. A form of retinitis pigmentosa may occur in older patients as well as papilloedema secondary to hydrocephaly both of which may lead to blindness. These patients also have a protuberant abdomen with hepatosplenomegaly. Although they develop kyphoscoliosis they do not develop the lumbar gibbus seen in Hurler syndrome. Stiffness of the joints occurs with the typical claw-hand deformity.

There is marked hypertrichosis, the hairs showing nodular or ridged thickening. Growth is retarded so that these patients become severely dwarfed. Mental retardation is slowly progressive and commonly associated with deafness. Patients with late onset type Hunter syndrome appear to preserve mathematical ability longer than they do verbal ability and some patients are known to retain a fair intelligence into adult life. They also have longer survival, usually up to the fourth decade, and occasionally up to the seventh. Patients with the juvenile type tend to die before they reach their teens. Most patients develop osteoarthritis of the hips in later life, and death is usually due to cardiac failure associated with pulmonary hypertension.

The condition is seen in caucasians, but is rare in other ethnic groups. Inheritance is X-linked recessive and occurs only in boys, although it has been described in girls with either inactivation of the normal X chromosome or with a balanced translocation of the X. The biochemical deficiency is in the activity of iduronate sulphatase and results in excessive excretion of dermatan sulphate and heparan sulphate, although the relative proportions of the two glycosaminoglycans is somewhat variable.

Mucopolysaccharidosis III (Sanfilippo syndrome)

The clinical features in this mucopolysaccharidosis are usually less marked than they are in Hurler syndrome. The skull is usually normal although the circumference may be increased early in life and tend towards normal circumference later. The nasal bridge is only slightly flattened and the facies often appear normal. The eyes are usually normal although corneal stippling may be seen on slit lamp examination, but this does not usually interfere with vision. The neck is short as in Type IH. The abdomen is only moderately enlarged and the spine is usually normal externally. The spleen is enlarged in about 20% of patients and inguinal herniae occur in about one third of males. Four different genotypes are now recognised, designated IIIA, IIIB, IIIC and IIID. Liver enlargement occurs in all patients with Type IIIA but does not appear to be as common in patients with the other varieties. All patients may show moderate contractures of various joints and genu valgum is often present. The hair is dry and coarse as seen in the other mucopolysaccharidoses.

Growth tends to be accelerated in infancy and patients maintain good height up until puberty, although bone age is retarded. Early neurological development is normal, but is followed by regression between the ages of 1 to 4 years, during which speech loss and associated deafness are common features. These patients seem to find speech control most difficult and develop stuttering. Dementia is not a cardinal feature of the disease early on and the neurological findings are not consistent. The deafness is of a conductive type in two-thirds of the patients, and approximately one-third learn to speak late. Mental retardation seems to be a more prominent feature of Type IIIB, whereas behaviour disturbances, sometimes associated with violence and hyperactivity, especially if the patient is restrained, are more common in Type IIIA. About half of the patients show abnormalities before the age of 3 years, although patients with Type IIIB may present later during their school years, and disturbances of sleep may be the first sign of the disorder.

The course of the disease is extremely variable, and the mean life expectancy is usually beyond adolescence, although patients with Type IIIA tend to die earlier. Cardiovascular problems are rare and death is usually due to respiratory difficulties, recurrent respiratory infection being a common feature. Other clinical features commonly seen are episodes of diarrhoea, polyphagy and pica.

Radiological features are less marked than they are in Hurler syndrome, tend to revert to normal in later childhood, and are not detectable before 18 months of age. Biconvex vertebral bodies are common in the thoracic region. The disease is mainly seen in caucasians and it is the commonest mucopolysaccharidosis in the United Kingdom and in Holland, where Type A exceeds Type B by fourfold, and Type A exceeds C by twofold. The incidence at birth has been calculated as 1:24 000.

The enzyme deficient in Type A is heparan sulphamidase; in Type B, N-acetyl-D-glucosaminidase; in Type C, acetyl CoA-glucosaminide-N-acetyl-transferase, and in Type D, N-acetylglucosamine-6-sulphate sulphatase. All patients excrete excessive amounts of heparan sulphate.

Mucopolysaccharidosis IV (Morquio syndrome)

Neurological abnormalities are not a prominent feature of this rare mucopolysaccharidosis in which skeletal abnormalities are more obvious. It is basically a spondyloepiphyseal dysplasia with extraskeletal features which may include corneal opacities, aortic valve disease, and rarely mental retardation. These patients have the broad mouth seen in Hurler syndrome with prominent maxillae, a short nose and widely spaced teeth. The neck is short and the abdomen may be protuberant. There is beaking of the lumbar vertebrae as seen in other mucopolysaccharidoses. The joints are hyperextensible, the wrists are enlarged and the shape of the hands is distinctly odd. Growth is markedly retarded so that these patients are strikingly dwarfed.

Development appears to be normal in the first year of life but between the ages of 2 and 3 years growth slows, and the patients usually present with abnormal gait. On examination flared ribs, large joints, knock-knees and a dorsal kyphosis are usually evident, and all of these become worse with age. The radiology is quite distinctive, particularly the marked platyspondyly in the lumbar spine. Patients excrete excessive amounts of keratan sulphate early in childhood although this excretion pattern may revert to normal in adulthood, and a similar pattern may be seen in other bone dysplasias.

Two types are now recognised, a severe condition with distinctive bone changes, cloudy corneae and aortic regurgitation (Type A) and a milder type (Type B). Both types of patients may excrete excessive amounts of keratan sulphate, but the enzyme defect is different being galactosamine-6-sulphatase in Type A and β-galactosidase in Type B.

Mucopolysaccharidosis VI (Maroteaux – Lamy syndrome)

Patients with this extremely rare disorder show similar skeletal changes to patients with Type IH mucopolysaccharidosis, but are usually of normal intellect, and bone changes are more severe. The most severe have a poor survival. Dwarfism is extremely marked and noticeable at the age of 2–3 years with growth ultimately ceasing at the age of 7 years.

The most striking radiological features occur in the pelvis. The acetabula are small with a sloping roof and the ilia are flared. Ossification of the femoral heads is irregular and this condition is often confused with Legg–Perthes disease. A distinctive feature is constriction of the metaphyses which is not seen in that condition or in other mucopolysaccharidoses.

Patients excrete excessive amounts of dermatan sulphate, and cytoplasmic inclusions are more common than they are in the other mucopolysaccharidoses, usually being seen in over 75% of peripheral blood leucocytes. The enzyme defect is in the activity of aryl sulphatase B (N-acetylgalactosamine 4-sulphatesulphatase) which is thought to result from a mutation on chromosome 5.

Mucopolysaccharidosis VII (Sly syndrome)

This rare mucopolysaccharidosis was described by Sly and colleagues in 1973. Their patient, a black infant, had odd facies with hypertelorism, small epicanthic folds, depressed nasal bridge, and an increased head circumference later in infancy. The cornea were clear, the abdomen was protuberant with enlargement of spleen and liver associated with diastasis recti and umbilical hernia. There was a marked lumbar gibbus, and radiological examination revealed a J-shaped sella turcica, flared ribs and hypoplastic odontoid. The enzyme which was defective was β-glucuronidase. Both parents and several other relations had intermediate activity of this enzyme, indicating autosomal recessive inheritance. The locus for this enzyme has been identified on the long arm of chromosome 7. Urinary mucopolysaccharide excretion was only increased in the early weeks of life, and consisted of chondroitin sulphate excretion in excess, and was therefore difficult to distinguish from excretion in some normal infants.

The principal enzyme defects in the mucopolysacharidoses are summarised in Figure 5.3.

Oligosaccharidoses

The common feature of this group of disorders is the excretion of oligosaccharides in the urine. They are difficult to classify at present since some of them result from faulty degradation of the oligosaccharide fragment of glycoproteins and others result from faulty degradation of the oligosaccharide fraction of gangliosides.[12] They include some conditions which have previously been classified as glycoproteinoses and others which have been classified as mucolipidoses. Since there is no evidence to suggest that the protein part of the glycoprotein is involved and since mucolipids as chemicals in the strict sense of the term do not exist, it seems preferable to use the term oligosaccharidoses which more directly reflects the abnormality of catabolism, although that too is deficient in the sense that it creates overlap between other classifications such as the ganglioside storage disorders. In the following paragraphs only those conditions affecting the oligosaccharide portion of glycopeptides or glycoproteins are discussed and the ganglioside storage disorders have been described under the heading of lipidoses.

Sialidosis

This disorder, or group of disorders, is due to failure to remove sialic acid residues from the oligosaccharide side-chains of both glycoproteins and gangliosides.[20] Two major types of this very rare condition are now recognised: a normosomatic type seen in infantile form in Japanese, with a later-onset juvenile presentation seen in Italians, and a dysmorphic type of variable clinical presentation usually seen in caucasians. The normosomatic types present with diminishing visual acuity associated with development of a red spot in the macular region of the fundus. The condition has previously been called cherry red spot myoclonus syndrome since a progressive action type myoclonus, which a wide range of therapeutic agents fails to control, is a distinctive feature seen in the majority of patients. Intelligence in this condition does not seem to be grossly impaired although it is difficult to measure because of the myoclonic spasms. A rare congenital form also exists, presenting at birth with hydrops and early death.

Only a small number of patients with dysmorphic sialidosis has been described and they show the same clinical signs as the normosomatic patients but associated with coarse facial featues of the Hurler type and a similar bone dysplasia, hepatomegaly and corneal opacities. Another variant, largely affecting the kidney, called nephrosialidosis has also been described.

Galactosialidosis presents in a similar manner and results from apparent

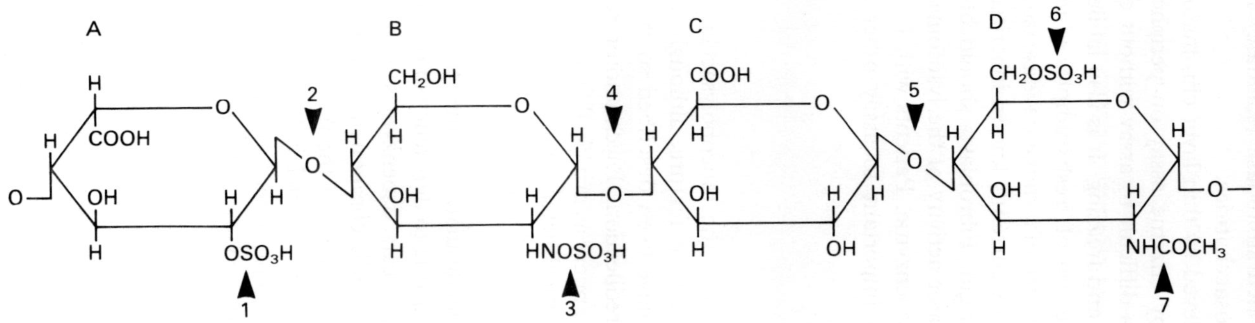

Fig. 5.3 Catabolism of heparan sulphate and associated lysosomal disease.
A – iduronic acid-2-sulphate, B – N-sulphated glucosamine, C – glucuronic acid, D – N-acetylglucosamine-6-sulphate.
1. iduronate sulphatase (MPS II Hunter)
2. iduronidase (MPS I Hurler or Scheie)
3. heparan-N-sulphamidase (MPS III Sanfilippo A)
4. N-acetylglucosaminidase (MPS IIIB Sanfilippo B)
5. glucuronidase (MPS VII Sly)
6. N-acetylglucosamine-6-sulphate sulphatase (MPS IIID Sanfilippo D)
7. acetyl CoA glucosaminide transferase (MPS IIIC Sanfilippo C)

1, 3 and 6: multiple sulphatase deficiency
1–7: 1-cell disease/pseudo-Hurler.

deficiency of both sialidase and galactosidase activity, due to the fact that these two enzymes exist in a complex with a protective protein and the latter is defective. Accumulation of a wide range of sialyloligosaccharides probably occurs in most tissues and many are found in the urine with a preponderance of those with sialyl linkages of the α-2-6 configuration. The defect is due to a deficiency of a neuraminidase (sialidase) isoenzyme required for degradation of sialyloligosaccharides.

Laboratory diagnosis may be achieved by thin layer chromatography of sialyloligosaccharides and verified by enzyme assay on peripheral blood leucocytes. However, this enzyme is difficult to assay without experience because it is unstable on sonication and freezing. It is also labile in whole blood at room temperature and the use of fresh samples is imperative. Further difficulty arises from the presence of a stable sialidase isoenzyme in leucocytes, which is not deficient in any currently known inherited disorder and is possibly non-lysosomal in origin. Fibroblasts should be used for confirmation since they contain greater activity of the lysosomal sialidase and negligible activity of the other isoenzyme. Patients with I-cell disease may show similar results and it is important to assay other lysosomal enzymes in dysmorphic patients.

Mannosidosis

This disorder is clinically reminiscent of the mucopolysaccharidoses but mucopolysacchariduria is not a prominent feature, although it has been recorded. Fewer than 100 patients have been described so far and there does not seem to be any ethnic predilection. Psychomotor retardation, coarse facies, ataxia and hearing loss appear as principal features associated with dysostosis multiplex. Marked clinical heterogeneity exists even within a family and it has been suggested that two forms of the disease exist with a mild form surviving into adulthood.

Mannose-rich oligosaccharides accumulate in the tissues and are excreted in the urine. The condition is due to deficiency of α-mannosidase and has been described in cattle and cats. Isoenzymes with acidic and neutral pH optima exist and it is the acidic component which is defective. Enzyme assay on serum is unreliable because of the relatively low content of the acidic lysosomal fraction, even in normal individuals, whereas in leucocytes that is the major component. Even so, activity varies with different leucocyte populations and may be influenced by infections. Definitive diagnosis relies on the combination of clinical features, demonstration of abnormal urinary oligosaccharides as well as enzyme assays under carefully controlled conditions. Heterozygote detection is not easy but prenatal diagnosis is feasible.

About 10% of the New Zealand stock of Aberdeen Angus cattle are heterozygous carriers of an abnormal α-mannosidase gene. Homozygous cattle show a similar progressive ataxic disease to that seen in humans and experimental enzyme replacement therapy has been tried but failed to normalise the neurological deficit. In spite of problems with isoenzymes, screening for heterozygotes has been successful using serum or plasma, followed by confirmatory studies on lymphocytes in borderline cases, provided that results are compared with age- and sex-matched controls.

A similar neurodegenerative disorder due to deficiency of β- mannosidase has been described in goats and has recently been found in man. Clinical presentation of the human disease is very heterogeneous, ranging from a mild Hurler-like syndrome to a condition presenting with mental retardation and scrotal angiokeratoma, but lacking dysmorphism or organomegaly.

Fucosidosis

Less than 100 patients, mainly of Italian descent, have been described with this condition which presents in either an infantile or a chronic form of similar presentation but slower progression.[21] Early hypotonia progresses to hypertonia and spasticity. Some infants have Hurler-like facies and most of them have hepatomegaly and cardiomegaly associated with progressive neurological deterioration and failure to thrive.

The disorder is due to the accumulation of fucoglycoconjugates such as fucose-containing glycopeptides, oligosaccharides, H isoantigen and keratan sulphate. Laboratory diagnosis is based on demonstration of vacuolated lymphocytes, raised sweat sodium chloride content, identification of abnormal urine oligosaccharide excretion and demonstration of α-L-fucosidase deficiency in leucocytes and fibroblasts. Serum assay is not reliable as about 6–10% of phenotypically normal individuals show diminished activity due to inheritance of a variant enzyme. Heterozygote detection is not easy in either leucocytes or fibroblasts because the enzyme activity appears to change with the growth cycle of the cells, but prenatal diagnosis is feasible nevertheless.

Aspartlyglucosaminuria

This disorder of glycoprotein metabolism is almost unknown in all races other than Finns where the incidence is about 1:26 000, rising to 1:2000 in a population of Finnish extraction now living in Northern Norway. Aspartylglycosamine residues form the linkage of the carbohydrate moeity to the polypeptide in many glycoproteins, including red cell membrane sialoglycoprotein, thyroglobulin, IgM and IgE, transferrin, ceruloplasmin, α_2-macroglobulin and chorionic gonadotrophin. The disorder is due to deficiency of the specific amidohydrolase required to hydrolyse the linkage, which results in accumulation and excretion of aspartylglucosamine (2-acetamido-1-(β-2-aspartamido)-1,2-dideoxy-β-D-glucose) and some higher asparagines.[22]

Clinical presentation may be confused with that of the mucopolysaccharidoses. Normal early development and facial appearance is complicated by episodes of unusual diarrhoea in about one-third of patients and recurrent infections in all of them during the first year of life. Gradual and progressive hypotonia and mental deterioration, heralded by loss of speech, occur with development of skeletal abnormalities similar to those seen in the mucopolysaccharidoses and almost indistinguishable from those seen in mannosidosis. The facial characteristics are also indistinguishable from those seen in Hurler syndrome but occur much later and eventually become quite grotesque as the mental handicap worsens. Over half of the patients have a systolic murmur possibly due to infiltration of the mitral valve which has been described in the few postmortem examinations recorded.

Deficiency of 1-aspartamido-β-N-acetylglucosamine amidohydrolase (AADGase) is demonstrable in leucocytes, serum and cultured fibroblasts; but the enzyme assay is not easy to do and requires long incubation times because the Morgan–Elsen reaction, used to measure the release of N-acetylglucosamine, is relatively insensitive and tissue enzyme activity, even in normal tissues, is very low. Aspartylglucosamine excretion can be detected in amino acid chromatograms stained with ninhydrin and heated to 120°C for 5 minutes to give a characteristic deep blue spot. One dimensional chromatography of urinary oligosaccharides stained with resorcinol yields a purple brown spot with associated minor components in the area of the chromatogram usually occupied by tetrasaccharides (i.e. low R_F).

There is no successful treatment currently available but heterozygotes may be detected by enzyme assay on lymphocytes. Prenatal diagnosis is feasible but rarely requested as most parents have completed their family by the time the index patient has been diagnosed.

Disorders of lysosomal enzyme transport

I-cell disease and pseudo-Hurler polydystrophy

I-cell disease and pseudo-Hurler polydystrophy (sometimes referred to as mucolipidosis II and III but for which multiple hydrolase deficiency seems a preferable term) are closely related diseases but clinically very different. Several acid hydrolases are absent from the lysosomes because the mannose-6-phosphate recognition marker has not been added to the pro-enzyme so that it can be pinocytozed into the lysosome.[23] The enzymes thus appear in the intracellular fluids and blood plasma, since they cannot be taken up by lysosomes. The macromolecules which they should have digested accumulate in the lysosomes, hence the name I-cell or inclusion cell disease. The enzymes so affected may also exhibit slightly different physicochemical properties since they have not undergone partial proteolytic digestion within the lysosome to convert them into their most active form.

Clinical presentation of I-cell disease may be difficult to distinguish from that of Hurler syndrome. I-cell disease is also difficult to differentiate biochemically from pseudo-Hurler polydystrophy but the latter exhibits a milder course, and is presumed to be due to a partial phosphorylation defect. The presentation of I-cell disease is usually neonatal with gargoyle facies and development of severe dysostosis multiplex with progressive neurological degeneration culminating in death in early infancy. Corneal opacities are usually present but difficult to demonstrate and the only distinguishing features from MPS I are the very early presentation and the development of very marked gingival hyperplasia.

Since many different lysosomal hydrolases may be involved the urine may contain abnormal oligosaccharides or mucopolysaccharides (particularly heparan sulphate) and either of these macromolecules as well as sphingolipids may accumulate in tissues. Diagnosis may be confirmed by demonstrating increased activity of β-hexosaminidase, iduronate sulphatase and arylsulphatase A in plasma or serum, associated with diminished activity of these, and other enzymes, in fibroblasts. The use of mixed leucocytes is fallible since enzymes are deficient in lymphocytes but not in granulocytes.

The primary enzyme defect is in UDP-N-acetylglucosamine glycoprotein-N-acetylglucosaminyl phosphotransferase responsible for phosphorylating mannose in the carbohydrate side-chain of the lysosomal hydrolases. The reaction catalysed by this enzyme still proceeds, but at a very low rate, in pseudo-Hurler polydystrophy fibroblasts so that partial phosphorylation, and hence enzyme uptake, probably occurs in that condition and accounts for its milder clinical presentation.

The direct assay of this phosphotransferase is now available using commercially available substrates.

Disorders of transport across the lysosomal membrane

Cystinosis

This condition is now confirmed as a rare lysosomal disorder with defective carrier-mediated transport of cystine across the lysosomal membrane[24] which leads to accumulation of free cystine, and crystal formation within the lysosomes resulting in progressive tissue damage, particularly in the corneae and kidneys.

Two clinical presentations are recognised, in a nephropathic form and a benign form, both inherited in an autosomal recessive manner with a few patients showing intermediate expression. Considerable genetic heterogeneity exists, with patients in the same family often showing variable expression.

Early development is normal but gradual onset of polyuria and polydypsia precedes the renal tubular damage which is a feature of the nephropathic form. Hyperpyrexia is a common and unusual early feature often associated with severe dehydration. As the renal tubular damage due to cystine accumulation worsens there is a progressive development of a Fanconi type syndrome with a potassium wasting acidosis, aminoaciduria and glycosuria associated with stunted growth and the development of hypophosphataemic rickets. Many children have fair hair, a fair complexion and exhibit photophobia with a poor melanotic response to sunlight. Cystine deposits may be demonstrated by slit-lamp examination of the anterior two-thirds of the cornea and, with an associated peripheral retinopathy, are pathognomonic of cystinosis. The renal disease progresses to renal failure before puberty. In the benign form, cystine deposits seem to be confined to the eyes, bone marrow and leucocytes and appear to lead to no disability.

Treatment is largely symptomatic with adequate fluid intake supplemented by potassium in the form of potassium citrate which helps to correct the acidosis, and vitamin D with or without phosphate to correct the rickets, always being mindful that excess phosphate with alkali may precipitate tetany. Prenatal diagnosis may be achieved by following the uptake of ^{35}S in cultured cells. The label usually appears in protein, cysteine and glutathione in normal cells but ends up as cystine in cystinotic cell lines.

Sialic acid storage disease

A large group of patients were described from Salla in Finland who presented with psychomotor retardation, ataxia and abnormal lysosomal inclusions[25].

Delayed development was first noted in the early years of life, followed by a gradual but definite deterioration beginning in the second or third decade, although life expectancy appeared normal. Increased free sialic acid (N-acetyl neuraminic acid, NANA) levels were found in urine and subsequently in liver and fibroblasts. In fibroblasts a range of lysosomal enzymes showed normal activities, as did several other enzymes involved with sialic acid synthesis or degradation. The disorder was named Salla disease, after the area from which the patients originated.

Other patients, from a wide range of ethnic backgrounds, presented in infancy with coarse facies, hepatosplenomegaly and profound inactivity. The clinical course was one of relentless neurological deterioration with death in early childhood. Urinary free SA was markedly increased. Accumulation of free NANA was demonstrated in brain, liver, kidney and fibroblasts, and again activities of sialidase and other enzymes relevant to SA turnover were found to be normal. This disorder was referred to as infantile sialic acid storage disease (ISSD).

Loading experiments demonstrated defective egress of NANA from lysosomes both of ISSD and of Salla fibroblasts[26]. It was found that the differences in clinical severity between these groups of patients broadly reflected different magnitudes of storage as evidenced by urinary NANA levels. The term sialic acid storage disease (SASD) is increasingly being applied across the clinical spectrum to avoid confusion. The recent identification of a proton-driven carrier for NANA in the lysosomal membrane, and its characterisation in reconstituted membrane systems, may be expected to lead to elucidation of the primary defects in sialic acid storage disorders of varying severity. Differences in residual transport activity have now been correlated with different clinical phenotypes. It is also now known that the same transporter carries glucuronic acid, and this also accumulates in SASD.

LABORATORY DIAGNOSIS OF LYSOSOMAL STORAGE DISEASE

It will not have escaped the reader's notice that there is considerable clinical heterogeneity within the presentation of any single lysosomal storage disorder and that there is an impressive degree of overlap in clinical presentation between diseases, even those due to accumulation of different macromolecules.[14]

Gargoyle-like facies, dysostosis multiplex and mental and motor retardation with visual loss are seen in nearly all of the mucopolysaccharidoses, oligosaccharidoses and GM_1 gangliosidosis, although they may be absent from variants of these conditions. Seizures are rare in all but the most severe disorders of glycoprotein catabolism but myoclonus should make one think of sialidase deficiencies. Hypotonia is usually the initial feature of fucosidosis, GM_1 gangliosidosis and Sandhoff disease with rapid progression to spasticity.

The laboratory investigations are very important[27] and a suspected clinical diagnosis of any one of these conditions should alert the biochemist to search more widely and carefully if the initial clinical diagnosis proves to be wrong. In the author's laboratory all of the patients diagnosed as having a mucopolysaccharidosis Type IV A (Morquio) had been thought to have Hurler syndrome at initial presentation below the age of 5 years, the diagnosis only being modified as the clinical picture and radiological changes unfolded and biochemical identification of abnormal keratan sulphate was made. Careful note should be made of specific clinical features such as a cherry red macula, corneal clouding or gingival hypertrophy which often helps as much to exclude a disorder as to confirm it.

Demonstration of vacuolated lymphocytes or foam cells in marrow are highly suggestive of a lysosomal disorder. Enzyme assays can be done on serum, plasma, tears, saliva, leucocytes, hair follicles and cultured fibroblasts.[28,29] Assay on cultured individual hair follicles may be useful in detection of carriers of X-linked disease based on the principle that some follicles will show normal enzyme activity and others will have very low activity depending on which X chromosome is active.

Simple urine screening tests are available for initial help in the diagnosis of the mucopolysaccharidoses but those such as filter paper spot tests which do not take urine concentration into account are likely to give false results.[30] A positive screening test can be confirmed by estimation of alcian blue precipitable material or the hexuronic acid precipitated by a suitable detergent. The excretion pattern may be discerned by two dimensional electrophoresis or sequential thin layer chromatography but considerable experience is required to identify abnormalities with certainty. Patients with Sanfilippo syndrome may only have moderately increased excretion and the abnormal heparan sulphate is sometimes difficult to identify by thin layer chromatography. Patients with I-cell disease excrete mucopolysaccharides and may be difficult to differentiate from MPS disorders, while the diagnosis of Morquio disease by detection of abnormal keratan sulphate excretion (also seen in GM_1 gangliosidosis and fucosidosis) is particularly difficult since it may not persist throughout the life of the patient.

Urinary oligosaccharide excretion may also be evaluated by simple thin layer chromatography[31–33] but careful examination of urine from healthy children reveals several oligosaccharides and interpretation of a chromatogram from a patient may require considerable experience. Simple chromatographic techniques can also suggest which enzymes should be studied in blood or tissues.

Looking for the right enzyme first time may be a problem. Because of this some laboratories operate a selective screening approach in which several of the lysosomal enzyme activities are estimated in any patient with progressive neurological handicap but no single feature to indicate a specific diagnosis. Such an approach may be valuable and often helps to diagnose the unexpected, but there are limitations since, unless the list of enzyme assays available is comprehensive, some conditions will inevitably be missed and a partial list of conditions which have been excluded, especially if lengthy, may give the clinician the idea that all possible lysosomal defects have been excluded and the opportunity for prenatal diagnosis in subsequent pregnancies is lost.

The laboratory staff offering a diagnostic service must ensure that they have experience of all the enzymes referred to in this text, as well as new ones which may be identified in the future, and have adequate information culled from their own experiments to identify optimal conditions for enzymes assay and provide adequate information on reference ranges. Special care may be required with those enzyme assays where isoenzymes are likely to interfere, or the enzyme is labile or affected by the stage of cell development or cultural growth conditions. It is becoming increasingly clear that, although many lysosomal enzyme assays appear to be as easy to perform as a serum alkaline or acid phosphatase assay, there are many pitfalls for the unwary and these tests should probably be done in specialised laboratories providing specific services for the investigation of inherited metabolic disease. This is an absolute requirement when prenatal diagnosis is being considered and adequate lists of suitable laboratories are available throughout the countries of Europe and in the United States.

Finally, both clinician and laboratory scientist should be alert to the increasing number of these disorders which may present as late-onset neurological disease in adults.[34]

TREATMENT OF LYSOSOMAL STORAGE DISEASE

Treatment of these conditions has been largely palliative and supportive, often requiring institutional care for the severely and progressively handicapped. Orthopaedic surgery plays an important part in some of the conditions where skeletal abnormalities predominate. Fusion of the atlantooccipital axis in Morquio disease is essential to prevent early death or quadriplegia and relief of carpal tunnel syndrome may be required in all the mucopolysaccharidoses. Corneal grafting may be temporarily helpful but the graft usually becomes opaque quite rapidly.

Recent attempts to replace the missing enzyme by marrow transplantation[5], although resulting in biochemical and clinical improvement, have been bedevilled by graft-versus-host disease.[6] Attempts to avoid this problem by using amniotic tissue transplants have produced temporary resolution of corneal clouding but little change in biochemical parameters. Any treatment is unlikely to reverse the neurological damage already sustained unless it can be given in utero. Such an approach would be possible since prenatal diagnosis of most of these conditions is feasible and widely available. However, termination of affected pregnancies is probably the more logical if not always ethically acceptable course. Where the condition has a specific ethnic predilection and heterozygous status can be readily identified, sound genetic advice may be given to help eradicate the disease. Success in the treatment of Gaucher disease[7] may provide the breakthrough required to treat other lysosomal storage diseases.

REFERENCES

1. Callahan J W, Lowden J A (eds) 1981 Lysosomes and lysosomal storage disease. Raven Press, New York
2. Haselik A, Neufeld E F 1980 Biosynthesis of lysosomal enzymes in fibroblasts: phophorylation of mannose residues. Journal of Biological Chemistry 255:4946–4950
3. Hers H G, Van Hoof F (eds) 1973 Lysosomes and storage disease. Academic Press, New York
4. O'Brien J S 1975 Molecular genetics of GM_1 galactosidase. Clinical Genetics 8:303–313
5. Hobbs J R (ed) 1989 Correction of certain genetic diseases by transplantation. The Cogent Fund, Westminster Hospital School Research Trust, London
6. O'Reilly J R, Brochstein J, Dinsmore R, Kirkpatrick D 1985 Marrow transplantation for congenital disorders. Seminars in Hematology 21:188–222
7. Fink J K, Correll P H, Perry L K, Brady R O, Karlsson S 1991 Correction of glucocerebrosidase deficiency after retroviral-mediated gene transfer into hematopoietic progenitor cells from patients with Gaucher disease. Proceedings of the National Academy of Science USA 87:2334–2338
8. Stoddart R W 1984 The biosynthesis of polysaccharides. Croom Helm, London
9. Varma R, Varma R S 1983 Mucopolysaccharides – Glycosaminoglycans of body fluids in health and disease. Walter de Gruyter, Berlin

10. McKusick V A 1972 Heritable disorders of connective tissues, 4th edn. C V Mosby, ST Louis
11. Leroy J G 1982 The oligosaccharidoses: Proposal of a new name and a new classification for the mucolipidoses. Birth Defects: Original Article Series 18:3–12
12. Cantz M, Ulrich-Bolt B 1990 Disorders of glycoprotein degradation. Journal of Inherited Metabolic Disease 13:523–537
13. McKusick V A 1992 Mendelian inheritance in man, 10th edn. Johns Hopkins University Press, Baltimore
14. Whiteman P, Young E 1977 The laboratory diagnosis of Sanfilippo disease. Clinica Chimica Acta 76:139–147
15. Hers H G 1973 The concept of inborn lysosomal disease. In: Hers H G Van Hoof F (eds) Lysosomes and storage diseases. Academic Press, New York, p 625–633
16. Beutler E 1991 Gaucher's disease. New England Journal of Medicine 325:1354–1360
17. Spence M W, Callahan J W 1989 The Niemann-Pick group of diseases. In: Scriver C R, Beaudet A L, Sly W S, Valle D (eds) The metabolic basis of inherited disease, 6th edn. McGraw – Hill, p 1655–1676
18. Suzuki K 1984 Gangliosides and disease: A review. Advances in Experimental Medicine and Biology 74:407–418
19. Roy A B 1976 Sulphatases, lysosomes and disease. Australian Journal of Experimental Biology and Medical Science 54:111–135
20. Lowden J A, O'Brien J S 1979 Sialidosis: A review of human neuraminidase deficiency. American Journal of Medical Genetics 31:1–18
21. Willems P J, Gatti R, Darby J K, Romeo G, Durand P, Dumon J E, O'Brien J S 1991 Fucosidosis revisited: A review of 77 patients. American Journal of Medical Genetics 38:111–131
22. Maury C P J 1982 Aspartyglucosaminuria: An inborn error of glycoprotein catabolism. Journal of Inherited Metabolic Disease 5:192–196
23. Sly W S, Sundaram V 1985 The I-cell model: the molecular basis for abnormal lysosomal enzyme transport in mucolipidosis II and mucolipidosis III. In: Lloyd J K, Scriver C R (eds) Genetics and metabolic disease in pediatrics. Butterworth, London, p. 91–110
24. Gahl W A, Bashan N, Tietze F, Bernardini I, Schulman J D 1982 Lysosomal cystine transport is defective in cystinosis. Science 217:1263–1265
25. Renlund M, Aula P, Raivio K, Sainio K, Rapala J, Koskala L 1983 Salla disease: a new lysosomal storage disorder with disturbed sialic acid metabolism. Neurology 33:57–66
26. Mancini G M S, Beerens C E M T, Aula P P, Verheijen F W 1991 Sialic acid storage diseases: a multiple lysosomal transport defect for acid monosaccharides. Journal of Clinical Investigation 87:1329–1335
27. Applegarth D A, Toone J R, Macleod P M 1983 Laboratory diagnosis of inborn errors of metabolism in children. Pediatric Pathology 1:107–130
28. Hall C W, Liebaers I, DiNatale P, Neufeld E F 1982 Enzymic diagnosis of genetic mucopolysaccharide storage disorders, In: Colowick S P, Kaplan N C (eds) Methods in Enzymology 83:439–455
29. Suzuki K 1982 Enzymic diagnosis of sphingolipidoses. In: Colowick S P, Kaplan N C (eds) Methods in Enzymology 83:456–488
30. Pennock C A 1980 Investigation of the mucopolysaccharidoses. Broadsheet 93: Association of Clinical Pathologists, British Medical Association, London, p 1–11
31. Humbel R, Collart M 1975 Oligosaccharides in urine of patients with glycoprotein storage diseases. Clinica Chimica Acta 60:143–145
32. Sewell A C 1980 Urinary oligosaccharide excretion in disorders of glycolipid, glycoprotein and glycogen metabolism. European Journal of Pediatrics 134:183–194
33. Sewell A C 1983 The simple detection of neuraminic acid-containing urinary oligosaccharides in patients with glycoprotein storage disease. Journal of Inherited Metabolic Disease 6:153–157
34. Baumann N, Federico A, Suzuki K (eds) 1991 Late onset neurometabolic genetic disoders. Karger, Basle

6. Peroxisomal disorders

R. B. H. Schutgens R. J. A. Wanders

INTRODUCTION

Peroxisomes (microbodies, glyoxysomes, glycosomes) were the last of the subcellular organelle structures to be detected in eukaryotic cells. They are widespread in nature as they are described in mammals, seeds and leaves of plants, protozoa and fungi. In mammals peroxisomes were first observed only in 1954 in the cytoplasm of mouse proximal kidney tubules and, originally, were classified as microbodies due to their size and because of lack of knowledge regarding their associated biochemistry. Later it became apparent, especially through the pioneering work of De Duve & Baudhuin[1] that the organelles were a metabolic entity.

Peroxisomes are present in every mammalian cell except for the mature erythrocyte. They are abundant in tissues active in lipid metabolism. In addition to the peroxisomes in liver (Fig. 6.1) and kidney, smaller peroxisomes (microperoxisomes) are present in other cell types, including chorionic villus cells, cultured fibroblasts and amniocytes from humans. Microperoxisomes seem to have essentially the same enzyme content and function as the larger sized peroxisomes in liver and kidney. Visualization is achieved by light or electron microscopy after staining with 3,3'-diaminobenzidine (DAB), employing the peroxidative activity of catalase at alkaline pH[2–4], or by immunocytochemistry or immunofluorimetry with specific antisera against peroxisomal matrix or membrane proteins. A biotin-streptavidin signal enhancement step can be employed in order to visualize the (micro)peroxisomes in cultured human skin fibroblasts. Incubations with these specific antibodies show a punctate fluorescent labelling pattern in peroxisome-containing cells and a diffuse pattern in peroxisome-deficient cells. Hypolipidaemic drugs like clofibrate, herbicides and phalate ester plasticisers induce proliferation of peroxisomes in hepatic parenchymal cells of rodents, but not in monkey and human cells.

Peroxisomes do not contain DNA. As a consequence all peroxisomal proteins are coded for by nuclear genes. This includes the peroxisomal matrix proteins and a set of specific peroxisomal integral membrane proteins (69/70 kDa, 53 kDa, and 22 kDa respectively). The 22 kDa

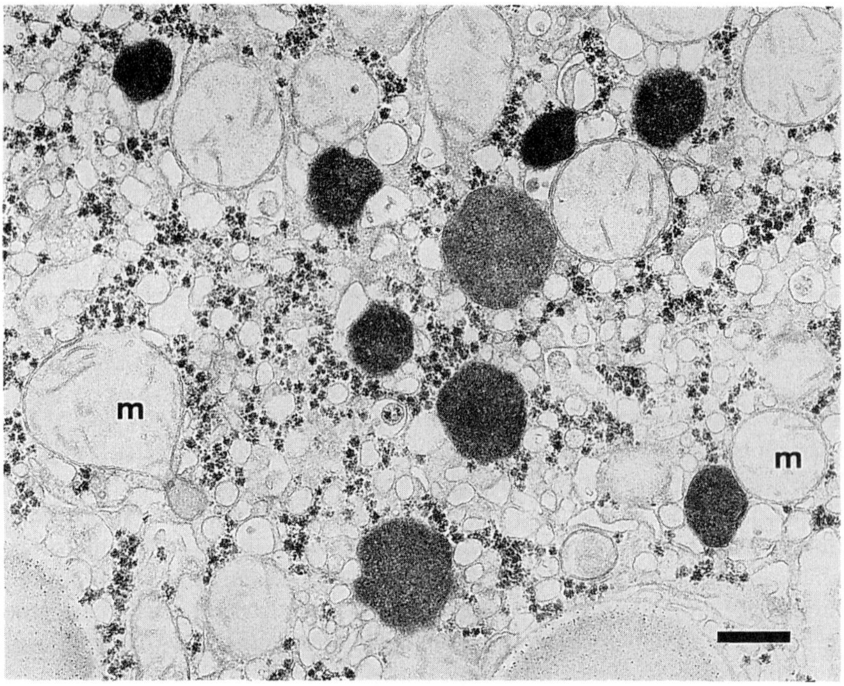

Fig. 6.1 Ultrastructure of a normal adult human liver cell. Peroxisomes are dark after cytochemical staining for catalase activity. Small block granules are glycogen rosettes; m – mitochondria marker = 0.5 μm. From Roels 1991[4], by courtesy of the publisher.

protein is believed to be involved in the permeability of peroxisomal membranes to small molecules.[5] Another protein that is most abundant in the peroxisomal membrane, the 35/36 kDa protein, is probably also present in the mitochondrial and the microsomal membrane.

Initially it was thought that the only function of mammalian peroxisomes was the detoxification of the hydrogen peroxide produced by the oxidases present. However, during the last few years it has become clear that peroxisomes constitute an indispensible compartment in mammalian cells in which a large number of specific metabolic functions occur.

Recently, a growing number of genetic disorders have been recognised that result from the impairment of one or more peroxisomal metabolic functions. As a group they are called 'peroxisomal disorders'.[6,7] An impressive amount of knowledge has accumulated about the clinical and biochemical characteristics of these disorders and the essential metabolic functions of peroxisomes.

The clinical heterogeneity of some of these disorders has been found to be surprisingly great. However, much has still to be learned about the relationship between pathophysiology and the metabolic defect(s) in most of these disorders, and about the primary defect in several of them.

Probably a growing number of peroxisomal disorders will be identified in the coming years.

FUNCTIONS OF MAMMALIAN PEROXISOMES

Table 6.1 summarises a selection of major metabolic functions in mammalian peroxisomes. The processes involved are discussed below.

Peroxisomal oxidation and respiration

The peroxisomal respiratory pathway, responsible for as much as 20% of oxygen consumption in rat liver, was originally identified by De Duve & Baudhuin.[1] Hydrogen peroxide, H_2O_2, is formed in this pathway by different oxidases reacting with substrates like acyl-CoAs, D- and L-aminoacids, L-pipecolic acid, L-α-hydroxyacids, glutaryl-CoA, oxalate, tri(di)hydroxycholestanoyl-CoA, pristanoyl-CoA and others. Subsequently H_20_2 is decomposed either peroxidatively, accepting substrates like ethanol, methanol, quinones, nitrite and formate, or catalatically by reaction of two molecules of H_2O_2 to form H_2O and O_2.

Peroxisomal β-oxidation

It has been shown, that mammalian cells contain a peroxisomal fatty acid β-oxidation system in addition to the mitochondrial β-oxidation pathway.[8] The peroxisomal system is not just a functional duplication of the mitochondrial system but it is involved in the β-oxidative chain shortening of a distinct set of compounds that cannot be handled by the mitochondrial system.

Table 6.1 Major metabolic functions of peroxisomes in man

Catabolic functions
Hydrogen peroxide-based cellular respiration
β-Oxidation
Long chain fatty acids (saturated/unsaturated)
Very long chain fatty acids (saturated/unsaturated)
Branched chain fatty acids
Prostaglandins
Xenobiotics
L-Pipecolic acid oxidation
Ethanol oxidation
Purine catabolism
Polyamine catabolism
Anabolic Functions
Plasmalogen biosynthesis
Cholesterol biosynthesis
Bile acid biosynthesis
Dolichol biosynthesis
Glyoxylate transamination

The activity of the peroxisomal system towards short-chain fatty acids is negligible. Activation of other saturated and (poly)unsaturated free fatty acids to CoA esters by a variety of specific acyl-CoA synthetases is the first obligatory step in the peroxisomal β-oxidation of these metabolites. A long-chain acyl-CoA synthetase has been identified at the peroxisomal membrane next to a second acyl-CoA synthetase which preferentially activates very long chain fatty acids (VLCFAs) such as tetracosanoic ($C_{24:0}$) and hexacosanoic ($C_{26:0}$) acid.[9–11] The latter enzyme activity is present in peroxisomes and the endoplasmic reticulum but not in mitochondria. Evidence was obtained for an obligatory coupling between the activation of VLCFAs on the peroxisomal membrane and their subsequent β-oxidation within the peroxisomes. Like the mitochondrial β-oxidation, the peroxisomal β-oxidation of saturated fatty acids proceeds via successive steps of dehydrogenation, hydratation, dehydrogenation and thiolytic cleavage (Fig. 6.2). The peroxisomal enzymes, acyl-CoA oxidases, a multifunctional polypeptide containing enoyl-CoA hydratase, L-3-hydroxyacyl-CoA dehydrogenase activity, enoyl-CoA isomerase activity (earlier known as bifunctional enzyme) and peroxisomal 3-ketoacyl-CoA thiolase are quite distinct from their mitochondrial counterparts. Antisera raised against the respective peroxisomal β-oxidation enzyme proteins do not cross-react with their mitochondrial counterparts.

Apart from the enzymes directly involved in β-oxidation of saturated fatty acids, peroxisomes also contain the auxiliary enzymes required for the degradation of unsaturated fatty acids and/or D-hydroxy fatty acids (for review, see Hiltunen[12]). Peroxisomes also possess medium-chain carnitine acyltransferase activity and carnitine acetyltransferase activity. It is assumed that these enzymes are involved in the transport of the end-products of peroxisomal β-oxidation of fatty acids to the mitochondria as carnitine esters.[13]

Cholic acid is formed from 3-α,7-α,12-α-trihydroxy-5-β-cholestanoic acid (THCA) via β-oxidation. Peroxisomes are probably the sole site of THCA oxidation.[14] Also, the β-oxidation of branched chain fatty acids, such as pristanic acid, appears to occur in peroxisomes[15, 16], and peroxisomes have been implicated in the β-oxidation of dicarboxylic acids, prostaglandins E_2 and $F_{2\alpha}$, and xenobiotics with an acyl side-chain (see review by Van den Bosch et al[17]). It is as yet uncertain, however, whether peroxisomes are the sole site of β-oxidation of these compounds.

Glyoxylate metabolism

In mammals glyoxylate can be metabolized by conversion to glycine in a reaction catalysed by alanine:glyoxylate aminotransferase (AGT). In man this enzyme is detected only in liver peroxisomes and to a lesser extent in kidney peroxisomes.[18,19] In this way glyoxylate enters the gluconeogenic pathway.

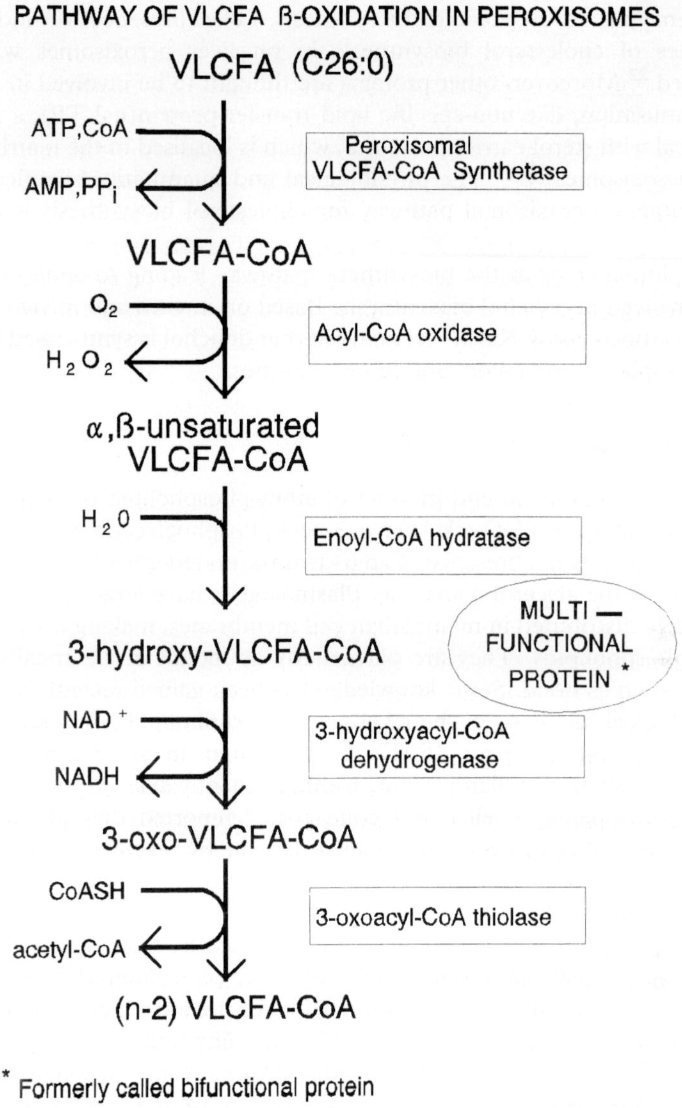

Fig. 6.2 The activation and subsequent β-oxidation of very long chain fatty acids in peroxisomes.

Cholesterol and dolichol metabolism

Mammalian peroxisomes have recently been implicated as a site of cholesterol biosynthesis. Immunoelectronmicroscopy and subcellular fractionation studies demonstrated that substantial amounts of 3-hydroxy-3-methylglutaryl-CoA reductase are present in peroxisomes.[20, 21] This enzyme, in the endoplasmic reticulum, is considered to be the key regulatory enzyme of isoprenoid biosynthesis. The presence of individual enzymes of cholesterol biosynthesis in rat liver peroxisomes was also reported.[22] Moreover, other proteins are thought to be involved in cholesterol utilisation, like non-specific lipid transfer protein(nsLTP), a protein identical with sterol carrier protein 2, which is localised in the matrix of rat liver peroxisomes.[23, 24] The physiological and quantitative significance of this putative peroxisomal pathway for cholesterol biosynthesis is not yet clear.

The initial steps in the biosynthetic pathway leading to cholesterol are also involved in dolichol biosynthesis. Based on in vitro and in vivo experiments, Appelkvist & Kalen[25] concluded that dolichol is synthesised both in the endoplasmic reticulum and in peroxisomes.

Ether lipid synthesis

In mammals the main end product of ether-phospholipid biosynthesis are the plasmalogens (1-O-alk-1'-enyl-2-acyl-phosphoglycerides), which are characterised by the presence of an α-,β-unsaturated ether bond at the *sn*-1 position of the glycerol backbone. Plasmalogens have long been known to be widely distributed in mammalian cell membranes, making up 5–20% of total phospholipids. They are particularly abundant in electrically active tissues such as brain. Some knowledge has been gained recently about the physiological functions of the alkyl-glycerophospholipids. It is known that platelet activating factor (PAF) is implicated in several pathological processes, such as inflammation, asthma, anaphylaxis, hypotension and thrombocytopenia. Zoeller and colleagues[26] reported that plasmalogens protect animal cell membranes against damage by reactive oxygen species such as singlet oxygen.

The initial steps in the biosynthesis of plasmalogens take place inside the peroxisomes, but subsequent steps are catalysed by microsomal enzymes. Peroxisomes play an essential role in ether-phospholipid biosynthesis, since the two enzyme activities responsible for the introduction of the ether bond in ether-phospholipids, i.e. acyl-CoA dihydroxyacetone phosphate acyltransferase (DHAPAT) and alkyldihydroxyacetone phosphate synthase (alkyl DHAP synthase), are almost exclusively localised in peroxisomes.[27]

Other metabolic functions of peroxisomes

Recently it was shown that the conversion of L-pipecolic acid to α-aminoadipic acid takes place in peroxisomes.[28] Wanders and coworkers[29] discovered that in man the first step in L-pipecolic acid degradation is catalysed by the peroxisomal enzyme L-pipecolic acid oxidase. Peroxisomes contain, also, an oxidase capable of oxidizing different polyamines. Finally, it has been established, that peroxisomes are involved in the metabolism of phytanic acid, as peroxisomes contain pristanoyl-CoA oxidase activity.[16, 30]

BIOGENESIS OF PEROXISOMES

It is now well established that peroxisomes arise by growth and division of pre-existing peroxisomes.[31] As peroxisomes contain no DNA, all peroxisomal proteins must be coded for by nuclear genes. The genes for several peroxisomal proteins have been cloned and characterized (see review by Van den Bosch et al[17]).

All peroxisomal proteins investigated so far, including soluble matrix proteins and integral peroxisomal membrane proteins, are synthesised on free ribosomes and imported post-translationally into peroxisomes. Almost all are synthesized at their final size (see review by Borst[32]).

Recent studies have shown that the targeting signal for a substantial number of peroxisomal proteins resides either in a carboxyterminal or an internally positioned tripeptide, Ser-Lys-Leu (SKL).[33] The targeting signal for the peroxisomal 3-oxoacyl-CoA thiolase is located at the N-terminal end that is removed upon maturation of the enzyme protein.[34] Accordingly, import of proteins into peroxisomes requires at least two receptors recognizing their respective targeting signals.

PEROXISOMAL DISORDERS

In humans the vital importance of peroxisomes for cellular metabolism received particular emphasis by the recognition of a number of inherited diseases involving either a defect in the biogenesis of peroxisomes or a deficiency of one or more peroxisomal enzymes. As a group they are known as peroxisomal disorders. So far at least 14 different peroxisomal disorders have been described and most of them are lethal diseases.

A tentative classification of the peroxisomal disorders is presented in Table 6.2. Three major classification groups are recognized. Group 1 includes the disorders in which functional peroxisomes are reduced in number or absent in all cell types studied, due to a defect at the level of the biogenesis of peroxisomes. In the second group disorders are listed with a normal or nearly normal peroxisome structure, at least in fibroblasts, but with multiple deficiencies of peroxisomal enzymes. The third group includes those disorders in which there is defective function of a single peroxisomal enzyme. In this group peroxisome structure is normal.

CLINICAL CHARACTERISTICS

1. Disorders of peroxisome biogenesis

Group 1 includes the peroxisome deficiency disorders. The disorders belonging to this category include autosomal recessively inherited disorders like the cerebrohepatorenal (Zellweger) syndrome (McKusick 214100, 214110); the neonatal type of adrenoleukodystrophy (NALD, McKusick 202370); the infantile type of Refsum disease (McKusick 266510), and

Table 6.2 Classification of peroxisomal disorders

1. Peroxisome deficiency disorders
   Zellweger (cerebrohepatorenal) syndrome
   Neonatal adrenoleukodystrophy
   Infantile Refsum disease
   Hyperpipecolic acidaemia
2. Disorders with loss of multiple peroxisomal functions and peroxisome structure in fibroblasts
   Rhizomelic chondrodysplasia punctata
   'Zellweger-like' syndrome
3. Disorders with an impairment of only one peroxisomal function and normal peroxisomal structure
   A. Disorders of peroxisomal β-oxidation
      Adrenoleukodystrophy (X-linked) and variants
      Acyl-CoA oxidase deficiency
      Bi(multi) functional protein deficiency
      Peroxisomal thiolase deficiency
   B. Other disorders
      Acyl-CoA: dihydroxyacetone phosphate acyltransferase (DHAP-AT) deficiency
      Primary hyperoxaluria Type I
      Acatalasaemia
      Glutaryl oxidase deficiency

hyperpipecolic acidaemia (McKusick 239400). In these disorders a severely reduced number or complete absence of functional peroxisomes is found in all cells, resulting in an almost complete loss of all peroxisomal functions.

Goldfischer and coworkers[35] were the first to recognize that morphologically distinguishable peroxisomes are absent in Zellweger patients. Recent immunofluorimetric studies in cultured fibroblasts from Zellweger patients have shown that some of the peroxisomal integral membrane proteins are present in these cells in unusual, largely empty, membrane structures called peroxisomal 'ghosts'.[36–38] It cannot be ruled out, however, that, these 'ghosts' are, in fact, peroxisomal membranes being degraded in autophagosomes.[39] Probably all peroxisomal enzyme proteins are synthesised normally in the cells of the patients belonging to this category, but most of them are degraded rapidly in the cytosol post-translationally, as the peroxisomal structures which are present are incapable of import of the newly synthesised enzyme proteins. A few enzyme proteins, like catalase and alanine: glyoxylate aminotransferase, escape rapid degradation in the cytosol and are still functionally active, although they are present in the cytosol and not in peroxisomes.

Zellweger syndrome

This is a usually lethal disease with severe clinical, pathological and biochemical abnormalities, including a typical craniofacial dysmorphism and neuronal migration disturbances present at birth. Major and minor clinical abnormalities are summarised in Table 6.3. The deterioration in this disorder starts prenatally, an important consideration with respect to treatment.

Some phenotypic variability has been noticed as a few patients survive the first year of life and exhibit some psychomotor development.[40,41] The 'classic' Zellweger syndrome is characterized by typical craniofacial abnormalities, severe neurological dysfunction including severe psychomotor retardation and hypotonia, neurosensory defects, progressive ocular manifestations, liver dysfunction and chondrodysplasia calcificans of the patellae and the acetabulum. Most patients die within the first 6 months of life. Pathological examination shows abnormalities in many different organs, notably in brain, liver and kidney. Neuropathological examination may reveal abnormalities in gyration, myelination and neuronal migration. The liver may show cholestasis, abnormal intrahepatic bile ducts and severe iron storage in the neonatal period, which slowly disappears after 20 weeks of age. In the same period progressive liver fibrosis may become manifest. In almost all patients renal cysts can be found although renal function is normal.

Neonatal adrenoleukodystrophy

The clinical manifestations in NALD patients resemble Zellweger syndrome, but are usually somewhat milder as patients mostly show some psychomotor development and reach certain milestones before regression sets in. Facial dysmorphia is less frequent in NALD. Computerized tomography may show contrast enhancement around demyelinating areas. As in Zellweger syndrome, neuropathological abnormalities in NALD are diverse, being dysontogenetic and degenerative in nature. This is reflected in the finding of demyelination in the cerebral hemispheres, cerebellum and brainstem, neuronal migration disturbances, neocortical microgyria

Table 6.3 Major and minor clinical characteristics of Zellweger syndrome

Major Symptoms	Hypotonia Psychomotor retardation Sensorineural deafness Abnormal ERG
Minor Symptoms	Wide open fontanelles/sutures Shallow supraorbital ridge Hypertelorism Epicanthus Flat occiput Foot deformity Hepatomegaly (1st year of life) Retinitis pigmentosa Redundant neck skinfolds

and perivascular lymphocytic infiltrates. Kelley and coworkers[42] have suggested criteria to discriminate between Zellweger patients and NALD patients. According to these criteria, NALD patients would demonstrate adrenal atrophy, cerebral demyelination, systemic infiltrations of lipid-laden macrophages and elevated levels of saturated very long chain fatty acids (VLCFAs), whereas Zellweger patients would have chondrodysplasia, glomerulocystic disease of the kidney, CNS dysmyelination rather than demyelination and elevated levels of both saturated and unsaturated VLCFAs. However, adrenal atrophy is also described in Zellweger patients.

Infantile Refsum disease (IRD)

The clinical course in this disease is milder than in Zellweger patients and NALD patients. Mental retardation, retinitis pigmentosa, failure to thrive and hypocholesterolaemia are characteristic clinical features in IRD patients. However, distinct abnormalities are absent in the neonatal period, dysmorphia is usually only minor and patients survive into the second decade of life. The patients described by Poll-Thé and coworkers[43] were able to explore objects bimanually and to walk independently. Autopsy findings in an IRD patient revealed no malformations of the cerebral cortex and no heterotopias of the cerebral or cerebellar white matter. Furthermore, there were no cortical cysts, skeletal changes or liver damage.

Hyperpipecolic acidaemia

There is a strong resemblance in clinical and biochemical presentation between the hyperpipecolic acidaemia patients and Zellweger patients. Whether hyperpipecolic acidaemia has to be considered as a distinct clinical entity is doubtful.

2. Disorders with loss of multiple peroxisome functions and peroxisome structures in cultured fibroblasts

Rhizomelic chondrodysplasia punctata

Rhizomelic chondrodysplasia punctata (RCDP) belongs to a genetically heterogenous group of bone dysplasias whose common feature is stippling of the epiphyses in infancy.[44] It is an autosomal recessive disorder, characterised by a disproportionate short stature primarily affecting the proximal parts of the extremities, a typical facial appearance, joint contractures, a palpable liver in a majority of the patients, normal liver function and architecture and severe mental and growth retardation. Roentgenological studies revealed marked metaphyseal changes, disturbed ossification of humeri and/or femora, and severe, symmetrical epiphysial and extraepiphysial calcifications. Survival is well into the second decade of life. In other types of chondrodysplasia punctata, like the milder, autosomal recessive Conradi–Hunermann and both the X-linked dominant and X-linked recessive, no peroxisomal abnormalities have been found so far.

Zellweger-like syndrome

Two patients are described with a clinical presentation indistinguishable from classical Zellweger syndrome but showing abundant peroxisomes in liver.[45,46] Both plasmalogen metabolism and the peroxisomal β-oxidation system are defective in these patients.

3. Disorders with impairment of one peroxisomal function and normal peroxisome structure

A. Peroxisomal β-oxidation disorders with one deficient enzyme activity

Adrenoleukodystrophy. (McKusick 300100.) In this X-linked recessively inherited disorder there is considerable phenotypic variability even within the same kindred. Approximately 50% of affected males develop neurological symptoms between 4 and 10 years of age. School failure, or attentional deficit disorders, may be the first manifestation, followed by seizures, visual disturbances or paralysis, leading to an apparently vegetative state and death. This phenotype is known as childhood adrenoleukodystrophy (ALD). Another 25% present in adulthood with paraparesis that is slowly progressive over decades (adrenomyeloneuropathy type), while the remainder may exhibit adrenocortical insufficiency without neurological involvement or a variety of other neurological symptoms (see review by Moser & Moser[47]). At least 20% of female heterozygotes develop mild or moderate progressive paraparesis in the fourth decade or later.

***Acyl-CoA oxidase deficiency (Pseudoneonatal adrenoleukodystrophy)* (McKusick 264470)**. This condition has been described in only a very limited number of patients. The patients described by Poll-Thé and coworkers[48] presented with early seizures, muscle hypotonia, progressive hearing loss, visual impairment due to retinopathy and latent adrenocortical insufficiency. Psychomotor development was severely delayed. Moreover, extinguished electroretinograms and absent flash-evoked visual responses were found. No dysmorphia is reported.

Bi (multi)functional protein deficiency. This rare disorder presented in a patient with hypotonia and macrocephaly at birth who subsequently demonstrated clonic movements of the upper extremities, depressed reflexes and developmental delay.[49] An EEG showed multifocal spikes; visual evoked response and brainstem evoked response were grossly abnormal. Brain biopsy at 6 weeks of age revealed polymicrogyria and abnormalities in both the grey and white matter.

Peroxisomal 3-oxoacyl-CoA thiolase deficiency (Pseudo-Zellweger syndrome) **(McKusick 261510.)** A patient was described with all the clinical and pathological features of Zellweger syndrome, including marked facial dysmorphia, muscle weakness and hypotonia at birth.[50] The patient died at the age of 11 months. However, morphological studies revealed that the liver contained abundant peroxisomes. Later studies using immunoblotting showed that the biochemical defect in this patient was at the level of a deficient peroxisomal 3-oxoacyl-CoA thiolase.[51]

B. *Other disorders*

Acyl-CoA dihydroxyacetone-phosphate acyltransferase (DHAP-AT) deficiency. Recently we identified several patients in which plasmalogen metabolism was disturbed due to a deficient DHAP-AT activity. Phytanic acid metabolism and the peroxisomal β-oxidation of fatty acids were both normal. The patients exhibited all the clinical signs and symptoms described for rhizomelic chondrodysplasia punctata patients.[52]

Primary hyperoxaluria Type I. (McKusick 259900.) This autosomal recessive disorder of glyoxylate metabolism shows considerable phenotypic variation. Patients usually present during the first decade of life with recurrent calcium oxalate nephrolithiasis and nephrocalcinosis. However, some patients present with only minimal renal damage while others suffer from an acute neonatal form with rapid progression and early death.[53]

Acatalasaemia. (McKusick 115500.) This disorder shows some genetic variation, but cases typically present with gangrenous oral ulcerations.

Other rare peroxisomal disorders. Those described in the literature are THCA-CoA oxidase deficiency[54] and glutaryl-CoA oxidase deficiency.[55] Moreover, in recent years several patients have been described with defects in peroxisomal beta β-oxidation of yet unknown aetiology. Finally, it has been suggested that the Dyggve–Melchior– Clausen syndrome (McKusick 223800, 304950) is a peroxisomal disorder.[56]

BIOCHEMICAL CHARACTERISTICS

1. Biochemistry of disorders of peroxisome biogenesis

Patients suffering from a peroxisome deficiency disorder show absence or a reduced number of catalase-positive particles (peroxisomes) in liver, in cultured fibroblasts and amniocytes. Catalase activity is found in the cytosol as can be shown in immunofluorimetric studies, in cell fractionation studies or by analysing catalase latency. This represents ways of demonstrating the loss of integrity of peroxisomal structure and is also of diagnostic value.

Surprisingly, it has been shown that the 22, 36 and 69 kDa peroxisomal membrane proteins were present at near-normal levels and were confined to a membraneous fraction both in a control liver as well as in the livers from Zellweger patients. These proteins are most probably contained in non-functional peroxisomal structures called peroxisomal ghosts.

Secondary to the defective peroxisome structure, patients show a characteristic set of biochemical abnormalities (Table 6.4). These include an impaired plasmalogen biosynthesis, a defective peroxisomal β-oxidation system and defective pipecolic acid and phytanic acid metabolism, resulting in characteristic abnormalities in plasma, urine, tissues and in cultured cells of the patients. A drastic decrease in the polyunsaturated fatty acid content in erythrocytes, kidney, liver and cerebrum of Zellweger syndrome patients was reported recently, suggesting an enzyme defect involving the desaturase system of long-chain polyunsaturated fatty acids.[57]

Diagnostic tests include measurement of the DHAP-AT activity in blood platelets, cultured skin or chorionic villus fibroblasts, or cultured amniotic fluid cells; fractionation of the very long (>C22) fatty acids and bile acids in plasma; analysis of the de novo plasmalogen biosynthesis in cultured cells; analysis of the intracellular localisation of catalase in cultured cells and measurement of the plasmalogen levels in cultured cells. Usually, biochemical abnormalities in Zellweger syndrome and in neonatal ALD are more severe than in infantile Refsum disease.

Heterozygote detection is not possible with these biochemical procedures, probably reflecting the fact that all these biochemical abnormalities

Table 6.4 Biochemical characteristics of the main peroxisomal disorders; n – normal, ↑ – elevated, ↑↑ – very elevated, ↓ – decreased, ↓↓ – very decreased

Parameter	Zellweger syndrome	RCDP	X-linked ALD
Metabolites in plasma			
Very long chain fatty acids	↑↑	n	↑
Bile acid intermediates (THCA/DHCA/C_{29} bile acid)	↑↑	n	n
Pipecolic acid	↑↑/↑	n	n
Phytanic acid	↑/↑↑	↑↑	n
Metabolites in urine			
Bile acid intermediates (THCA/DHCA)	↑↑	n	n
Pipecolic acid	↑[1]	n	n
Phytanic acid	↑[1]	↑↑	n
Fibroblasts/amniocytes			
DHAPAT activity	↓↓	↓	n
De novo plasmalogen synthesis	↓	↓↓	n
Plasmalogen content	↓	↓↓	n
Very long chain fatty acids	↑↑	n	↑
VLCFA β-oxidation	↓↓	n	↓
Phytanic acid α-oxidation	↓	↓↓	n

[1] May sometimes be normal depending on age and diet.

are phenomena secondary to an as yet unidentified primary defect at the level of the biogenesis of peroxisomes.

Prenatal diagnosis can be done for Zellweger syndrome, NALD and IRD[58] as specific and sensitive diagnostic biochemical tests are available (Table 6.5).

Complementation analysis with cultured skin fibroblast cell lines from patients belonging to this category has revealed a remarkable genetic heterogeneity. In these studies cultured fibroblasts from different patients are fused and the resulting multinucleated cells are studied for complementation. The studies have revealed the existence of at least nine different complementation groups among the patients with disorders of peroxisome biogenesis.[59] It is presumed that each of the complementation groups represents a distinct genotype, each presumably involving a separate defect in peroxisome biogenesis.

Primary defect

Experimental evidence suggests that the primary defect in the different complementation groups of the peroxisome deficiency disorders results in an inability to import proteins into peroxisomes. These defects can be at the level of the peroxisomal proteins themselves, but are most probably at

Table 6.5 Diagnostic tests for the prenatal diagnosis of peroxisomal disorders; CB – chorion biopsy material, CVF – chorionic villus fibroblasts, AC – cultured amniocytes, VLCFA – very long chain fatty acids, RFLP – restriction fragment length polymorphism

Peroxisomal disorder	Material	Type of analysis
Peroxisome deficiency disorders	CB	DHAPAT, peroxisomes
	CVF, AC	VLCFA, DHAPAT, plasmalogen biosynthesis particle-bound catalase, phytanic acid oxidase
Rhizomelic chondrodysplasia punctata	CB	DHAPAT, plasmalogens, thiolase
	CVF, AC	DHAPAT, de novo plasmalogen biosynthesis, thiolase (immunoblotting), plasmalogens
Adrenoleukodystrophy	CB	RFLP studies
	CVF, AC	VLCFA, $C_{26:0}$ β-oxidation, RFLP studies
Acyl-CoA oxidase deficiency	CVF, AC	VLCFA, $C_{26:0}$ β-oxidation, acyl-CoA oxidase (immunoblotting)
Thiolase deficiency	CVF, AC	VLCFA, $C_{26:0}$ β-oxidation, thiolase (immunoblotting)
Hyperoxaluria Type I	Fetal liver biopsy	Alanine: glyoxylate aminotransferase

the level of the mechanism required for binding the peroxisomal proteins to the peroxisomal membrane and/or the translocation of peroxisomal proteins across the membrane. Information about the uptake mechanism of peroxisomes, is at present sparse.

Tsukamoto and coworkers[60] have recently succeeded in restoring peroxisome biogenesis in a Chinese hamster ovary (CHO) mutant by transfecting the cells with rat liver cDNA. They have identified the correction factor as a 35 kDa peroxisomal membrane protein (peroxisome assembly factor-1). Shimozawa and colleagues subsequently found that a cell line of a Japanese Zellweger patient did not complement with this CHO mutant, indicating that both cell lines belong to the same complementation group. Analysis at the gene level resulted in the identification of the mutation in the gene for the 35 kDa peroxisomal membrane protein in this patient. Further studies on the primary defect in Zellweger syndrome, IRD and NALD patients are in progress.

2. Disorders with multiple peroxisomal function loss: biochemical features

Rhizomelic chondrodysplasia punctata (RCDP) is characterised biochemically by a deficiency of the peroxisomal enzymes of plasmalogen biosynthesis (DHAP-AT but especially alkyl-DHAP synthase), by defective phytanic acid metabolism and by a defect in the processing of the peroxisomal 3-oxo-acyl-CoA thiolase enzyme protein. Residual DHAP-AT activity in platelets and in fibroblasts can be near the low normal range in some patients. In all RCDP patients the plasmalogen levels in erythrocytes and in fibroblasts are very low; de novo plasmalogen biosynthesis, measured in cultured cells, is severely deficient and plasma phytanic acid levels are elevated (Table 6.4). Other peroxisomal functions are normal.

There is no functional deficiency of the peroxisomal β-oxidation in RCDP and no accumulation of VLCFAs and intermediates of bile acid biosynthesis are found.

Heterozygote detection is not possible with the biochemical procedures described above. This is due to the fact that the characteristic biochemical abnormalities in RCDP are probably secondary to an as yet unknown primary defect.

Prenatal diagnosis is possible and good experience has been gained in specialised laboratories. First trimester prenatal diagnosis can be achieved by measurement of the plasmalogen levels in chorionic biopsy samples by immunoblotting with anti-peroxisomal thiolase in cultured chorionic villus fibroblasts or amniotic fluid cells, and by assay of de novo plasmalogen biosynthesis in cultured cells (Table 6.5).

Primary defect in RCDP. This is not yet known. It has been postulated that the defect is at the level of a specific receptor at the peroxisomal membrane or at the level of the import of a specific set of peroxisomal proteins.

3. Disorders with impairment of a single peroxisomal function: biochemical features

Adrenoleukodystrophy (X-linked)

This disorder can be diagnosed biochemically by the finding of elevated levels of the very long chain fatty acids $C_{26:0}$ and $C_{24:0}$ in plasma or cultured cells, or by demonstrating the impaired β-oxidation of very long chain fatty acids (VLCFAs) in the liver or cultured cells of patients. The disorder has been mapped to Xq28, the terminal segment of the long arm of the X chromosome.

Heterozygote detection for X-linked ALD can be performed using plasma VLCFA analysis and/or by restriction length polymorphism studies using the DNA probe St14.[61] Prenatal diagnosis for X-linked ALD is done by analysing the VLCFAs in cultured chorionic cells or in cultured amniotic fluid cells (Table 6.5) or by molecular biology techniques.[62]

Primary defect in ALD. This has been localised at the level of a deficient peroxisomal VLCFA-CoA synthetase. This enzyme normally activates VLCFAs to CoA-esters that subsequently enter the peroxisomal β-oxidation system.

Acyl-CoA oxidase deficiency; bifunctional protein deficiency; peroxisomal 3-oxo-acyl-CoA thiolase deficiency

These disorders can be diagnosed biochemically by the finding of elevated levels of VLCFAs in plasma and cultured cells, resulting from an impaired peroxisomal β-oxidation, and the finding of normal results in the analyses of other peroxisomal functions. Intermediates of bile acid biosynthesis like THCA and DHCA accumulate in plasma both in bi (multi) functional protein deficiency and peroxisomal thiolase deficiency, but not in acyl-CoA oxidase deficiency. Detailed biochemical studies are necessary to localise the biochemical defects more precisely. In some patients the diagnosis can be established by immunoblot studies with antisera raised against the respective enzyme proteins. However, in others, in which normal immunoresponses are found with all three antisera, time consuming complementation studies are necessary to localise the defect.

Heterozygote detection has not yet been performed successfully. Theoretically it should be possible to detect heterozygotes by analysing the respective peroxisomal enzyme activities. Prenatal diagnosis has been achieved successfully in several pregnancies at risk for recurrence of one of these disorders.

Primary hyperoxaluria Type I

This disorder is caused by a deficiency of the enzyme alanine:glyoxylate aminotransferase (AGT). The enzyme can only be detected in liver and, to a lesser extent, kidney. In humans the enzyme is exclusively present in peroxisomes. More mildly affected patients usually have higher residual AGT activities compared to patients exhibiting the severe neonatal form, in which no residual liver enzyme activity can usually be detected. Danpure and coworkers[63] identified several patients with a trafficking defect resulting in diversion of newly synthesised AGT to the mitochondria. This mitochondrial AGT apparently is functionally inactive in these patients.

Patients can be identified biochemically by the finding of elevated urinary excretion levels of both oxalate and glycolate. However, this can be unreliable when the patient is in renal failure. In addition, there exist hyperoxaluric variant patients who have only mild hyperoxaluria but significant hyperglycolic aciduria, or significant hyperoxaluria with urinary glycolate being raised only slightly or not at all. A more specific diagnostic test is the detection of deficient AGT activity in liver samples from patients. Recently, the gene for AGT has been cloned and cDNA isolated. Detection of the disorder by molecular genetic studies will be available soon. Primary hyperoxaluria Type I is genetically distinct from the clinically similar, but rarer disease, primary hyperoxaluria Type II (D-glycerate dehydrogenase deficiency, McKusick 260000), which is characterised biochemically by hyperoxaluria and hyper-l-glyceric aciduria.

Prenatal diagnosis for primary hyperoxaluria Type I has been achieved in a few patients by measuring the AGT activity in a fetal liver biopsy specimen. Molecular genetic studies will facilitate the prenatal diagnosis of this disorder in the near future. Earlier attempts to identify the disorder prenatally by measuring oxalate and glycolate in amniotic fluid were unsuccessful.[64]

TREATMENT

It is now possible to normalise the plasma VLCFA levels in patients with X-linked ALD by a dietary regimen combining fat restriction and supplementation with glycerol trioleate and glycerol-trierucate.[65] This approach has been shown to improve peripheral nerve function in adrenomyeloneuropathy patients, but long-term effects are as yet undetermined. Unfortunately this dietary regimen does not seem to be beneficial in the childhood ALD variant.

Recent reports indicate that bone marrow transplantation can have promising therapeutic effects in mildly affected childhood ALD patients. However, in more advanced X-linked ALD, bone marrow transplantation was found to hasten neurological deterioration.[66] It is suggested that X-linked ALD may be an excellent candidate for gene therapy.

Therapeutic interventions for the disorders of peroxisome biogenesis are more limited because of the abnormalities that are already present at birth.

Treatment with pyridoxine can be effective in a minority of patients with primary hyperoxaluria Type I. This compound is metabolised to pyridoxal phosphate which is an essential cofactor for AGT activity. For the other patients treatment has been largely symptomatic. Low oxalate diet and high fluid intake are of limited use. Haemodialysis is necessary during end-stage renal failure, not only to relieve uraemia but also to decrease the body burden of oxalate, which increases to very high levels when the glomerular filtration rate falls below 20 ml/min.[67] Surgical removal of renal oxalate obstructions is usually necessary but, eventually, combined liver and kidney transplantation is required.[68] A case can be made for transplanting the liver earlier, before end-stage renal failure. This may prevent significant oxalate accumulation and possibly preclude the necessity for kidney transplantation.

X-LINKED ALD

Until recently it was assumed, that the gene coding for VLCFA CoA synthetase could be a candidate gene for X-linked ALD. Recently Mosser et al[69] reported the identification of a gene in the Xq28 region that was found to be partially deleted in 6 of 85 independent patients with X-linked ALD. Surprisingly the deduced amino acid sequence shows 78.9% sequence similarity with human and rat 70K a peroxisomal membrane protein that is involved in peroxisome biogenesis and belongs to the 'ATP-binding' superfamily of transporters which include for example the cystic fibrosis transmembrane conductance regulator.

The putative ALD protein seems to be a protein involved in transport of newly synthesized VLCFA-CoA synthetase into the peroxisomal membrane or a protein that is functionally associated with VLCFA-CoA synthetase in the peroxisomal membrane. Phenotypic variability of ALD is probably due to secondary factors or the influence of still unidentified modifier genes.

REFERENCES

1. De Duve C, Baudhuin P 1966 Peroxisomes/microbodies and related particles. Physiological Reviews 46:323–357
2. Novikoff A B, Goldfischer S 1968 Visualisation of peroxisomes (microbodies) for light and electron microscopy. Journal of Histochemistry and Cytochemistry 16:507
3. Fahimi H D 1968 Cytochemical localisation of peroxidase activity in rat hepatic microbodies (peroxisomes). Journal of Histochemistry and Cytochemistary 16:547–550
4. Roels F 1991 Peroxisomes. A personal account. VUB Press, Brussels
5. Van Veldhoven P P, Just W W, Mannaerts G P 1987 Permeability of the peroxisomal membrane to cofactors of β-oxidation. Evidence for the presence of a pore-forming protein. Journal of Biological Chemistry 262:4310–4318
6. Schutgens R B H, Heymans H S A, Wanders R J A, Van den Bosch H, Tager J M 1986 Peroxisomal disorders: a newly recognized group of genetic diseases. European Journal of Pediatrics 144:430–440
7. Lazarow P B, Moser H W 1989 Disorders in peroxisome biogenesis. In: Scriver C R, Beaudet A L, Sly W S, Valle D (eds) The metabolic basis of inherited disease 6th edn McGraw–Hill, New York, p 1479–1509

8. Lazarow P B, de Duve C 1976 A fatty acyl-CoA oxidizing system in rat liver peroxisomes: enhancement by clofibrate, a hypolipidemic drug. Proceedings of the National Academy of Sciences USA 73:2043–2046
9. Bhushan A, Singh R P, Singh I 1986 Characterisation of rat brain microsomal acylcoenzyme A ligase: different enzymes for the synthesis of palmitoyl-CoA and lignoceroyl-CoA. Archives of Biochemistry and Biophysics 246:374–380
10. Wanders R J A, van Roermund C W T, van Wijland M J A et al 1987 Peroxisomal fatty acid β-oxidation in relation to the accumulation of very long-chain fatty acids in cultured skin fibroblasts from patients with Zellweger syndrome and other peroxisomal disorders. Journal of Clinical Investigations 80:1778–1783
11. Singh H, Derwas N, Poulos A 1985 β-Oxidation of very long chain fatty acids and their coenzyme A derivatives by human skin fibroblasts. Archives of Biochemistry and Biophysics 359:382–390
12. Hiltunen J K 1991 Peroxisomes and β-oxidation of long chain unsaturated carboxylic acids. Scandinavian Journal of Laboratory Investigations 51 (Suppl 204): 33–46
13. Farrell S O, Bieber L L 1983 Carnitine octanoyl transferase of mouse liver peroxisomes: properties and effects of hypolipidemic drugs. Archives of Biochemistry and Biophysics 222:123–132
14. Kase B F, Björkhem I, Pedersen J I 1983 Formation of cholic acid from 3α,7α,12α trihydroxy-5β-cholestanoic acid by rat liver peroxisomes. Journal of Lipid Research 24: 1560–1567
15. Singh H, Usher S, Johnson D, Poulos A 1990 A comparative study of straight chain and branched chain fatty acid oxidation in skin fibroblasts from patients with peroxisomal disorders. Journal of Lipid Research 31:217–225
16. Wanders R J A, ten Brink H, van Roermund C W T, Schutgens R B H, Tager J M, Jakobs C 1990 Identification of pristanoyl-CoA oxidase activity in human liver and its deficiency in the Zellweger syndrome. Biochemical and Biophysical Research Communications 172:490–495
17. Van den Bosch H, Schutgens R B H, Wanders R J A, Tager J M 1992 Biochemistry of peroxisomes. Annual Reviews of Biochemistry 61:157–197
18. Noguchi T 1987 Amino acid metabolism in animal peroxisomes. In: Fahimi H D, Sies H (eds) Peroxisomes in biology and medicine. Springer, Berlin, p 234–243
19. Danpure C 1989 Recent advances in the understanding, diagnosis and treatment of primary hyperoxaluria type I. Journal of Inherited Metabolic Disease 12:210–224
20. Keller G A, Barton M C, Shapiro D J, Singer S J 1985 3-Hydroxy-3-methylglutaryl coenzyme A reductase is present in peroxisomes in normal rat liver cells. Proceedings of the National Academy of Sciences USA 82:770–774
21. Krisans S K, Pazirandeh M, Keller G A 1987 Localisation of 3-hydroxy-3-methylglutaryl-coenzyme A reductase in rat liver peroxisomes. In: Fahimi H D, Sies H (eds) Peroxisomes in biology and medicine. Springer, Berlin, p 40–52
22. Appelkvist E-L, Reinhart M, Fischer R, Billheimer J, Dallner 1990 Presence of individual enzymes of cholesterol biosynthesis in rat liver peroxisomes. Archives of Biochemistry and Biophysics 282:318–325
23. Van Amerongen A, van Noort M, van Beckhoven J R C M, Rommerts F F G, Orly J, Wirtz K 1989 The subcellular distribution of the nonspecific lipid transfer protein (sterol carrier protein 2) in rat liver and adrenal gland. Biochimica et Biophysica Acta 1001: 243–248
24. Suzuki Y, Yamaguchi S, Orii T, Tsuneoka M, Tashiro Y 1990 Nonspecific lipid transfer protein (sterol carrier-2) defective in patients with deficient peroxisomes. Cell Structure and Function 15:308–310
25. Appelkvist E-L, Kalén A 1989 Biosynthesis of dolichol by rat liver peroxisomes. European Journal of Biochemistry 185:503–509
26. Zoeller R A, Morand O H, Raetz C H R 1988 A possible role for plasmalogens in protecting animal cells against photosensitized killing. Journal of Biological Chemistry 263:11590–11596
27. Hajra A K, Bishop J E 1982 Glycerolipid biosynthesis in peroxisomes via the acyl dihydroxy-acetone phosphate pathway. Annals of the New York Academy of Sciences 386:170–182
28. Mihalik S J, Rhead W J 1989 L-Pipecolic acid oxidation in the rabbit and cynomolgus

monkey: evidence for differing organellar locations and cofactor requirements in each species. Journal of Biological Chemistry 264:2509–2517
29. Wanders R J A, Romeyn G-J, van Roermund C W T, Schutgens R B H, van den Bosch H, Tager J M 1988 Identification of L-pipecolic acid oxidase in human liver and its deficiency in the Zellweger syndrome. Biochemical and Biophysical Research Communications 154:33–38
30. Vanhove G, Van Velthoven P P, Vanhoute F, Parmentier G, Eyssen H J, Mannaerts G P 1991 Mitrochondrial and peroxisomal β-oxidation of the branched chain fatty acid 2-methylpalmitrate in rat liver. Journal of Biological Chemistry 266: 24670–24675
31. Lazarow P B, Fujiki Y 1985 Biogenesis of peroxisomes. Annual Reviews of Cell Biology 1:489–530
32. Borst P 1989 Peroxisome biogenesis revisited. Biochimica et Biophysica Acta 1008:1–13
33. Gould S J, Keller G A, Hasken N, Wilkinson J, Subramani S 1989 A conserved tripeptide sorts proteins to peroxisomes. Journal of Cell Biology 108:1657–1664
34. Swinkels B W, Gould S J, Bodnar A G, Rachubinski R A, Subramani S 1991 A novel, cleavable peroxisomal targetting signal at the animo-terminus of the rat 3-ketoacyl-CoA thiolase. EMBO Journal 10:3255–3262
35. Goldfischer S, Moore C L, Johnson A B et al 1973 Peroxisomal and mitochondrial defects in the cerebro-hepato-renal syndrome. Science 183:62–64
36. Santos M J, Imanaka T, Shio H, Small G M, Lazarow P B 1988 Peroxisomal membrane ghosts in Zellweger syndrome – aberrant organelle assembly. Science 239:1536–1538
37. Wiemer E A C, Brul S, Just W W et al 1989 Presence of peroxisomal membrane proteins in liver and fibroblasts from patients with Zellweger syndrome and related disorders: Evidence for the existence of peroxisomal ghosts. European Journal of Cell Biology 50:407–417
38. Gärtner J, Chen W W, Kelley R I, Mihalik S J, Moser H W 1991 The 22-kd peroxisomal integral membrane protein in Zellweger syndrome – presence, abundance and association with a peroxisomal thiolase precursor protein. Pediatric Research 29:141–146
39. Heikoop J C, van den Berg M, Strijland A, Weijers P J, Just W W, Meijer A J, Tager J M 1992 Turnover of peroxisomal vesicles by autophagic proteolysis in cultured fibroblasts from Zellweger patients. European Journal of Cell Biology 57:165–171
40. Barth P G, Schutgens R B H, Wanders R J A et al 1987 A sibship with a mild variant of Zellweger Syndrome. Journal of Inherited Metabolic Disease 10:253–259
41. Bleeker-Wagemakers E M, Oorthuys J W E, Wanders R J A, Schutgens R B H 1986 Long term survival of a patient with cerebro-hepato-renal (Zellweger) syndrome. Clinical Genetics 29:160–164
42. Kelley R I, Datta N S, Dobyns W S et al 1986 Neonatal adrenoleukodystrophy: new cases, biochemical studies and differentiation from Zellweger and related peroxisomal polydystrophy syndromes. American Journal of Medical Genetics 23:869–901
43. Poll-Thé B-T, Saudubray J M, Ogier H A M et al 1987 Infantile Refsum disease: an inherited peroxisomal disorder; comparison with Zellweger syndrome and neonatal adrenoleukodystrophy. European Journal of Pediatrics 146:477–483
44. Spranger J W, Opitz J M, Bidder U 1971 Heterogeneity of chondrodysplasia punctata. Human Genetics 11:190–212
45. Paterneau-Jouas M, Taillard F, Gansmuller A, Mikol J, Aigrot M S, Sereni C 1987 Clinical, biochemical and pathological aspects of a ‘Zellweger-like’ peroxisomal disorder. In: Salvayre R (ed) Lipid storage disorders. Nato-Inserm. Toulouse, p 133–134
46. Suzuki Y, Shimozawa N, Orii T, Igarashi N, Kono N, Hashimoto T 1988 Molecular analysis of peroxisomal β-oxidation enzymes in infants with Zellweger syndrome and Zellweger-like syndrome: further heterogeneity of the peroxisomal disorders. Clinica Chimica Acta 172:65–76
47. Moser H W, Moser A B 1989 X-linked adrenoleukodystrophy. In: Scriver C R, Beadet A L, Sly W S, Valle D (eds) The Metabolic basis of inherited disease 6th edn. McGraw–Hill New York, p 1511–1532
48. Poll-Thé B-T, Roels F, Ogier H et al 1988 A new peroxisomal disorder with enlarged peroxisomes and a specific deficiency of acyl-CoA oxidase (pseudo neonatal adrenoleukodystrophy). American Journal of Human Genetics 42:422–434

49. Watkins P A, Chen W W, Harris C J et al 1989 Peroxisomal bifunctional enzyme deficiency. Journal of Clinical Investigations 83:771–777
50. Goldfischer S, Collins J, Rapin I et al 1986 Pseudo-Zellweger syndrome: deficiencies in several peroxisomal oxidative activities. Journal of Pediatrics 108:25–32
51. Schram A W, Goldfischer S, van Roermund C W T et al 1987 Human peroxisomal 3-oxoacyl-coenzyme A thiolase deficiency. Proceedings of the National Academy of Sciences USA 84: 494–2496
52. Wanders R J A, Heikoop J, Schutgens R B H, Schumacher H, Tager J M 1992 Human dihydroxyacetone phosphate acyltransferase (DHAP-AT) deficiency: A new peroxisomal disorder. Journal of Inherited Metabolic Disease 15: 389–391
53. Williams H E, Smith L H 1983 Primary hyperoxaluria. In: Stanbury J B, Wyngaarden J B, Fredrickson D S, Goldstein J L, Brown M S (eds) The metabolic basis of inherited disease, 5th edn. McGraw-Hill, New York, p 204
54. Christensen E, van Eldere J, Brandt N J, Schutgens R B H, Wanders R J A, Eyssen H J 1990 A new peroxisomal disorder: di- and trihydroxy cholestanaemia due to a presumed trihydroxycholestanoyl-CoA oxidase deficiency. Journal of Inherited Metabolic Disease 13:363–366
55. Bennet M J, Pollitt R J, Hale D E, Goodman S I, Vamecq J 1991 Deficiency of glutaryl-CoA oxidase. A new peroxisomal disorder. Pediatric Research 29:127A Abstract 746
56. Roesel R A, Carroll J E, Rizzo W B, van der Zalm T, Hahn D A 1991 Dyggve–Melchior – Clausen syndrome with increased pipecolic acid in plasma and urine. Journal of Inherited Metabolic Disease 14:867–880
57. Martinez M 1989 Polysaturated fatty acid changes suggesting a new enzymatic defect in Zellweger syndrome. Lipids 24:261–264
58. Schutgens R B H, Schrakamp G, Wanders R J A et al 1989 Prenatal and perinatal diagnosis of peroxisomal disorders. Journal of Inherited Metabolic Disease 12 Suppl 1:118–134
59. Shimozawa N, Tsukamoto T, Suzuki Y et al 1992 A human gene responsible for Zellweger syndrome that affects peroxisome assembly. Science 225: 1132–1134
60. Tsukamoto T, Miura S, Fujiki Y 1991 Restoration by a 35 kDa membrane protein of peroxisome assembly in a peroxisome deficient mammalian cell mutant. Nature 350:77–81
61. Aubourg P R, Sack G H, Meyers D A, Lease J J, Moser H W 1987 Linkage of adrenoleukodystrophy to a polymorphic DNA probe. Annals of Neurology 21:349–342
62. Boue J, Oberle I, Heilig R et al 1985 First trimester prenatal diagnosis of adrenoleukodystrophy by determination of very long chain fatty acid levels and by linkage analysis to a DNA probe. Human Genetics 69:272–274
63. Danpure C J, Cooper P J, Wise P J, Jennings P R 1989 A enzyme trafficking defect in two patients with primary hyperoxaluria type 1: Peroxisomal alanine/glyoxylate aminotransferase rerouted to mitochondria. Journal of Cell Biology 108:1345-1352
64. Leumann E, Matasovic A, Niederwieser A 1986 Primary hyperoxaluria type I. Lancet 2:340
65. Rizzo W B, Leshner R T, Odone A et al 1989 Dietary erucic acid therapy for X-linked adrenoleukodystrophy. Neurology 30:1415–1422
66. Moser H W 1991 Peroxisomal disorders. Clinical Biochemistry 24:343–351
67. Morgan S H, Purkiss P, Watts R W E, Mandell M A 1987 Oxalate dynamics in chronic renal failure. A comparison with normal subjects and patients with primary hyperoxaluria. Nephron 46:253–257
68. Watts R W E, Calne R Y, Rolles K et al 1987 Successful treatment of primary hyperoxaluria Type I by combined hepatic and renal transplantation. Lancet 1:474–475
69. Mosser J, Douar A-M, Sarde C-O et al 1993 Putative X-linked adrenoleukodystrophy gene shares unexpected homology with ABC transporters. Nature 361: 726–730

7. Defects of the mitochondrial respiratory chain

L. A. Bindoff   D. M. Turnbull

INTRODUCTION

Defects of the mitochondrial respiratory chain produce a diverse clinical spectrum of disease ranging from fatal infantile lactic acidosis to late-onset myopathy and/or dementia. The last ten to 15 years have seen a dramatic increase in interest in disorders associated with respiratory chain dysfunction. This has been stimulated by an increased awareness that defects of the respiratory chain are not rare disorders of purely academic interest, but should now be considered in the differential diagnosis of many neurological and other diseases. Despite these undoubted advances there is still much to learn about the clinical presentations, pathogenesis and treatment of these disorders. The aim of this chapter is to provide a general understanding of the biochemistry and molecular genetics of the respiratory chain, the investigation of defects of this pathway and to describe the clinical features seen in these disorders.

BIOCHEMISTRY AND GENETICS OF THE RESPIRATORY CHAIN

Background biochemistry

All higher eukaryotic cells require a constant supply of energy to maintain a basic integrity and whatever specialised function they subserve. Cellular energy, in the form of ATP, is predominantly generated by oxidative metabolism within the mitochondria. Energy required to drive ATP production is provided by the breakdown of metabolic fuels, principally glucose, fatty acids, ketone bodies and amino acids. The breakdown of metabolic fuels (substrate oxidation) generates reduced cofactors – NADH and reduced flavoproteins – which must continually be reoxidised for metabolism to proceed. This reoxidation is achieved by the respiratory chain (Fig. 7.1).

The balance of metabolism, which fuels are oxidised under which conditions, depends on the tissue and the prevailing environment, i.e. whether the individual is fed or fasted, the hormonal balance and the degree of activity. For example, the main metabolic fuels oxidised in skeletal muscle

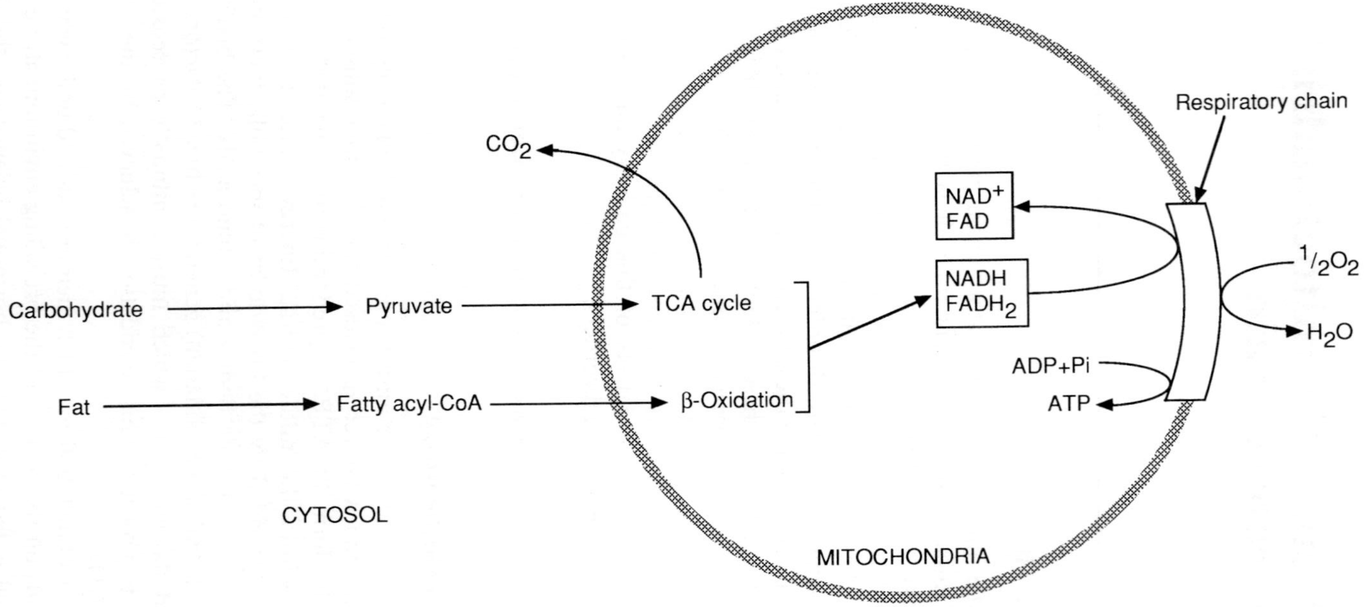

Fig. 7.1 The oxidation of the principal metabolic fuels, carbohydrate and fatty acids, occurs within the mitochondrial matrix and results in the formation of reduced cofactors NADH and $FADH_2$. These are reoxidised by the respiratory chain and the energy released harnessed to convert ADP + Pi to ATP.

mitochondria are pyruvate, long-chain fatty acids, ketone bodies (acetoacetate, 3-hydroxybutyrate) and some amino acids. Following a meal, the main substrates oxidised are glucose and fatty acids; during fasting, especially if prolonged, the major metabolic fuels are fatty acids released from body stores. Exercise will also change this balance: during intense, short-duration activity, glucose from the blood and released from glycogen stores within the muscle provides energy mainly via glycolysis. The lactate formed by this process is converted back to glucose in the liver when exercise ceases. During prolonged, submaximal exercise fatty acids are consumed. The acetyl-CoA generated from the breakdown of metabolic fuels is further metabolised by the tricarboxylic acid (TCA) cycle with the concurrent production of carbon dioxide and water. Each of these processes will generate large quantities of NADH and reduced flavoproteins necessitating therefore the continued activity of the respiratory chain for the continued breakdown of metabolic fuels.

The respiratory chain components

The mitochondrial respiratory chain is a series of five multisubunit complexes situated within the inner mitochondrial membrane: complex I (NADH-ubiquinone oxidoreductase), complex II (succinate-ubiquinone oxidoreductase), complex III (ubiquinol-cytochrome c oxidoreductase), complex IV (cytochrome c oxidase) and complex V (ATP synthase). In addition to these five complexes, there are two small, mobile electron carriers namely ubiquinone and cytochrome c. The nature of the inner mitochondrial membrane itself is important for the function of the respiratory chain. This membrane has a large cardiolipin content which is thought to provide good electrical insulation and is impermeable to all but a few small non-polar molecules. Substrates destined for the intramitochondrial compartment usually cross the membrane by specific carriers.[1]

The reoxidation of NADH and reduced flavoproteins is achieved by the transfer of electrons from reduced cofactor to respiratory chain complexes (Figs 7.2 and 7.3). Electrons from NADH are transferred to complex I whilst electrons from flavoproteins are passed either directly to ubiquinone (from glycerol-3-phosphate dehydrogenase), to ubiquinone via complex II (through succinate dehydrogenase), or via electron transfer flavoprotein (ETF) and ETF dehydrogenase (from several dehydrogenases including the fatty acyl-CoA, isovaleryl and sarcosine dehydrogenases). The respiratory chain complexes act as a series of graded, redox couples. Electrons are passed from complex I to complex III and from complex II to complex III via the mobile electron carrier ubiquinone. From complex III, electrons are transferred to complex IV via cytochrome c. Complex IV donates electrons directly to molecular oxygen. Sufficient energy is generated at three steps (at complexes I, III and IV) to drive the extrusion of protons (H^+) across the inner mitochondrial membrane and out of the mitochondria. Because of

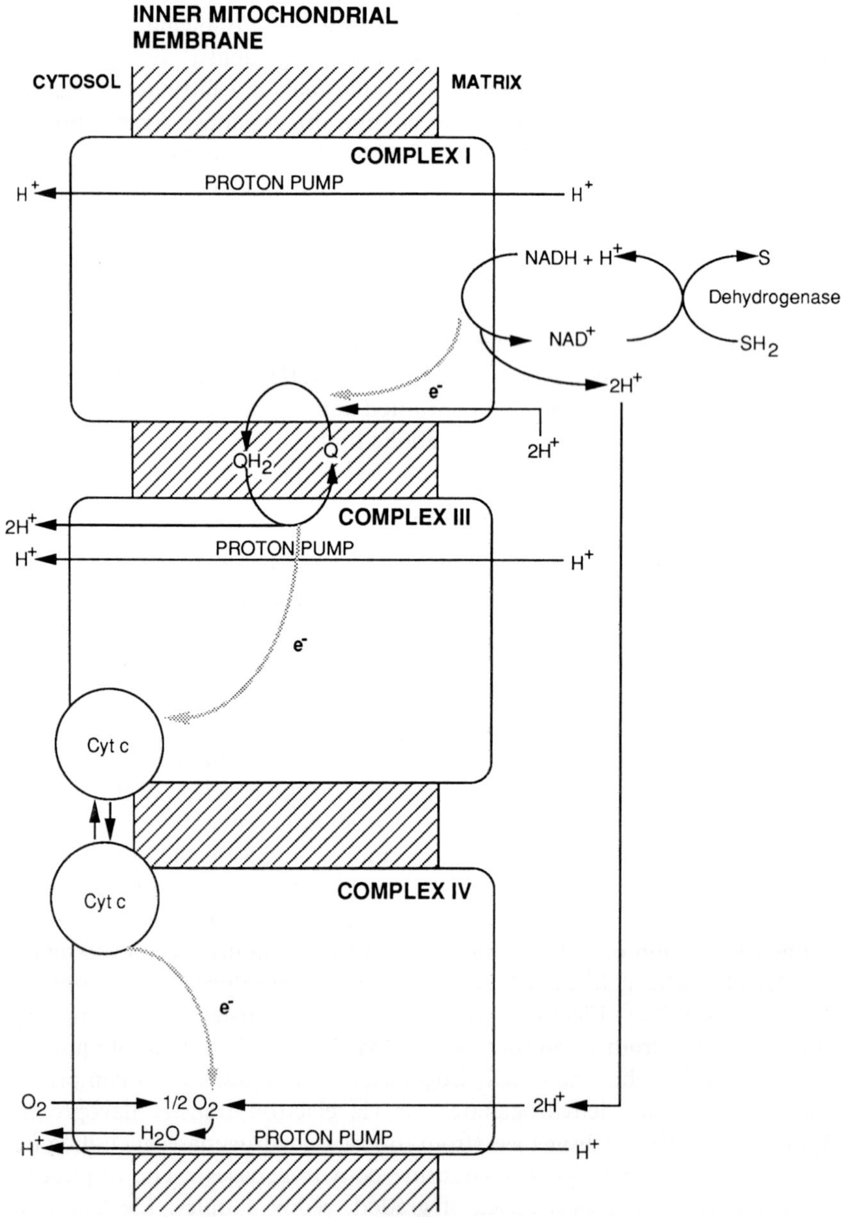

Fig. 7.2 Electron flow from NAD^+-linked dehydrogenase to molecular oxygen. NADH is reoxidised by donating two electrons to complex I. These electrons are passed through several iron–sulphur clusters to ubiquinone (UQ) to form ubiquinol (UQH_2). Ubiquinol is reoxidised by complex III and the electrons are transferred to cytochrome c (Cyt c). Cytochrome c transfers the electrons via cytochrome c oxidase (complex IV) to molecular oxygen which combines with $2H^+$ to form water. At all three complexes the energy derived from the electron transfer is used to pump protons across the inner mitochondrial membrane.

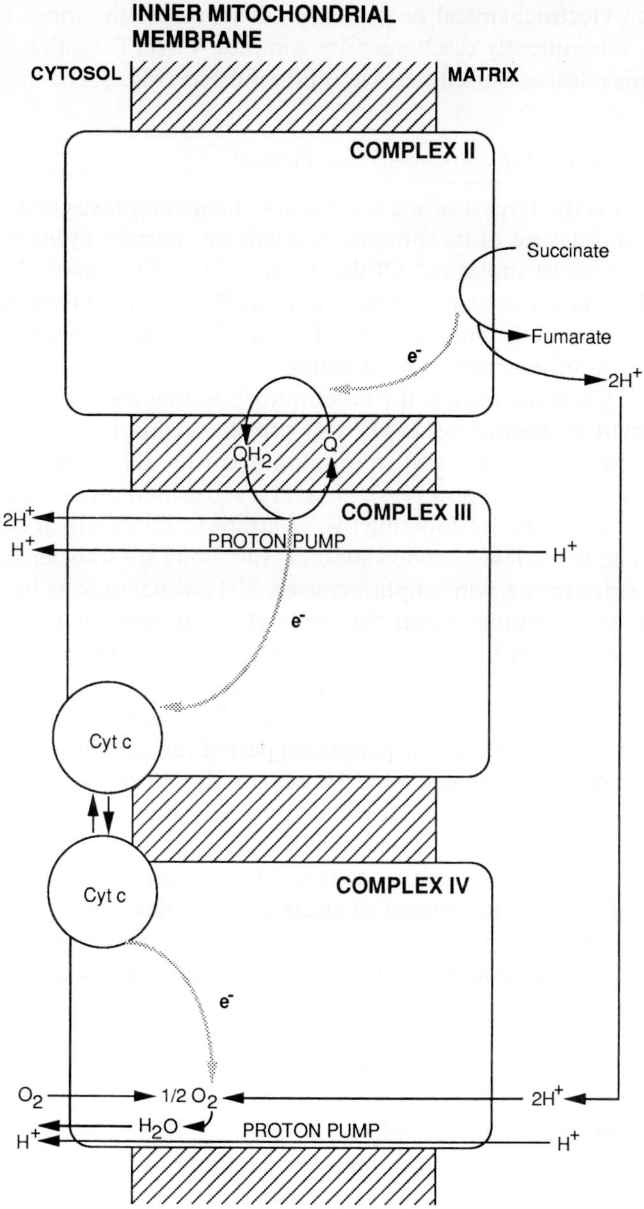

Fig. 7.3 Electron flow from succinate to molecular oxygen. Succinate is converted to fumarate by the succinate dehydrogenase component of complex II. Electrons are transferred to ubiquinone via a covalently bound FAD and iron–sulphur clusters. The reduced ubiquinone is reoxidised by complex III and electron flow follows an identical path to that described for the NAD^+-linked dehydrogenases. The detailed pathway of electron flow and the stoichiometry of proton pumping are given in the text.

the insulating properties of the inner mitochondrial membrane, these protons cannot return to the matrix side of the inner membrane. This creates an electrochemical or proton gradient across the inner membrane which is subsequently discharged by complex V (ATP synthase), and the energy this releases is used to drive ATP synthesis (Fig. 7.4).

Complex I (NADH ubiquinone-oxidoreductase)

Complex I is the largest of the respiratory chain complexes and, whilst the number and nature of its subunits is unknown, current opinion estimates approximately 30 subunits.[2] Of the 30 or so subunits, seven (ND1-6) are encoded by DNA actually within the mitochondria (mtDNA, see below) and this dual genetic control is one of the unique and complicating features of this series of enzymes. The function of most of the subunits is largely unknown. Complex I spans the inner mitochondrial membrane, contains a single flavin mononucleotide (FMN) prosthetic group and several iron–sulphur clusters: a [2Fe–2S] iron–sulphur cluster (N-2) and three [4Fe–4S] clusters (N-1, N-3 and N-4). NADH is reoxidised on the matrix side of the inner membrane by donating two electrons to FMN which is associated with a 51 kDa nuclear encoded subunit. Electrons are transferred in single electron steps to the iron–sulphur cluster, N-1, which may be ligated to the same 51 kDa subunit. Again via single electron steps, it is thought that electrons are passed to N-3 and N-4 ligated with a 75 kDa nuclear encoded subunit. Electrons may now pass to an internal quinone, the presence of which has not been proven unequivocally. The pathway described so far takes place entirely within the peripheral part of the complex. It is proposed that the electron pathway now passes to the hydrophobic membrane domain by the passage of electrons from the internal quinone to N-2 (liganded with the ND5 protein encoded by mtDNA) and finally to the substrate ubiquinone which is stabilised by binding to the ND1 subunit. Associated with the movement of electrons, complex I pumps protons out of the mitochondrial matrix. The exact number of protons translocated by complex I is still uncertain. However, available data suggest that four protons are translocated for each two electrons.

Complex II (succinate ubiquinone-oxidoreductase)

Structurally, this is the simplest and smallest of the five complexes. It comprises four subunits, the largest two going to form succinate dehydrogenase (SDH) whilst the smaller two anchor this enzyme to the membrane and provide a ubiquinone binding site.[3] The simplicity of this complex belies its unique importance since the enzyme functions in two major metabolic pathways – the respiratory chain and the TCA cycle.

The succinate dehydrogenase component of the enzyme contains a covalently bound flavin adenine dinucleotide (FAD) group. It also contains

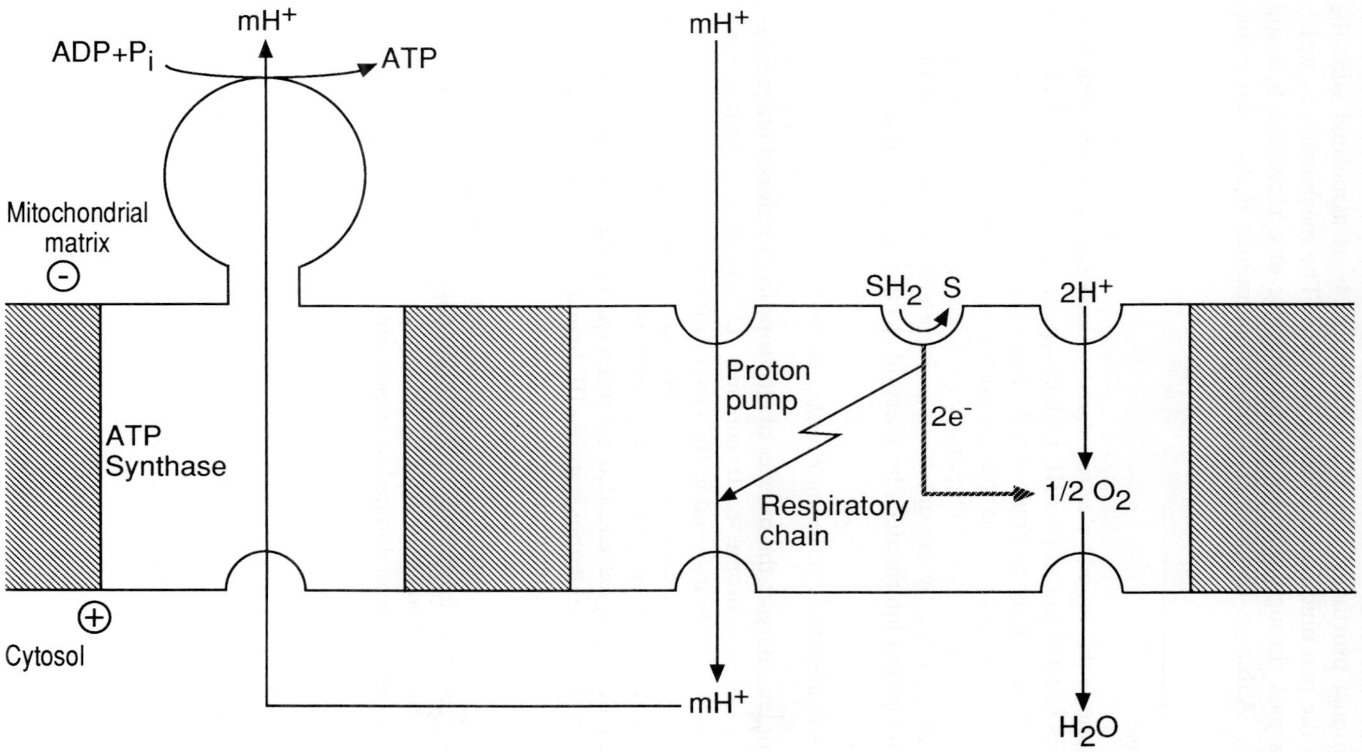

Fig. 7.4 Generation of electrochemical gradient and synthesis of ATP. The energy released by electron transfer along the respiratory chain is used to pump protons across the mitochondrial inner membrane. This creates an electrochemical gradient or proton-motive force which is discharged through complex V (mitochondrial ATP synthase). Complex V uses the energy derived from the protomotive force to convert ADP + Pi to ATP.

an iron–sulphur protein which probably contains all three iron–sulphur clusters ([2Fe–2S], [3Fe–4S] and [4Fe–4S]) associated with this enzyme. An additional prosthetic group, a cytochrome b, is associated with the larger of the two ubiquinone-binding proteins. The mechanism by which electrons pass through complex II and the role of cytochrome b is still uncertain. Although complex II is transmembranous it does not pump protons.

Ubiquinone

Ubiquinone is the mobile electron carrier which transfers electrons from complexes I and II to complex III. Ubiquinone (coenzyme Q) is a quinone derivative with a long isoprenoid tail. The number of isoprene units in ubiquinone depends upon the species, the most common form in mammals contains ten isoprene units (ubiquinone$_{10}$). Ubiquinone is reduced to a free radical semiquinone by the uptake of a single electron; reduction of this membrane-bound intermediate by a second electron gives ubiquinol.

Complex III (ubiquinol-cytochrome c oxidoreductase)

This complex catalyses the transfer of electrons from reduced ubiquinone, ubiquinol, to cytochrome c. It contains 11 subunits including three proteins known to be involved in the electron transfer: cytochrome c_1, the Rieske iron–sulphur protein and cytochrome b, a single polypeptide that contains two b-type haem groups.[4] The apocytochrome b subunit is the only protein of this complex encoded by mtDNA. Probably more is known about electron transfer within complex III than any of the other complexes. Studies have shown that transfer of two electrons is associated with the extrusion of four protons. An explanation for this unbalanced stoichiometry was provided by Mitchell in 1976 in the form of the Q-cycle, a mechanism whereby the formation of a semiquinone intermediate and the movement of electrons within the b cytochrome permits the extrusion of two protons per electron donated to cytochrome c.

Cytochrome c

Cytochrome c transfers electrons from complex III to complex IV. Cytochrome c is a single polypeptide with a covalently bound haem group. It is situated on the outer face of the inner mitochondrial membrane and may be readily solubilised from intact mitochondria.

Complex IV (cytochrome c oxidase)

Complex IV is the final electron-transferring complex of the respiratory chain. It catalyses the transfer of electrons from reduced cytochrome c to oxygen, the terminal electron acceptor, resulting in the production of H_2O. Cytochrome c oxidase is the third respiratory chain complex in which electron transfer is linked to proton pumping and ATP synthesis. The complex consists of 13 subunits and contains two haems (a-type cytochromes) and at least two copper atoms which act as electron-transferring prosthetic groups.[5] The three largest subunits (CO I, II and III) are all mitochondrially encoded and are responsible for the catalytic and proton pumping activities of the complex. The prosthetic groups (haems a and a_3) and coppers (Cu_A and Cu_B) are known to be liganded to subunits I and II. Subunit II also contains the cytochrome c binding site and subunit III is thought to be involved in proton pumping. The additional subunits of complex IV are all nuclear-encoded and some exist as tissue-specific isoforms. The function of these subunits is uncertain although some may be involved in the structure of the complex and others in the control of electron flow. The presence of developmental isoforms has been inferred as a result of studies of a rare clinical phenotype (see below under benign infantile lactic acidosis).

Complex V (ATP synthetase)

The production of ATP from ADP+ P_i is catalysed by complex V. This complex contains approximately 14 subunits, two of which (ATPase 6 and ATPase 8) are encoded by mitochondrial DNA. ATP synthetase is divisible into F_0 and F_1 moeities which are responsible for proton conduction and catalysis respectively.[6] The F_1 sector appears as a 'knob' protruding from the membrane into the matrix. The highly hydrophobic F_0 sector is embedded in the membrane, and the two moeities are connected by a narrow stalk-like structure. The movement of protons through the channel in F_0 appears to cause conformational change in the F_1 subunit which is associated with concerted synthesis and release of ATP.

Genetics

Mitochondrially-encoded subunits

Two genomes are involved in the production of respiratory chain proteins, the nuclear genome, and a separate cytoplasmic DNA found within the mitochondria (Fig. 7.5). Mitochondrial DNA (mtDNA) is circular, contains 16 569 base pairs and encodes 13 polypeptides, 22 transfer RNA (tRNA) and 2 ribosomal RNA (rRNA).[7] The 13 proteins are all subunits of the respiratory chain complexes: seven are complex I proteins (ND genes), one is the apocytochrome b protein of complex III, three are cytochrome c oxidase subunits (CO I–III) and two are involved in ATP synthetase (ATPase 6 and 8). These proteins are synthesised within the mitochondria using the tRNA and rRNA encoded by mtDNA. MtDNA shows remarkable economy of organisation with only a short section, the D loop, not containing assignable coding information. The D loop has evolved as the control centre for both transcription and replication of mtDNA. Apart from being the only DNA found outside the nucleus in higher eukaryote cells, mtDNA has several further unique features:

1. *It is predominantly inherited from the mother.* Mitochondria are present in both sperm and ova, but less than 0.1% of mtDNA in the offspring is contributed by the sperm.

2. *There is more than one copy of mitochondrial DNA per mitochondrion.* In skeletal muscle, the number may be as high as ten and therefore there may be many thousands of copies per cell.

3. *Transcription of mtDNA produces large polycistronic transcripts from both strands.* These transcripts are processed (literally cut up) into their component RNA by enzymes imported into the mitochondrion.[8] Unlike nuclear genes there are no intervening sequences (introns) and the mechanism for recognising the junction between the coding regions is thought to be a combination of secondary structure formation by tRNA and possibly sequence recognition.

The two strands of mtDNA (see Fig. 7.5) can be separated on the basis of buoyant density. The heavy (H) strand contains the majority of coding information whilst the light (L) strand encodes only a single polypeptide and 8 tRNA. The D loop, the only non-coding region (about 1 kb), contains the promoters for transcription of both H- and L-strands plus the origin of replication of the H-strand (ORI_H). MtDNA contains little or no intervening sequence between coding regions and most protein-coding genes are separated by tRNA. Transcription of both strands produces large polycistronic species which are cleaved subsequently into their component tRNA, mRNA and rRNA. Replication of mtDNA begins with the H-strand; L-strand replication does not proceed until ORI_L is exposed by the oncoming H-strand synthesis.

Figure 7.5 shows several of the commoner abnormalities found in mtDNA. The demarcated area between ND5 and ATPase 8 is the region involved in the so-called 'common' deletion. As shown, there are 13 base pair repeats at each break point and these are thought to be involved in the process of deletion although the precise mechanism is still unknown. The majority of deletions occurring in CPEO/KSS (see clinical syndromes section) are found in the same region but are smaller or larger and not always flanked by large repeats. The MELAS syndrome is most commonly associated with a mutation within $tRNA^{Leu(UUR)}$ at position 3243. This particular tRNA appears to be a 'hot-spot' since several different mutations, with both MELAS and other phenotypes, have been identified here. The MERRF mutation occurs in $tRNA^{Lys}$ (single letter code K), whilst Leber's optic neuropathy is most commonly associated with mutations in ND4 and ND1.

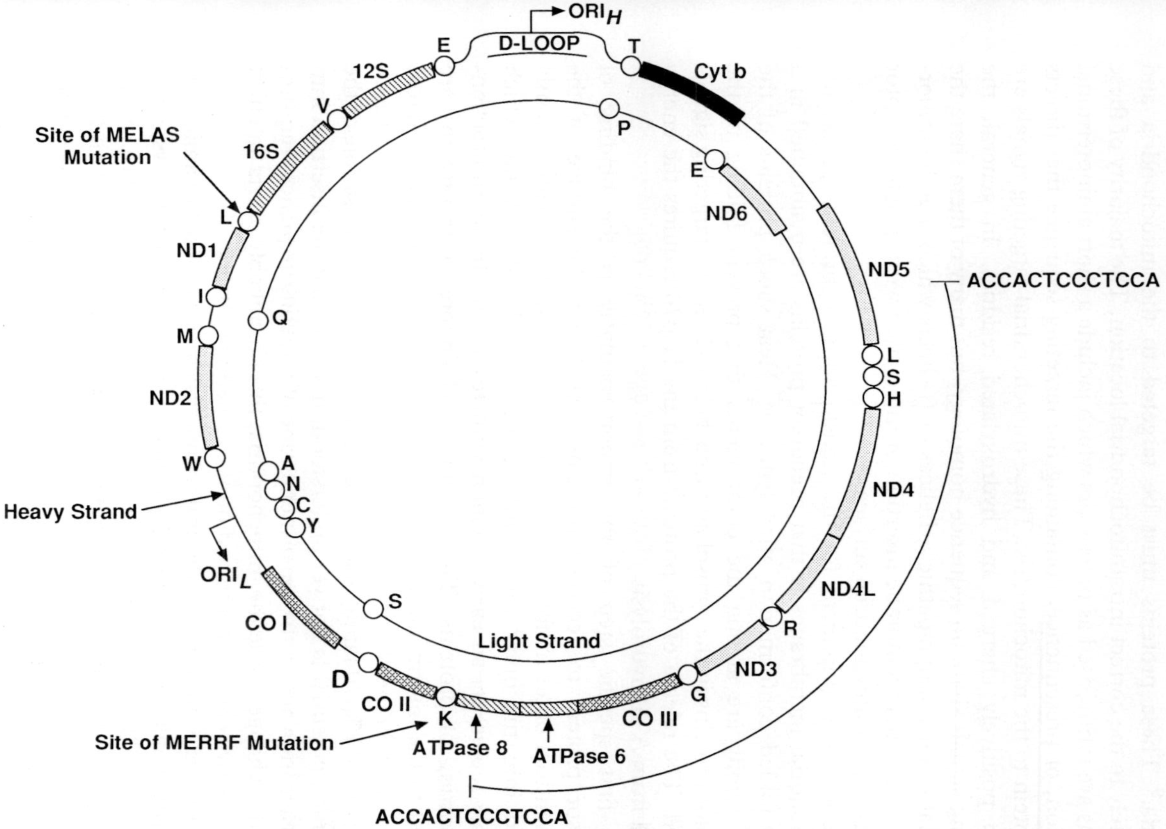

Fig. 7.5 Schematic representation of mitochondrial DNA. Mitochondrial DNA is circular and encodes 13 proteins: seven subunits of complex I (ND 1–6); three subunits of cytochrome oxidase (CO I–III); two subunits of complex V (ATPase 6 and 8), and one from complex III (cytochrome b). There are two ribosomal RNA (16S and 12SrRNA) and 22 tRNA (shown as circles with single letter code identification).

Nuclear-encoded subunits

The nuclear-encoded respiratory chain proteins are synthesised on cytosolic ribosomes and are post-translationally imported into mitochondria.[9] These proteins must be targeted to the mitochondria and ultimately to the correct intramitochondrial location. The majority of these proteins are synthesised as precursors which include a short aminoterminal extension, or presequence, containing the targeting sequence that directs the protein to the mitochondria. These mitochondrial targeting signals are rich in positively charged and hydroxylated residues. In general, the targeting signals share no sequence homology, but many of them share the potential to form amphipathic α helices or β-sheets which may be important for the initial membrane insertion or interaction with specific receptor proteins at the mitochondrial surface.

An essential requirement for the translocation of proteins across the mitochondrial membranes is that precursor proteins are maintained in a loosely folded conformation after synthesis. Heat shock proteins of the Hsp70 family are among the components that prevent folding of the precursor proteins in the cytosol and thus help to keep the targeting signals exposed. The release of the proteins from the Hsp70 requires the energy derived from ATP hydrolysis.

The first specific step of the import pathway is the binding of precursor protein to receptor proteins present on the surface of the mitochondrial outer membrane. The precursor proteins are subsequently inserted into the outer membrane at the general insertion site which probably represents an early junction with respect to the intramitochondrial sorting of proteins. The respiratory chain precursor proteins are exposed to the intermembrane space and the translocation into or across the inner membrane requires a membrane potential and another heat shock protein of the Hsp70 family within the matrix. Whilst the precise role of the membrane potential is not yet understood, it seems that the insertion into or translocation across the inner membrane of targeting sequences requires a negative change inside the mitochondria; this presumably exerts an effect on the positive charges contained on the targeting sequence.

Once translocated across the mitochondrial membranes, the aminoterminal presequences are cleaved by a highly specific processing system in the matrix. This proteolytic processing requires two structurally related components, the mitochondrial processing peptidase itself, and the processing-enhancing protein. A final important component occurring within the mitochondrial matrix is the refolding of proteins and the formation of oligomeric complexes. It has been proposed that an additional chaperonin, a mitochondrial Hsp60, is responsible for these processes.

Whilst it is thought that most proteins destined for the inner membrane or intermembrane space are transported into the mitochondrial matrix and then directed to the appropriate mitochondrial compartment, a few proteins are known that do not conform to this pattern. For example, cytochrome c seems to have an unusual entry into the intermembrane space. The precursor, apocytochrome c, is made without a cleavable presequence and does not seem to interact with a receptor protein at the surface of the mitochondria. Crossing the outer membrane seems to occur directly, and completion of this translocation is probably mediated by interaction with cytochrome c-haem lyase at the inner face of the outer mitochondrial membrane and by covalent attachment of the haem.

INVESTIGATION OF DEFECTS OF THE RESPIRATORY CHAIN

The causation of disease by defects of mitochondrial energy metabolism is a relatively recent concept. Indeed, although first documented in 1962 when Luft and colleagues identified a woman with hypermetabolism due to abnormal mitochondrial coupling, it was not until the early 1970s that methods had progressed sufficiently for us to move from purely morphological description to biochemical definition of such diseases. Due to the complexity of this pathway, both in biochemical and molecular terms, difficulties still surround the identification and classification of respiratory chain disease. In the following section, the clinical, biochemical and genetic abnormalities found in patients with respiratory chain disease will be described. Methods of investigation will be discussed in general terms and a more detailed description provided in the references. Clearly, the findings on simple history and examination will first suggest the possibility of respiratory chain disease and secondly help define its extent, i.e. which tissues might be involved.

Clinical

The search for an elevated venous lactate is perhaps the commonest screening investigation used. The increase may be modest (2–3 mmol/l) or extreme (concentrations of 28 mmol/l are recorded). In some individuals, basal levels may be normal, so that some form of provocation e.g. fasting, carbohydrate load or exercise is necessary. Occasionally, in patients with predominantly CNS symptoms, abnormal elevation of lactate is confined to, or maximal, in the cerebrospinal fluid (CSF). Therefore, in these patients we tend to measure both venous and CSF lactate after provocation, such as following a formal period of fasting. Spurious elevations of venous lactate concentration are common due to venous stasis and/or an upset child; venous samples should be obtained after removal of a tourniquet. Alternatively arterial samples are obtained.

Computerized tomographic scanning (CT) and the more sensitive magnetic resonance (MR) imaging are both useful methods for detecting disease within the central nervous system (CNS). In some cases characteristic lesions are present, e.g. low density slit-like areas in the basal ganglia seen in Leigh's syndrome (see later). Nevertheless, both these techniques will still only define the site of abnormality. Electrophysiological studies including electromyography (EMG) and electroencephalography (EEG) may also be of value. These studies are relatively non-invasive methods which again help define the extent of the disease. For example, in some patients with purely cardiac or myopathic involvement, an abnormal EEG strongly suggests CNS involvement. NMR spectroscopy will add further information, although the changes seen, low phosphocreatine and impaired conversion of ADP to ATP, are fairly non-specific and do not allow differentiation between different biochemical defects or clinical syndromes.[10] One major advantage of NMR spectroscopy is that it allows use of a non-invasive method of studying the biochemical effects of treatment. PET scanning is also informative since it is possible to show uncoupling of the normal ratio of oxygen consumed per molecule of glucose metabolised. When uncoupling occurs it suggests that anaerobic metabolism is being used to provide energy in cells where normal respiratory chain function is deficient. In certain centres, whole body investigation measuring metabolic rate, fuel consumption, energy turnover etc. has provided a great deal of information concerning the general metabolism in patients with respiratory chain disease. These facilities are not widely available so most centres screen using, predominantly, assessment of the clinical features, lactate concentration and CNS imaging.

Morphological studies

Owing to the frequency with which it is involved, as well as the low morbidity associated with biopsy, skeletal muscle is the preferred tissue for study. Historically, morphological abnormalities in skeletal muscle mitochondria provided one of the earliest indications that disease may be caused by altered mitochondrial function. Muscle fibre necrosis and atrophy may be seen in patients with respiratory chain disease. More specifically, qualitative and quantitative abnormalities of mitochondria have been found in these patients. Perhaps the most well known finding is the 'ragged-red fibre' which describes the abnormal accumulation of normal and abnormal mitochondria beneath the muscle cell membrane giving it a ragged edge. When stained by the Gomori trichrome method, accumulated mitochondria are stained red hence the 'ragged-red fibre'.[11] Such changes are, however, more specifically demonstrated by use of specific mitochondrial enzyme markers such as succinate dehydrogenase (SDH) and cytochrome oxidase (Fig. 7.6).

Qualitative differences in mitochondria are best seen using electron microscopy. A variety of abnormalities have been described including intramitochondrial inclusions. However, whilst more marked in muscle from patients with respiratory chain disease, they are also found in other conditions.

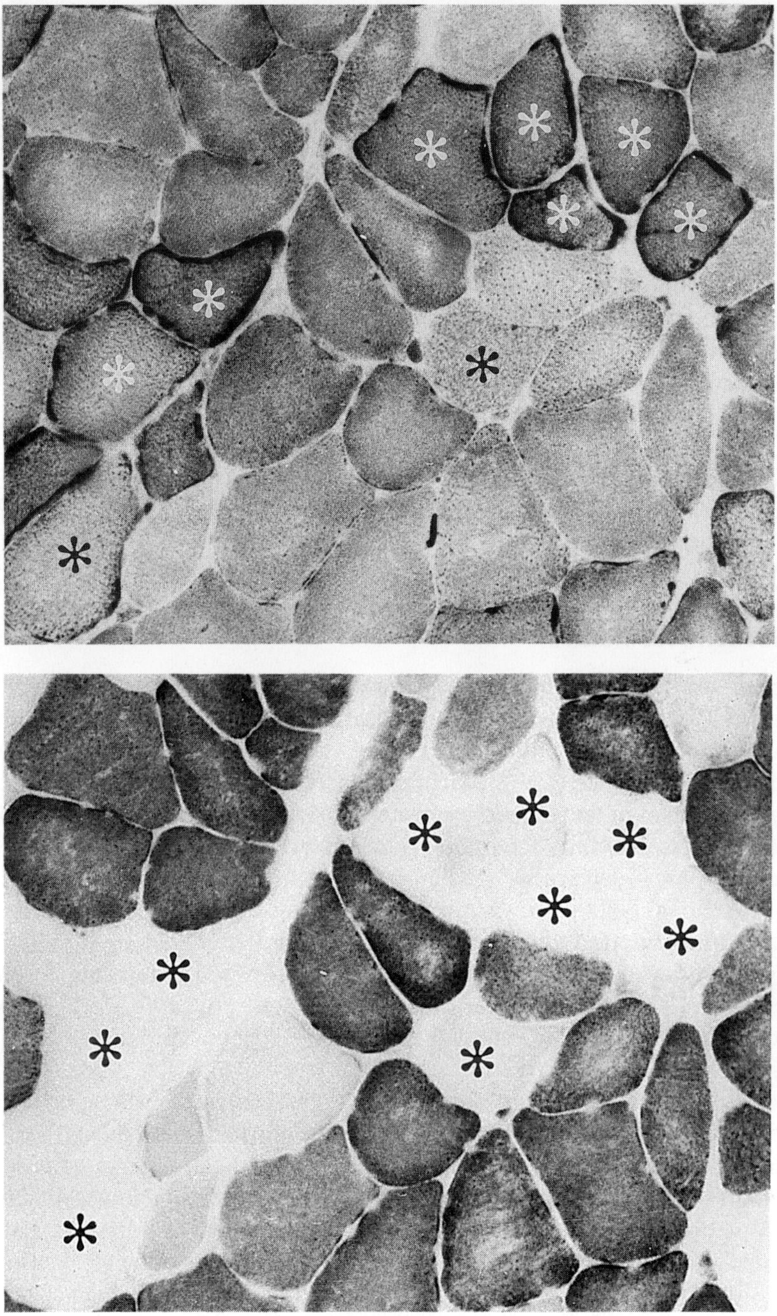

Fig. 7.6 Cross-sections of skeletal muscle from a patient with a defect of the mitochondrial respiratory chain. **A** Succinate dehydrogenase showing peripheral accumulations of mitochondria in many muscle fibres ('ragged red fibres') e.g. the group of 5 starred fibres, top right. **B** Cytochrome oxidase in serial section: fibres which are cytochrome oxidase-negative usually show mitochondrial aggregates(*).

In addition to the changes in mitochondrial number and structure, several other observations can be made using tissue sections:

1. Direct enzyme measurement is possible. The activity of succinate dehydrogenase, part of complex II, and cytochrome c oxidase may both be measured in tissue sections.[12]

2. Abnormal storage of lipid is a frequent finding in patients with defects of the respiratory chain and is due to a secondary effect on mitochondrial β-oxidation.

3. Immunocytochemistry allows detection and localisation of specific proteins involved in the respiratory chain. This is of great importance since it shows whether decreased activity is associated with decreased or normal concentration of a particular protein.[13]

4. In situ hybridisation involves the use of specific single stranded DNA or RNA probes to detect the presence/absence of mRNA for the proteins of the respiratory chain. The same technique may be used to detect mtDNA and demonstrate the site and concentration of any abnormal population of this genome.[14]

Biochemical studies

These are essential to define precisely the nature and extent of the defect(s). In addition, correlation of the biochemical defect to the genetic abnormality and the clinical phenotype will help us understand the pathogenesis of these diseases. Biochemical studies may involve whole cells (measurement of lactate and pyruvate ratios and ATP production) or more frequently isolated mitochondria. Since muscle is commonly involved, the majority of biochemical studies have involved muscle mitochondria. Further advantages of using muscle are that it is often affected and contains many mitochondria which can be isolated and prepared by a variety of homogenisation and centrifugation procedures. Since respiratory chain defects are systemic, however, there has been a desire to use less invasive techniques and this has included the use of platelets, lymphocyte cell lines and fibroblasts to provide mitochondrial fractions. Whilst these cells (or platelets) are easy to obtain, they have the disadvantage of not being heavily dependent on oxidative metabolism (fibroblasts and platelets) or not present in large numbers (lymphocytes). The removal of large volumes of blood (at least 60 ml) required for platelet studies, although acceptable in adults, precludes the use of platelets from infants and children, an important clinical group. Immortalisation of WBC by EBV-transformation is possible, but such expertise is not often available and transformed cells may not necessarily reflect the biochemical phenotype of the original cells. Skin fibroblast cell lines however do have many advantages, including the ready availability of controls, the possible investigation of family members and that such cells can be easily transported between centres.

It is important to recognise when investigating a clinically non-affected tissue that the biochemical defect may not be apparent. This is due to several factors including tissue-specific differences in nuclear-encoded subunits, differences between tissues in mRNA processing and translation, and, also, the control strength of individual complexes on mitochondrial oxidations. Thus, the tissue chosen for biochemical analysis is important, and whilst muscle is usually affected it may be entirely normal in patients with only CNS symptoms.

Studies on whole cells. The ratio of lactate to pyruvate measured in fibroblast culture medium reflects the internal redox state of the cell and therefore has been used to indicate disruption of the mitochondrial respiratory chain.[15] Other methods include comparison of substrate utilisation by complexes I and II by the measurement of carbon dioxide release or ATP production.

Studies on isolated mitochondria. Overall flux through the pathway can be measured polarographically using an oxygen electrode. This has the advantage that the coupling of substrate oxidation to the amount of ADP and oxygen may also be measured.[16] Polarographic studies have the disadvantage that they use relatively large amounts of mitochondria, although these can be saved and used for other studies. Alternative methods of measuring overall flux by spectrophotometric techniques use artificial electron acceptors whose light absorption in the visible region of the spectrum changes during oxidation–reduction reactions. The structural organisation of the respiratory chain in the inner mitochondrial membrane allows suitable acceptors to 'tap off' electrons at the level of cytochrome c (III).[16] Although both polarographic and spectrophotometric methods ultimately reflect electron flux through the respiratory chain, the actions of several other systems are necessary: uptake mechanisms, NAD^+ and FAD-linked dehydrogenases, the adenine nucleotide translocator and the electrochemical gradient. These assays are not, therefore, entirely specific for respiratory chain activity and results (abnormal or normal) must be interpreted with caution.

Spectrophotometric assays are used to identify defects of individual complexes. The widely used NADH-cytochrome c and succinate-cytochrome c reductase assays measure flux through two complexes. There are problems associated with these assays in that a partial defect of one complex may not be detected. It is best, therefore, to measure the activity of the individual complexes directly.[17]

In addition to measuring enzyme activity, it is possible to determine the steady-state concentration of individual protein subunits of the respiratory chain complexes by immunoblotting. This involves the separation of the proteins on the basis of molecular weight and their detection using antibodies specific to individual subunits. The concentration of the important redox proteins, the cytochromes, can also be determined since they contain iron-porphyrin rings which have characteristic absorption spectra. This enables them to be detected in mitochondrial membranes by the technique of difference spectroscopy.[16]

Molecular studies

Thus far, the molecular investigation of respiratory chain disease has concentrated on finding abnormalities of the mitochondrial genome. Nuclear gene defects occur and are obvious by clear autosomal inheritance, however, the precise nature of these defects has yet to be defined. The major abnormalities of mtDNA are rearrangements (either deletion or duplication), mtDNA depletion and point mutations. Deletions and duplications may be detected by either Southern blotting or by using the polymerase chain reaction (PCR). Although the latter is extremely sensitive, quantification is difficult. MtDNA depletion is detected by Southern blotting. Known point mutations can be detected either by sequencing the region of interest or, if the mutation creates or destroys a restriction endonuclease site, by PCR amplification and restriction digest. Since mtDNA exists in multiple copies and not all may be involved, the appearance of two populations, one normal and one abnormal, is possible. This situation has been termed *heteroplasmy*.

A new and exciting technique for investigating mitochondrial myopathies has been the development of cells which completely lack mtDNA (rho° cells).[18] These rho° cells depend entirely on glycolysis for their energy requirements and are, in addition, dependant on uridine for growth. Mitochondria from cells containing defective mtDNA can be transferred into rho° cells; this is achieved by enucleation of the donor cells (ie those containing mutant mtDNA) in the presence of cytocholasin B, followed by fusion of the resulting cytoplasts with the rho° cells. The molecular and biochemical defect can then be studied in detail in the resulting cells which contain the mutant DNA. Use of this technique permitted the clear demonstration that abnormal mtDNA alone was the cause of a biochemical defect.[19]

CLASSIFICATION OF RESPIRATORY CHAIN DEFECTS

Attempts at classifying respiratory chain defects have been based on clinical, biochemical or more recently genetic criteria. Difficulties arise with each and in the following section we shall explore some of these problems.

Clinical

Initially, mitochondrial respiratory chain diseases were described in muscle and this led to the generic term mitochondrial myopathies. Involvement of other tissues, especially brain, has led to a broader clinical spectrum. The systemic nature of some defects has meant, however, that there are a number of descriptive titles that provide little basis for rational classification. Progress made in the molecular definition of these diseases has allowed for some improvement.

Defects of the respiratory chain produce several broad categories of disease: isolated myopathy; eye movement disorder (ophthalmoplegia) with or without myopathy and occasionally with CNS dysfunction such as ataxia; multisystem disease with the brunt of the abnormality falling within the CNS; fatal lactic acidosis of infancy; apparent single organ dysfunction such as cardiomyopathy. No clear relationship between the biochemical defect of the respiratory chain and clinical phenotype has emerged. Some correlation between genotype and phenotype has been possible, nevertheless it remains true to say that the same apparent (reported) biochemical defect may be associated with very different phenotypes and that the same genetic abnormality can be associated with very different biochemical findings.

Biochemical

Definition of respiratory chain diseases by the enzyme(s) involved presupposes that measurement of these activities is uniform. This is not the case. In a previous review[20] we did group cases according to which complex or complexes were reported as affected, but acknowledged that in many instances more than one complex activity was lowered. Certainly, our own observations suggest that the commonest finding is of multiple abnormal respiratory chain complexes in any single patient.

In many instances biochemical evaluation of the respiratory chain is both inadequate and incomplete. This in part reflects the difficulty of this evaluation and the variety of the different techniques used in different laboratories. Because of this it is not possible to construct a rational classification based on which enzyme or enzymes are affected.

Genetic

Deletions of mtDNA were discovered in 1988[21] and this finding was quickly followed by the identification of duplications and point mutations. These genetic abnormalities show greater congruence with clinical subtypes than biochemical findings. Thus, the majority of patients with the syndrome of MELAS (see later) have a particular point mutation in $tRNA^{Leu(UUR)}$. There is, however, undoubted overlap in the clinical features observed and the different genetic defects. In addition, there are still many patients in whom the molecular defect has not been identified making genetic classification alone inadequate. Therefore, until more information provides a clearer understanding of the disorders, a combination of all three parameters should be used. In the following section (Clinical syndromes) the recognised syndromes have been grouped according to the broad categories described earlier. Information concerning the biochemical and genetic findings will be given for each category.

CLINICAL SYNDROMES

Isolated myopathy

Despite the early concentration on muscle-related disease, isolated myopathy is surprisingly uncommon. These patients do not have ophthalmoplegia, ptosis or retinopathy. Patients present with non-specific symptoms such as cramp-like pain, burning discomfort in the muscles, weakness and fatigue. The distribution of weakness is proximal/axial and may also involve the face giving a fascioscapulohumeral picture. Neck flexion weakness is almost uniform. The weakness in these patients may be progressive and ultimately result in death due to respiratory muscle weakness.

Clinical investigation often shows elevation of serum lactate at rest which increases markedly on exercise. Electromyography (EMG) demonstrates myopathic changes. Morphological examination of muscle shows the typical subsarcolemmal mitochondrial accumulation and histochemical analysis will in most cases show cytochrome oxidase negative fibres. Biochemical analysis of mitochondrial fractions isolated from muscle biopsy have shown multiple respiratory chain defects and no consistent molecular abnormality has been identified.

Chronic progressive external ophthalmoplegia

Chronic progressive external ophthalmoplegia (CPEO) is one of the commonest adult presentations of respiratory chain dysfunction. It may occur as an isolated finding or in association with myopathy, pigmentary retinopathy and/or CNS disease, particularly ataxia. Presentation is with ptosis, double vision, fatigue or unsteadiness. Lactate levels in blood are often normal or only mildly elevated. CT/MRI may show atrophy confined to the cerebellum or occasionally more generalised involvement. Muscle histochemistry shows subsarcolemmal accumulation of mitochondria and cytochrome c oxidase-deficient fibres. Biochemical analysis of mitochondrial fractions shows that, whilst a defect of complex IV is the most frequently reported, multiple respiratory chain defects are common.

Genetic analysis shows that the majority of patients with CPEO have a rearrangement of mtDNA.[21] Deletions vary from approximately 1 kb to over 7 kb and are invariably heteroplasmic. Many of the deletions occur in the same region of mtDNA, the so-called 'common' deletion. Studies have shown that in many instances, and this is particularly true of the common site, the deleted region is flanked by repeated sequences and it has been suggested that recombination between these regions cause the loss of intermediary mtDNA.[22]

Encephalopathies

A number of clearly recognisable syndromes manifest with predominantly CNS disease. However distinct these syndromes appear, there is overlap and it is not always possible to fit patients into one category.

Kearns–Sayre syndrome (KSS)

This disorder, which is also called the oculocraniosomatic syndrome, is characterised by progressive external ophthalmoplegia, pigmentary retinopathy and heart block, but may include a number of other distinctive features (Table 7.1). It is by definition a disorder with onset of symptoms before the age of 20 years. What is of interest, however, is the similarity between this syndrome and CPEO which may also manifest deafness, ataxia, etc. Clinical investigation often demonstrates a range of features; lactate is usually elevated in blood and CSF, and muscle histology characteristically shows mitochondrial accumulation and cytochrome c oxidase-negative fibres. Biochemical studies again commonly show multiple defects (complexes I, III and IV), although isolated complex I or complex IV deficiency has been frequently reported.

Table 7.1 Clinical, biochemical and molecular features of defects of mitochondrial genome. KSS – Kearns – Sayre syndrome, MERFF – myoclonic epilepsy and 'ragged red' fibre disease, MELAS – myopathy, encephalopathy, lactic acidosis and stroke-like episodes, Depletion – mtDNA depletion syndrome, NARP – neurogenic weakness, ataxia and retinitis pigmentosa, M – maternal transmission, A – autosomal recessive

Clinical feature	KSS	MERRF	MELAS	Depletion	NARP
Ophthalmoplegia	+	–	–	–	–
Retinal degeneration	+	–	–	–	+
Heart block	+	–	–	–	–
CSF protein >100 mg/dl	+	–	–	–	–
Myoclonus	–	+	–	–	–
Ataxia	+	+	–	–	+
Weakness	+	+	+	+	+
Episodic vomiting	–	–	+	–	–
Cerebral blindness	–	–	+	–	–
Hemiparesis, hemianopia	–	–	+	–	–
Seizures	–	+	+	+	+
Dementia	+	+	+	+	+
Short stature	+	+	+	–	+
Sensorineural hearing loss	+	+	+	–	–
Lactic acidosis	+	+	+	+	–
Family history	–	M	M	A	M
Ragged red fibres	+	+	+	+	–
Leigh's phenotype	–	–	–	–	+
mtDNA deletion	+	–	–	–	–
mtDNA depletion	–	–	–	+	–
mtDNA point mutation	–	$tRNA^{lys}$	$tRNA^{LEU(UUR)}$	–	ATPase 6^{8993}

At the genetic level, almost all cases of KSS have a major rearrangement of mtDNA; in the majority this is a deletion and once again the majority of these cases have the so called 'common' deletion. In rare, but an increasing number of cases, duplication of mtDNA has been documented.[23]

Myoclonus epilepsy with ragged red fibres (MERRF)

As the name suggests, myoclonus is a major feature of this disorder. Weakness, ataxia, deafness and dementia are also found (Table 7.1). The finding of morphological abnormalities in skeletal muscle (the 'ragged red fibre') gave the initial clue that this disorder may be due to mitochondrial dysfunction and indeed this has been confirmed. Biochemical studies usually show multiple defects suggesting once again that mtDNA is affected. MERRF was one of the first of the mitochondrial disorders to be linked with a point mutation in the mitochondrial genome.[24] This mutation affects a tRNA (that for lysine) and is found in a high proportion of, but not all, cases with this syndrome. Additional reports are appearing of patients initially diagnosed as having MERRF but who later develop stroke-like episodes (see MELAS below). As would be expected for a mitochondrial genetic disorder, maternal transmission is found in many of the cases.

Myopathy, encephalopathy, lactic acidosis and stroke-like episodes (MELAS)

The feature that distinguishes this syndrome is the occurrence of stroke-like episodes. These are so termed because although they mimic stroke clinically, their nature is uncertain. Whilst they may be due to vascular insufficiency an alternative possibility is that they result from metabolic insufficiency within the CNS. Characteristic lesions are seen on CT and MRI; these lesions may resolve rapidly or proceed to an established neurological defect. The onset of symptoms is before the age of 15 years in most patients. Cortical blindness and hemianopia are present in virtually all patients and stroke-like episodes may be preceded by a migraine-like headache together with nausea and vomiting.[25] Focal and generalised seizures are common, as is dementia (Table 7.1). There may be overlap between MELAS and other mitochondrial encephalopathies with some patients having myoclonus, ophthalmoplegia, retinopathy and ptosis.

Lactate levels are often high, especially within the CSF. The MELAS syndrome has been associated with different biochemical findings, although complex I deficiency appears by far the most common. As in the MERRF syndrome, a mutation in mtDNA has been demonstrated but this affects a different tRNA from that in MERRF. The majority of mutations occur within the tRNA for leucine (UUR)[26] but a mutation in the tRNA for isoleucine has also been associated with this phenotype. In several instances, maternal inheritance has been recorded although sporadic disease is also described.

Neurogenic weakness, ataxia and retinitis pigmentosa (NARP)

This clinical syndrome is inherited in a maternal manner and the predominant clinical features are retinitis pigmentosa, epilepsy, ataxia, neurogenic weakness and peripheral neuropathy[27] (Table 7.1). In one family a severely affected child had the clinical and pathological features of Leigh's disease[28] (see below). Unlike the syndromes described above there are no morphological changes in skeletal muscle. There is a point mutation in the ATPase-6 gene, which does not seem to affect ATP hydrolysis by this enzyme but presumably affects ATP synthesis.

Leigh's syndrome

Also called subacute necrotising encephalomyopathy, this syndrome is essentially diagnosed by the neuropathological findings of symmetrical necrotic lesions, glial reaction and vascular proliferation in the mid-brain, pons, basal ganglia, thalamus and optic nerves. It usually presents as a devastating encephalopathy in infancy or childhood. The major findings are of failure to thrive associated with vomiting, motor and intellectual retardation and respiratory problems, especially irregularity in the pattern of respiration with hyper- and hypoventilation (Table 7.1). Additional features include ophthalmoplegia, optic atrophy, nystagmus and dystonia. The disease may present in children from birth to late teenage but is commonest in infants from 6 months to around 4 years.

No single biochemical abnormality is linked with Leigh's syndrome and defects of the respiratory chain, pyruvate dehydrogenase complex and biotinidase have been described. Lactate and pyruvate concentrations are frequently elevated in blood and CSF; CT/MRI scans show very characteristic (but not pathognomonic) low density areas within the basal ganglia or, less commonly, cerebellum. In those individuals with respiratory chain disease as the underlying defect, single complex deficiency (rather than multiple) appears to be more common than in other syndromes. This, together with the systemic nature and occasional autosomal recessive pattern of inheritance, has led us to presume that in most patients Leigh's syndrome may be caused by a nuclear gene rather than a mitochondrial gene defect. Having said this, however, cases with Leigh's syndrome phenotype have been found where the patients had a mutation in mtDNA (see above).

Other encephalopathies

As stated earlier, it is often difficult to fit individuals into the above categories. We have seen a number of patients presenting with features such as dementia, eye movement disorder (ophthalmoplegia or disorders of conjugate gaze), epilepsy, muscle weakness and peripheral neuropathy.

The majority of these patients have shown multiple defects of respiratory chain complexes suggesting once again that mtDNA is affected.

Leber's hereditary optic neuropathy (LHON)

Although not strictly an encephalopathy, this disorder warrants special attention because it is one of the commonest inherited causes of blindness in young men, and is clearly maternally inherited suggesting that it is due to a disorder of mtDNA. In 1988 this was confirmed. Mutations in several of the mitochondrial protein coding genes have now been identified, the commonest being in ND4 (11 778)[29] and ND1 (3460)[30], although involvement of non-complex I genes has also been reported.

In addition to blindness, several individuals within Leber's pedigrees manifest non-ophthalmological features; these include encephalopathy, deafness and dystonia. Moreover, cardiac conduction defects have been reported in some families. The finding of a point mutation in mtDNA may not be the complete story since it is clear from genetic analysis that the disease predominantly affects men. Evidence that a gene on the X chromosome may be linked with this disorder is accumulating, but is yet to be established.

Biochemical studies, using either skeletal muscle or platelet mitochondria, have shown that there is a defect in respiratory complex I in some of these patients. The clearest demonstration of this is in individuals carrying the ND1 mutation, although a more subtle defect in those with the ND4 mutation has been found.

Syndromes with non-neuromuscular presentation

Gastrointestinal involvement. Although relatively uncommon compared with other manifestations, gastrointestinal disease is recognised and probably underreported. Anorexia and vomiting may be general indicators of disease whilst abdominal pain is seen in many patients with systemic lactic acidosis. All can be found in a multisystem disorder such as MELAS. Liver dysfunction has been reported and occasionally may be the major disease component. Indeed, hepatic failure was the presenting feature in one recorded case later found to have a very low concentration of mtDNA (see below, Disorders presenting in infancy).

Myo-, neuro-, gastrointestinal encephalopathy syndrome (MNGIE). This name has been coined to describe a single case presenting with external ophthalmoplegia, muscular atrophy, peripheral neuropathy, malabsorption and a disorder of white matter within the brain. A partial decrease in cytochrome oxidase activity was reported as the cause.

Cardiomyopathy. Heart involvement occurs in the KSS/CPEO phenotype. The cardiac conduction system is predominantly affected and these patients often develop complete heart block. This is thought to be a significant cause of mortality and should be actively sought and treated by pacemaker insertion. In other patients, there is involvement of the heart muscle itself and this may lead to heart failure.[31] Apparently, the biochemical diagnosis in these patients was still made using skeletal muscle mitochondria suggesting, therefore, that the disease is widespread. Clearly this must be carefully evaluated when considering treatment, which may include transplantation, for the cardiac failure.

Renal disease. Generalised aminoaciduria (De Toni Fanconi Debré syndrome) has been described in several patients with respiratory chain disease. The majority of these had cytochrome c oxidase deficiency, diagnosed in skeletal muscle mitochondria, and almost all seem to have presented with a Leigh's phenotype or with profound lactic acidosis. Renal impairment or renal failure has rarely, if ever, been documented alone. The abnormality of the respiratory chain is identifiable in the kidney, although this tissue is rarely used for diagnostic purposes. Deletions of mitochondrial DNA have also been found in renal tissue in cases of the Kearns–Sayre syndrome.

Haematological. Haematological disease is a rare presentation of respiratory chain dysfunction. Abnormalities of mtDNA are frequently sought and identified in white blood cells (WBC) in individuals with disorders such as KSS, MELAS, etc. although they are often at a lower frequency (i.e. there is a greater percentage of wild type mtDNA) in these cells. This is thought to reflect the rapid turnover of white cells compared with stable cell types such as skeletal muscle. This is in turn thought to increase the selection pressure against the mutant DNA, although it must be stated that this has not been formally established. No abnormalities of WBC function (or of other blood cell type) have been identified in individuals with disorders such as KSS or MELAS.

Pearson's syndrome. This is a disorder which presents at birth or in early infancy with refractory sideroblastic anaemia, thrombocytopenia, neutropenia, metabolic acidosis, pancreatic insufficiency and hepatic dysfunction. Renal dysfunction, diarrhoea, steatorrhoea and ill-defined skin lesions are also reported. Children usually die due to liver failure. Deletions of mtDNA have now been identified in a significant proportion of children with this syndrome.[32] Furthermore, there are recorded cases of children presenting initially with Pearson's syndrome who later develop a disease identical to the Kearns–Sayre syndrome. These too carry a deletion of the mitochondrial genome. Clearly, Pearson's syndrome is a systemic disorder with its major manifestation in the haematological system.

Disorders of the respiratory chain presenting in infancy

Whilst many of the above syndromes may present in the very young, several conditions appear to be confined to infants and it is worthwhile discussing this group in isolation. It is important to remember that due to their lack of motor and intellectual development, especially lack of language, presentation of disease in infants follows different patterns to that seen in children and adults, for example, muscle weakness will manifest as a floppy infant, systemic disease may cause failure to thrive, whilst acidosis will provoke vomiting which is itself a common feature of disease in infancy.

Fatal infantile lactic acidosis

Profound lactic acidosis presenting from birth to around 3 months of age is highly suggestive of a respiratory chain defect. Hypotonia, vomiting and ventilatory distress are all commonly associated features, and death from respiratory failure is the usual outcome, often before the age of 6 months. Apart from the elevated blood lactate, several reports have mentioned generalised amino aciduria (De Toni Fanconi Debré syndrome); seizures, elevated calcium, liver dysfunction and hypoglycaemia have also been reported. Defects of complexes I, III and IV have been found.

Benign infantile lactic acidosis

Benign infantile lactic acidosis presents a similar initial picture.[33] Failure to thrive, hypotonia and ventilatory difficulty are all features of this condition, and lactic acid levels may be as high in this disorder as in the fatal form. Despite this, the condition gradually remits and by 12–18 months these infants are often normal. Biochemical studies have shown that all reported cases have been due to an initial, severe defect of cytochrome oxidase. This deficiency improves with age and it has been postulated that the defect involves a fetal isoform of a nuclear-encoded subunit of complex IV, the switch to the adult form being associated with the resolution of the disease. Immunohistochemical studies have suggested that it may be possible to differentiate fatal and benign forms.

The mtDNA depletion syndrome

This recently described syndrome affects neonates and infants.[34] Weakness, hypotonia and ventilatory difficulty are once again common, and renal involvement and seizures may occur (Table 7.1). The family history in some cases is suggestive of an autosomal recessive pattern of inheritance, indicating that the disease may itself be due to a nuclear gene defect. Interestingly, the degree of mtDNA depletion may vary between tissues in the same individual and this has led to clinical presentation outside the neuromuscular system, e.g. with liver disease. Biochemical studies have shown that complexes I, III and IV are affected, with the major deficiency apparently involving cytochrome c oxidase. The condition is fatal in the majority of cases, usually before the age of 12 months.

Other conditions

Luft's disease

Historically, this was the first condition to be linked with abnormal mitochondrial function. Paradoxically, it is extremely rare and only a single case has been added to that described by Luft and colleagues in 1962. Mitochondria in this disorder show poor respiratory control but normal phosphorylation capacity – a state termed 'loose coupling'. It is suggested that the cause of this disorder is an inability of mitochondria to retain calcium ions so that the constant recycling of calcium results in sustained, maximal respiration and hypermetabolism. The two individuals described presented with euthyroid hypermetabolism.

Ubiquinone deficiency

This encephalomyopathic disorder has been described only in two individuals who were sisters.[35] No particular clinical features appear to differentiate this condition although the presence of morphological mitochondrial abnormalities has directed the biochemical evaluation. Laboratory analysis demonstrates that flux through the respiratory chain is slow, whilst activity in the individual complexes measured with artificial electron acceptors, is normal. This paradox gave the first indication that it may be a disorder of ubiquinone rather than one of the individual complexes. Confirmation is by direct measurement of ubiquinone concentration.

Multiple mtDNA deletions

Whilst this syndrome clearly has a similar phenotype to KSS, the molecular basis is different.[36] The patients described had chronic progressive external ophthalmoplegia, proximal myopathy, sensorineural deafness, cataracts and peripheral neuropathy. Muscle histology shows subsarcolemmal accumulation of mitochondria, decreased cytochrome c oxidase activity and some neurogenic changes. Biochemical studies showed multiple respiratory chain defects and molecular studies showed multiple DNA deletions. Most deletions spanned a mtDNA region of several kilobases between the end of the D loop and the region encompassing genes for ATPase 8 and 6, and CO I. The syndrome is inherited in an autosomal dominant manner and implies a mutation in a nuclear-encoded gene. The mechanism by which this nuclear gene defect results in the multiple deletions is unknown. A similar syndrome has also been reported in two brothers, but the transmission in these cases was probably autosomal recessive.

Defects of complex II

These defects are unique in that they must all be inherited autosomally, since each complex II subunit is nuclear-encoded. They are probably fairly uncommon compared with defects of the other complexes. One family presented with myopathic and central nervous system features. The activity of complexes I–IV was low but the most severe defect involved complex II. A further patient has been described with a pure myopathy in whom again there were multiple respiratory chain deficiencies, but specific lowering of the iron–sulphur protein of complex II and the iron–sulphur (Rieske) protein of complex III. A further patient had myopathic symptoms with muscle pain and myoglobinuria on exercise.

Neurodegenerative disease

There is considerable debate as to the possible involvement of defects of the respiratory chain in neurodegenerative disease.[37] The link between neurodegenerative disease and the respiratory chain was provided by the finding that 1-methyl-4-phenyl-1,2,3,6-tetrahydropyridine (MPTP) caused a condition identical to Parkinson's disease.[38] A metabolite of MPTP was subsequently shown to be a profound inhibitor of complex I. Since this discovery, a variety of respiratory chain defects have been identified in a number of tissues from patients with Parkinson's disease. At this stage it is not possible to be certain which defects are primary or secondary, or whether mtDNA abnormalities are involved.

Following the findings in Parkinson's disease, the role of respiratory chain dysfunction has been investigated in other neurodegenerative disorders. In both Alzheimer's disease and Huntington's chorea respiratory chain abnormalities have been reported. However, the role of these defects in the neurodegenerative diseases is even more controversial.

Ageing

Studies on human muscle mitochondria have suggested that there is an age-related decline in respiratory chain activity.[37] It has been postulated that this decline causes impairment of cell viability and that it is due to the accumulation of mtDNA mutations. The initial damage to mtDNA may be caused by free radical damage, known to occur at a much greater frequency than to nuclear DNA. Since most mitochondria have a half-life of days to a few weeks, the mitochondrial population may reproduce itself several hundred times during the lifetime of an individual. If this abnormality also has a selective advantage, for example, a deletion would give rise to a smaller genome which replicates faster than the larger, normal one, then it may become the dominant form in the cell. There is some evidence to support the theory of increasing mtDNA mutations with age.

Low levels of a specific mtDNA deletion, previously only found in patients with mitochondrial encephalomyopathies, have been found in normal heart, muscle and brain from adult humans but not in fetal brain or liver.[39]

TREATMENT

The treatment of patients with respiratory chain defects is difficult and in our experience often unsuccessful. This difficulty is partly due to the nature of the biochemical defect. Since it involves the final common pathway of oxidative metabolism it is impossible to bypass by giving alternative metabolic fuels. In addition, we still understand relatively little about the biochemistry of these conditions and there have been conflicting results of treatment in patients with apparently similar biochemical abnormalities. Most success has been achieved with substances that act as artificial electron acceptors: vitamin C (ascorbate 4 g per day), vitamin K_3 (menadione, up to 80 mg per day)[40] and ubiquinone (up to 150 mg per day).[41] Objective increases in muscle strength have been reported with ascorbate and menadione and with ubiquinone. Improvements in electron transfer have been suggested by NMR studies in these patients. No improvement in the ophthalmoplegia or ptosis has been reported.

Other attempts at treating respiratory chain disorders include the use of thiamine, biotin, carnitine, riboflavin and dichloracetate. For many of these treatments there are either single case reports or anecdotal evidence of clinical improvement, but none has been consistently shown to be of therapeutic benefit. The mitochondrial respiratory chain generates free radicals, and their production may be increased in the presence of respiratory chain disease. Therefore, the use of free radical scavengers such as vitamin E could, in theory, help prevent further damage but there is little evidence, as yet, to justify their use.

An important aspect of patient care is rehabilitation and supportive care, since at present many of these conditions are progressive and associated with significant disability. Patients with respiratory muscle involvement may need ventilatory support.

Access to genetic counselling is important for patients and their families, especially since many of these disorders are inherited in a maternal manner. Prenatal diagnosis of some of the most severe presentations is now possible in a very few instances, by either identifying a biochemical abnormality in cultured cells from a chorionic villus biopsy or amniocentesis, or by genetic analysis of fetal material.

ACKNOWLEDGEMENTS

The authors are grateful to Dr Margaret Johnson for the morphology figures and Miss J Leggett for help with the manuscript. Our work on defects of the respiratory chain has been supported by the Muscular

Dystrophy Group of Great Britain, Action Research for the Crippled Child and the National Institutes of Health (USA).

REFERENCES

1. Sherratt H S A, Turnbull D M 1990 Mitochondrial oxidations and ATP synthesis in muscle. In: Harris J B, Turnbull D M (eds) Metabolic myopathies. Ballière–Tindall, London p 523–560
2. Weiss H, Friedrich T, Hofhaus G, Preis D 1991 The respiratory chain NADH dehydrogenase (complex I) of mitochondria. European Journal of Biochemistry 197:563–576
3. Ackrell B A C, Johnson M K, Gunsalus R P, Cecchini G 1992 Structure and function of succinate dehydrogenase and fumarate reductase. In: Muller F (ed) Chemistry and biochemistry of flavoproteins. Bocka Raton, Florida, CRC Press, vol 3, p 229–297
4. Weiss H 1987 Structure of mitochondrial ubiquinol-cytochrome c reductase (complex III). Current Topics in Bioenergetics 15:67–89
5. Capaldi R A 1990 Structure and assembly of cytochrome c oxidase. Archives of Biochemistry and Biophysics 280:252–262
6. Senior A E 1988 ATP synthesis by oxidative phosphorylation. Physiological Review 68:177–230
7. Anderson S, Bankier A T, Barrell B G et al 1981 Sequence organisation of the human mitochondrial genome. Nature 290:457–465
8. Clayton D A 1984 Transcription of the mammalian mitochondrial genome. Annual Review of Biochemistry 53:573–594
9. Hartl F-U, Neupert W 1990 Protein sorting to mitochondria: evolutionary conservations of folding and assembly. Science 247:930–938
10. Arnold D L, Taylor D J, Radda G K 1985 Investigation of human mitochondrial myopathies by phosphorus magnetic spectroscopy. Annals of Neurology 18:189–196
11. Olsen W, King-Engel W, Walsh G O, Einangler R 1972 Oculocraniosomatic neuromuscular disease with 'ragged-red' fibres. Archives of Neurology 26:193–211
12. Old S L, Johnson M A 1989 Methods for microphotometric assay of succinate dehydrogenase and cytochrome c oxidase activities for use on human skeletal muscle. Histochemical Journal 21:545–556
13. Johnson M A 1991 Cytochemical and immunocytochemical investigation of respiratory chain complexes in individual fibres of human skeletal muscle. In: Gorrod J W, Albano O, Ferrari E, Papa S (eds) Molecular basis of neurological disorders and their treatment. Chapman and Hall, London p 40–56
14. Mita S, Schmidt B, Schon E A et al 1989 Detection of 'deleted' mitochondrial genomes in cytochrome c oxidase deficient muscle fibres of a patient with Kearns–Sayre syndrome. Proceedings of National Academy of Sciences USA 86:9509–9513
15. Robinson B H, Glerum D M, Chow W, Petrova-Benedict R, Lightowlers R, Capaldi R 1990 The use of skin fibroblasts in the detection of respiratory chain defect in patients with lactic acidemia. Pediatric Research 28:549–555
16. Sherratt H S A, Watmough N J, Johnson M, Turnbull D M 1988 Methods used for the study of normal and abnormal skeletal muscle mitochondria. Methods in Biochemical Analysis 33:243–335
17. Birch-Machin M A, Jackson S, Singh Kler R, Turnbull D M 1993 Study of skeletal muscle mitochondrial dysfunction. Methods in Toxicology 2: 51–69
18. King M P, Attardi G 1989 Human cells lacking mtDNA: repopulation with exogenous mitochondria by complementation. Science 246:500–503
19. Chomyn A, Meola G, Bresolin N, Lai S T, Scarlato G, Attardi G 1991 In vitro genetic transfer of protein synthesis and respiration defect to mitochondrial DNA-less cells with myopathy-patient mitochondria. Molecular and Cellular Biology 11:2236–2244
20. Bindoff L A, Turnbull D M 1990 Defects of the respiratory chain. In: Harris J B, Turnbull D M (eds) Metabolic myopathies, Ballière–Tindall, London p 583–619
21. Holt I J, Harding A E, Morgan-Hughes 1988 Deletions of muscle mitchondrial DNA in patients with mitochondrial myopathies. Nature 331:717–719

22. Schon E A, Rizzuto R, Moraes C T, et al 1989 A direct repeat is a hot spot for large-scale deletion of human mitochondrial DNA. Science 244:346–349
23. Poulton J, Deadman M E, Gardiner R M 1989 Duplications of mitochondrial DNA in mitochondrial myopathy. Lancet: 236–240
24. Shoffner J M, Lott M T, Lezza A M S et al 1990 Myoclonic epilepsy and ragged-red fibre disease (MERRF) is associated with a mitochondrial DNA $tRNA^{Lys}$ mutation. Cell 61:931–937
25. Ciafaloni E, Ricci E, Shanske S et al 1992 MELAS: clinical features, biochemistry, and molecular genetics. Annals of Neurology 31:391–398
26. Goto Y-I, Nonaka I, Horai S 1990 A mutation in the $tRNA^{Leu(UUR)}$ gene associated with the MELAS subgroup of mitochondrial encephalopathies. Nature 348:651–653
27. Holt I J, Harding A E, Petty R K H, Morgan-Hughes J A 1990 A new mitochondrial disease associated with mitochondrial DNA heteroplasmy. American Journal of Human Genetics 46:428–433
28. Tatuch Y, Christodoulou J, Feigenbaum A et al 1992 Heteroplasmic mtDNA mutation (T-G) at 8993 can cause Leigh Disease when the percentage of abnormal mtDNA is high. American Journal of Human Genetics 50:842–848
29. Wallace D C, Singh G, Lott M T et al 1988 Mitochondrial DNA mutation associated with Leber's hereditary optic neuropathy. Science 242:1427–1430
30. Howell N, Bindoff L A, McCullough D A et al 1991 Leber's hereditary optic neuropathy: identification of the same ND1 mutation in six pedigrees. American Journal of Human Genetics 49:939–950
31. Zeviani M, Gellera C, Antozzi C et al 1991 Maternally inherited myopathy and cardiomyopathy: association with mutation in mitochondrial DNA $tRNA^{Leu(UUR)}$. Lancet 338:143–147
32. Rotig A, Colonna M, Bonnefont J P et al 1989 Mitochondrial DNA deletion in Pearson's marrow/pancreas syndrome. Lancet: 902–903
33. DiMauro S, Nicholson J F, Hays A P et al 1983 Benign infantile mitochondrial myopathy due to reversible cytochrome c oxidase deficiency. Annals of Neurology 14:226–234
34. Moraes C T, Shanske S, Tritschler H-J et al 1991 Mitochondrial DNA depletion with variable tissue specificity: a novel genetic abnormality in mitochondrial diseases. American Journal of Human Genetics 48:492–501
35. Ogasahara S, Engel A G, Frens D, Mack D 1989 Muscle coenzyme Q deficiency in familial mitochondrial encephalomyopathy. Proceedings of the National Academy of Sciences USA 86:2379–2382
36. Zeviani M, Servidei S, Gellera C, Bertini E, DiMauro S, DiDonato S 1989 An autosomal dominant disorder with multiple deletions of mitochondrial DNA starting at the D-loop region. Nature 339:309–311
37. Wallace D C 1992 Mitochondrial genetics: a paradigm for ageing and neurodegenerative diseases? Science 256:628–632
38. Langston J W, Ballard P, Tetrud J W, Irwin I 1983 Chronic parkinsonism in humans due to a product of meperidine-analog synthesis. Science 219:979–980
39. Cortopassi G A, Arnheim N 1990 Detection of a specific mitochondrial DNA deletion in tissues of older humans. Nucleic Acid Research 18:6927–6933
40. Argov Z, Bank W J, Maris J et al 1986 Treatment of mitochondrial myopathy due to complex III deficiency with vitamins K_3 and C: a ^{31}P-NMR follow-up study. Annals of Neurology 19:598–602
41. Ogasahara S, Nihikawa Y, Yoritugi S et al 1986 Treatment of Kearns–Sayre syndrome with coenzyme Q_{10} Neurology 36:45–53

8. Purine and pyrimidine disorders

H. A. Simmonds

INTRODUCTION

In today's age of molecular biology purines and pyrimidines are probably best known as the basic constituents of the polynucleotides DNA and RNA. Of predominant importance are the ribo- and deoxyribonucleotide forms of the five purine and pyrimidine bases adenine, guanine, uracil, cytosine and thymine. However, in addition to this, purines and pyrimidines constitute the basis of at least 50 other important compounds which serve equally vital but separate roles as integral components of intracellular mononucleotide pools; the purine ribonucleotide triphosphates, ATP and GTP, and the pyrimidine disphosphate sugars, UDP-glucose and CDP-choline (Figs 8.1 and 8.2) being of particular significance. Cellular purines and pyrimidines are derived almost exclusively from endogenous sources. The function of purine and pyrimidine metabolism is to maintain the supply of these basic components to the different nucleotide pools, largely through an extremely efficient mechanism involving the degradation and recycling of the daily waste products of normal cell turnover, derived during red cell senescence, muscle work, wound healing, etc.

The year 1990 marked a milestone in the treatment of human disease with the commencement of the first-ever human gene therapy experiments in the inherited purine disorder, adenosine deaminase deficiency.[1] Such achievements are even more remarkable considering that, although the nephrotoxicity of purines has been known for more than a century, their potential cellular toxicity became evident only over the past 20 years because of the associated clinical manifestations when one of the steps involved in the above processes was defective, or missing. The first inherited purine disorder, xanthine oxidase deficiency, was reported as a clinical entity in 1954. The biochemical basis was identified in 1959. A total of nine purine disorders with a proven genetic basis are now known; six of them have been described since 1970. The first inherited pyrimidine disorder was also identified in 1959 and five other defects have now been recognised. Genetic deficiencies of several other enzymes with no currently apparent clinical consequence have been identified, either in the erythrocytes

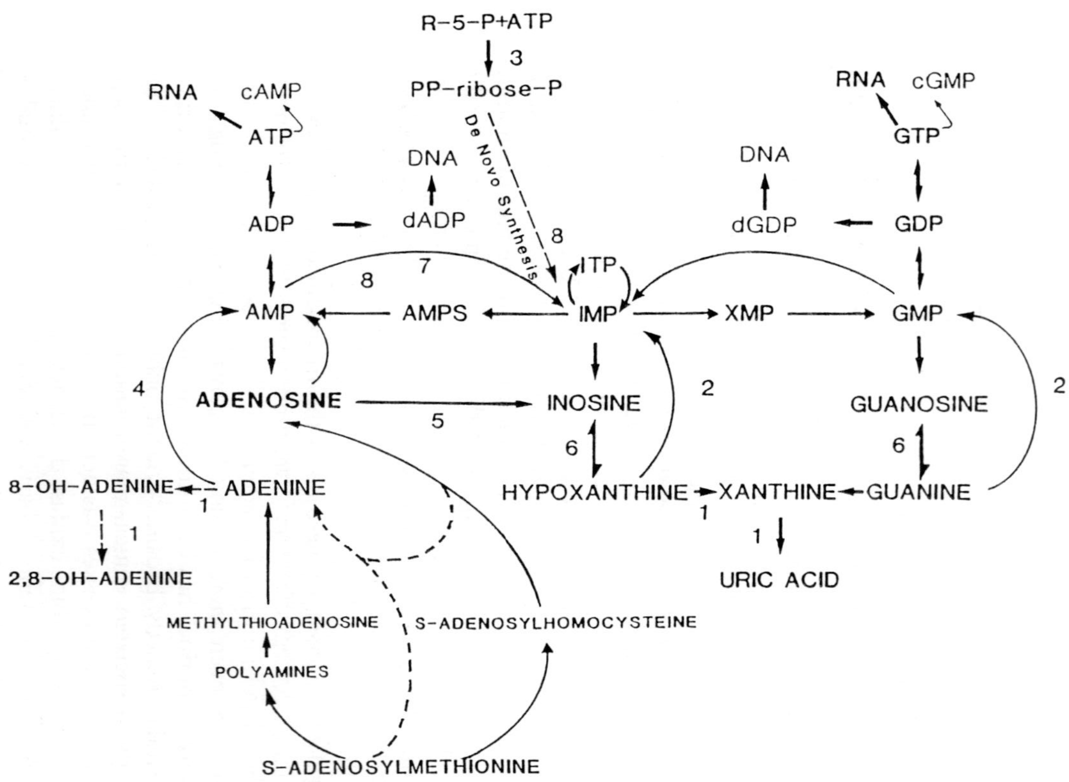

Fig. 8.1 Routes of synthesis, catabolism and salvage of the different intracellular purine mono- and polynucleotides in man, indicating the close associations with other metabolic pathways. The dotted lines indicate alternative metabolic routes when a particular enzyme is defective or absent. See text for abbreviations. The numbers indicate the specific enzyme involved in the different genetic metabolic purine disorders identified to date as follows: 1 – xanthine oxidase (XOD); 2 – hypoxanthine phosphoribosyltranferase (HPRT) 3 – phosphoribosylpyrophosphate synthetase (PRPS); 4 – adenine phosphoribosyltransferase (APRT); 5 – adenosine deaminase (ADA); 6 – purine nucleoside phosphorylase (PNP); 7 – myoadenylate deaminase (AMPDA); 8 – adenylosuccinase (ADS).

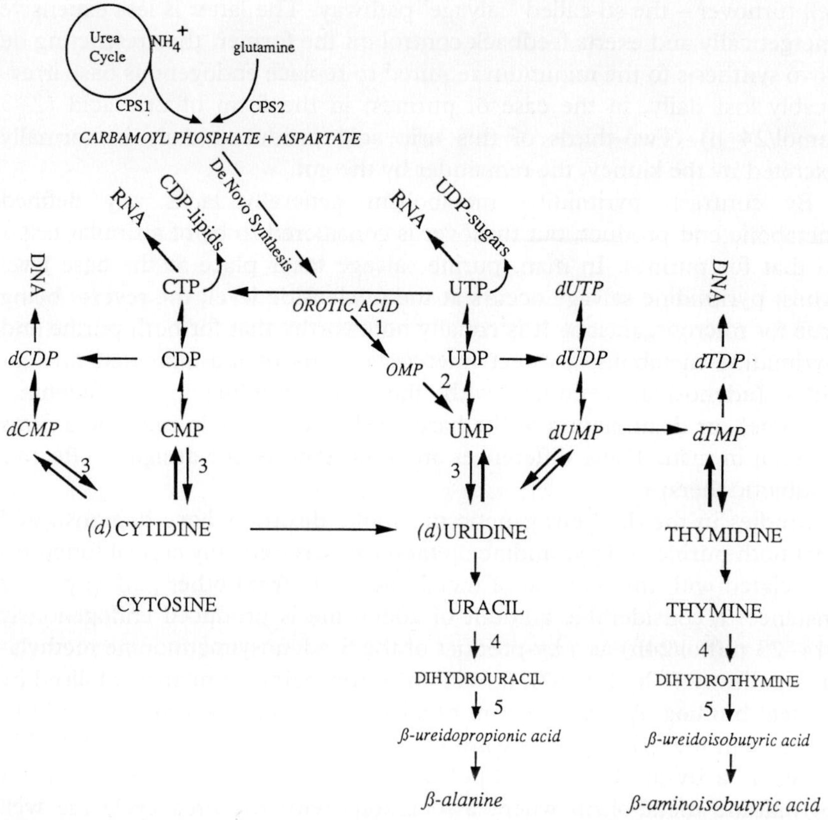

Fig. 8.2 Routes of synthesis, catabolism and salvage of the different intracellular pyrimidines in man. The potential for stimulation of the de novo pathway when the enzymes of the urea cycle are defective is indicated, as is the importance of pyrimidine nucleotides to carbohydrate and lipid metabolism as well as nucleic acid synthesis. See text for abbreviations. The numbers indicate the different enzymes implicated in the genetic metabolic pyrimidine disorders identified to date, as follows: 1 – orotic acid phosphoribosyltransferase (OPRT); 2 – orotidine-5'-monophosphate decarboxylase (ODC); 3 – pyrimidine-5-nucleotidase (UMPH 1); 4 – dihydropyrimidine dehydrogenase (DHPD); 5 – dihydropyrimidinase (DHPA).

of seemingly healthy subjects or during therapy with purine analogues, or investigation for another disorder.[2]

Purine and pyrimidine metabolic pathways

Purine and pyrimidine ribo- and deoxyribonucleotides may be synthesised de novo from simple molecules by energetically expensive, multistep pathways. (Figs 8.1 and 8.2). Alternatively, and more generally, these ribo- and deoxyribonucleotide pools are sustained by the recycling of the basic components derived from their catabolism during the normal process of cell turnover – the so-called 'salvage' pathway. The latter is less expensive energetically and exerts feedback control on the former, thus restricting de novo synthesis to the minimum required to replace endogenous base irrevocably lost daily; in the case of purines, in the form of uric acid (2–3 mmol/24 h). Two-thirds of this uric acid produced daily is normally excreted by the kidney, the remainder by the gut.

By contrast, pyrimidine metabolism generally lacks any defined metabolic end-product, but turnover is considered to be of a similar order to that for purines. In man, purine salvage takes place at the base level whilst pyrimidine salvage occurs at the nucleoside level; the reverse being true for microorganisms. It is equally noteworthy that for both purine and pyrimidine metabolism, direct interconversions of the aminated nucleosides (adenosine, cytidine) with the corresponding bases (adenine, cytosine), or deamination at the base level, occur only in microorganisms and not in man. These differences are important for the design of effective antibiotic therapy.

Studies in the different genetic metabolic disorders have demonstrated that both purine and pyrimidine metabolism serve equally crucial functions associated with the removal of metabolic waste from other pathways. For instance, a considerable amount of adenosine is produced endogenously (14–23 mmol/24h) as a by-product of the S-adenosylmethionine methylation pathway (Ch. 3 p. 82), a fraction of this being compartmentalised by protein binding. A small amount of adenine may also be produced via this route[2], but the bulk of adenine produced endogenously, about 1 mmol/24 h, arises as a by-product of the polyamine pathway. The same is true for pyrimidine metabolism where associations with the urea cycle are well documented (Ch. 3, p. 89).

It has also become apparent that the original concept of purine metabolism and its overall control does not apply to all cells, but is governed by a tissue- or cell-specific complement of enzymes and/or controls on them, depending on the function of that cell or tissue. An example is the human erythrocyte, which lacks adenylosuccinate synthetase and thus cannot use synthesis or salvage to maintain its ATP levels, requiring adenosine for this.[2] It also lacks guanase. The tissue-specific aspect of purine metabolism will be discussed with the different inherited disorders. Although not dealt with in this chapter, it is now evident that not all reactions involving purines take place intracellularly at the nucleotide level. An extensive literature now encompasses their biological effects exerted outside cells, mediated by externally directed membrane receptors.[2] Defects involving these processes have yet to be identified.

Clinical and biochemical consequences of disorders of purine and pyrimidine metabolism

It is not always appreciated that genetic metabolic defects of both purine and pyrimidine metabolism can present neonatally. Although most manifest in infancy or adolescence, considerable genetic heterogeneity is now evident, and some disorders can present at any age up to the sixth or eighth decade. The importance of the normal recycling of purine bases to the feedback control of purine synthesis is demonstrated by the gross overproduction found in the disorders where this is defective: hypoxanthine-guanine phosphoribosyltransferase (HPRT) deficiency, aberrant phosphoribosylpyrophosphate synthetase (PRPS) activity, purine nucleoside phosphorylase (PNP) and adenylosuccinase (ADS) deficiencies. Patients with the aberrant synthetase and HPRT deficiency may present with gout, uric acid stones or renal failure (Table 8.1). The potential nephrotoxicity resulting from the relative insolubility of the purine bases is also demonstrated in xanthine oxidase (XOD) and adenine phosphoribosyltransferase (APRT) deficiencies, which can present with kidney stones and/or renal failure.

In their severest form HPRT, PNP and ADS deficiencies and PRPS superactivity present in the first weeks of life with neurological deficits of varying severity, whilst seizures in the neonatal period are characteristic of combined XOD/sulphite oxidase (SO) deficiency. Additionally, XOD deficiency may be associated with myopathy, which is the presenting symptom in myoadenylate deaminase (AMPDA) deficiency.

Patients with PNP deficiency can also present neonatally with immunodeficiency, as do homozygotes for adenosine deaminase (ADA) deficiency. Low lymphocyte ecto 5'-nucleotidase (5'-NT) activity has been reported in different immunodeficiency syndromes.[3] Recent studies suggest that 5'-NT may have an important function as an 'accessary molecule' in facilitating the interaction of T cells with antigen-presenting cells. Since 5'-NT activity is five times higher in peripheral B cells than T cells and it is not certain whether low activity reflects a failure of lymphocyte maturation or is the primary cause of the hypogammaglobulinaemia, it is not listed as a genetic purine disorder.

The five pyrimidine disorders may present in the first weeks of life also; all are associated with retarded growth and development, three of them with anaemia. They comprise genetic deficiencies of uridine monophosphate synthase (UMPS), dihydropyrimidine dehydrogenase (DHPD), dihydropyrimidinase (DHPA) and uridine monophosphate hydrolase 1 (UMPH1); the genetic basis for CDP choline phosphotransferase (CDPC-P) deficiency is proposed but not proven[4]. UMPS deficiency is also characterised by hypochromic megaloblastic anaemia, while UMPH1 and CDPC-P deficiency, present with chronic haemolytic anaemia.

DISORDERS OF PURINE METABOLISM

Our knowledge of the number of disorders of purine metabolism associated with a specific enzyme defect has grown rapidly in the past two decades.

Table 8.1 Characteristic clinical signs relative to the importance of early diagnosis in the different inherited purine and pyrimidine disorders.
↑ – can present at any time from birth upwards; ? – insufficient data currently available

Defect	Early diagnosis	Clinical signs
XOD	Can present in acute renal failure in 1st year	Hypouricaemia, radiolucent stones, acute renal failure, myopathy
XOD/SO*	Essential – lethal	Neonatal fitting, dislocated lenses
APRT	Essential – benign or lethal Responds to treatment	Birth ↑: acute renal failure, crystalluria, recurrent urinary tract infection, haematuria, radiolucent stones
HPRT*	Essential – benign or lethal	Infant: Birth ↑: acute renal failure, ARF, crystalluria, haematuria, recurrent urinary tract infection, gout, radiolucent stones; delayed motor development, 3 months upwards; CNS involvement, 8 months upwards Adult: Gout radiolucent stones, acute renal failure
PRPS Super activity	Essential – benign or lethal	Infant: Birth ↑: head drops, delayed motor development 3 months upwards, nerve deafness, crystalluria, recurrent urinary tract infection, radiolucent stones Adult: gout, radiolucent stones
PNP*	Essential – generally lethal	Birth ↑: delayed motor development 3 months upwards, viral infections, lymphopenia, T cell dysfunction
ADA*	Essential – generally lethal	Birth ↑: failure to thrive, diarrhoea, thrush, lymphopenia, severe combined immunodeficiency (SCID)
ADS	Essential – potentially lethal	Birth ↑: severe psychomotor retardation, axial hypotonia, epilepsy, autism
AMPDA	Generally benign	Infant: hypotonia, cardiomyopathy Adult: exercise intolerance, myopathy
UMPS*	Essential – lethal Responds to treatment	Birth↑: hypochromic megablastic anaemia, crystalluria, retarded development
UMPH 1	Benign	Non-spherocytic haemolytic anaemia with basophilic stippling, haemoglobinuria
DHPD*	Essential – benign or lethal	Birth ↑: developmental retardation, epilepsy, microcephaly Adult: 5-fluorouracil toxicity
DHPA	Essential ? Responds to treatment	Birth ↑: seizures, developmental retardation, microcephaly
?CDPCP	? Relatively benign	Child/adult: haemolytic anaemia

*indicates defect for which prenatal diagnosis is essential/currently available

However, although primary gout is still the most prevalent purine disorder and has been known to mankind since ancient times, no underlying metabolic basis has been recognised as yet. A specific genetic defect of purine metabolism has been identified in less than 1% of patients presenting with gout.

Primary gout

This disorder, which afflicts predominantly middle-aged males, has been the subject of many excellent reviews.[5] In summary it is a disease manifest during times of plenty, associated generally with overindulgence in dietary purine, but may involve other factors affecting the renal clearance of uric acid. The basic problem lies in a markedly reduced ability of the gouty kidney to excrete uric acid. The fractional uric acid clearance (FE_{ur}) (clearance of uric acid divided by the creatinine clearance × 100) of patients with primary gout is reduced to about 5%, compared with that of healthy male controls, matched for age and sex, of 8%. This is not due to reduced renal function per se. In the majority of middle-aged males with primary gout glomerular filtration rate (GFR) is normal for age.[2]

Gout in hereditary disorders

Two genetic purine disorders (HPRT deficiency and aberrant PRPS activity) are associated with uric acid overproduction and gout[5], but unlike primary gout they present in childhood or adolescence and are X-linked (see below).

There are reports of at least two other rare forms of gout presenting at a young age which also appear X-linked, but in which activity of the above enzymes is normal. One of these is characterised by a chronic compensated non-anaemic haemolytic syndrome of unknown aetiology.[2] Gout is also a frequent complication of the recessively inherited disorder glycogenosis Type 1 (Ch.2, p. 26). Glycogenesis Types III, V and VII are also associated with exercise-induced hyperuricaemia. Hyperuricaemia in these glycogen storage diseases is attributed to rapid utilisation of ATP during muscular activity in excess of the ability to regenerate it.

Secondary gout

Gout may be precipitated during rapid tissue breakdown or accelerated cell turnover, whether occuring spontaneously or during aggressive therapy for malignant or haematological disorders. Gout may also develop in any situation which effectively reduces the clearance of uric acid; for example, volume depletion, starvation, ketoacidosis or drug therapy for an alternative condition. Thiazide diuretics now account for up to 50% of new patients presenting with gout.[2]

Familial juvenile gout (McKusick 162000)

Familial juvenile hyperuricaemic nephropathy (FJHN) is dealt with in detail because of its relatively recent recognition and, in contrast to 'primary gout' or the X-linked disorders, because of its presentation in young females as well as males and its potentially fatal nature.[6,7] Activity of the two enzymes associated with juvenile gout, HPRT and PRPS are normal. The biochemical defect is unknown. It may not be a single disorder.

Clinical presentation

In all instances there is a strong family history, with at least one member presenting with a single attack of gout, generally in the big toe, which has drawn attention to the disorder, often previously designated as a 'familial renal disease'.[7] The hallmark of FJHN is hyperuricaemia associated with extreme renal hypoexcretion of uric acid, the mean FE_{ur} of 4.7% being even lower than in primary gout. The age of presentation is generally around puberty and up to the third decade, although affected infants have been detected. FJHN may be distinguished from primary gout, or the X-linked disorders, by four factors: the occurrence of gout in such a young age group; the fact that young females as well as males are affected equally; the grossly reduced FE_{ur} for the young age and sex, and the frequent association with a rapidly declining renal function, leading to death unless recognised and treated sufficiently early.[6,7]

Inheritance and incidence

FJHN was considered hitherto to be a rare disorder. However, increased clinical awareness has resulted in the detection of over 150 cases from some 48 kindreds. The defect is inherited in an autosomal dominant fashion with high penetrance. There is considerable debate as to whether this is not a primary renal disease. However, the identification of children in FJHN kindreds with hyperuricaemia associated with a grossly reduced FE_{ur} and normal renal function is considered to be evidence against this.[6, 7]

Molecular defect

At present the genetic basis for this disorder, or disorders, is unknown. It is possible that there may be two separate defects linked on the same gene, or a single defect associated with the abnormal functioning of a pathway which results in the accumulation of a nephrotoxic metabolite which also reduces uric acid clearance. Alternatively a genetically determined lesion involving the urate transporter in either the brush-border, or basal membrane of the proximal tubule, could be the basis of the renal urate hypoexcretion. A secretory defect has been reported in gouty chickens[4], whilst pigs and rabbits lack the brush-border anion-exchanger recently identified in the proximal tubule.[2]

Diagnosis

Hyperuricaemia associated with an FE_{ur} grossly reduced for the young age, sex and GFR, generally in the absence of hypertension, is the hallmark of FJHN. A single gouty attack may be a fortuitous event in drawing attention to the disorder. Hyperuricaemia, with or without impaired renal function before the age of 25, plus a strong family history involving both sexes, requires immediate investigation of all kindred members. By this means early stages of the disease have been found in seemingly healthy subjects in several kindreds.[7] Mild hyperuricaemia will not be detected unless the plasma uric acid is evaluated against the appropriate control ranges for age, sex, GFR and for the country of origin, since diet varies considerably in different countries. Uric acid excretion is generally normal (2–3 mmol/24 h), as is the activity of the purine enzymes HPRT and PRPS in red cells.

A markedly reduced urinary concentrating capacity, disproportionately low for the reduction in GFR, is typical. Characteristic histological findings have been reported at renal biopsy in some cases, but generally a non-specific interstitial nephritis is found.[6,7]

Treatment and prognosis

Treatment involves the use of allopurinol, but at lower dosage relative to the reduction in GFR when renal function is impaired and also relative to the FE_{ur} since oxypurinol, the active metabolite of allopurinol, is cleared in a similar fashion to uric acid. Early recognition is important, as is good compliance, since allopurinol appears to have halted the rapid decline in renal function in some patients now studied for up to 20 years. The necessity for early recognition is underlined by the fact that the indicators of poor prognosis are the severity of the renal failure at diagnosis and the presence of hypertension. Consequently, adequate control of hypertension is equally vital.

Hereditary xanthinuria (McKusick 278300)

Biochemical disorder

The enzyme xanthine oxidase (EC 1.2.3.2) or, more correctly, xanthine dehydrogenase (EC 1.2.1.37), since in human tissue NAD^+ is the electron acceptor, catalyses the degradation of hypoxanthine and xanthine to uric acid (Fig. 8.3), the normal end-product of purine metabolism in man. It has an absolute requirement for molybdenum, FAD and iron. In man, activity is concentrated mainly in the liver and intestinal mucosa.

In homozygotes for XOD deficiency, xanthine and, to a lesser extent,

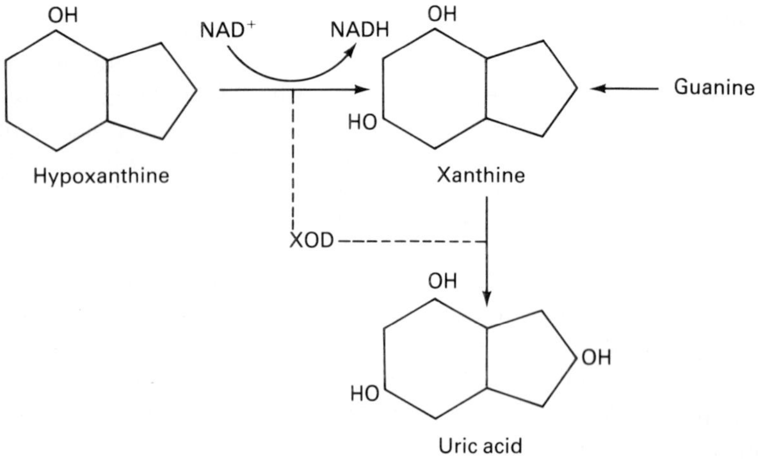

Fig. 8.3 The formation of uric acid from hypoxanthine and xanthine catalysed by xanthine oxidase (XOD).

hypoxanthine accumulate in place of uric acid. The preferential excretion of xanthine is due to the extensive normal recycling of hypoxanthine by the salvage pathway for which xanthine is not an effective substrate in vivo. Excess xanthine in the defect results from guanine nucleotide catabolism via guanase (Fig. 8.1).

Recently, combined XOD/sulphite oxidase (SO) deficiency has been described due to a congenital absence of a molybdenum cofactor essential for both enzymes, in which the clinical features of sulphite oxidase deficiency overshadow those of the xanthine oxidase defect (see Ch. p. 88).

Clinical presentation

The single enzyme defect may present in infancy, or in adults as late as the eighth decade and, although rare, can be an unsuspected cause of acute renal failure[2]. A total of 40% of patients have presented with symptoms which could be attributed directly to the defect: urinary tract infection, renal failure colic and/or xanthine calculi. The nephrotoxicity of xanthine is due to its extreme insolubility, coupled with a high renal clearance. Unlike uric acid, xanthine solubility in urine at pH 5.0 (0.5 mmol/l) is not greatly enhanced by alkalinisation of the urine (0.9 mmol/l at pH 7.0). In some cases the renal damage has been severe, and complications have included clubbing of the calyces of the kidney, hydronephrosis, nephrectomy, chronic renal failure, or even death.

More than 50% of homozygotes are asymptomatic and detected only by the very low plasma uric acid found during screening for a presumably unrelated disorder. Eight cases with myopathy have been reported, associated with crystalline deposits of xanthine and hypoxanthine in skeletal muscle in four of them.

Xanthine nephropathy and acute renal failure can also be precipitated by aggressive therapy for malignant disorders treated concomitantly with the xanthine oxidase inhibitor allopurinol to reduce the risk of uric acid nephropathy.[8]

The combined defect, XOD/SO deficiency, generally presents neonatally with seizures, extensive neurological dysfunction, dysmorphic features, and ocular lens dislocation. Description of a milder form, presenting in an adolescent with normal uric acid but raised xanthine and hypoxanthine[9], underlines the considerable heterogeneity of phenotypic expression in genetic metabolic disorders and the constant need to evaluate several parameters.

Inheritance and incidence

Xanthine oxidase deficiency has been identified in more than 100 cases, both male and female, of caucasian, Asian, oriental and negroid descent. Studies in several kindreds are consistent with an autosomal recessive mode of inheritance.

There is a strong element of consanguinity in cases presenting with the combined defect.

Molecular defect

Genetic heterogeneity in XOD deficiency has been demonstrated by the fact that some patients can convert allopurinol to oxypurinol, whilst others do not.[10] This has been found in 4 of 9 xanthinuric patients and has been related to a deficiency of the associated enzyme, aldehyde oxidase (EC 1.2.3.1), suggesting the combined deficiency of XOD and aldehyde oxidase might be relatively common. Since the molybdenum cofactor is also required for aldehyde oxidase, patients with the combined defect are likewise aldehyde oxidase deficient.

The genetic locus for XOD is on chromosome 2. The structural genes for XOD and aldehyde oxidase are closely linked on the same chromosome in *Drosophila*. A similar linkage has been proposed in humans, arising from a common progenitor by gene duplication.[2]

Diagnosis

The defect may generally by identified by the low to undetectable concentrations of uric acid in plasma. On a purine-free diet uric acid is virtually undetectable in plasma or urine, being replaced by xanthine and to a lesser extent hypoxanthine, with an approximate ratio in urine of 4–5:1. Total oxypurine excretion on a low purine diet is generally reduced (1–2 mmol/24 h compared to the normal of 2–3 mmol/24 h). Renal clearances of both purines (unlike uric acid) are high, hypoxanthine clearance approximating to the GFR, but tubular secretion of xanthine also occurs.[2] Raised urinary levels of xanthine and hypoxanthine have been reported in some heterozygotes. The enzyme defect cannot be detected in red cells, as XOD is confined to the liver and intestinal mucosa. Biopsy is thus essential if proof of homozygosity for the deficiency is required.

Xanthine stones are generally brownish orange, smooth and oval. They are easily cut and show a laminated appearance. Except for those with a calcium oxalate core, the stones are radiolucent. They give a positive murexide test, but can be distinguished from uric acid or 2,8-dihydroxyadenine stones by the UV spectrum at pH 2.0 and 10.0, by infra-red or mass spectrometry and by X-ray crystallography.

Prenatal diagnosis for combined XOD/SO deficiency is available in the first trimester.[11]

Treatment and prognosis

Because of the poor solubility of xanthine at any pH, alkalinisation of the urine is ineffective and a high fluid intake on a low purine diet is the only therapy. The importance of this is indicated by the nephropathy and the frequent necessity for nephrectomy in xanthinurics from arid climates, particularly those from countries bordering the Mediterranean[2]. The nephrotoxicity of xanthine is supported by experimental studies in the pig which demonstrated that even short periods of crystal deposition could precipitate acute renal failure, resulting in severe and permanent renal damage.

Different treatment regimes have also been tried in the combined defect without success and the prognosis is generally poor.[12]

Adenine phosphoribosyltransferase deficiency (McKusick 102600)

Biochemical disorder

Adenine phosphoribosyltransferase (APRT, EC 2.4.2.7) catalyses the conversion of adenine to AMP, a reaction requiring magnesium and PP-ribose-P (Fig. 8.4). APRT is ubiquitously distributed in all human cells, with the highest concentration in nucleated cells. The prime metabolic function of APRT is the removal of adenine arising as a metabolic waste product from the polyamine pathway.

Two types of defect are now recognised, a complete deficiency, Type 1,

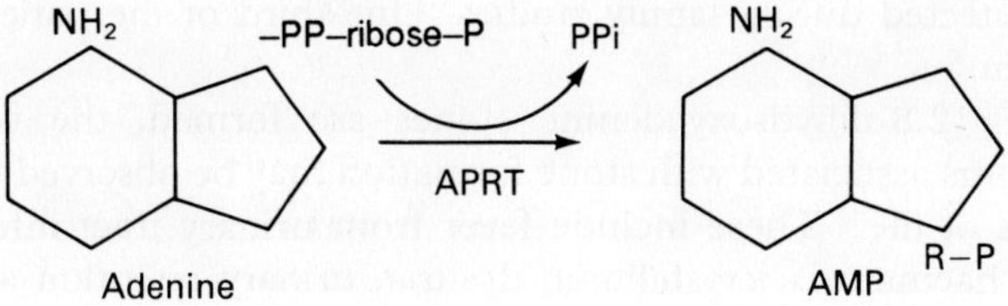

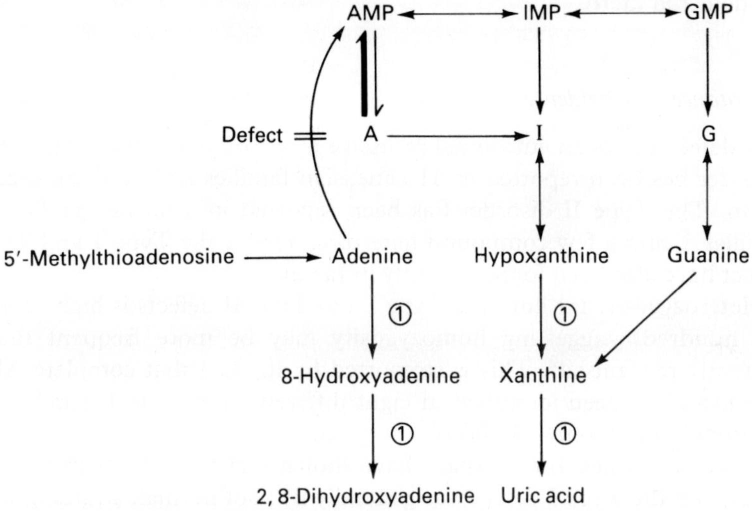

Fig. 8.4 The normal function of adenine phosphoribosyltransferase (APRT) is the removal of adenine derived as metabolic waste from the polyamine pathway and the alternative route of adenine metabolism to the extremely insoluble 2,8-dihydroxyadenine, which is operative when APRT is inactive. The alternative pathway is catalysed by xanthine oxidase (1).

found predominantly in caucasians[2], and Type II, found exclusively to date in Japanese, where the enzyme has a reduced affinity for PP-ribose-P, leading to a tenfold increase in the K_m for PP-ribose-P.[13]

In both types of APRT deficiency, adenine, as it cannot be salvaged normally, is catabolised by xanthine oxidase via 8-hydroxyadenine to the extremely insoluble 2,8-dihydroxyadenine.

Clinical presentation

Several cases have presented in infancy with acute renal failure.[8] However, the clinical spectrum is broad, and while the defect may be life-threatening and can present from birth, it may also be benign, presenting as late as the seventh decade. Some few cases remain completely asymptomatic and are only detected during family studies. One-third of the patients have been children.

When 2,8-dihydroxyadenine stones are formed, the whole scale of symptoms associated with stone formation may be observed within the first 2 years of life.[2] These include fever from urinary tract infection, macroscopic haematuria, crystalluria, dysuria, urinary retention and abdominal colic. Purine production and excretion is otherwise normal, as are the general biochemistry, other purine enzymes and immunology. The occurrence of spontaneous abortions in one family may represent expression of the defect in utero.

Inheritance and incidence

The defect shows an autosomal recessive mode of inheritance. The Type I disorder has been reported in 51 caucasian families and in 30 kindreds in Japan. The Type II disorder has been reported in a further 51 Japanese families[13], and a few compound heterozygotes for the Type 1 and Type 2 defect have also been found recently in Japan.

Heterozygosity for both the Type I and Type II defects is high (0.4–1.1 per hundred) suggesting homozygosity may be more frequent than is currently recognised[2]. This is supported by the fact that complete APRT deficiency has been identified in eight different families in Iceland, where the population is only 256 000.[14]

Detailed studies in caucasians have shown that the activity in heterozygotes with the Type I defect was generally 25% of normal, a finding which has been attributed to the fact that the enzyme is a dimer and that protein–protein interaction of two normal subunits is required for expression of normal activity.

Molecular defect

APRT is coded for by alleles at a gene locus on chromosome 16 (16q.24). The normal APRT gene is 2.8 kb in length and contains five exons. Analysis of mutant alleles in Japanese has shown that only three mutations account for the defective alleles in most patients[13]: 68% have an ATG to ACG mis-sense mutation at codon 136, 21% have a TGG to TGA mis-sense mutation at codon 98 and 7% have a duplication of a 4bp sequence in exon 3. The most common mutation involves a substitution of methionine for threonine at position 136, which is part of the putative PP-ribose-P binding site of human APRT. A splice donor mutation altering the exon four-intron four splice donor site from TG:GTAA to TG:GTTAA is a common mutation among caucasians.[14] This results in an A to T transversion at the third base downstream from the cleavage site resulting in aberrant splicing and deletion of exon 4 from mRNA. However, a variety of mutations, frequently involving different nucleotide sequences on each allele, mainly single base changes and small deletions, are found in other caucasians.

Diagnosis

The defect should be suspected where there is a history of recurrent urinary tract infection and 'uric acid' crystalluria or lithiasis, but normal uric acid levels. Renal ultrasound drew attention to the underlying nephropathy in a child presenting in coma.[8] The 2,8-dihydroxyadenine stones have previously been erroneously diagnosed as uric acid because of an identical reactivity in colorimetric reactions, the murexide test and thermogravimetric analysis.[2] The stones are radiolucent, like uric acid and xanthine stones, but are soft, creamy-grey and crush with ease: they may be distinguished by the UV spectrum at pH 2.0 and pH 10.0, infra-red and mass spectrometry and the lack of action of uricase which degrades uric acid to allantoin. The defect is established by the high levels of adenine, 8-hydroxyadenine and 2,8-dihydroxyadenine found in the urine by HPLC, in the approximate ratio of 1:0.03:1.5.[15] The combined excretion usually equals 20–30% of the total purines.

The diagnosis may be confirmed in the Type I defect by the absence of APRT activity in intact or lysed red cells[2], but APRT activity may be falsely raised if transfusion has been essential on admission, and it may take 6 months before homozygosity can be confirmed. Significant APRT activity is found in the majority of Type II Japanese cases of 2,8-dihydroxyadenine lithiasis and these represent kinetic mutants with a reduced affinity for PP-ribose-P.[13] Intact cell studies are thus essential to distinguish Type II homozygotes from carriers for the Type I and Type II defect. Elevated APRT activity due to the high percentage of young red cells has been noted in newborns, in renal failure, megaloblastic anaemia with reticulocytosis and in fetal blood.

Prenatal diagnosis is not required because, with early recognition, this is a treatable disorder.

Treatment and prognosis

Dietary purine restriction, together with high fluid is advised in asymptomatic homozygotes. In stone-formers, allopurinol (5–10 mg/kg, depending on age and renal function), but without alkali, will prevent further stone formation. Unlike uric acid, 2-8-dihydroxyadenine solubility is not improved by alkali and in several cases stone formation increased, suggesting the use of alkali is contraindicated. Allopurinol inhibits conversion of adenine to 2,8-dihydroxyadenine, but adenine does not normally accumulate because it is secreted and cleared rapidly by the human kidney.

Extracorporeal shock wave lithotripsy has been performed for renal or ureteric calculi.

At least six cases have required chronic haemodialysis and five of them have progressed to successful renal transplantation. Early diagnosis is thus important because this is a treatable disorder and such serious complications should be avoidable.

Hypoxanthine-guanine phosphoribosyltransferase deficiency
(McKusick 308000)

Biochemical disorder

Hypoxanthine-guanine phosphoribosyltransferase (HPRT, EC 2.4.2.8) catalyses the transfer of the phosphoribosyl moiety of PP-ribose-P to the 9 position of the purine ring of the bases hypoxanthine and guanine to form inosine monophospate (IMP) and guanosine monophosphate (GMP) respectively (Fig. 8.5). HPRT is a cytoplasmic enzyme present in virtually all tissues, with highest activity in brain and testes.[16] The enzyme does not

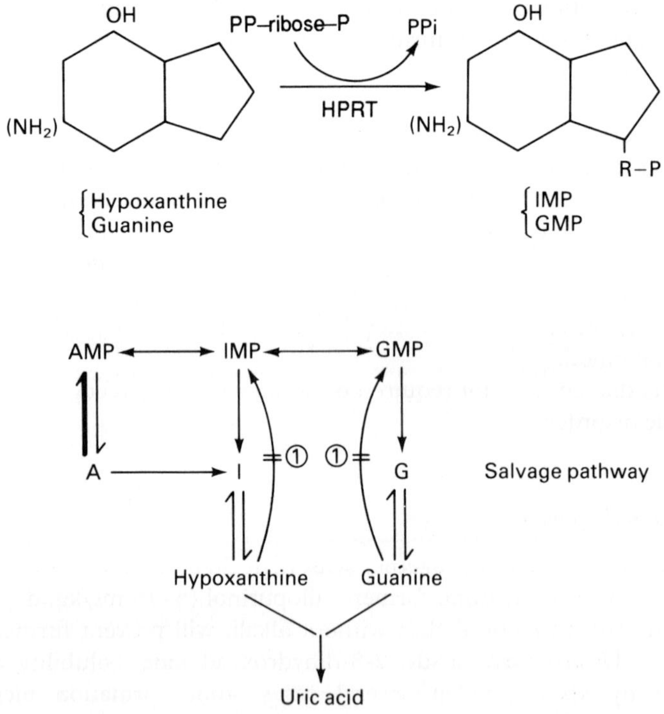

Fig. 8.5 The salvage pathway of the purine bases, hypoxanthine and guanine, to IMP and GMP, respectively, catalysed by HPRT (1) in the presence of PP-ribose-P. The defect in HPRT is shown.

react with xanthine in vivo in man. HPRT is one of the three enzymes involved in the so-called 'inosinate cycle', the nucleotides so formed exerting strong feedback control on de novo synthesis.[2]

The importance of HPRT in the normal interplay between synthesis and salvage is demonstrated by the biochemical and clinical consequences associated with HPRT deficiency. Gross uric acid overproduction results from the inability to recycle either hypoxanthine or guanine, which interrupts the inosinate cycle producing a lack of feedback control of synthesis, accompanied by rapid catabolism of these bases to uric acid (Fig. 8.1). PP-ribose-P not utilised in the salvage reaction of the inosinate cycle is considered to provide an additional stimulus to de novo synthesis and uric acid overproduction.

Clinical presentation

The defect may present in the first weeks of life with crystalluria, acute renal failure and gout.[8] As in other metabolic disorders there is considerable genetic heterogeneity and HPRT deficiency can present as any one of five different clinical phenotypes, the broad spectrum of presentation reflecting the severity of the genetic defect. Gross uric acid overproduction occurs in all instances.

The most extreme deficiency is found in the severely incapacitating Lesch–Nyhan syndrome, characterised by bizarre symptoms which include spasticity with pyramidal tract signs, compulsive self-mutilation, choreoathetosis and developmental retardation.[16] The pyramidal tract lesion may be the consequence of cervical cord compression, the basic motor abnormality being generalised muscular hypotonia. Lack of pubertal development and pre- as well as postnatal growth failure are striking features. Patients do not walk or sit without assistance. Evaluation of the apparent mental handicap may be complicated by lack of suitable intelligence tests. Some patients have shown megaloblastic anaemia, but immunodeficiency is not a problem: although lung and urinary tract infections are frequent, they can be secondary to aspiration or nephropathy.

The four other variant forms of clinical presentation may be characterised according to the severity of the neurological involvement: a Lesch–Nyhan type syndrome but without self-mutilation; ability to walk but with a spastic gait and choreoathetosis; mild neurololgical abnormalities of late onset, and patients with no neurological problems, the so-called partial defect, who usually present in their teens or early adulthood with hyperuricaemia, gout, renal failure, or kidney stones.[2,5,16]

Inheritance and incidence

HPRT deficiency is an X-linked recessive disorder. Although rare, the incidence is higher than for the other purine disorders. One-third of cases may be new mutations. The defect has recently been reported in a girl with classic Lesch–Nyhan symptoms (see below). A variety of studies have demonstrated altered kinetic, catalytic, electrophoretic and immunochemical properties, as well as in vitro or in vivo instability, with different mutants.

Molecular defect

The HPRT gene is located on the long arm of the X-chromosome (Xq26–q27.2). The nucleotide sequence of the nine exons within a 44 kb stretch of normal genomic DNA has been determined. Cloning of mutant cDNA from different patients has revealed significant heterogeneity involving over 50 different point mutations, substitutions, deletions and duplications occuring over the whole coding region of the protein.[17] These, in turn, could have important structural consequences, such as disrupting protein folding thereby affecting the nucleotide or PP-ribose-P binding domain, or rendering the enzyme more susceptible to proteolysis. A survey of the mutation in patients with differing degrees of neurological involvement has, disappointingly, not revealed any correlation with the molecular defect. The molecular mechanisms in the female Lesch–Nyhan patient relate to a total maternal gene deletion, coupled with inactivation of the paternal gene by methylation of a site on the first intron. The parents are both healthy.

Diagnosis

All patients with either partial or complete HPRT deficiency exhibit gross uric acid overproduction and excretion, but plasma uric acid may not appear raised until puberty because of the higher renal clearance in children. In the absence of renal failure[8], uric acid excretion on a creatinine basis in children is increased two- to fourfold (normal level, less than 1.0 mmol/mmol creatinine). In normal adults after puberty the plasma uric acid rises, more in males than in females, and the urine uric acid is correspondingly lower (normally less than 0.3 mmol/mmol creatinine). By contrast in HPRT-deficient adults with normal renal function, uric acid excretion is markedly raised on a creatinine basis. Urinary hypoxanthine excretion on a creatinine basis is also elevated in HPRT-deficient patients.

However, excessive uric acid excretion on a creatinine basis will be masked[8] in both children and adults presenting in acute renal failure. The diagnostic criterion in this situation is a grossly raised plasma uric acid (in excess of 1 mmol/l) in any patient presenting in acute renal failure. Renal ultrasound provided the clue to the correct diagnosis in two neonates. Uric acid stones may be the sole manifestation in some cases. They are radiolucent and generally yellowish, smooth, hard and crush with difficulty.

HPRT deficiency may be confirmed by the low to undetectable levels of HPRT in lysed red cells, generally associated with raised APRT activity.[5] Lesch–Nyhan patients have virtually no detectable enzyme in any cell type, intact or lysed. Patients with the partial deficiency, frequently have no detectable activity in lysed red cells, but have significant activity (5–25% of normal) in intact red cells or fibroblasts, indicating a mutation leading to an unstable enzyme in disrupted cells.[17]

Heterozygotes cannot be detected reliably from enzyme activity in lysed red cells, probably due to random Lyonisation of one X-chromosome (Ch.1, p. 16). (The female Lesch–Nyhan patient was thus unique in having no detectable HPRT activity in erythrocytes, T-lymphocytes and fibroblasts). The fact that up to 30% of cases can be new mutations has presented problems for carrier detection and some carriers cannot be recognised with certainty by the well established comparative HPRT/APRT ratio in hair roots, and at present only 85% can be identified using DNA probes.[18]

DNA technology and enzyme analysis have been applied to prenatal diagnosis of HPRT deficiency in the first trimester using chorionic biopsy material.[18-20] The possible pitfalls of using enzyme analysis have also been underlined.[20] Cultured amniotic fluid cells and fetal blood may be used for prenatal diagnosis in the second trimester.[19]

Associated findings

The basic defect underlying the neurological complications remains undefined.

Much lower concentrations of brain free amino acids may restrict precursors vital for neurotransmitter or protein synthesis, as well as contributing to the decrease in catecholamine levels noted in basal ganglia.[2] The severe GTP depletion,[21] accompanied by grossly raised NAD^+ levels, noted in red cells from Lesch–Nyhan patients, compared with normal GTP concentrations in the partial deficiency and varying degrees of depletion in the intermediate types, may reflect a similar deficit in neuronal tissues. Such tissues, like the erythrocyte, appear to be uniquely dependent on salvage for sustaining GTP at levels compatible with normal protein and DNA synthesis. Additionally, restriction of the supply of GTP which normally interacts via the regulatory G protein with the dopamine D_1 receptor may be related to dopaminergic receptor sensitivity and self-mutilation.[2]

Treatment and prognosis

The elevated uric acid levels in either the complete or partial deficiencies may be controlled by a high fluid intake, alkali and allopurinol. The latter should be used with care since urinary oxypurine excretion in

Lesch–Nyhan patients appears to be exquisitely sensitive to allopurinol and both xanthine and oxypurinol calculi have been reported.[8] As in patients with renal failure, the allopurinol dose must be carefully monitored and reduced, if necessary to no more than 5 mg/kg in children, or 100 mg/24 h in adults, to prevent xanthine nephropathy, or in renal disease the accumulation of oxypurinol, the active drug metabolite, with its attendant risk of other side-effects.

The prognosis is good in the partial defect, but patients with the Lesch–Nyhan syndrome rarely survive beyond adolescence, death being due to aspiration and pneumonia or renal failure. No successful treatment has been devised for the severe neurological complications. Exchange transfusion, or bone marrow transplantation as a source of enzyme replacement[22] and pharmacological approaches to therapy with tryptophan, 5-hydroxytryptophan or glutamate, etc., have failed to reverse the biochemical or neurological complications in the syndrome.[2,5] The defect is a prime candidate for gene transfer experiments. Success will undoubtedly lie in ensuring recombinant gene expression within the central nervous system (CNS). To date animal models have not proved successful.

Phosphoribosyl pyrophosphate synthetase superactivity (McKusick 311850)

Biochemical defect

Phosphoribosyl pyrophosphate synthetase (PRPS, EC 2.7.6.1) catalyses the transfer of the pyrophosphate group of ATP to ribose-5-phosphate to form PP-ribose-P (Fig. 8.6). The enzyme exists as a complex aggregate of up to 32 subunits, only the 16 and 32 subunits having significant activity. It requires $Mg,^{2+}$ is activated by inorganic phosphate, and is subject to complex regulation by different nucleotide end-products of the pathways for which PP-ribose-P is a substrate, particularly ADP and GDP.[23]

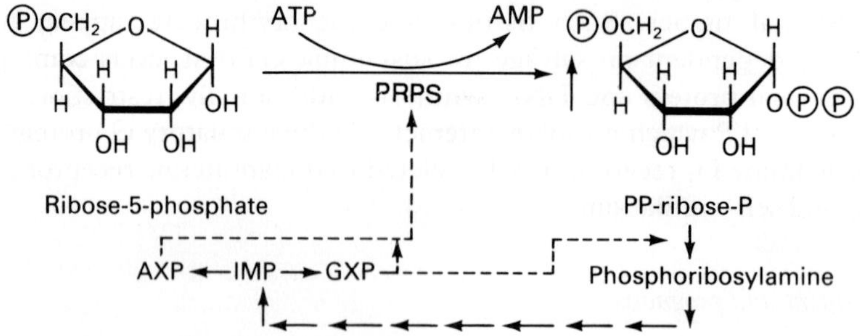

Fig. 8.6 The role of PP-ribose-P in the de novo synthesis of IMP and adenosine (AXP) and guanosine (GXP) nucleotides, and the feedback control normally exerted by these nucleotides on de novo purine synthesis.

PP-ribose-P acts as an allosteric regulator of the first specific reaction of de novo purine biosynthesis (Fig. 8.1), in which the interaction of glutamine and PP-ribose-P is catalysed by amidophosphoribosyl transferase, producing a slow activation of the amidotransferase by changing it from a large, inactive dimer to an active monomer.[2] Purine nucleotides cause a rapid reversal of this process, producing the inactive form.

Variant forms of PRPS have been described, insensitive to normal regulatory functions, or with a raised specific activity. This results in continuous PP-ribose-P synthesis which stimulates de novo purine production, resulting in accelerated uric acid formation and overexcretion.[23]

Clinical presentation

The majority of cases with this X-linked disorder have presented with severe gout or kidney stones in adolescence or early adulthood.[5] An association between the kinetic defect and the severity of the phenotypic expression, as in HPRT deficiency, is suggested by the finding of patients presenting neonatally with severe neurodevelopmental retardation, hypotonia, a left convergent squint and inherited nerve deafness.[2] There is a family history of repeated attacks of bronchopneumonia and death in early infancy, in addition to gross purine overproduction. Families with metabolic and neurologic abnormalities between these two extremes have been identified.[23] Female heterozygotes also show purine overproduction and generally develop gout, and, in the severe form, have sensorineural deafness.

Inheritance and incidence

This is an extremely rare X-linked disorder described in some 20 families to date.[23] Several variant forms of the enzyme have been identified, which show either a reduced sensitivity to the nucleotide inhibitors ADP or GDP, increased specific activity per enzyme molecule, increased affinity for ribose-5-phosphate, or a combination of these.

Molecular defect

X-linked inheritance was originally suggested and the gene for this enzyme assigned to the long arm of the X-chromosome (Xq22–q26) just above that for HPRT. Recent studies have identified two distinct X-linked loci for PRPS, PRPS 1 and PRPS 2, using cDNA cloning. PRPS 1 maps to the Xq21–qter region, PRPS 2 to the short arm of X (Xp22.3–p22.3). The latter escapes X-chromosome inactivation. The presence of two PRPS1-related genes assigned to chromosomes 7 and 9 have also been reported.[2] Studies of cDNA of two patients with neurological defects and feedback-resistant superactivity have revealed that while PRPS 2 was identical with normal, a single point mutation, distinct in each case, was present in PRPS 1 cDNA, which altered the amino acid sequence.[24]

Diagnosis

The defect should be suspected in any child or young adult of either sex with marked hyperuricaemia and/or hyperuricosuria 2–4 times normal, but with normal HPRT and APRT activity in lysed red cells. Reported values for PRPS activity have varied widely with the method used. Patients with variant enzymes have activity 2–4 times normal.[23] Erythrocyte PP-ribose-P levels are also generally elevated, but in the more severe form this may only be evident in the youngest red cells, due to enzyme instability. Raised PP-ribose-P levels have also been found in lymphoblasts and fibroblasts. In the severe form another characteristic feature has been the inability of intact red cells to increase the incorporation of either hypoxanthine or adenine into the corresponding nucleotide at high phosphate concentrations (PP-ribose-P stimulating conditions), as do normal red cells.[2]

Low red cell NAD^+ and GTP levels have been reported in two patients with the severe defect.[21] The former relate to a decreased formation at the initial step involving the nicotinamide and nicotinic acid phosphoribosyltransferases. The finding of low erythrocyte GTP in the patients with severe neurological deficits, as in HPRT deficiency, suggests a similar inability to sustain GTP at levels compatible with normal physiological function in the CNS.

Prenatal diagnosis has not been performed, but may be possible in severe cases by karyotyping if the abnormal nucleotide pattern is present in fetal blood.

Treatment and prognosis

Prognosis for patients presenting in adolescence is good. Allopurinol, again used with care to avoid xanthine nephropathy[8], will control plasma and uric acid levels in patients with normal renal function and gout or kidney stones. A high fluid intake and alkalinisation of the urine may help. In any case with associated gouty nephropathy, the dose must be reduced even further in parallel with the degree of reduction in renal function. To date, no successful therapy for the associated neurological complications in the severe cases has been devised, and death in infancy is frequent.

Purine nucleoside phosphorylase deficiency (MuKusick 164050)

Biochemical defect

Purine nucleoside phosphorylase (PNP, EC 2.4.2.1) catalyses the degradation of the nucleosides inosine, guanosine or their deoxyanalogues to the corresponding base. Although this is essentially a reversible reaction, base formation is favoured because intracellular phosphate levels normally exceed those of either ribose-, or deoxyribose-1-phosphate. The enzyme is a vital link in the 'inosinate cycle' of the purine salvage pathway (Fig. 8.7) and has a wide tissue distribution.

Homozygotes for PNP deficiency are unable to catabolise these nucleosides, or deoxynucleosides, which consequently accumulate in body fluids. Enzyme-deficient patients have in effect a double defect, since the next step in the inosinate cycle involving HPRT is unable to operate through the absence of substrate.[25] Gross purine overproduction results, due to lack of nucleotide formation and feedback inhibition of de novo synthesis, as in the Lesch–Nyhan syndrome (Fig. 8.1). Red cells and fibroblasts from PNP-deficient patients incorporate hypoxanthine and guanine into the nucleotide more rapidly than normal cells, indicating HPRT is active though normally inoperative: but, in contrast to normal cells, IMP and GMP are rapidly degraded to the nucleoside, leading to the suggestion that the enzyme defect unmasked a normal cyclic process.[2]

The associated toxicity to the immune system has been related to the conversion of deoxyguanosine to dGTP, by either deoxycytidine kinase or a specific kinase in T but not B cells[26] with subsequent inhibition of ribonucleotide reductase and DNA synthesis. The presence of some T-helper cell function is considered to explain the relatively normal B cell

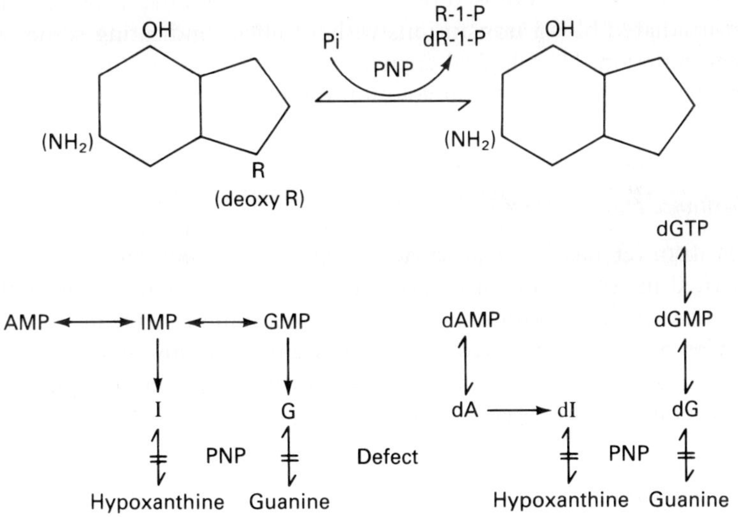

Fig. 8.7 The necessity of purine nucleoside phosphorylase (PNP) for the normal catabolism and salvage of both nucleosides and deoxynucleosides, resulting in the accumulation of dGTP, exclusively, in the absence of the enzyme, since kinases do not exist for the other nucleosides in man. The lack of functional HPRT activity, through absence of substrate, in PNP deficiency is also apparent.

function. Kinases for the other three nucleosides accumulating in PNP deficiency do not exist in human cells.

Clinical presentation

The age of presentation has varied, but it has generally occurred in the first 4 years of life, associated with neurological or immunological problems, or both.[27] Neurological symptoms, as in HPRT deficiency, show a broad spectrum, the most severe presentations occuring in patients with complete deficiency and including head-lag and excessive irritability, noted as early as 3 months. Severely deficient patients have remained extremely hypotonic and developmentally retarded; some have manifest spastic tetraparesis.

The most severely affected also present neonatally with lymphopenia and defective cell-mediated (T cell) immunity: phytohaemagglutinin responses may be normal at birth but diminish rapidly. Although actual B cell numbers may be low, as a percentage of total lymphocytes they are normal. Immunoglobulin levels are normal or increased. Some cases have developed autoimmune disease and have been identified by the hypouricaemia noted during screening for Coombes positive haemolytic anaemia; anaemia has been reported in 30% of cases. Long-term survivors have some PNP activity and lack neurological involvement.

Infections are less frequent than in ADA deficiency but otitis media is common. Patients become increasingly susceptible to varicella, vaccinia or cytomegalovirus and the majority have died from such viral infections. Many have been immunised prior to diagnosis with live vaccines, or given non-irradiated blood transfusions without effect, indicating some residual T cell function. Histological changes in the thymus at autopsy have been considered consistent with involution rather than a congenital absence of the thymus.

Inheritance and incidence

This disorder has been described in at least 30 patients. The defect is inherited in an autosomal recessive manner and in many families there is evidence of consanguinity. Studies of the mutant enzyme in different families have demonstrated varying amounts of immunologically reactive protein with altered kinetic parameters, isoelectric points and electrophoretic mobility.

Molecular defect

The enzyme is coded for by a gene located on the long arm of chromosome 14 (14q13.1). The human PNP gene, as characterised by Southern blot analysis, includes six exons dispersed across 10 kb of DNA. Molecular analysis of the different mutations in PNP deficiency has produced two major findings: an unexpected repetition of point mutations leading to amino acid substitutions in unrelated patients, and a novel splicing defect.[27]

Diagnosis

The finding of undetectable, or extremely low, blood and urine uric acid levels in a child with neurological defects, or recurrent viral infection, is suggestive of PNP deficiency.[25] The biochemical abnormality may be established by the presence of grossly raised amounts of inosine, guanosine, deoxyinosine and deoxyguanosine in plasma (50, 10, 5 and 5 μmol/l respectively) compared with normally undetectable levels. In urine the same compounds are excreted in excess in the same relative proportions, total purine excretion (in the form of nucleosides) being increased two- to fourfold on a creatinine basis. In severe cases no uric acid is detectable in any body fluid, but significant levels have been found in late presenters. Hypoxanthine or guanine may be found in urine in late presenters, or due to nucleoside degradation by bacterial contamination or collection into acid.[15]

The defect may be confirmed by the finding of low-to-undetectable PNP activity in lysed erythrocytes. Heterozygotes have intermediate levels but are clinically normal. Red cell APRT activity is twice normal, possibly, as in HPRT deficiency, due to stabilisation by the raised PP-ribose-P levels also present. Increased PP-ribose-P levels have likewise been noted in fibroblasts and lymphoblasts.

Raised levels of dGTP (normally undetectable) have been found in red cells, accompanied in developmentally retarded patients by severe GTP depletion and three times normal NAD^+ levels, and, as in HPRT deficiency, these specific findings are diagnostic of the defect.[21] One interpretation of the consistent finding of low erythrocyte GTP levels in three different defects, all associated with neurological deficits, is that a guanylate cycle exists, similar to the inosinate cycle, essential for the control of purine synthesis, which is of particular importance to the human CNS.

Prenatal diagnosis is available in both the first and second trimester.[19]

Treatment and prognosis

One case of successful haploidental bone marrow transplantation has been reported.[2] Therapeutic interventions (transfusion with irradiated erythrocytes) were not effective in the long-term. Approaches using alternative substrates, such as deoxycytidine provided no further benefit, and specific metabolites such as hypoxanthine or guanine (alone or with allopurinol) proved equally ineffective, confirming that salvage of dietary purines is of little significance in man. No satisfactory therapy has yet been found for the majority of these patients and the most severely affected have invariably died within the first 5 years.

Adenosine deaminase deficiency (McKusick 102700)

Biochemical disorder

Adenosine deaminase (ADA, EC 3.5.4.4) catalyses the deamination of adenosine and 2'-deoxyadenosine to inosine or 2'-deoxyinosine respectively (Fig. 8.8). Most of the adenosine derived endogenously is normally phosphorylated rather than deaminated because the K_m for adenosine kinase (1 μM) is an order of magnitude lower than that for ADA (25 μM).[2] Moreover, a series of rigorous controls ensures that AMP is normally deaminated at the nucleotide level in most tissues by AMP deaminase and there should generally be little flux through the ADA degradative pathway (Fig. 8.1). However, unlike AMP, 2'-deoxy AMP (dAMP) is not a substrate for AMPDA and must first be degraded to 2'-deoxyadenosine and then further catabolised by ADA. The occurrence of the highest ADA activity in lymphoid tissues has highlighted the importance of ADA for the catabolism of toxic deoxynucleotides.[28] In contrast to microorganisms, human cells lack the ability to convert adenosine to adenine via purine nucleoside phosphorylase, or to deaminate adenine at the base level.[2] Recent histological studies have invoked an extracellular function for ADA, the enzyme being associated with, and located on, the extracellular surface of the plasma membrane.[29]

In patients homozygous for ADA deficiency, 2'-deoxyadenosine accumulating during the rapid turnover of cells rich in DNA is converted

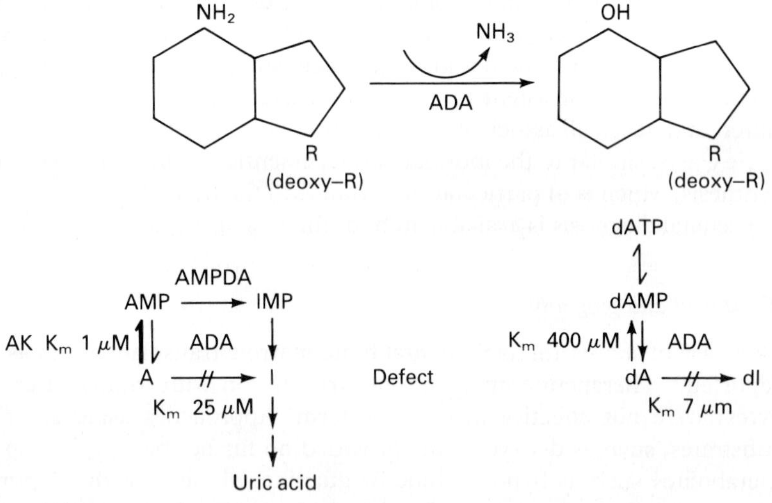

Fig. 8.8 The importance of adenosine deaminase (ADA) for the catabolism of dA, but not A, and the resultant accumulation of dATP when ADA is defective. A is normally salvaged by adenosine kinase (see K_m values of A for ADA and the kinase, AK) and deficiency of ADA is not significant in this situation.

back to dATP, either by adenosine kinase or deoxycytidine kinase.[2] Many hypotheses have been advanced to explain the specific toxicity to the immune system in ADA deficiency.[28,30,31] The apparently selective accumulation of dATP in thymocytes and peripheral blood B cells, with resultant inhibition of ribonucleotide reductase and DNA synthesis is probably the principal mechanism. Action of 2'-deoxyadenosine directly through irreversible binding to, and inhibition of, S-adenosylhomocysteine hydrolase, and hence inactivation of methylation reactions vital to normal cell function, may also be important.

Clinical presentation

ADA deficiency has been identified as the metabolic basis for 20–30% of cases with recessively inherited severe combined immunodeficiency (SCID). Affected infants are subject to recurrent chronic viral, fungal, protozoal, and bacterial infections and frequently present with persistent diarrhoea, failure to thrive and candidiasis.[28] Severely affected cases present neonatally with no detectable lymphocytes in peripheral blood or bone marrow and both cell-mediated and humoral immunity is defective. T cells are generally absent, agammaglobulinaemia is the rule and lymphocyte proliferative and specific antibody responses are lacking. The age of onset has varied from birth to 5 years of age, but is usually within the first 2 years of life. In later presenters the defect may not be easily recognised; lymphocyte numbers are not reduced, cellular immunodeficiency may not be so profound and immunoglobulin levels are normal. Histopathological studies have shown the presence of Hassals corpuscles and other criteria suggesting involution of a previously differentiated thymus. Some patients have had associated bony and hair growth abnormalities and occasionally non-specific neurological disorders, attributed to malnutrition or viral infection.

Partial ADA deficiency, due to mutations leading to absence of detectable ADA in erythrocytes but residual activity in other cell types, is usually associated with normal immune function. However, at least two such patients have presented with late onset immunodeficiency.

Inheritance and incidence

ADA deficiency is an autosomal recessive disorder. More than 100 cases have been identified. The defect has been described in caucasians, negroes and Asians. The enzyme is genetically polymorphic in the normal population and three phenotypes have been recognised on electrophoresis: ADA 1, ADA 2 and ADA 2/1, ADA 2 being much less common. ADA exists in two forms having different molecular masses: the small form is present in red cells and the large form in other cells and tissues where ADA is complexed to a high molecular weight binding protein, one molecule of which binds two molecules of ADA. The small form is considered to be the catalytically active form. Severely affected children have no detectable ADA isoenzymes in any tissues, but binding protein is normal. Late presenters have had low but detectable activity in mononuclear cells.

Molecular defect

The structural gene for ADA is encoded as a single 32 kb locus containing 12 exons[30,31] on the long arm of chromosome 20 (20q13.2–qter). Studies of the molecular defect in ADA-deficient patients have shown that mRNA is usually detectable in normal or supranormal amounts. Specific point mutations have been detected in the majority of cases with the complete deficiency. A C-to-T point mutation in exon 11 accounts for a high proportion of these, whilst a few patients are homozygous for large deletions encompassing exon 1.[30] A common point mutation resulting in a heat-labile ADA has been characterised in some patients with partial ADA deficiency, a disorder with an apparently increased prevalence in the Caribbean.[31]

Diagnosis

Raised erythrocyte dATP levels are a diagnostic feature, accompanied by varying degrees of ATP depletion depending on the severity of the genetic disorder. The finding of 2'-deoxyadenosine in urine (0.01–0.26 mmol/mmol creatinine) is an equally characteristic feature[28] and it is also present in plasma in severely affected infants (3–14 µmol/l). Adenosine has been found in plasma (2–10 µmol/l) and urine (0–0.06 mmol/mmol creatinine) in some, but not all, cases. Purine production as well as uric acid and other purine and pyrimidine levels are normal in the defect.

Because of the considerable variation in expression, ADA deficiency may not always be suspected as a cause of SCID, but should be considered in any child or adult presenting with generalised candidiasis, particularly where there is evidence of autosomal recessive inheritance. The defect may be confirmed by the finding of undetectable ADA levels in lysed red cells. As ADA is unstable at –20°C, blood must be transported at room temperature and stored at –70°C. S-adenosylhomocysteine hydrolase activity is also grossly reduced in lysed red cells. At least 11 cases exist with undetectable ADA activity in lysed red cells which are not immunodeficient[31] and have detectable ADA activity in lymphocytes, lymphoblasts and fibroblasts, and intact erythrocytes. Heterozygosity for the defect can be difficult to detect, since many obligate heterozygotes have ADA levels at the lower limit of the normal range.[28]

Prenatal diagnosis is possible using chorionic villus sampling,[19] enzyme and nucleotide levels in fetal blood[28] and in cultured amniotic fluid cells, but in some affected cases the amniotic fluid cells may fail to grow. Analysis of fetal blood in the second trimester has demonstrated severe lymphopenia, with complete absence of T cells and T cell subsets, and raised dATP levels, indicating the early onset of lymphocytotoxicity.

Treatment

As yet no totally effective therapy for ADA deficiency has been reported, except in those few cases where bone marrow from an HLA/MLR compatible sibling donor was available.[31] Many different regimes have been tried, including enzyme replacement with irradiated red cells, thymic hormone, and pharmacological approaches employing deoxycytidine. All have had minimal success, except in late presenters with residual ADA activity in mononuclear cells.[32] Two therapeutic approaches have provided long-term benefit in specific instances. First, reconstitution using T cell depleted mismatched sibling marrow has been encouraging[28], particularly in early presenters completely deficient in ADA. Secondly, therapy with polyethylene glycol-modified adenosine deaminase (PEG-ADA) for more than 5 years has produced a sustained increase in lymphocyte numbers and mitogen responses together with evidence of in vivo B cell function. Success has generally been achieved in late presenters with residual ADA activity in mononuclear cells.[32]

ADA deficiency has been chosen as the candidate disease for gene replacement therapy and the first human experiment commenced in 1990. Although the therapy appears to be boosting resistance to infection,[33] the protocol requires the concomitant use of PEG-ADA, which makes the results difficult to evaluate. There is much research activity in this area and many other models for improving retroviral delivery are currently under investigation. The clinical consequences of overexpression of ADA activity – one of the potential hazards of gene implant – are known and take the form of an hereditary haemolytic anaemia associated with a tissue-specific increase in ADA activity. The genetic basis for the latter autosomal dominant disorder seemingly relates to markedly increased levels of structurally normal ADA mRNA.[2]

Myoadenylate deaminase deficiency (McKusick 254750)

Biochemical disorder

Adenylate deaminase (AMPDA EC: 3.5.4.6) catalyses the deamination of AMP to IMP. Four isoenzymes of AMPDA have been noted in human tissues. The enzyme consists of four identical subunits with a molecular mass of approximately 69–76 kDa each and is widely distributed in different tissues, with maximal activity in skeletal muscle. AMPDA is normally subject to a variety of tissue-specific controls, being inhibited in some tissues by GTP and inorganic phosphate (P_1) and stimulated by ATP. In most tissues (heart being the prime exception) the predominant route of AMP catabolism is deamination via AMPDA, rather than dephosphorylation, and only when the adenylate energy charge has fallen below 0.6 does the latter route become significant.[2]

The muscle enzyme is considered to form part of an important cycle, the adenine nucleotide cycle[34] involving two other enzymes which act in concert to reconvert IMP to AMP: adenylosuccinate (AMPS) synthetase which requires GTP and aspartate, and adenylosuccinate lyase (adenylosuccinase:ADS), which releases fumarate from AMPS (Fig. 8.9).

A deficiency of AMPDA is the most common enzyme defect found in skeletal muscle, with activity being less than 5% of normal, which has stimulated much debate about the significance of the above cycle for normal muscle function. Intense muscular exercise, at or near fatigue, depletes total adenine nucleotides by approximately 15%, associated with an increase in IMP and AMPDA activity. The latter could promote local ammonia production which would, in turn, buffer hydrogen ions and stimulate glycolysis. Alternatively the increased AMPDA activity may be simply a response to high ATP turnover coupled with a low phosphocreatine level. A third hypothesis involves the increase in fumarate during reconversion of IMP to AMP in the cycle. This could provide a mechanism whereby citric acid cycle intermediates could be replenished during muscle work.

Clinical presentation

The majority of patients have presented with muscle cramps or myalgias following exercise and 67% of them had their first symptoms in childhood or adolesence. Muscle weakness has been found in 27% of patients,

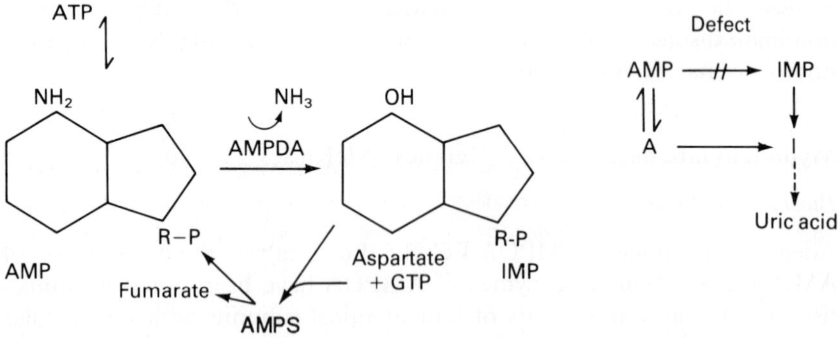

Fig. 8.9 The role of AMPDA in the deamination of AMP to IMP, and the reconversion of the latter to AMP via AMPS, thus completing the purine nucleotide cycle which is of particular importance in muscle.

but muscle wasting has not been reported. Hypotonia has developed in only 8%. Some studies have failed to find an association between the enzyme deficiency and exertional myalgia or cramps. Such discrepancies may relate to the fact that the defect may be primary (inherited) or secondary to an associated muscular disorder. In one family the defect was associated with progressive muscle weakness and fatal cardiomyopathy.

A complete deficiency of the erythrocyte AMPDA has been reported recently, but no clinical associates have been noted. The availability of appropriate genetic probes may uncover other tissue-specific defects.

Inheritance and incidence

Muscle AMPDA deficiency shows equal sex distribution and the mode of inheritance in the primary defect is considered to be autosomal recessive, although in a single family with a fatal cardiomyopathy it appeared to be dominant. This defect is specific to skeletal muscle and, as demonstrated below, may be one of the commonest genetic defects, with a heterozygosity as high as 1 in 5. In affected patients AMPDA activity is normal in other tissues and cells, including erythrocytes, leucocytes and fibroblasts, supporting the existence of a separate genetic locus for the isoenzymes demonstrated in different tissues.

The muscle defect has been described in more than 30 patients but, in addition, three separate studies of 770 muscle biopsies from patients with muscle weakness or poor exercise tolerance, revealed histological and biochemically confirmed AMPDA deficiency in 2% of cases.

Molecular defect

AMPDA is encoded for by a multigene family which controls the tissue-specific pattern of expression. Of the four isoforms of AMPDA found in human tissues E1 and E2 exist in erythrocytes, the L form in liver and the M form in muscle. A stage-specific progression during human skeletal muscle development has also been demonstrated, which led to the postulate that AMPDA-deficient patients might lack the adult isoform.

The AMPDA1 gene encoding the predominant isoform in adult human skeletal muscle has been cloned.[34] It is located on the short arm of chromosome 1. Point mutations have been identified in patients, one a non-sense mutation involving the last nucleotide in exon 2, the second an amino acid substitution in exon 3. Both mutations have been identified in one of two genomic libraries and random screening of caucasians identified 2 of 10 volunteers as heterozygotes for this mutant allele, suggesting a very high frequency in the normal population.[34] It was speculated that the late onset and relatively mild symptoms in homozygotes may relate to alternative splicing of exon 2 that removes the deleterious non-sense mutation during muscle development.

Diagnosis

A simple test is used in diagnosis which measures the lactate/ammonia exercise ratio during ischaemic exercise.[2] Exercise does not lead to NH_3 production, or an increase in plasma inosine and hypoxanthine as in normal individuals, whilst plasma adenosine shows no significant changes, although the adenosine content of end-exercise muscle is greater in patients. Muscle ATP and total purine content fall following exercise to a greater extent than in controls. Increased serum creatinine kinase has been found in some 60% of patients. AMPDA activity (determined histochemically or enzymatically) is low-to-undetectable in muscle samples from all patients, but is normal in other types of cell. Intermediate levels have recently been reported in muscle biopsies from carriers for the defect. Levels of purine metabolites such as uric acid, xanthine and hypoxanthine have not generally been reported, so it is not known whether total purine production and excretion is altered in this defect. However, gout and/or hyperuricaemia has been noted in three patients.

Treatment

The prognosis in most instances is good, with no evidence of progressive debilitation or structural damage. Oral ribose has been used successfully to alleviate symptoms in some but not all patients.[2]

Adenylosuccinase deficiency (McKusick 103050)

Biochemical disorder

Adenylosuccinate lyase (adenylosuccinase ADS: EC 4.3.2.2) catalyses the eighth step in the ten-step de novo synthetic pathway, and also the second step in the formation of ATP from IMP in the adenine nucleotide cycle (Fig. 8.10). The substrate for the first reaction is succinylaminoimidazole carboxamide ribotide (SAICAR); the product is aminoimidazole carboxamide ribotide (AICAR). In the second reaction the substrate is adenylosuccinic acid (AMPS) and the product is AMP, with fumarate also being released in both instances.

A defect of this enzyme results in the accumulation of the two substrates for these enzymes in the form of their nucleoside derivatives.[35]

Pathophysiological mechanisms relating to a deficiency of this enzyme are unknown. Impairment of the purine nucleotide cycle may play a role in the pathogenesis of the brain dysfunction and in the growth retardation. The defect has been demonstrated in liver and kidney, but not red cells,

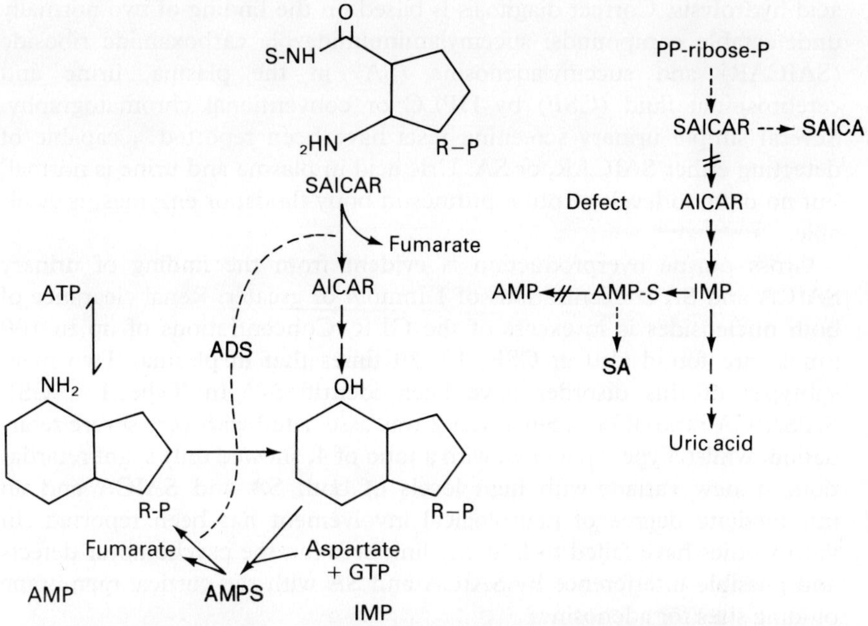

Fig. 8.10 The dual role of adenylosuccinate lyase (ADS) in catalysing the eighth step of the de novo pathway, the conversion of succinylaminoimidazole carboxamide ribotide (SAICAR) to aminoimidazole carboxamide ribotide (AICAR), as well as the second step in the conversion of IMP to AMP via adenylsuccinic acid (AMPS), with the release of fumarate. The formation of both succinylaminoimidazole carboxamide riboside (SAICA) and succinyl adenosine (SA) occurs when ADS is defective.

granulocytes or skeletal muscle, suggesting that, as with AMPDA deficiency, there may be several isoenzymes in human tissue.

Clinical presentation

Affected children are normal at birth, but psychomotor retardation, the principal symptom of this defect, becomes evident in the first 2 years. There is considerable genetic heterogeneity in clinical expression. Five patients have had epilepsy, whilst autistic features were evident in the first three reported patients. Some cases show severe mental retardation, self-mutilation, involuntary movements of the extremities, hypertonicity, muscle wasting, growth failure and cerebellar hypoplasia on CT scan.

Diagnosis

The diagnosis may be suspected from the presence of raised levels of aspartic acid and glycine detected in body fluids by TLC or GLC following acid hydrolysis. Correct diagnosis is based on the finding of two normally undetectable compounds: succinylaminoimidazole carboxamide riboside (SAICAR) and succinyladenosine (SA) in the plasma, urine and cerebrospinal fluid (CSF) by HPLC or conventional chromatography. Several simple urinary screening tests have been reported[36], capable of detecting either SAICAR, or SA. Uric acid in plasma and urine is normal, but no data on levels of other purines in body fluids, or enzymes, is available.

Gross purine overproduction is evident from the finding of urinary SAICA and SA concentrations of 1 mmol/l or greater. Renal clearance of both nucleosides is in excess of the GFR. Concentrations of up to 100 μmol/l are found also in CSF, 10–20 times that in plasma. Two main subtypes of this disorder have been identified.[35] In Type 1 a CSF SA/SAICA ratio of between 1 and 2 was associated with very severe retardation, whilst Type 2 patients, with a ratio of 4, showed only slight retardation. A new variant with high levels of both SA and SAICA and an intermediate degree of neurological involvement has been reported. In vitro studies have failed to find any link between the psychomotor defects and possible interference by SAICA and SA with the cortical membrane binding sites for adenosine.

The enzyme deficiency may be demonstrated in liver, kidney, muscle, fibroblasts and lymphocytes, but not red cells. Studies using intact fibroblasts have shown that only a profound deficiency will lead to the accumulation of succinyl purines, confirming the considerable heterogeneity in the defect. These findings underline the need for systematic screening for this disorder in mild psychomotor retardation, whether or not accompanied by epilepsy or behavioural disturbances.

Treatment

The pathophysiological mechanism is unknown and no specific treatment is available. Further epidemiological studies are needed to identify other patients and improve understanding of the metabolic basis for this condition.

Inheritance and incidence

ADS deficiency has been reported in 12 patients (seven female, five male), three of whom have died. The disorder has been identified in patients of different nationalities, principally in the Netherlands and Belgium and is possibly autosomal recessive. The occurrence of the defect in two siblings of different sex belonging to related parents, supports this.

Efficient screening in at-risk population groups is obviously needed to establish more data about this disorder, but not a single case was reported as a result of the Massachusetts Metabolic Disorder Screening Program, suggesting a higher incidence in specific ethnic groups.[37]

Molecular defect

The gene for ADS is located on chromosome 22. Enzyme investigations indicate the existence of isoenzymes in human tissues. Molecular analysis has now been reported. Preliminary data indicate a sequence similarity in all enzymes which liberate fumarate. A point mutation involving a T to C substitution has been identified in one kindred.

DISORDERS OF PYRIMIDINE METABOLISM

Hereditary orotic aciduria (**UMP synthase deficiency**) (McKusick 258900)

Biochemical defect

Orotic acid is the fourth intermediate in the de novo pyrimidine synthetic pathway which commences with carbamoyl phosphate (CP). CP may be synthesised by CP synthetase 1 (CPS 1), an enzyme present in the mitochrondria, which is essential for the urea cycle (Ch. 3) and confined almost exclusively to the liver, with low activity in kidney, intestinal mucosa and leucocytes. CP may also be synthesised by CPS 2, a cytosolic enzyme widely distributed throughout the body which forms a multienzyme complex with the next two enzymes of pyrimidine biosynthesis, and is subject to complex feedback regulatory processes (Fig. 8.2). However, CPS 1 may be a significant source of liver pyrimidines since, even at optimal conditions, a third of the CP synthesised by this route is reportedly exported to the cytosol, with 80% being incorporated into hepatic pyrimidines. The fourth enzyme, dihydroorotate dehydrogenase, is located on the outer surface of the inner membrane of the mitochondrion.

The activities of the last two enzymes of the de novo synthetic pathway, orotic acid phosphoribosyltransferase (OPRT: EC 2.4.2.10) and orotidine-5'-monophosphate decarboxylase (ODC: EC 4.1.1.23), are contained in a bifunctional protein, UMP synthase (UMPS).[38,39] These enzymes catalyse the conversion of orotic acid to UMP via the transitory intermediate OMP, the first step requiring PP-ribose-P (Fig. 8.11).

UMPS deficiency, otherwise known as hereditary orotic aciduria, results in the accumulation of orotic acid, which is excreted in quantity.[38] The clinical features are assumed to be related to pyrimidine nucleotide depletion. Depletion of CDP-ethanolamine and CDP-choline, necessary for phospholipid synthesis, or UDP sugars necessary for galactose utilisation and glycogen formation, have been proposed as the basis for the skeletal muscle weakness in some cases.

Clinical presentation

The onset of symptoms has usually occurred in the first few months of life.

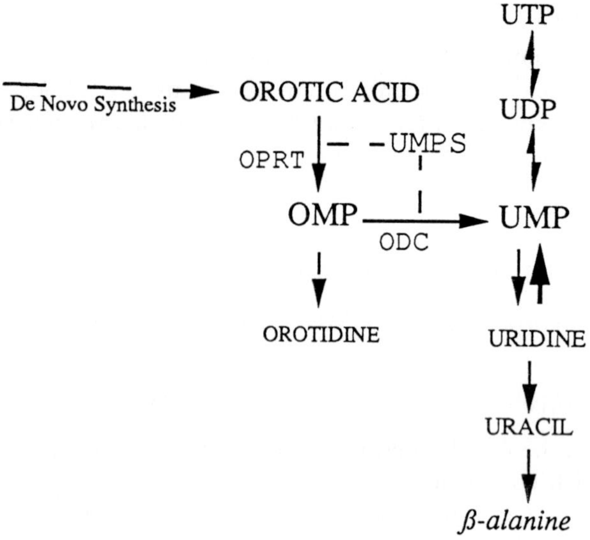

Fig. 8.11 The UMP synthase (UMPS) complex, a bifunctional protein comprising the enzymes orotic acid phosphoribosyltransferase (OPRT) and orotidine-5'-monophosphate decarboxylase (ODC), which catalyse the last two steps of de novo pyrimidine synthesis, resulting in the formation of UMP. Overexcretion of orotic acid results when the enzyme complex is defective. Orotidine formation can occur by the alternative pathway indicated during therapy with ODC inhibitors.

All patients have had a macrocytic hypochromic megaloblastic anaemia unresponsive to the usual forms of therapy (iron, folic acid and B_{12}), and sometimes leucopenia. Failure to thrive, developmental retardation, cardiac malformations, bilateral strabismus, sparse hair, inability to sit unaided, and gross crystalluria, occasionally with ureteric obstruction, have been general findings. Renal function is generally normal. Infections have occurred in some instances, associated with abnormalities of immune function. Heterozygotes show mild orotic aciduria but are otherwise unaffected.

Inheritance and incidence

This is an extremely rare disorder and has been identified in 14 cases widely distributed geographically, including caucasians, orientals, Polynesians, American Indians and negroes. The enzyme defect is inherited in an autosomal recessive fashion and has been confirmed in liver, fibroblasts, lymphoblasts, erythrocytes and leucocytes from affected individuals.

The molecular defect

The activities for OPRT and ODC reside in separate domains of a single polypeptide coded for by a single gene located on the long arm of chromosome 3 (3q13). The UMPS gene has been cloned and the nucleotide sequence of the complete coding region determined.[39] Cells from patients with the mutant enzyme express the UMPS gene at normal levels and produce a stable mRNA transcript identical in size and quantity to mRNA of control cells. It has been proposed that UMPS deficiency results from the production of a structurally abnormal protein due to an altered amino acid sequence which changes the ability of the subunits to form the 5.6-S altered dimer conformation necessary for optimal ODC activity.

Metabolites derived from a variety of pharmacological agents producing secondary oroticaciduria and orotidinuria (see below) are specific inhibitors of ODC and can lead to a coordinate increase in UMPS activity, secondary to amplification of the UMPS gene.

Diagnosis

Homozygotes may be detected by the severe refractory megaloblastic anaemia and the high levels of orotic acid in the urine of up to 10 mmol (2g)/24 h, compared with normal values of less than 10 μmol (2 mg)/24 h. Urinary orotic acid may be measured colorimetrically, but blanks must be included since falsely raised values can be produced by histidine, septrin etc.[38] HPLC methods specific for orotic acid measurement in plasma and urine are available[15] and plasma orotic acid concentrations of 40 μmol/l, compared to the normal of less than 0.1 μmol/l, have been reported. The fractional clearance of orotic acid exceeds the GFR which indicates active secretion and explains why plasma levels are not raised unless accumulation is excessive.

The defect may be confirmed by the low-to-undetectable levels of OPRT and ODC in lysed erythrocytes. However, OPRT is unstable even in frozen erythrocytes, and although ODC is less so, both enzyme activities decrease with erythrocyte age. The majority of patients have low but detectable activity of both OPRT and ODC in fibroblasts. The erythrocyte enzyme levels in heterozygotes overlap the lower end of the normal range. Consequently, definitive diagnosis of heterozygosity requires both a low enzyme level coupled with a slightly raised urinary excretion of orotic acid.

Purine metabolism is normal but uric acid clearance is high, probably due to the uricosuric effect of orotic acid. Purine enzymes are likewise normal, apart from APRT which is raised. This is not due to stabilisation by raised PP-ribose-P levels as in HPRT deficiency, since PP-ribose-P levels are normal in orotic aciduria; increased enzyme synthesis has been demonstrated.

Methods for early prenatal diagnosis using chorionic villus sampling have been reported, as has the exclusion of the defect by this means.[19]

Secondary orotic aciduria

Orotic acid excretion and UMPS activity may be affected by a variety of factors, such as haematological status, reticulocytosis, iron, and pharmacological agents such as 5-azauridine, 5-azaorotic acid, or allopurinol. These agents, or their metabolites, are converted to inhibitors of ODC which produce an increase in orotic acid excretion and may confuse the diagnosis, unless orotidine is measured. The increment in orotidine, exclusive to secondary oroticaciduria, is due to the rapid degradation of the OMP accumulating following ODC inhibition by an OMP-specific nucleotidase. Conversely, pharmacological agents have produced near-normal OPRT/ODC levels in enzyme deficient fibroblasts in vitro and a reduction in orotic acid excretion in vivo in hereditary orotic aciduria.[38]

Treatment and prognosis

Replacement therapy with large doses of oral uridine (150 mg/kg or 0.5 mmol kg^{-1} 24 h^{-1} in three divided doses) has been effective in most cases and has reduced orotic acid excretion to below 1 g or 5 mmol/24 h. One patient (now treated successfully for 30 years) relapsed immediately when compliance was poor during adolescence, indicating a lifelong requirement for therapy. Uracil was ineffective,[38] confirming that, unlike purines, pyrimidine salvage takes place at the nucleoside level. Despite the high level of orotic acid and uric acid in the urine, renal function is not impaired, but a high water intake is advisable. The long-term prognosis in uncomplicated cases is thus good. However, other features, such as immunodeficiency or congenital malformations, may adversely affect this.

Orotic aciduria in other genetic metabolic defects

Urea cycle defects. Orotic aciduria secondary to genetic metabolic defects involving four of the six enzymes associated with the urea cycle, results from stimulation of de novo pyrimidine biosynthesis following overflow of mitochondrial-derived CP into the cytoplasm. The orotic aciduria can equal that in the hereditary disorder, but can be distinguished by the raised blood ammonia levels and the grossly raised levels of uridine and uracil in plasma and urine. However, in some hemizygotes or carriers for ornithine carbamoyltransferase (OCT) deficiency, orotic acid excretion may be normal, the only detectable abnormality being raised urinary uracil levels.[40] The orotic aciduria is considered secondary to PP-ribose-P depletion in consequence of the greatly increased flux through the de novo pathway. The degree of orotic aciduria seen in the urea cycle defects can also be mimicked in patients with *dietary deficiencies of essential amino acids*, *Reyes' syndrome*, *hereditary protein intolerance*, or on *parenteral nutrition*.

A new carrier detection test for OCT deficiency (and possibly other urea cycle defects), based on the orotic aciduria and orotidinuria produced following a single allopurinol dose has recently been introduced. The test appears more sensitive and also avoids the unpleasantness and attendant hazards of protein loading tests.[41]

Dihydropyrimidine dehydrogenase deficiency (McKusick 274270)

Biochemical disorder

Pyrimidine metabolism, unlike purine metabolism, normally lacks an identifiable end-product (Fig. 8.2). The bases uracil and thymine produced following nucleotide catabolism are normally further degraded in three additional steps to the amino acids β-alanine and β–aminoisobutyric acid, respectively, and CO_2 (Fig. 8.12). The enzyme dihydropyrimidine dehydrogenase (DHPD: EC 1.3.1.2) catalyses the first and rate-limiting NADPH-dependent step in this process, producing the dihydro derivatives of uracil and thymine. The rate-limiting nature of this step possibly accounts for the exclusive accumulation of uracil in some cases of OCT deficiency. The enzyme is also responsible for the breakdown of the

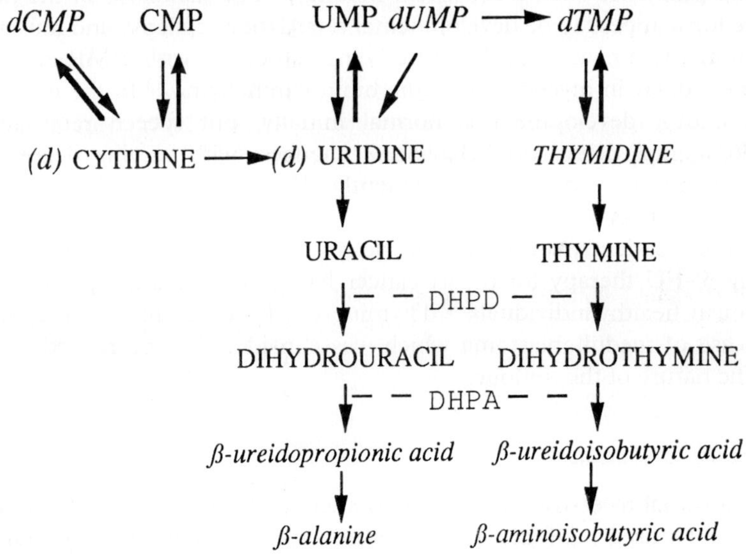

Fig. 8.12 Dihydropyrimidine dehydrogenase (DHPD) is responsible for the catabolism of the end-products of pyrimidine metabolism (uracil and thymine) to dihydrouracil and dihydrothymine. A deficiency of DHPD leads to accumulation of uracil and thymine. Dihydropyrimidine amidohydrolase (DHPA) catalyses the next step in the further catabolism of dihydrouracil and dihydrothymine to amino acids. A deficiency of DHPA results in the accumulation of small amounts of uracil and thymine together with larger amounts of the dihydroderivatives.

antineoplastic agent 5-fluorouracil (5'-FU), thereby limiting its effectiveness.

DHPD has been identified in most tissues, the highest activity being found in lymphocytes, and may exist in more than one isozymic form. The liver enzyme is considered to be a dimer of two identical subunits, each containing four molecules of FAD and three molecules of iron. Early reports of failure to detect activity in extrahepatic tissues may have related to assay problems, including substrate inhibition and the absence of the next enzyme in some tissues.

A deficiency of DHPD leads to the unusual overexcretion of uracil and thymine in the urine. In all instances a defect in DHPD was demonstrated.[42] Two cases exhibiting uraciluria without thyminuria, but with normal DHPD activity were also reported. Since uraciluria without orotic aciduria has been identified recently in male and female infants with OCT deficiency, the latter should be excluded when uraciluria alone is found.[40]

Clinical presentation

There is considerable genetic heterogeneity in clinical expression. The defect has been described in children and adults. The paediatric patients so far reported have not exhibited a characteristic clinical picture. Microcephaly has been a consistent finding.[42] The hallmarks of the more severe form appear to be developmental retardation, epilepsy and muscular hypotonia, this neurological picture being associated with NMR evidence of severe delay in myelination of the brain parenchyma.[43] In the majority, psychomotor development is normal initially, but speech retardation, developmental delay and behavioural changes, with varying degrees of involvement, may develop subsequently. Four cases have had atypical epileptic seizures of late onset.

In adult patients, severe neurotoxicity associated with pyrimidinaemia during 5'-FU therapy for breast cancer has been a presenting feature in previously healthy individuals.[43] Thymine-uraciluria has also been reported in a case of medulloblastoma which was considered to be related to the specific nature of the tumour.

Inheritance and incidence

An autosomal recessive mode of inheritance has been demonstrated in two separate kindreds. Of the 13 paediatric cases, 12 have been of Dutch origin. The defect has also been identified in an adolescent and four adults, and in three of the latter it was the metabolic basis for drug-induced toxicity during 5'-FU therapy, suggesting this defect may not be as rare as previously thought. Heterozygotes may be difficult to detect; although some have reduced activity in fibroblasts, there is overlap with the normal range. The molecular defect is unknown.

Diagnosis

High levels of thymine and uracil are found in the urine by GC-MS or HPLC. Plasma ammonia, plasma and urinary amino acids and other routine clinical chemistry are normal. DHPD deficiency may be confirmed by demonstrating the enzyme defect in cultured fibroblasts and leucocytes.[42,43] Oral loading with uracil or thymine, resulting in the recovery of more than 70% of the load in urine, may also be used to confirm the defect. Normal levels of uric acid and pseudouridine have been reported, indicating that tissue breakdown is not enhanced; neither orotic acid nor orotidine have been elevated consistently in the defect, Prenatal diagnosis has been reported.[44]

Treatment and prognosis

There is no established treatment for this disorder and the long-term outcome is unknown. However, patients with DHPD deficiency, and the defect described below, should not be given 5'-FU.

Dihydropyrimidinase deficiency (McKusick 222748)

Biochemical defect

Dihydropyrimidinase (5,6-dihydropyrimidine amidohydrolase DHPA; EC 3.5.2.2), the second enzyme in the breakdown of the pyrimidine bases, catalyses the degradation of dihydrouracil and dihydrothymine to β-ureidopropionic acid and β-ureidoisobutyric acid respectively (Fig. 8.12). DHPA is a tetramer and has been isolated and characterised from the liver of various mammalian species. Although no detectable activity has been found in tissues other than the liver, including lymphocytes, high enzyme activity has been demonstrated in all solid tumours, as distinct from their normal tissue counterparts.

A deficiency of this enzyme has been assumed from the accumulation and excretion in the urine of the substrates for the enzyme, dihydrouracil and dihydrothymine.[45] A putative neurotransmitter function has been ascribed to the end-product of pyrimidine catabolism, the amino acid β-alanine, of which the pyrimidine catabolic pathway is the only known source. Defective functioning of this pathway may thus provide a biochemical basis for some of the clinical symptoms in both dihydropyrimidinase and DHPD deficiency.

Clinical presentation

Although pregnancy and delivery were unremarkable and early development was initially normal, the two young male patients identified both presented at 6–8 weeks.[45,46] The first case developed feeding difficulties with convulsions and lowered consciousness, and was the 5th child of consanguineous parents. The second case presented with a febrile illness and seizures at 6 weeks, and suffered frequent generalised seizures at approximately 2-monthly intervals thereafter. When first investigated at $2\frac{1}{2}$ years of age, gross microcephaly as well as developmental retardation was evident, with signs of spastic quadriplegia. Jerky choreoform movements of the upper limbs were observed and the child could not sit without support.

Inheritance and incidence

The identification of the defect in a Turkish and a Pakistani kindred with evidence of consanguinity in both instances would be consistent with an autosomal recessive mode of inheritance. The recent description of the disorder, coupled with the fact that the underlying biochemical defect is not readily identifiable by HPLC (see below), means it could easily be missed and might not be so rare. The molecular defect is unknown.

Diagnosis

The detection of the unusual components, dihydrothymine and dihydrouracil, in the urine in quantity (0.5–1.0 mmol/l) during organic acid screening by GC-MS will alert the investigator to the possible diagnosis. Identification by HPLC is difficult because the maximal UV-absorbance of both compounds is below 230 nm, but their presence may be established by monitoring with diode-array and UV-detection from 200–320 nm. Moderate amounts of uracil and thymine are also excreted (0.1–0.5 mmol/l). Oral loading tests with uracil, dihydrouracil, thymine and dihydrothymine (1 mmol/kg) have been used to distinguish the defect from DHPD deficiency.[45] A simple confirmatory test involving conversion of these dihydropyrimidines to amino acids by acid hydrolysis has been published.[47]

The enzyme defect is difficult to establish. Normal erythrocytes, leucocytes and fibroblasts are apparently devoid of activity, as are most other tissues. Liver appears obligatory for definitive proof of the presence or absence of activity. Exclusion of a deficiency of DHPD in leucocytes and fibroblasts, has been used as an indirect confirmation of diagnosis.[46]

Treatment and prognosis

No further episodes have occurred in the first case and physical and mental development at 19 months have been reported as normal. The more severely affected Pakistani infant was treated with sodium valproate with good effect, but was lost to subsequent follow-up.

Pyrimidine-5'-nucleotidase deficiency (UMP hydrolase deficiency) (McKusick 266120)

Biochemical defect

Pyrimidine-5'-nucleotidase (EC: 3.1.3.5) is the first degradative enzyme of the pyrimidine salvage cycle (Fig. 8.13) and catalyses the specific hydrolysis of pyrimidine-5'-nucleotides. It is a cytosolic enzyme requiring Mg^{2+} for activity, while lead, copper and mercury are markedly inhibitory. Activity is due to two isoenzymes, designated uridine monophosphate hydrolase 1 and 2 (UMPH 1 and 2), which have overlapping substrate specificities and pH optima. UMPH 1 hydrolyses UMP, CMP and dCMP preferentially, whereas UMPH 2 prefers dUMP and dTMP as substrates and has a wide pH optimum. UMPH 1 and 2 activities have been demonstrated in a wide range of human tissues, including lymphoblasts, and there is evidence for tissue specificity of isoenzyme composition. The major part of this activity, 90–95%, resides in UMPH 1, the remainder is due to overlapping specificity of UMPH 2.

Deficiency of UMPH 1[48] results in the accumulation of high levels of pyrimidine nucleotides in the erythrocytes of homozygotes and it was proposed originally that these were derived from RNA degradation in maturing erythrocytes, trapped through the enzyme defect. However, demonstration of active uptake of orotic acid into pyrimidine nucleotides by both normal and deficient erythrocytes, implies an important role for the erythrocyte in pyrimidine transport and hence an alternative explanation for the raised nucleotide levels. Although only the erythrocyte shows pathological effects of this disorder, UMPH 1 is selectively deficient in patients' mononuclear and lymphoblastoid cells and accumulation of slightly raised levels of UTP and UDP sugars has also been noted.

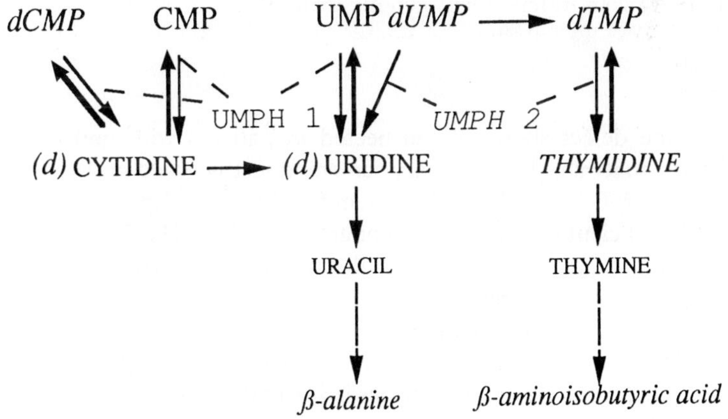

Fig. 8.13 The role of uridine monophosphate hydrolases (UMPH) 1 and 2 in the catabolism of UMP, CMP, and dCMP (UMPH 1), and dUMP and dTMP (UMPH 2).

Clinical presentation

Homozygotes present with non-spherocytic haemolytic anaemia characterised by marked basophilic stippling in their erythrocytes.[48] The age of presentation has varied widely. Other characteristic findings include reticulocytosis, anisocytosis, splenomegaly and sometimes cholelithiasis. Increased levels of indirect bilirubin, increased erythrocyte levels of reduced glutathione, with reduced activity of PP-ribose-P synthetase may also be found. In addition, two recent cases showed intravascular haemolysis, haemoglobulinuria, urinary iron loss and enlarged kidneys. Biopsy showed iron in the epithelium of the proximal tubules. Heterozygotes are clinically and haematologically normal.

Inheritance and incidence

This is an autosomal recessive disorder. The defect has been reported in a number of families, affecting both children and adults, showing a wide distribution around the world. Individuals of Jewish or African ancestry may be particularly susceptible. Heterozygotes may be difficult to detect. Studies in a large Dutch kindred showed an increased amount of UDP sugars in both apparent and questionable heterozygotes, indicating the importance of analysis of red cell ribonucleotide patterns in combination with UMPH activity for heterozygote detection.[48]

Electrophoretic analysis of erythrocytes, lymphocytes and lymphoblasts from patients with the disorder have shown a complete deficiency of the major isoenzyme UMPH 1. In some cases the abnormal UMPH 1 has been reported to have different electrophoretic characteristics, pH optima and heat stability, and increased K_m. Normal levels of UMPH 2 have been found, both by assay and electrophoresis. The fact that this isozyme appears unaffected by the genetic deficiency of UMPH 1 suggests it may be determined by an independent genetic locus.

Diagnosis

The enzyme defect should be suspected in patients with non-spherocytic haemolytic anaemia. A preliminary screening test is based on the characteristic UV absorption profile at 280 nm and 254 nm for deproteinised extracts of enzyme deficient erythrocytes, compared with normal cells. Enzyme levels in lysed erythrocytes by conventional assay have shown activity approximately 10% of the normal range of 8–15 nmol $mgHb^{-1}$ h^{-1}. Most of the residual activity in affected individuals is undoubtedly attributable to the deoxypyrimidine nucleotidase UMPH 2. Electrophoretic analysis coupled with staining for the different isozymes is a useful confirmatory test.

HPLC should be used to demonstrate the characteristically increased pyrimidine nucleotide concentrations in the erythrocytes, principally

UDP-glucose, UDP-N-acetylglucosamine and CDP-choline, UTP and CTP. In the normal erythrocyte, adenine nucleotides comprise over 90% of the total nucleotide pool and, apart from low levels of UDP-glucose, pyrimidine nucleotides are undetectable. In UMPH 1 deficiency the concentration of pyrimidine nucleotides may exceed those of the adenine nucleotides, although the former may vary, possibly due to the episodic nature of the disease.

Studies using ^{31}P, NMR spectroscopy have shown that the additional pyrimidine triphosphates are Mg^{2+} bound and there is a nearly proportional increase in erythrocyte Mg^{2+}. The near doubling of the triphosphate pool results in a low intracellular pH, which is thought to explain a low oxygen affinity and altered levels of glycolytic intermediates in the deficient cells, despite a normal 2,3-diphosphoglycerate concentration.

Erythrocyte PP-ribose-P synthetase activity is 30% of that for normal cells of comparable age, related to a decrease in enzyme protein. Whether production or degradation is altered is uncertain. Impairment of pentose phosphate shunt activity may contribute to the pathogenesis of the haemolysis and the reduced PP-ribose-P synthetase activity in the defect. Glutathione reductase activity has been reported normal or increased. Unfortunately, neither pyrimidine nor purine levels have been reported in the body fluids in this defect.

Treatment

The disease is relatively benign. Anaemia in the defect has usually been moderate with transfusion rarely necessary. Splenectomy has not proved beneficial.

Acquired pyrimidine-5'-nucleotidase deficiency

Severe lead intoxication is associated with a similar syndrome which may include haemolytic anaemia and marked erythrocyte basophilic stippling. All subjects with lead intoxication have shown substantial reductions in erythrocyte enzyme activity. However, only in severe cases has significant accumulation of erythrocyte pyrimidine nucleotides been demonstrated, associated with anaemia and prominent basophilic stippling. Lead-induced deficiency mimics the genetic disorder at concentrations of blood lead in excess of 200 μg/100 ml.

CDP-choline phosphotransferase deficiency (McKusick ?)

Biochemical disorder

The last two steps in lecithin synthesis are mediated by CDP-choline synthetase (CTP:cholinephosphate cytidyltransferase; EC 2.7.7.15)

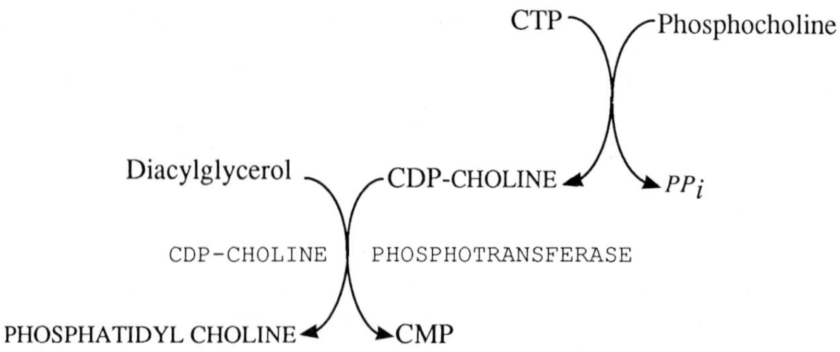

Fig. 8.14 CDP-choline phosphotransferase catalyses the last step in the synthesis of phosphatidyl choline. A deficiency of this enzyme is proposed as the metabolic basis for the selective accumulation of CDP-choline in the erythrocytes of rare patients with an unusual form of haemolytic anaemia.

and choline phosphotransferase (CDP-choline:1,2-diacylglycerol choline-phosphotransferase; EC 2.7.8.2). The first step results in the formation of CDP-choline and pyrophosphate (Fig. 8.14). Although potentially readily reversible, the presence of an active inorganic pyrophosphatase in human erythrocytes makes CDP-choline formation irreversible.

The accumulation of high levels of CDP-choline in erythrocytes has been attributed to a deficiency of the latter enzyme.[4] It has been hypothesised that the associated chronic haemolysis in the defect may be related to ineffective erythropoiesis due to intramarrow death of erythroid precursors during maturation.

Clinical presentation

Patients have invariably presented with haemolytic anaemia and jaundice with evidence of splenomegaly. There is considerable heterogeneity in clinical expression ranging from presentation at birth, requiring exchange transfusions, to a relatively benign presentation in late adolescence. The erythrocytes have shown significant basophilic stippling, as well as polychromasia. Reticulocytosis has generally been modest (up to 8%), with a low haemoglobin (6–8 g). One case had a past history of bilateral dislocated lenses and possible fits.

Inheritance and incidence

Only four patients with this defect (which is presumed, not proven) have been diagnosed, two of them from a large consanguineous Asian kindred, one of which was identified only during the family study. Another Asian case was also from a first-cousin marriage, results which would be compatible with an autosomal recessive mode of inheritance.[49] The first reported case was of Irish/Scottish/Dutch ancestry, indicating a wide ethnic distribution. The molecular defect is unknown.

Diagnosis

The defect may be diagnosed from the selective accumulation of CDP-choline in the erythrocytes in a patient with a history of chronic anaemia and jaundice. It may be suspected from the unusual shift in the UV absorption spectra in the screening test used for UMPH 1 deficiency. The absence of high levels of the pyrimidine nucleotides and presence of normal UMPH 1 activity, will distinguish this disorder from pyrimidine-5'-nucleotidase deficiency. The selective nucleotide accumulation is assumed to be related to a deficiency of CDP-choline phosphotransferase in erythroid precursors, but is not yet proven, since the enzyme is not present in mature erythrocytes.

No other abnormalities of purine or pyrimidine metabolism have been found in this defect. Purine production and excretion is normal.

Treatment and prognosis

Episodes of brisk haemolysis have required several successive transfusions, but subsequent growth in a case with neonatal onset has been normal. One adult, studied for 9 years, has recently required splenectomy for splenomegaly and hypersplenism.

Secondary defects

Secondary accumulation of CDP-choline is found in the erythrocytes of some patients with chronic renal failure. The fact that it is not found in all cases raises the question as to whether such patients might be heterozygotes for a similar deficiency which is manifest in the uraemic state.

LABORATORY DIAGNOSIS OF PURINE AND PYRIMIDINE DISORDERS

All the above defects (apart from AMPDA deficiency) may be detected by altered levels of metabolites in plasma, urine or erythrocytes.[15] For a summary of findings see Table 8.2. In HPRT deficiency and aberrant PRPS activity, uric acid levels are grossly raised in urine relative to creatinine in patients with normal renal function[8], as are hypoxanthine levels; total purine excretion on a creatinine basis is elevated in PNP and ADS deficiency. XOD and PNP deficiency should be suspected in any patient with low-to-undetectable plasma urate levels on routine screening, and appropriate clinical manifestations.

Table 8.2 List of abnormal metabolites which may accumulate (or show alteration in normal levels) in body fluids and red cells, in the inherited disorders of purine and pyrimidine metabolism which have been identified to date, or secondary to OCT deficiency

Disorder	Juvenile gout	HPRT a/b	PRPS↑ a/b	APRT I/II	PNP	ADA	XOD XOD/SO	AMPDA	ADS	UMPS	DHPD DHPA	UMPH	OCT
Blood													
Red blood cells (RBC)													
Enzyme(s)	N	–/–+	/	–/25%	—	—	No	N	No	—	No	—	No
Nucleotide++	N	↓GTP/N	↓GTP/N	N	↑dGTP/↓GTP	↑dATP	N	N	N	↑UDPG	?	↑UTP/CTP	?
PPRP	N	↑	↑	N	↑	N	N	?	?	N	?	?	N
Carrier													
RBC enzyme	N	N	N	25%/25%	50%	50%/–	No	?	No	±	No	±	No
Prenatal diagnosis CVS	?	√	?	NR	√	√	√SO	NR	?	√	√/ ?–	?	√
Plasma													
Uric acid	↑	↑	↑	N	—	N	—	?	N	N	N	N	N
Other Purine	N	*	*	N	*	N/*	*	?	*	N	N	*	N
Orotic acid	—	—	—	—	—	—	—	—	—	↑	—	?	↑OA/U/UR
Urine													
Uric acid	N	↑↑	↑↑	N	—	N	—	?	N	↑	N	?	N
X	N	—	—	N	—	N	↑↑	?	N	N	N	?	N
H	N	↑	↑	N	—	N	↑	?	N	N	N	?	N
A													
8-HA													
2,8-DHA	—	—	—	↑↑	—	—	—	—	—	—	—	—	—

Table 8.2 *Contd*

Disorder	Juvenile gout	HPRT a/b	PRPS↑ a/b	APRT I/II	PNP	ADA	XOD XOD/SO	AMPDA	ADS	UMPS	DHPD DHPA	UMPH	OCT
HR GR	—	—	—	—	↑↑	—	—	—	—	—	—	—	—
dHR dGR	—	—	—	—	↑	—	—	—	—	—	—	—	—
dAR	—	—	—	—	—	↑↑	—	—	—	—	—	—	—
SAR SAICAR	—	—	—	—	—	—	—	—	↑↑	—	—	—	—
Orotic acid	—	—	—	—	—	—	—	—	—	↑↑	—	?	↑↑
U	—	—	—	—	—	—	—	—	—	—	↑↑/↑	?	↑↑U/UR
T	—	—	—	—	—	—	—	—	—	—	↑↑/↑	?	—
Total purine	N	x (2–4)↑	x (2–4)↑	N	x 4 *↑	N	N	?	x (2–4)↑	N	N	?	N

a – severe   b – partial   I – Type 1   II – Type II   - - Below limit of detection   ↓ – decreased   ↑ – increased
N – normal   ? – Not known   NR – not required   * – as for urine   ++ – abnormal nucleotide pattern   No – enzyme not expressed in RBC
–+ – sometimes detectable   ± – overlap heterozygote/normal range   √ – methods available

XOD deficiency may be distinguished from renal hypouricaemia (tubular reabsorption defect) by the absence of uric acid from both plasma and urine[2], with replacement predominantly by xanthine. In PNP deficiency, inosine, guanosine and their deoxyanalogues, deoxyinosine and deoxyguanosine replace uric acid in plasma and urine. In ADA deficiency the abnormal metabolite excreted is deoxyadenosine and in APRT deficiency, adenine 8-hydroxyadenine and 2,8-dihydroxyadenine.

These purine defects can be confirmed by enzyme assay in lysed erythrocytes, cultured lymphoblasts or fibroblasts, except for XOD (IM, liver) and AMPDA (muscle) where biopsy alone will confirm the diagnosis. In HPRT, ADA and PNP deficiencies and aberrant PRPS activity, characteristic alterations in erythrocyte nucleotides are also found using HPLC techniques.[15] These techniques may also be employed, where indicated, for rapid prenatal diagnosis using fetal blood.

In the pyrimidine disorders HPLC is also used to detect the grossly raised orotic acid levels in urine and plasma found in UMPS deficiency and the uracil plus thymine excreted in DHPD deficiency. Dihydrouracil and dihydrothymine, identified by GC-MS, with lesser amounts of uracil and thymine, are found in DHPA deficiency.

Uracil alone may be indicative of OCT deficiency where there is residual hepatic activity.[40] In symptomatic patients orotic acid, orotidine and uridine are also grossly elevated (Table 8.2).

UMPS, and UMPH 1 deficiencies may be confirmed by enzyme assay either in lysed erythrocytes, leucocytes or fibroblasts. However the enzyme is not present in erythrocytes, and leucocytes or fibroblasts are required for DHPD deficiency. DHPA is not present in tissues other than liver, and biopsy is thus essential for confirmation of DHPA deficiency.

In UMPH 1 deficiency and CDP-choline phosphotransferase deficiency, high levels of unusual pyrimidine nucleotides are found in erythrocyte extracts (Table 8.2). An increment in pyrimidine nucleotides is also found in UMPS deficiency.

REFERENCES

1. Kelley W N 1991 Gene therapy in humans: a new era begins. Annals of Internal Medicine 114:697–698
2. Stone T W, Simmonds H A 1991 Purines: basic and clinical aspects. Kluwer, London
3. Thompson L F 1991 5'-Nucleotidase: an overview of the last three years. Advances in Experimental Medicine and Biology 309B:145–150
4. Paglia D E, Valentine W N, Nakatani M, Rauth B J 1983 Selective accumulation of cytosol CDP-choline as an isolated erythrocyte defect in chronic haemolysis. Proceedings of the National Acadademy of Sciences USA 80:3081–3085
5. Wyngaarden J B, Kelley W N 1976 Gout and hyperuricaemia. Grune and Stratton, New York
6. Calabrese G, Simmonds H A, Cameron J S 1990 Precocious familial gout with reduced fractional urate clearance and normal purine enzymes. Quarterly Journal of Medicine 277:441–450
7. Moro F, Ogg C, Cameron J S, Simmonds H A, Duley J A, McBride M B, Davies P M

1991 Familial juvenile gouty nephropathy with renal urate hypoexcretion preceding renal disease. Clinical Nephrology 35:263–269

8. Simmonds H A, Cameron J S, Barratt T M, Dillon M J, Meadow S R, Trompeter R S 1989 Purine enzyme defects as a cause of acute renal failure in childhood. Pediatric Nephrology 3:433–437
9. Johnson J L, Wuebbens M M, Mandell R, Shih V E 1988 Molybdenum cofactor deficiency in a patient previously characterised as deficient in sulphite oxidase. Biochemical Medicine Metabolism and Biology 40: 86–93
10. Reiter S, Simmonds H A, Zollner N, Braun S, Knedel M 1990 Demonstration of a combined deficiency of xanthine oxidase and aldehyde oxidase in xanthinuric patients not forming oxipurinol. Clinica Chimica Acta 187:221–234
11. Desiacques P, Mousson B, Vianey-Llaud C, Boulieu R, Bory C, Baltassat P, Divry P, Zabot M T, Cotte J, Lagier P, Philip N 1985 Combined deficiency of xanthine oxidase and sulphite oxidase : diagnosis of a new case followed by an antenatal diagnosis. Journal of Inherited Metabolic Disease 8:117–118
12. Fujitaka M, Sakura N, Ueda K, Konishi, H, Yoshida S, Yamasaki T 1991 Attempt at treatment with tetrahydrobiopterin in combined deficiency of xanthine oxidase and sulphite oxidase. Journal of Inherited Metabolic Disease 14:843–845
13. Kamatani N, Hakoda M, Otsuka S, Yoshikawa H, Kashiwazaki S 1992 Only three mutations account for almost all defective alleles causing adenine phosphoribosyltransferase deficiency in Japanese patients. Journal of Clinical Investigation 90:130–136
14. Chen J, Sahota A, Laxdal T, Scrine M, Bowman S, Cui C, Stambrook P J, Tischfield J S 1991. Identification of a single missense mutation in the adenine phosphoribosyltransferase gene from five Icelandic patients and a British patient. American Journal of Human Genetics 49:251–255
15. Simmonds H A, Duley J A, Davies P M 1991 Analysis of purines and pyrimidines in blood, urine and other physiological fluids. In: Hommes F (ed) Techniques in diagnostic human biochemical genetics: a laboratory manual. Wiley–Liss, New York, p 397–424
16. Watts R W E, Harkness R A, Spellacy E, Taylor N F 1987 Lesch-Nyhan syndrome: growth delay, testicular atrophy and a partial failure of the 11β-hydroxylation of steroids. Journal of Inherited Metabolic Disease 10:210–223
17. Davidson B L, Tarle S A, van Antwerp M, Gibbs D A, Watts R W E, Kelley W N, Palella T D 1991 Identification of 17 independent mutations responsible for human hypoxanthine-guanine phosphoribosyltransferase (HPRT) deficiency. American Journal of Human Genetics 48:951–958
18. Gibbs R A, Nguyen P H, McBride L J, Koepf S M, Caskey C T 1989 Identification of mutations leading to the Lesch – Nyhan syndrome by automated direct sequencing of in vitro amplified cDNA. Proceedings of the National Academy of Sciences USA 86 : 1919–1923
19. Perignon J L, Durandy A, Peter M O, Freycon F, Dumez Y, Griscelli C 1987 Early prenatal diagnosis of inherited severe immunodeficiencies linked to enzyme deficiencies. Journal of Pediatrics 111:595–598
20. Page T, Broock R L 1990 A pitfall in the prenatal diagnosis of Lesch – Nyhan syndrome by chorionic villus sampling. Prenatal Diagnosis 10:153–157
21. Simmonds H A, Fairbanks L D, Duley J A, Micheli V 1990 Importance of the human erythrocyte in the diagnosis of inherited purine and pyrimidine disorders. Biomedicine Biochimica Acta 49:259–264
22. Endres W, Helmig M, Shin Y S, Albert E, Wank R, Ibel H, Weiss M, Hadorn, H-B, Hass R 1991 Bone marrow transplantation in Lesch – Nyhan disease. Journal of Inherited Metabolic Disease 14:270–271
23. Becker M A, Puig J G, Mateos F A, Jiminez M L, Kim M, Simmonds H A 1988 Inherited superactivity of phosphoribosylpyrophosphate synthetase: association of uric acid overproduction and sensorineural deafness. American Journal of Medicine 85:383–390
24. Roessler B J, Golovoy N, Palella T D, Heidler S, Becker M A 1991 Identification of distinct PRPS1 mutations in two patients with X-linked phosphoribosylpyrophosphate synthetase superactivity. Advances in Experimental Medicine and Biology 309B:125–128

25. Simmonds H A, Fairbanks L D, Morris G S, Morgan G, Watson A R, Timms P, Singh B 1987 CNS dysfunction and erythrocyte GTP depletion in purine nucleoside phosphorylase deficiency. Archives of Disease in Childhood 62:385–391
26. Fairbanks L D, Taddeo A, Duley J A, Simmonds H A 1990 Mechanisms of deoxyguanosine lymphotoxicity: human thymocytes but not peripheral blood lymphocytes accumulate deoxy GTP in conditions simulating purine nucleoside phosphorylase deficiency. Journal of Immunology 144:90–96
27. Markert M L, Andrews L G, Aust M R, Barrett M J, Norby-Slycord C J, Jakos T J 1991 Molecular analysis of mutations in three patients with purine nucleoside phosphorylase deficiency. Journal of Purine and Pyrimidine Research 2 Suppl 1:63
28. Morgan G, Levinsky R J, Hugh-Jones K, Fairbanks L D, Morris G S, Simmonds H A 1987 Heterogeneity of biochemical, clinical and immunological parameters in severe combined immunodeficiency due to adenosine deaminase deficiency. Clinical and Experimental Immunology 70:491–499
29. Franco R, Aran J M, Colomer D, Matutes E, Vive-Corrons J L 1990 Association of adenosine deaminase with erythrocyte and platelet plasma membrane: an immunological study using light and electron microscopy. Journal of Histochemistry and Cytochemistry 38:653–658
30. Markert M L, Norby-Slycord C, Ward F E 1989 A high proportion of ADA point mutations associated with a specific alanine-to-valine substitution. American Journal of Human Genetics 45:354–361
31. Hirshorn R, Tzall S, Ellenbogen A, Orkin S H 1989 Identification of a point mutation resulting in a heat-labile adenosine deaminase (ADA) in two unrelated children with partial ADA deficiency. Journal of Clinical Investigation 83:497–501
32. Hershfield M S, Chafee S, Koro-Johnson L, Mary A S, Smith A A, Short S A 1991 Use of site-directed mutagenesis to enhance the epitype-shielding effect of covalent modification of proteins with polyethylene glycol. Proceedings of the National Academy of Sciences USA 88:7185–7189
33. Marwick C 1991 Two more cell infusions on schedule for gene replacement therapy patient. Journal of the American Medical Association. 265:2311–2312
34. Mahnke-Zizelman D K, Bausch-Jurken M T, Sabina R L 1993 The AMP-deaminase multigene family in rats and humans. In: Gresser U (ed) Molecular genetics, biochemical and clinical aspects of inherited disorders of purine and pyrimidine metabolism. Springer Verlag, Heidelberg (in press)
35. Jaeken J, Wadman S K, Duran M, Van Sprang F J, Beemer F A, Holl R A, Theunissen P M, de Cock P, van den Berghe F, Vincent M F, van den Berghe G 1988 Adenylosuccinase deficiency: an inborn error of purine nucleotide synthesis. European Journal of Paediatrics 148:126–131
36. De Bree P K, Wadman S K, Duran M, Fabery de Jonge H 1986 Diagnosis of inherited adenylosuccinase by thin layer chromatography of urinary imidazoles and by automated cation exchange column chromatography of purines. Clinica Chimica Acta 156:279–288
37. Levy H L, Coulombe J T, Benjamin R 1984 Massachusetts metabolic disorders screening program. Pediatrics 74:509–513
38. Becroft D M O, Webster D R, Simmonds H A, Fairbanks L D, Wilson J D, Phillips L I 1986 Hereditary orotic aciduria: further biochemistry. Advances in Experimental Medicine and Biology 195A:67–70
39. Qumsiyeh M B, Valentine M B, Suttle D P 1989 Localisation of the gene for uridine monophosphate synthase to human chromosome region 3q13 by in situ hybridization. Genomics 5:160–162
40. Rabier D, Guillois B, Bardet J, Deprun C, Parvy P, Kamoun P 1991 Ornithine carbomyltransferase deficiency with subnormal enzyme activity. Journal of Inherited Metabolic Disease 14:842–843
41. Hauser E R, Finkelstein J E, Valle D, Brusilow S W 1990 Allopurinol-induced orotidinuria: a test for mutations at the ornithine carbamoyltransferase locus in women. New England Journal of Medicine 322:1641–1645
42. Braakhekke J P, Renier W O, Gabreels F U M, De Abreu R A, Bakkeren J A J M, Sengers R C A 1987 Dihydropyrimidine dehydrogenase deficiency: neurological aspects. Journal of Neurological Sciences 78:71–77
43. Brockstedt M, Jakobs C, Smit L M E, van Gennip A H, Berger R 1990 A new case of

dihydropyrimidine dehydrogenase deficiency. Journal of Inherited Metabolic Disease 13:121–124
44. Jakobs C, Stellaard F, Smit L M, van Vugt J M, Duran M, Berger R, Rovers P 1991 The First prenatal diagnosis of dihydropyrimidine dehydrogenase deficiency. European Journal of Paediatrics 150:291
45. Duran M, Rovers P, de Bree P K, Schreuder C H, Beukenhorst H, Dorland L, Berger R 1991 Dihydropyrimidinuria: a new inborn error of pyrimidine metabolism. Journal of Inherited Metabolic Disease 14:367–370
46. Ward K, Henderson M J, Simmonds H A, Duley J A, Davies P M 1993. A second case of dihydropyrimidinuria in a severely retarded child. Journal of Inherited Metabolic Disease (in press)
47. Van Gennip A H, Busch S, Scholten E G, Abeling N G G M 1991 Simple method for the quantitative analysis of dihydropyrimidines and N-carbamyl-β-amino acids in urine. Advances in Experimental Medicine and Biology 309B:15–21
48. De Korte D, Sijstermans J M, Seip M, van Doorn C C, van Gennip A H, Roos D 1989 Pyrimidine 5'-nucleotidase deficiency: improved detection of carriers. Clinica Chimica Acta 1989 184:175–180
49. Smith A, Kelley S J, Simmonds H A, Duley J A 1992 CDP – choline accumulation in erythrocytes of patients from two kindreds with chronic haemolytic anaemia: an inborn error of pyrimidine metabolism?, in preparation

9. The porphyrias

G.H. Elder

INTRODUCTION

The porphyrias are a group of disorders of haem biosynthesis in which characteristic clinical features are associated with specific patterns of overproduction of haem precursors. The clinical features are of two types: acute attacks of porphyria which are neurological in origin and are always associated with increased excretion of the porphyrin precursors, porphobilinogen (PBG) or 5-aminolaevulinic acid (ALA), and skin lesions which are caused by photosensitization by porphyrins. The seven main types of porphyria are listed in Table 9.1. Each results from partial deficiency of a different enzyme of haem biosynthesis and the specific patterns of haem precursor overproduction that characterises each disorder reflects accumulation of the substrate of the deficient enzyme. In Table 9.1 the porphyrias are divided into two groups according to the concentration of porphyrin in erythrocytes. This is a useful practical division that serves to separate those conditions in which detectable accumulation of haem precursors is restricted to the liver, the hepatic porphyrias, from those in which porphyrin concentrations are increased in erythroid cells and the liver with one or other of these sites predominating.

Table 9.1 The main types of porphyria. (McKusick numbers in parentheses)

Disorder	Clinical presentation	
	Acute porphyria	Photocutaneous
1. Erythrocyte porphyrin concentration increased		
a. Congenital erythropoietic porphyria (263700)	–	+
b. Erythropoietic protoporphyria (177000)	–	+
c. Porphobilinogen synthase deficiency (125270)	+	–
2. Erythrocyte free porphyrin concentration normal (hepatic porphyrias)		
a. Acute hepatic porphyrias		
(i) Acute intermittent porphyria (176000)	+	–
(ii) Hereditary coproporphyria (121300)	+	+
(iii) Variegate porphyria (176200)	+	+
b. Porphyria cutanea tarda (176090 and 176100)	–	+

Very occasionally other porphyrias are encountered; a number of these rare variants have been identified in recent years and are described later. In addition, more than one type of porphyria may occur independently in the same family[1] and mixed or dual porphyrias which combine the features of two separate disorders have been described.[2,3]

HAEM BIOSYNTHESIS

Haem is synthesised in all mammalian cells, although erythroid cells lose this capacity as they mature into erythrocytes. Normal adults produce about 7 μmol of haem/kg body weight each day, of which 80–85% is used for the formation of haemoglobin. Most of the remaining 15–20% is synthesised in the liver. In the rat about 70% of haem produced in the liver is incorporated into microsomal haemoproteins of the cytochrome P_{450} series which catalyse the oxidative metabolism of a wide range of endogenous compounds, drugs and other foreign substances. In humans, the amount of haem that is synthesised for this purpose is probably lower because cytochrome P_{450} constitutes a smaller proportion of the total haem concentration in hepatocytes.

The pathway of haem biosynthesis

The pathway of haem biosynthesis consists of a series of irreversible reactions which are outlined in Figure 9.1. The formation of the first committed haem precursor, 5-amino-laevulinate, from glycine and succinyl CoA, is catalysed by the mitochondrial enzyme, ALA synthase (EC 2.3.1.37). ALA then enters the cytosol where two molecules condense to form the colourless monopyrrole, porphobilinogen (PBG). Next PBG deaminase (uroporphyrinogen I synthase; hydroxymethylbilane synthase; EC 4.3.1.8) catalyses the formation of the symmetrical, linear tetrapyrrole, hydroxymethylbilane from four molecules of PBG. This compound is very unstable and, particularly in the presence of acid, undergoes rapid non-enzymatic cyclisation to the symmetrical porphyrinogen, uroporphyrinogen I. However, in normal physiological circumstances, uroporphyrinogen III synthase catalyses a reaction in which cyclisation occurs with reversal of the order of the side-chains on ring D so that the asymmetrical series III isomer, uroporphyrinogen III, is formed. As a consequence, normally less than 1% of hydroxymethylbilane is diverted to the formation of series I porphyrinogens, which cannot be metabolised to haem (Fig. 9.1).

In the subsequent series of reactions the side-chains of uroporphyrinogen III are progressively modified to form protoporphyrinogen IX. Uroporphyrinogen decarboxylase (EC 4.11.37) catalyses the sequential decarboxylation of the four acetic acid substituents of uroporphyrinogen to produce coproporphyrinogen with the formation of hepta-, hexa- and

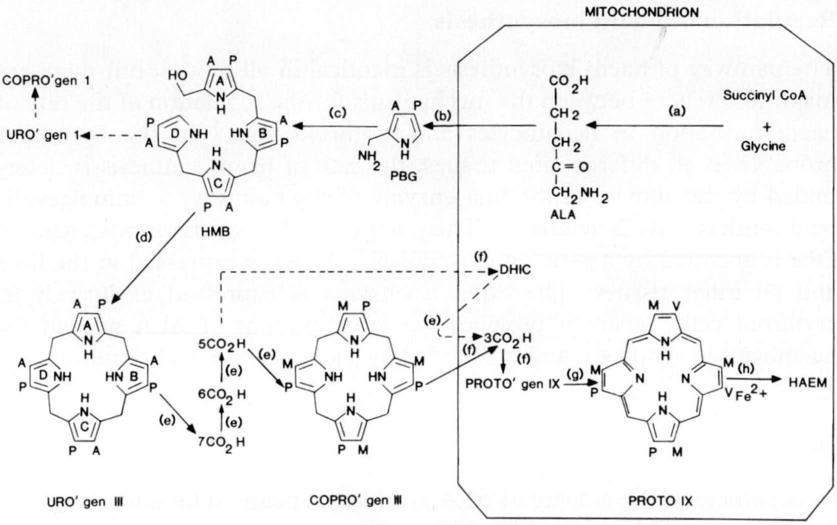

Fig. 9.1 The pathway of haem biosynthesis. Substituents in pyrrole rings A – CH_2CO_2H; P – $CH_2CH_2CO_2H$, M – CH_3, V – $CH{=}CH_2$. HMB – hydroxymethylbilane; DHIC – dehydroisocoproporphyrinogen; ALA – 5-aminolaevulinic acid; PBG – porphobilinogen, URO'gen – uroporphyrinogen. COPRO'gen – coproporphyrinogen; PROTO'gen – protoporphyrinogen; 3-, 5-, 6-, $7CO_2H$ – tri-, penta-, hexa-, heptacarboxylic porphyrinogen. Reactions are catalysed by ALA synthase (a), PBG synthase (b), PBG deaminase (c), uroporphyrinogen III synthase (d), uroporphyrinogen decarboxylase (e), coproporphyrinogen oxidase (f), protoporphyrinogen oxidase (g) and ferrochelatase (h). In normal circumstances, the alternative pathway via DHIC is unlikely to function to any extent; accumulation of $5CO_2H$, as in porphyria cutanea tarda, leads to increased production of DHIC and the isocoproporphyrins derived from it.

pentacarboxylic porphyrinogens as intermediates. Coproporphyrinogen III is then converted to protoporphyrinogen IX by coproporphyrinogen oxidase (EC 1.3.3.39). Since this enzyme does not metabolise coproporphyrinogen I, the pathway becomes isomer-specific at this stage. Finally, protoporphyrinogen IX undergoes enzymatic aromatization to protoporphyrin IX before ferrochelatase (EC 4.99.1.1) catalyses the insertion of ferrous iron to form protohaem. Like ALA synthase, the last three enzymes of the pathway are located in the mitochondrion. Although in theory transport of substrates and haem across the inner mitochondrial membrane provides potential regulatory sites for the control of haem metabolism, there is no evidence to suggest that these processes are important in the pathogenesis of the porphyrias.

It is important to appreciate that, apart from protoporphyrin IX, porphyrinogens rather than porphyrins are intermediates of the pathway (Fig. 9.1). These compounds are colourless, unstable hexahydro derivatives of porphyrins that readily autoxidise to porphyrins within tissues, especially when they accumulate in pathological conditions and during excretion.

Regulation of haem biosynthesis

The pathway of haem biosynthesis is identical in all tissues, but there are major differences between the mechanisms for the regulation of the rate of haem formation in hepatocytes and erythroid cells.[4] In the liver, and probably in all differentiated tissues, the rate of haem synthesis is determined by the activity of the first enzyme of the pathway, 5-aminolaevulinate synthase (ALA synthase). There are two ALA synthase isoenzymes.[5] One is encoded by a gene on chromosome 3 that is expressed in the liver and all other tissues. The other isoenzyme is expressed exclusively in erythroid cells, where it provides the large amount of ALA needed for haemoglobin synthesis, and is encoded by a gene on the X chromosome.

Regulation in liver

In hepatocytes, the activity of ALA synthase appears to be under negative feedback control by haem.[4] Depletion of a regulatory free haem pool leads to an increase in ALA synthase activity which can be prevented by administration of haem. Haem acts by depressing the synthesis of ALA synthase, rather than through direct inhibition of the enzyme. This provides an effective mechanism for the short-term regulation of enzyme activity because the turnover of ALA synthase in mammalian liver is rapid; the half-life of the enzyme in rat liver being about 70 minutes. Haem blocks the synthesis of ALA synthase by two main mechanisms: by inhibiting transcription and by preventing the processing of a precursor form of the enzyme for insertion into mitochondria. The relative importance of these different actions remains uncertain.

The induction of ALA synthase can also be modified by compounds other than haem. Thus, induction is prevented by loading with carbohydrate, while glucocorticoids and possibly other hormones may be required for maximum induction.

A large variety of drugs, chemicals and endogenous compounds, including various steroid metabolites, induce ALA synthase activity in liver cells.[6,7] Many of these substances decrease the concentration of free haem in the regulatory pool and promote the synthesis of new enzyme. Most of the drugs that have this action, for example phenobarbitone, induce microsomal cytochromes of the P_{450} series and the accompanying increase in ALA synthase activity appears to be related to the need to supply the additional haem required for this purpose. Drugs of this type primarily stimulate the synthesis of apocytochrome P_{450} which, by combining with available free haem, depletes the regulatory haem pool and leads to secondary induction of ALA synthase. This mechanism ensures close coordination between haem and apoprotein synthesis. In contrast, a small number of drugs and chemicals produces a much more marked increase in ALA synthase, with massive overproduction of porphyrin by the liver and experimental porphyria. Compounds in this group, for example 2-allyl-2-isopropylacetamide, 3,5-dicarboxyethyl-1, 4-dihydrocollidine and griseofulvin, have two properties: they are lipophilic and stimulate apocytochrome P_{450} synthesis, and they deplete haem by acting as 'suicide' substrates of the cytochrome P_{450} system that undergo oxidative metabolism to compounds that react with the haem moiety to form N-alkylprotoporphyrins, some of which are specific inhibitors of ferrochelatase. Similar enhanced induction of hepatic ALA synthase occurs when a drug that induces apocytochrome P_{450} synthesis is given together with an inhibitor of haem synthesis.

Thus, in the liver, haem synthesis is regulated in a way which enables the supply of haem for microsomal haemoprotein synthesis to change rapidly in response to a wide variety of external stimuli. Impairment of the supply of haem enhances the sensitivity of ALA synthase to induction by a wide variety of common drugs that are metabolised in the liver by the cytochrome P_{450}-dependent monooxygenase system.

Regulation in erythroid cells

The regulation of haem synthesis in erythroid cells appears to be less flexible.[4] Alterations in the rate of haem formation largely reflect changes in the number of cells that differentiate to produce haem. ALA synthase activity increases early in erythroid differentiation and the few factors that stimulate erythroid ALA synthase activity – erythropoietin, hypoxia and some steroid metabolites – may act through promoting differentiation rather than by increasing enzyme activity in individual cells. In reticulocytes, haem inhibits ALA synthase activity directly. In less differentiated cells, haem may also act post-transcriptionally to regulate ALA synthase activity, but the mechanism and significance of this action is unclear. Synthesis of erythroid ALA synthase may also be regulated by iron at the level of translation since its mRNA contains a 5' sequence that is very similar to the iron-responsive elements of ferritin subunit mRNAs.

Co-ordination of haem and globin synthesis in erythroid cells is achieved by a mechanism which involves initiation of globin chain synthesis by haem. The efficiency of the process that terminates haem synthesis when the cell is fully haemoglobinised is such that, in mature erythrocytes, haem is in 26 000-fold molar excess of porphyrin, which is present as zinc-protoporphyrin.

Metabolism and excretion of haem precursors

Under normal circumstances, the total daily excretion of haem precursors represents less than 2.5% of the amount of ALA used for haem synthesis. There is little or no alternative metabolism so the quantities excreted indicate the extent of loss of intermediates from the pathway. Table 9.2

Table 9.2 Haem precursors in normal urine, faeces and blood

	Urine	Faeces	Plasma	Erythrocytes
Porphobilinogen (PBG) (μmol/day)	0–11			
5-aminolaevulinic acid (ALA) (μmol/day)	0–46			
Total porphyrin (nmol/1)	40–320	0–200*	0.5–5.0	90–1690
Porphyrins (mean % of total)				
Proto-	—	72.5		>90
Copro-	76.8	23.5		<10
(% isomer Type III)	(50–60)	(5–15)		
Isocopro-	—	0.03		—
Pentacarboxylic ($5CO_2H$)	2.3	1.7		—
Hexacarboxylic ($6CO_2H$)	0.8	0.6		—
Heptacarboxylic ($7CO_2H$)	4.5	0.2		—
Uro-	15.3	1.0		—

* nmol/g dry weight

shows the reference ranges of haem precursors and their oxidised derivatives in urine, faeces, erythrocytes and plasma.

ALA and PBG are excreted in the urine while porphyrins and porphyrinogens are excreted in the urine and the bile. Hydrophilic porphyrins with more than four acidic side-chains, such as uroporphyrin and heptacarboxylic porphyrin, are preferentially excreted in the urine, while the relatively water-insoluble di- and tricarboxylic porphyrins are restricted to the bile (Table 9.2). Coproporphyrin is excreted by both routes with preferential excretion of the series I isomer in the bile. Impairment of biliary excretion by cholestasis leads to increased urinary excretion of corproporphyrin I. Part of the dicarboxylic 'protoporphyrin' fraction of faeces is formed within the gut, particularly by the action of microorganisms on haem from the diet and other sources. In addition, protoporphyrin is converted to other dicarboxylic porphyrins by the action of the gut flora.[8]

BIOCHEMICAL AND MOLECULAR GENETICS

Enzyme deficiencies

Each type of porphyria results from a partial deficiency of one of the enzymes of haem biosynthesis.[7] The sites of the enzyme defects are listed in Table 9.3. All are inherited, with the exception of some abnormalities of uroporphyrinogen decarboxylase (Table 9.3).

In all the autosomal dominant porphyrias, except erythropoietic protoporphyria, enzyme activities are decreased by approximately 50% (Table 9.3), consistent with the view that most or all of the residual enzyme activity reflects expression of a normal gene allelic to a mutant gene which

Table 9.3 Enzyme deficiencies in the porphyrias. AD – autosomal dominant, AR – autosomal recessive

Defective enzyme	Activity in porphyria (% normal)	Condition	Inheritance	Chromosomal location of defective gene
1. PBG synthase	1–12	PBG synthase deficiency	AR	9q
2. PBG deaminase (uroporphy-rinogen-I-synthase)	47	Acute intermittent porphyria	AD	11q
	17	Homozygous variant		
3. Urophorphyrinogen-III-synthase)	16	Congenital erythropoietic porphyria	AR }	Unknown
4. Uroporphyrinogen decarboxylase	41–65	Type II PCT	AD	1
	40*	Type I PCT	Pathogenesis unknown	
	5–24	Hepatoerythropoietic porphyria	See text	1
	not measured	Toxic PCT	Acquired	
5. Coproporphyrinogen oxidase	48–53	Hereditary coproporphyria	AD	9
	2–10	Homozygous variants		
6. Protoporphyrinogen oxidase	43–55	Variegate porphyria	AD	(?)14
	14	Homozygous variant		
7. Ferrochelatase	28	Erythropoietic protoporphyria	AD	18q

* Decreased activity restricted to the liver

produces little or no active enzyme. Patients who appear to be homozygous for the enzyme deficiencies that underly the autosomal dominant porphyrias have also been described.[7] All have very low enzyme activities (Table 9.3) and some have clinically affected heterozygous relatives, indicating that at least some of the mutations in the autosomal dominant porphyrias depress but do not abolish enzyme activity. In erythropoietic protoporphyria, enzyme activity is lower than would be expected for an autosomal dominant condition (Table 9.3). Activities are closer to 50% of normal in asymptomatic carriers of the gene for erythropoietic protoporphyria and it is possible that some additional factor is needed for clinical expression. An autosomal recessive form of erythropoietic protoporphyria that is clinically indistinguishable from the autosomal dominant type has also been described[9]; its prevalence has yet to be determined.

Consequences of enzyme deficiencies

Metabolic consequences

The pattern of haem precursor overproduction that is typical of each type of porphyria reflects accumulation of substrate proximal to the primary enzyme defect. This response to the enzyme deficiency is brought about through operation of the system for negative feedback control of ALA synthase by haem. In normal circumstances, the K_m values of the enzymes of the pathway of haem biosynthesis are higher than the concentrations of their substrates (Table 9.4). Thus an increase in substrate production, secondary to increased ALA synthase activity, will compensate for

Table 9.4 Enzymes of haem biosynthesis in human liver: activities, K_m values and substrate concentrations. Activities are expressed as nmol ALA or ALA equivalents produced or utilized per hour per mg protein. One mole of porphyrin is equivalent to 8 mole ALA. Mean values or ranges are shown

	Activity (nmol h^{-1} mg^{-1})	Substrate concentration (nmol/g wet weight.)	Apparent K_m (μM)
ALA synthase	0.22	—	11^2 2500^3
PBG synthase	9.8–15.9	0.04 (rat liver)	270
PBG deaminase	0.15	1.0	6.0
Uroporphyrinogen decarboxylase	11.0^1	0.01–0.05 (rat liver)	1.5
Coproporphyrinogen oxidase	13.0	0.04–0.11	0.9
Protoporphyrinogen oxidase	—	—	—
Ferrochelatase	16.6	0.13–0.62	1.8^4 17^5

[1]Pentacarboxylate porphyrinogen III as substrate; [2] Succinyl-CoA; [3]Glycine; [4] Protoporphyrin IX; [5] Fe^{2+}

decreased enzyme activity and restore the rate of haem synthesis to normal. Accumulation of substrate, with its clinical consequences, appears to be the price that is paid for maintaining normal, or near-normal, rates of haem synthesis in the porphyrias.

These compensatory changes do not occur in all tissues in which there is an enzyme defect. In the hereditary hepatic porphyrias, haem precursor accumulation can be detected in the liver but not in the bone marrow, and the liver appears to be the main source of the increased quantities of porphyrins and porphyrin precursors that are excreted. Similarly, increased ALA synthase activity has been detected only in the liver and peripheral blood leucocytes. In spite of the absence of compensatory changes in erythroid cells, anaemia is not a clinical feature of the hepatic porphyrias and haemoglobinisation appears to be unimpaired by the 50% decrease in enzyme activity that is present in these conditions.

The severe enzyme defects that are present in homozygous individuals (Table 9.3) appear to invariably produce accumulation of haem precursors. With the quantitatively less severe defects that are found in the autosomal dominant conditions (Table 9.3), the metabolic consequences vary widely between individuals. Thus similar deficiency of the same enzyme may be associated with marked overproduction of haem precursors in one individual and with no detectable accumulation in another. Much of this variation between individuals seems to be determined by interaction between enzyme defects and acquired factors. In the acute hepatic porphyrias, drugs and steroid hormones are important in this respect, while the role of alcoholic liver disease in the development of overt porphyria cutanea tarda is well-established. However, interaction with other genes may also be important.

Clinical consequences

The clinical consequences of enzyme deficiencies in the haem biosynthetic pathway are directly related to overproduction of haem precursors. Acute porphyria is always associated with overproduction of PBG and ALA: predominantly PBG in the acute hepatic porphyrias (Table 9.1), and predominantly ALA in the very rare PBG synthase (EC 4.2.1.24) deficiency (Table 9.3). PBG and ALA excretion are normal in those conditions in which acute attacks never occur (Table 9.1). The relationship between the biochemical and clinical features of acute porphyria is discussed later.

Skin lesions are seen in all porphyrias in which there is overproduction of porphyrins, or their unstable porphyrinogen or hydroxymethylbilane precursors. Porphyrins are potent photosensitizers so that lesions develop in areas of skin exposed to sunlight. This photodynamic effect of porphyrin requires oxygen and has an action spectrum that resembles the electronic absorption spectrum of porphyrin with a major peak around 400 nm.

Irradiation of porphyrin with light at these wavelengths in the presence of oxygen leads to the formation of singlet oxygen, and possibly other oxygen radicals, that are capable of causing local oxidative damage in skin, perhaps through peroxidation of membrane lipids and the release of hydrolytic enzymes from lysosomes. Histological changes include the presence of PAS-staining material in and around subpapillary capillaries, and non-specific deposition of IgG. In some patients with porphyria cutanea tarda or congenital erythropoietic porphyria, sclerodermatous plaques may occur in either light-exposed or light-protected areas; a change that may be related to stimulation of collagen formation by uroporphyrin.

Latent porphyria

In all types of autosomal dominant porphyria, individuals who have inherited the enzyme defect but have not developed symptoms (latent porphyrics) are much commoner than those with clinically overt porphyria. Many individuals remain asymptomatic throughout life and in a patient who presents with one of these conditions lack of a family history is common and of no diagnostic significance. Some latent porphyrics may show abnormalities of haem precursor excretion or have increased tissue porphyrin concentrations (subclinical porphyria) but others show no detectable biochemical abnormality apart from enzyme deficiency. At present, there is little evidence to suggest that those latent porphyrics with detectable overproduction of haem precursors are more likely to develop symptoms.

Molecular genetics

Each of the enzymes listed in Table 9.3 is encoded by a single autosomal gene that is expressed in all tissues. In recent years, cDNAs have been isolated for all the human enzymes of haem biosynthesis, except coproporphyrinogen and protoporphyrinogen oxidases, and the complete gene structure has been determined for porphobilinogen deaminase, uroporphyrinogen III synthase and uroporphyrinogen decarboxylase.[10–12] Expression of porphobilinogen deaminase is tissue-specific but the other enzymes appear to be identical in all tissues. Thus, with the exception of one type of acute intermittent porphyria, the enzyme deficiencies that produce porphyria are present in all tissues, although the mitochondrial enzymes are absent from mature erythrocytes.

Acute intermittent porphyria

The human porphobilinogen deaminase gene contains 15 exons spread over 10 kb of DNA. Through use of separate tissue-specific promoters and differential RNA splicing, it gives rise to two different mRNAs that encode erythroid and ubiquitous isoenzymes that differ by 17 amino acids at their NH_2 termini.[10] The larger, ubiquitous mRNA is present in all tissues and contains exon 1 and the sequence from exon 3 to exon 15 that is common to both mRNAs. The smaller mRNA is expressed only in erythroid cells, where it is far more abundant than the ubiquitous mRNA, and contains exon 2, which is not translated, and the common sequence.

Acute intermittent porphyria can be divided into three main types by biochemical and genetic studies.[11] In about 85% of patients, the disorder is cross-reacting immunological material (CRIM)-negative with the decrease in catalytic activity of the erythrocyte enzyme being paralleled by a decrease in enzyme mass, as determined immunochemically. Most of the remainder have a CRIM-positive enzyme defect, except for a small number of families in which porphobilinogen deaminase activity and concentration are normal in erythrocytes but decreased in other tissues. Occurrence of this last type of acute intermittent porphyria has been neatly explained by the identification of mutations that produce aberrant splicing of exon 1.[11]

At least 12 different mutations have now been identified by DNA analysis of the other types of acute intermittent porphyria.[12–14] Two point mutations in exon 10 that produce CRIM-positive defects appear to be common in this form of the disease but the mutations responsible for CRIM-negative acute intermittent porphyria are highly heterogeneous: none having been found in more than one family[12], with the exception of the mutation that is responsible for the unusually high frequency of the condition in Lapland.[13]

Other porphyrias

Investigation of the molecular basis of the enzyme deficiencies in other porphyrias has also revealed heterogeneity at the DNA level. Initially, the search for mutations in the uroporphyrinogen decarboxylase gene that cause the autosomal dominant, Type II form of porphyria cutanea tarda (PCT) focused on its presumed homozygous counterpart, hepatoerythropoietic porphyria. All patients with Type II porphyria cutanea tarda appear to have a CRIM-negative enzyme defect but enzymatic and immunochemical studies have shown a range of different enzyme defects in hepatoerythropoietic porphyria.[15] Two different point mutations have now been identified in this condition.[16] Although both produce a CRIM-negative defect in heterozygotes, neither has yet been found in a family with Type II PCT. Direct investigation of patients with Type II PCT has revealed other uroporphyrinogen decarboxylase mutations, one of which was present in 5 of 22 unrelated families that were tested.[17]

A number of different, disease-specific point mutations have also recently been identified in erythropoietic protoporphyria,[9,18] and in the two autosomal recessive porphyrias, porphobilinogen synthase deficiency[19] and congenital erythropoietic porphyria.[20,21]

Bacterial expression systems have been used to investigate the functional effects of a number of missense mutations that have been described.[19–21] In view of the emerging evidence for extensive heterogeneity of mutations in the porphyrias, classification of mutations by their functional effects will probably be required, in addition to clinical studies, if the phenotypic variation between families that is seen in some porphyrias is to be correlated with a particular type of mutation.

THE ACUTE PORPHYRIAS

Acute hepatic porphyrias

The most important clinical feature of the three acute hepatic porphyrias (Table 9.1) is the occurrence of episodic attacks of acute porphyria, which may end fatally. In acute intermittent porphyria, (McKusick 176000) acute attacks are the only clinical manifestation. In hereditary coproporphyria (McKusick 121300) and variegate porphyria (McKusiack 176200), skin lesions, which are indistinguishable from those of porphyria cutanea tarda, also occur (Table 9.1). Almost all patients with hereditary coproporphyria present with acute porphyria; about one-third also have mild skin lesions. In variegate porphyria, the mode of presentation shows some geographical variation. About 60% of South African patients present with skin lesions alone; about 20% have skin lesions and acute porphyria, while the remainder have acute attacks only. A similar pattern is found in the United Kingdom, but in Finland acute attacks predominate.

The acute hepatic porphyrias occur throughout the world. In Europe the prevalence of acute attacks of porphyria is about 2–3 per 100 000 of the population. Most of these attacks are caused by acute intermittent porphyria, with variegate porphyria accounting for no more than one-third and hereditary coproporphyria being uncommon. Since most carriers of the gene for acute intermittent porphyria are asymptomatic, the gene frequency may approach 0.5–1 per 10 000. In South Africa, variegate porphyria provides a classical example of a founder effect with a prevalence as high as 1 : 250 among the White Afrikaans speakers of the Eastern Cape.

Clinical features of acute porphyria

The clinical features of acute porphyria show remarkable constancy, whether they are caused by acute intermittent porphyria, variegate porphyria or hereditary coproporphyria.[22,23] The frequency of acute attacks tends to be lower in hereditary coproporphyria and variegate porphyria than in acute intermittent porphyria.

Acute porphyria is about three times commoner in women than in men, and is most frequent during the third decade in women and the fourth decade in men. Attacks are very uncommon before puberty and do not appear to have been reported before the age of 6 years. At the other extreme, attacks have occurred for the first time after the age of 80. The main symptoms and signs are listed in Table 9.5. Over 90% of patients present with the sudden onset of severe abdominal pain. Some abdominal tenderness is usually present but is much less than expected from the amount of pain. About 60% of patients develop a predominantly motor peripheral neuropathy, usually after the onset of pain. Convulsions are common and, in a patient with abdominal pain, may provide the first indication of the diagnosis. Presentation with a neuropathy that is neither accompanied nor preceded by pain is very rare. Although mental confusion and other psychiatric disorders are common (Table 9.5), they rarely, with the exception of depression, persist beyond the acute phase. Vomiting may be severe, and is one factor contributing to the hyponatraemia, which is a frequent feature. Another cause is inappropriate secretion of antidiuretic hormone which is one of several hypothalamopituitary abnormalities that have been described.[24]

Attacks usually subside after several days but they occasionally persist for weeks or even months. The pattern of attacks is variable. Most patients have fewer than three but they may be multiple or even merge with intermittent exacerbations against a background of chronic pain over many months. Attacks may occur in relation to the menstrual cycle and a few women have regular, disabling premenstrual attacks. About 5% of attacks that are severe enough to require hospitalization end fatally, usually through respiratory paralysis. Weakness, and other neurological sequelae, may remain for years. Persistent hypertension and premature death from chronic renal failure have been reported.

A number of factors are known to precipitate acute porphyria and are implicated in the onset of about 75% of attacks. The list of known precipi-

Table 9.5 Acute porphyria: signs and symptoms. (Adapted from Bonkowsky & Schady[23].)

Symptoms	% of cases	Signs	% of cases
Abdominal pain	95	Tachycardia	80
Extremity pain/paraesthesia	50	Dark urine	74
Constipation	48	Peripheral motor neuropathy	60
Nausea, vomiting	43	Bulbar involvement	46
Mental changes	40	Mental confusion/hallucinations	40
Back pain	29	Hypertension (diastolic > 90 mmHg)	36
Chest pain	12	Absent reflexes	29
Diarrhoea	5	Peripheral sensory neuropathy	26
		Postural hypotension	21
		Palpable dilated loops of bowel	21
		Convulsions	20
		Bladder distension	12
		Coma	10

tants includes more than 100 drugs, hormone preparations, including oral contraceptives, alcohol and low calorie weight-reducing diets.[6] The development of acute attacks is also facilitated by endogenous steroid hormones. Thus some women suffer cyclical premenstrual attacks, and various abnormalities of androgen metabolism, particularly impaired 5-α-hydrogenation of C_{19} and C_{21} metabolites, have been described in symptomatic patients with acute intermittent porphyria.

Biochemical features and pathogenesis of acute porphyria

Attacks of acute hepatic porphyria are accompanied by a number of characteristic biochemical changes. There is a marked increase in urinary PBG and, to a lesser extent, ALA excretion with increased activity of ALA synthase in the liver. Formation of cytochrome P_{450} in the liver is impaired. These changes are similar to those produced in laboratory animals by the combination of inhibition of haem synthesis and induction of apocytochrome P_{450}. Many of the drugs and other compounds that provoke attacks of acute hepatic porphyria are known to induce both cytochrome P_{450} and ALA synthase. It appears that in the acute hepatic porphyrias, the increased demand for haem imposed by these drugs cannot be met because enzyme defects are present that either directly or indirectly limit haem synthesis at the level of PBG deaminase.

All the clinical features of acute porphyria, including the abdominal pain, are neurological in origin, the main histological lesion being axonal degeneration with secondary demyelination. The relationship between the biochemical and neurological abnormalities is unexplained. Of several theories that have been proposed[23], a direct neurotoxic effect of ALA seems to be supported by the most evidence. ALA can cross the blood – brain barrier and is known to have various neuropharmacological actions, while manoeuvres that depress ALA production may be effective therapeutically. In addition, other conditions in which there is excessive formation of ALA, but not PBG, for example PBG synthase deficiency, hereditary tyrosinaemia[25] and lead poisoning are associated with identical or similar neurological syndromes. Nevertheless, little is known about haem metabolism in nervous tissue and the possibility that the enzyme deficiency, which is presumably present in this tissue, has a direct effect within neurones cannot be discounted. It is also unclear whether the mental disturbances arise in the same way as the neuropathy. Haem is a major determinant of tryptophan pyrrolase activity in the liver and disordered tryptophan metabolism has been implicated in the pathogenesis of affective disorders.

Diagnosis of the acute hepatic porphyrias

The diagnosis of an acute attack of acute intermittent porphyria, variegate porphyria or hereditary coproporphyria is established by demonstrating a coincidental increase in urinary PBG excretion (Table 9.6). Virtually all patients with abdominal pain caused by porphyria excrete sufficient PBG to give a positive result with the simple Watson – Schwartz screening test, or one of its modifications, which detect PBG by the red colour given with Ehrlich's reagent (p-dimethylaminobenzaldehyde in acid).[8] However, false positive results may occur and it is essential that all positive tests are confirmed by a specific, quantitative test. In all three conditions PBG excretion is higher during acute attacks than during remission. In both variegate porphyria and hereditary coproporphyria, PBG excretion may fall very rapidly after the onset of symptoms and usually returns to normal in remission. Return to normal is less common in acute intermittent porphyria, but may occur. The diagnosis of acute porphyria cannot be excluded, therefore, particularly when patients present late in the attack,

Table 9.6 Laboratory diagnosis of acute hepatic porphyrias and PBG synthase deficiency. N – no increase in concentration of PBG, ALA or porphyrin. Figures in parentheses give approximate positions of fluorescence emission maxima in aqueous solution at neutral pH

Condition	Increased concentrations			
	Urine	Faeces	Erythrocytes	Plasma
Acute intermittent porphyria (acute attack)	PBG>ALA Porphyrin (mainly due to polymerisation of PBG to uroporphyrin)	N (very occasionally slight increase)	N	PBG ±uroporphyrin (615 nm)
Hereditary coproporphyria (acute attack)	As for acute intermittent porphyria Coproporphyrin III	Coproporphyrin III	N	Coproporphyrin III (615 nm)
Variegate porphyria (acute attack)	As for hereditary coproporphyria	Coproporphyrin III Protoporphyrin (Proto>copro) Porphyrin-X	N	Unidentified porphyrin (626 nm)
Variegate porphyria (cutaneous phase)	±PBG (often normal) Coproporphyrin III (occasionally normal)	As above	N	As above
PBG synthase deficiency	ALA>PBG Coproporphyrin III	N	Zinc-protoporphyrin	

unless PBG and faecal porphyrin excretion are both shown to be normal. In this situation it is important to quantify PBG because the Watson – Schwartz screening test does not detect small, but diagnostic, increases in PBG concentration. Urine containing large amounts of PBG is normal in colour, but darkens to reddish-brown on standing due to the polymerisation of PBG to porphyrins and the brown pigment, porphobilin. These changes may occur before micturition, especially if the urine is acid.

Acute intermittent porphyria, variegate porphyria and hereditary coproporphyria are differentiated by measuring faecal porphyrin concentrations (Table 9.6).[8] In acute intermittent porphyria, faecal porphyrin concentrations are usually normal. Occasional small increases are probably caused by constipation. In both hereditary coproporphyria and variegate porphyria, there is a marked increase in total faecal porphyrin excretion. This increase is caused by coproporphyrin III in hereditary coproporphyria while in variegate porphyria the faeces contain increased concentrations of protoporphyrin IX, coproporphyrin III and a mixture of hydrophilic dicarboxylic porphyrin conjugates of uncertain origin, which have been called peptide-porphyrins or porphyrin-X (Table 9.6; Fig. 9.2). Similar conjugates may be responsible for the presence in plasma of a porphyrin with a fluorescence emission peak at 624–626 nm which is characteristic of variegate porphyria .[8]

There are three main methods for the detection of latent acute intermittent porphyria: measurement of urinary PBG excretion, measurement of erythrocyte PBG deaminase activity and DNA analysis.[8] PBG deaminase measurement is currently the most widely used method because it is able to detect latent acute intermittent porphyria before puberty, when PBG excretion is normal, and in the 70% of adult gene carriers who have normal excretion. However, not all putative gene carriers can be unequivocally assigned by enzyme measurement, because, even for families where the mutation decreases erythrocyte PBG deaminase activity, there is some overlap between the ranges of enzyme activities in normal and affected individuals.[26] In addition, PBG deaminase activity is very dependent on the age distribution of circulating erythrocytes. For this reason, the test is unreliable before the age of 6–8 months and in individuals who are haematologically abnormal. More accurate identification of gene carriers can be achieved by gene tracking, using restriction fragment length polymorphisms (RFLPs) within the PBG deaminase gene[27] or by direct detection of mutations, but these approaches are restricted to the 50% or so of families in which the RFLPs are potentially informative and to those families in which the mutation can be identified. Although the latter approach is complicated by the extensive molecular heterogeneity of the disorder, it seems likely to become the method of choice. Prenatal diagnosis of acute intermittent porphyria is practicable but is rarely indicated.

Latent variegate porphyria and hereditary coproporphyria are most simply detected by measurement of faecal porphyrin concentrations;

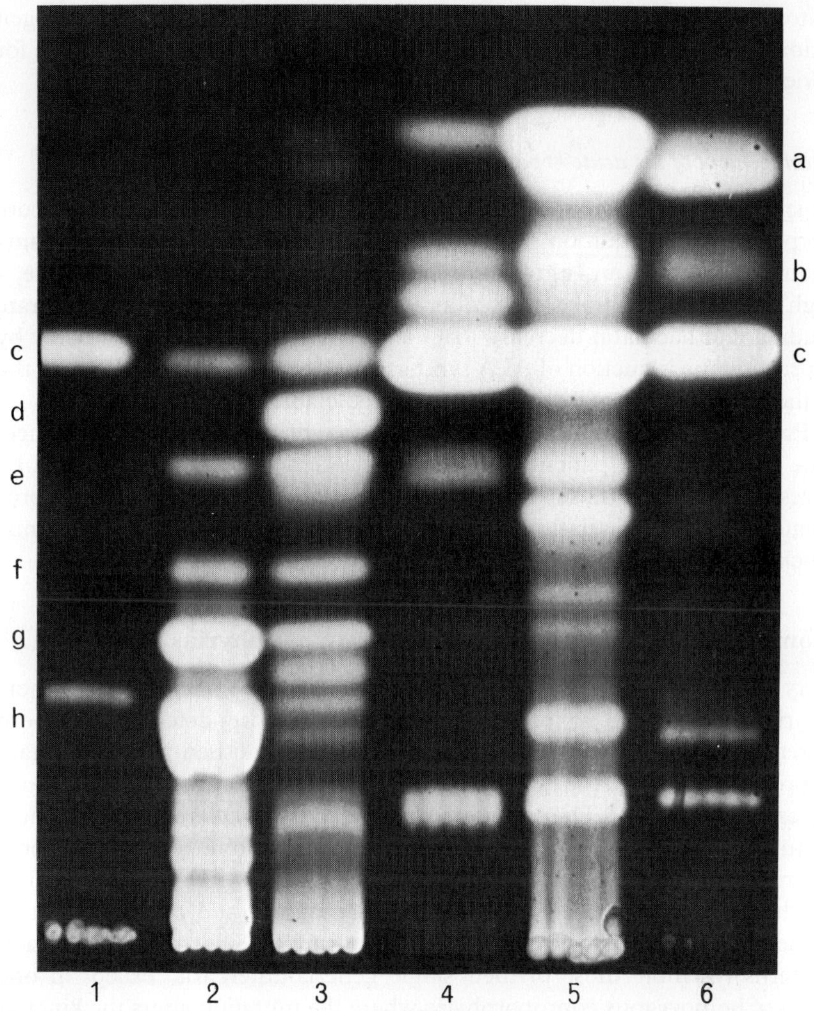

Fig. 9.2 Porphyrin excretion patterns. Thin-layer chromatogram of the methyl ester derivatives of porphyrins from urine and faeces. Tracks show porphyrins from: 1 normal urine; 2 porphyria cutanea tarda urine; 3 porphyria cutanea tarda faeces; 4 hereditary coproporphyria faeces; 5 variegate porphyria faeces; 6 normal faeces. a protophyrin and other dicarboxylic porphyrins; b tricarboxylic porphyrin; c coproporphyrin; d isocoproporphyrin; e–g penta-, hexa- and heptacarboxylic porphyrin; h uroporphyrin. The silica gel plate was developed with toluene:ethylacetate:ethanol (80:15:3, by volume) and photographed in uv light.

urinary PBG and porphyrin excretion are usually normal (Table 9.6). However, in both conditions, faecal porphyrin excretion is normal before puberty and in at least 20% of adult carriers of the genes. Identification of latent porphyria in putative gene carriers in these categories, or when faecal analyses are equivocal, requires measurement of the appropriate mitochondrial enzyme in lymphocytes or fibroblasts: coproporphyrinogen oxidase for hereditary coproporphyria and protoporphyrinogen oxidase for variegate porphyria (Table 9.3).

Management of the acute hepatic porphyrias

In spite of recent improvements, there is still no reliable therapy for acute porphyria.[22] In addition to general supportive measures, precipitants should be removed and intravenous haem arginate or, if this is unavailable, a high carbohydrate intake, started as soon as possible.[28] Both carbohydrate loading and haematin decrease PBG and ALA production, presumably by repressing the induction of ALA synthase in the liver; but their effect on the clinical progression of the attack is less predictable.

Prevention of the acute attack remains of paramount importance. The relatives of all patients who present with acute porphyria should be investigated so that those identified as latent porphyrics can be given appropriate advice, particularly about the need to avoid known precipitants. Cyclical premenstrual attacks may be prevented by LH-RH inhibitors.[29]

Homozygous variants of the acute hepatic porphyrias

Very rarely patients are encountered who have inherited coproporphyrinogen oxidase or protoporphyrinogen oxidase defects from both parents (Table 9.3).[30] These conditions are distinguished from hereditary coproporphyria and variegate porphyria by the appearance of skin lesions in early childhood. They are otherwise clinically heterogeneous. Short stature has been reported in some patients with homozygous coproporphyria and in homozygous variegate porphyria, while a neurological syndrome of mental retardation, ocular nystagmus and fits is present in some cases of homozygous variegate porphyria. Porphyrin excretion patterns resemble those of their single gene counterparts, except in one form of homozygous coproporphyria where the mutation alters the kinetics of the enzyme so that a tricarboxylic porphyrinogen intermediate of the reaction, harderoporphyrinogen, accumulates.

Compound homozygotes for mutations that cause acute intermittent porphyria have also been described recently.[31,30] Of three affected children from two families, two had different developmental abnormalities of the brain but typical attacks of acute porphyria have not yet been reported.

PBG synthase deficiency porphyria (McKuisick 125270)

This condition has been described in four unrelated families (Table 9.3).[19] Clinical manifestations included failure to thrive in infancy, attacks of abdominal pain and polyneuropathy during adolescence, closely resembling those seen in the acute hepatic porphyrias, and subacute polyneuropathy during the seventh decade. Attacks were accompanied by a marked increase in the urinary excretion of ALA and coproporphyrin III with only a minimal increase in PBG excretion, and increased zinc-protoporphyrin in erythrocytes.

Two other conditions are known in which there is severe inhibition of PBG synthase: lead poisoning and hereditary tyrosinaemia (tyrosinosis). In lead poisoning, the pattern of haem precursor overproduction is very similar to that found in PBG synthase deficiency but the two conditions can be distinguished by measuring the blood lead concentration and by family studies. In hereditary tyrosinaemia (p. 183), where PBG synthase is specifically inhibited by the abnormal metabolite, succinylacetone, increased excretion of ALA is unaccompanied by any abnormality of porphyrin metabolism. These differences have not been explained.

PORPHYRIA CUTANEA TARDA AND RELATED SYNDROMES

Porphyria cutanea tarda is the commonest type of porphyria in Europe and North America. Unlike other types of porphyria it is not a distinct entity with a well-defined pattern of inheritance but an aetiologically diverse group of conditions that share the same primary enzyme defect: decreased activity of uroporphyrinogen decarboxylase in the liver (Table 9.3).

All types of porphyria cutanea tarda, and the rarer allied conditions that also result from uroporphyrinogen decarboxylase deficiency (Table 9.3), have certain characteristics in common. Their sole clinical features are cutaneous and, although their severity may vary, the skin lesions that result from porphyrin accumulation are indistinguishable from those in congenital erythropoietic porphyria, variegate porphyria, and hereditary coproporphyria. Acute attacks of porphyria do not occur and patients do not react adversely to barbiturates and the other lipophilic compounds that precipitate acute porphyria. All have a similar pattern of overproduction of haem precursors which is characteristic of uroporphyrinogen decarboxylase deficiency. Uroporphyrin and other acetic acid substituted porphyrins derived from the substrate and intermediates of the uroporphyrinogen decarboxylase reaction (Fig. 9.1), are excreted in excess and accumulate in the liver. Typically, the urine contains large amounts of uroporphyrin and heptacarboxylic porphyrin, while isocoproporphyrin and heptacarboxylic porphyrin predominate in faeces (Fig. 9.2). Uroporphyrin is mainly the Type I isomer; heptacarboxylic porphyrin is almost entirely Type III. PBG excretion is always normal.

Porphyria cutanea tarda

Classification

Porphyria cutanea tarda can be divided into two main types by measuring uroporphyrinogen decarboxylase in erythrocytes.[31] In Type I, or sporadic, porphyria cutanea tarda (McKusick 176090), erythrocyte uroporphyrinogen decarboxylase activity is normal and there is no family history of overt porphyria. In Type II, or familial, porphyria cutanea tarda (McKusick 176100), which accounts for 20–30% of patients in most parts of the world, uroporphyrinogen decarboxylase activity is decreased to about 50% of normal in erythrocytes and all other tissues that have been investigated. This defect is inherited as an autosomal dominant characteristic, and is frequently latent. In addition, there are rare families in which porphyria cutanea tarda affects more than one individual yet erythrocyte uroporphyrinogen decarboxylase activity is normal. There is also a toxic form of porphyria cutanea tarda which results from exposure to polyhalogenated aromatic hydrocarbons, notably hexachlorobenzene and 2,3,7,8-tetrachlorodibenzo-p-dioxin.

Clinical features

Porphyria cutanea tarda usually presents during the fourth to sixth decades and is commoner in men. The familial type tends to occur at a younger age. Onset before the age of 20 is a strong indicator of the familial type but otherwise, in the absence of a family history, the familial and sporadic types cannot be distinguished clinically. The commonest clinical feature is increased fragility of the skin with superficial erosions, most characteristically on the backs of the hands, following trivial trauma. The next most frequent symptom, and the usual reason for seeking medical advice, is the appearance of subepidermal vesicles and bullae. These break to form erosions which heal slowly and often leave atrophic scars. Milia are common in areas which suffer repeated trauma. Other common features are hypertrichosis, pigmentation and scleroderma-like lesions.

Many patients with porphyria cutanea tarda show some evidence of iron overload. About 85% of those undergoing liver biopsy have some degree of hepatic siderosis with stainable iron in parenchymal cells. Siderosis is usually no more than moderate; deposition of iron to the extent seen in haemochromatosis is unusual. Total body iron stores are slightly to moderately increased in about three-quarters of European patients. However, although porphyria cutanea tarda has been recorded in association with idiopathic haemochromatosis and other iron storage disorders, it is a very rare complication of these conditions and experimental iron does not appear to be a direct consequence of iron overload.

Most adults with porphyria cutanea tarda have some associated conditions, usually affecting the liver.[31] The commonest is alcoholic liver disease, but porphyria cutanea tarda has been reported in many other types of liver disease, including chronic active hepatitis, infective hepatitis, haemochromatosis and various granulomatous conditions. Liver disease is usually mild and only revealed by investigation, although in some series as many as 30% of patients have been reported to have cirrhosis. Only a minority present with liver disease and are then found to have porphyria cutanea tarda. After alcohol, the most important aetiological factor is oestrogen therapy. In recent years, the widespread use of oestrogens in oral contraceptive and other preparations has led to an increased prevalence of porphyria cutanea tarda in women. Even in this group the liver may be histologically abnormal with some peripheral inflammation and focal hepatocellular necrosis. Porphyria cutanea tarda is also associated with systemic lupus erythromatosus and occurs with increased frequency in patients undergoing long-term haemodialysis. About 15% of patients have diabetes mellitus. Hepatoma may develop in long-standing cases of porphyria cutanea tarda, and there is some evidence that the incidence of this complication is greater than in other types of long-standing liver disease. In general, the prognosis of porphyria cutanea tarda is largely related to the severity of the underlying liver disease.

Subclinical porphyria cutanea tarda appears to be more frequent than the overt condition. Surveys of patients with chronic liver disease and of chronic alcoholics have shown that abnormalities of porphyrin metabolism, of the type found in patients with porphyria cutanea tarda who have gone into clinical remission, may be present in 10–20%. Although some of these patients undoubtedly have subclinical porphyria cutanea tarda, there is no direct evidence that the abnormalities in the majority, particularly those in which coproporphyrin excretion predominates, are related to porphyria cutanea tarda.

Laboratory diagnosis of porphyria cutanea tarda

Porphyria cutanea tarda and other uroporphyrinogen decarboxylase defects can be distinguished from all other types of porphyria by demonstrating the characteristic pattern of porphyrin excretion in urine and faeces, and by showing that erythrocyte porphyrin concentration is normal (Table 9.7; Fig. 9.2).[8] Omission of faecal porphyrin analysis may lead to misdiagnosis, since a few patients with variegate porphyria have a urinary porphyrin excretion pattern that is indistinguishable from porphyria cutanea tarda. Urinary, faecal and plasma porphyrin concentrations decrease during remission, eventually returning to normal. The abnormal porphyrin excretion pattern persists after total urinary and faecal porphyrin concentrations have become normal, until in prolonged remission the pattern also eventually becomes normal. The liver contains high concentrations of uroporphyrin and heptacarboxylic porphyrin. Needle biopsy samples show bright red fluorescence due to porphyrin when viewed in long-wave ultraviolet light, and hepatocytes contain needle-like inclusions, resembling uroporphyrin crystals, which appear to be a specific feature of porphyria cutanea tarda.

A small number of patients with a condition that is clinically indistin-

Table 9.7 Laboratory diagnosis of the cutaneous porphyrias. Figures in parentheses give approximate positions of fluorescence emission maxima in aqueous solution at neutral pH. N – no increase in concentration of PBG, ALA or porphyrin; 5-, 6-, 7–CO_2H – penta-, hexa-, heptacarboxylic porphyrinogen

	Increased concentrations			
Condition	Urine	Faeces	Erythrocytes	Plasma
Porphyria cutanea tarda (PCT)	Uroporphyrin (30% III) $7CO_2H$ (>90% III) (uro>7 CO_2H) Smaller amounts of 6-, 5-CO_2H, and copro	Isocoproporphyrin $7CO_2H$ Smaller amounts of copro, 6-,5-CO_2H and uro	N	Uroporphyrin (615 nm)
Congenital erythropoietic porphyria (CEP)	Uroporphyrin (>80% I) Coproporphyrin (>80% I) (Uro>copro)	Coproporphyrin I	Uroporphyrin I Coproporphyrin I ±Zinc-protoporphyrin	Uroporphyrin I (615 nm)
Protoporphyria (PP)	N	Protoporphyrin IX, about 40% of patients	Protoporphyrin IX (Proto>> Zn-proto)	Protoporphyrin IX (634 nm)

guishable from porphyria cutanea tarda have been shown to have porphyrin-producing hepatic tumours.[32]

Treatment

Porphyria cutanea tarda is the only form of porphyria for which specific and effective treatments exist.[33] The treatment of choice is reduction of total body iron stores to the verge of iron-deficiency by repeated venesection. This manoeuvre is invariably followed by remission which may be prolonged for many years or even be permanent. Treatment with low-dose chloroquine is as effective for producing clinical remission, but relapse may be more frequent and the theoretical possibility of exacerbating the underlying liver cell damage has not been entirely excluded. Neither treatment is dependent on withdrawal of aetiological agents, such as alcohol and oestrogens, although this should be encouraged and may in itself lead to prolonged remission.

Pathogenesis of porphyria cutanea tarda

The low activity of uroporphyrinogen decarboxylase in the liver during the symptomatic phase of porphyria cutanea tarda appears to be caused by a process that specifically inactivates the enzyme without decreasing its concentration.[31] This process is reversible, so that hepatic uroporphyrinogen decarboxylase activity eventually returns to normal in Type I porphyria cutanea tarda after prolonged clinical remission. It is likely that the same process operates in the autosomal dominant, Type II form of the disorder, although here susceptibility to develop symptoms is enhanced because the level of the target enzyme in hepatocytes is already decreased to half-normal by mutation.

The nature of the inactivation process is uncertain.[31] It appears to be iron-dependent, and experiments on the analogous porphyria that is produced in animals by polycyclic aromatic hydrocarbons suggest that it requires an intermediate of haem biosynthesis and is enhanced by induction of microsomal cytochromes of the P_{4501A} subfamily. One current theory is that uroporphyrinogen is oxidised by a cytochrome P_{450}-dependent reaction that, in the presence of iron, produces a catalytic site-directed inhibitor of uroporphyrinogen decarboxylase. However, at present there is no direct evidence for such a mechanism in humans.

The apparent predisposition of certain patients with common disorders such as alcoholic liver cell damage to develop porphyria cutanea tarda is also unexplained; particularly as it is now clear that the existence of an autosomal dominantly inherited enzyme deficiency provides only a partial explanation for the minority of patients with Type II disease. The predisposition may be explained by postulating that a number of factors contributing to the inactivation process need to come together in an individual patient [31] or, alternatively, the possibility has not been excluded that patients with porphyria cutanea tarda have inherited an enzyme variant that is susceptible to inactivation in the liver.

Other uroporphyrinogen decarboxylase defects

Hepatoerythropoietic porphyria (McKusick 176100)

A total of 11 cases of hepatoerythropoietic porphyria have been reported since its first description in 1969. The condition presents in early childhood with skin lesions similar to those of porphyria cutanea tarda.[15,30] In older children and adults, the persistence of severe skin lesions with associated infection, scarring and atrophy may lead to photomutilation. Porphyrin is deposited in bone, and the teeth may show red fluorescence in ultraviolet light, although they do not become as visibly discoloured by porphyrin as in congenital erythropoietic porphyria. Liver disease is absent or minimal, and patients may survive to the age of 60 or more.

The porphyrin excretion pattern is variable but in general closely resembles that of porphyria cutanea tarda. However, in hepatoerythropoietic porphyria, the concentration of zinc-protoporphyrin and, to a lesser extent, free protoporphyrin is moderately increased in erythrocytes. Erythrocyte uroporphyrinogen decarboxylase activity is decreased to less than 10% of normal (Table 9.3) and a similarly severe enzyme defect appears to be present in nucleated cells.

Uroporphyrinogen decarboxylase deficiency and dyserythropoiesis

A patient with severe photomutilation, a porphyria cutanea tarda-like pattern of porphyrin excretion, an inherited 50% reduction of erythrocyte uroporphyrinogen decarboxylase activity, minimal increase in liver proporphyrin concentration and dyserythropoietic anaemia has been described by Kushner et al.[34]

OTHER CUTANEOUS PORPHYRIAS

Congenital erythropoietic porphyria (McKusick 263700)

Clinical features

Congenital erythropoietic porphyria is an uncommon, severe, cutaneous disorder that was first described in 1874.[35] Most patients present in early infancy, either with severe skin lesions of the type seen in porphyria cutanea tarda, or because red urine, due to the presence of large amounts of porphyrin, is noted before the onset of skin symptoms. Photosensitisation is severe and frequently leads to gross photomutilation. Erythrodontia, a brown discoloration of the teeth due to deposition of porphyrin, is common. Haemolytic anaemia, probably caused by the action of light on porphyrin-containing erythrocytes in superficial capillaries, is a frequent complication. Its severity varies greatly both with time in individual patients and from patient to patient; in many patients it contributes to the poor prognosis with few patients surviving beyond the age of 40 years. A mild, late-onset, type of congenital erythropoietic porphyria, which presents in late childhood or adult life and is clinically indistinguishable from porphyria cutanea tarda, has been described.[35]

Biochemical features and laboratory diagnosis

Deficiency of uroporphyrinogen III synthase is the primary inherited enzyme defect in congenital erythropoietic porphyria. Activity is decreased to the same extent in the classical and late-onset forms (Table 9.3). The low activity of uroporphyrinogen III synthase leads to massive overproduction of uroporphyrinogen I which is presumably formed by non-enzymatic cyclisation of accumulated hydroxymethylbilane (Fig. 9.1). Uroporphyrinogen I is decarboxylated to coproporphyrinogen I but cannot be metabolised further. The main site of overproduction is the bone marrow. Erythroid cells contain large amounts of porphyrinogens, and porphyrins derived from them by oxidation, and thus show characteristic red autofluorescence in ultraviolet light. Formation of haem from uroporphyrinogen III is not decreased, and in many patients may be considerably increased due to the presence of haemolytic anaemia.

The diagnosis of congenital erythropoietic porphyria is established by analysis of the isomer type of the excreted porphyrins and by measurement of porphyrins in erythrocytes (Table 9.7).

Management

The treatment of congenital erythropoietic porphyria is aimed at preventing exposure to sunlight and at controlling the haemolytic anaemia.[35] However, such measures do no more than ameliorate the condition. The severe photomutilation, restricted lifestyle, and relatively poor prognosis, make congenital erythropoietic porphyria probably the only porphyria in which prevention by termination following prenatal diagnosis should be considered for all families. Measurements of uroporphyrinogen III synthase in cultured amnion cells and of uroporphyrin I in amniotic fluid have been used for this purpose[35] but are likely to be superseded by DNA techniques.

Erythropoietic protoporphyria (McKusick 177000)

In most countries, protoporphyria (erythropoietic protoporphyria) is less common than porphyria cutanea tarda. Many individuals who inherit the gene for protoporphyria show no abnormality other than decreased ferrochelatase activity, and the risk of a gene carrier developing symptoms has been estimated at less than 10%.

Clinical features

In contrast to all other cutaneous porphyrias, the dominant feature of protoporphyria is acute photosensitivity.[36] Onset usually occurs during early childhood but may be delayed until adult life. Exposure to sunlight provokes burning, itching or painful sensations in the skin which are accompanied by slight oedema and reddening. Vesicle formation is uncommon. Repeated episodes of oedema and erythema may lead to some thickening and lichenification, particularly over the bridge of the nose and the backs of the hands. Skin fragility, hypertrichosis and pigmentation do not occur. Patients may be very pale due to many years of assiduous avoidance of sunlight. Some patients have a mild hypochromic, microcytic anaemia, and there is an increased incidence of cholelithiasis with the formation of stones that contain protoporphyrin IX. However, the most important complication is liver disease. Minor abnormalities of biochemical liver function tests and deposits of protoporphyrin in the liver are common; but a small minority of patients develop cirrhosis and hepatic failure which is rapidly fatal.[37]

Biochemical features and laboratory diagnosis

Erythropoietic protoporphyria is characterised biochemically by an increased concentration of free protoporphyrin IX in erythrocytes. Erythrocyte protoporphyrin concentrations may also be increased in lead poisoning, in iron deficiency and in some anaemias.[38] However in these conditions, as in normal subjects, virtually all the protoporphyrin is present as its zinc chelate, whereas in erythropoietic protoporphyria free, uncomplexed protoporphyrin predominates. In addition, plasma protoporphyrin concentrations are increased in erythropoietic protoporphyria but not in the other conditions. Urinary porphyrin excretion is normal but faecal protoporphyrin concentrations are increased in about 40% of patients (Table 9.7).

Identification of the major site of protoporphyrin production in this condition has been controversial. In most patients, erythroid cells appear to be the main source of excess protoporphyrin. Porphyrin accumulates during the later stages of erythroid maturation but, as circulating erythrocytes mature, some leaks into the plasma to be excreted by the liver into the bile. However production of protoporphyrin by the liver may also be increased. Most of this probably enters the bile, although some plasma porphyrin may be of hepatic origin. The source of the protoporphyrin that accumulates in the liver as crystalline deposits, and which may cause liver cell damage leading to hepatic failure, is unclear.

Management

Photosensitivity in protoporphyria can usually be controlled by administration of sufficient β-carotene to produce photoprotective pigmentation of the skin.[39] The management and prevention of liver disease has been less successful. At present, there is no reliable method for predicting which patients are likely to develop this complication. Patients with abnormal liver function tests, or very high red cell and plasma protoporphyrin concentrations, should undergo liver biopsy. Cholestyramine has been used to interrupt the enterohepatic circulation of protoporphyrin, and thus lessen accumulation in the liver, and may reverse early hepatic damage in some patients. This and other approaches to treatment of the liver disease, including transplantation, have been reviewed.[37]

REFERENCES

1. Doss M 1988 New dual form of porphyria. Lancet 1:945–6
2. Day R S, Eales L, Meissner D 1982 Coexistent variegate porphyria and porphyria cutanea tarda. New England Journal; of Medicine 307:36–41
3. Qadiri M R, Church S E, McColl K E L et al 1986 Chester porphyria – a clinical study of a new form of acute porphyria. British Medical Journal 292:455–9
4. Dierks P 1990 Molecular biology of eukaryotic 5-amino-levulinate synthase. In: Daley H (ed) Biosynthesis of heme and chlorophylls. McGraw– Hill, New York, p 201–233

5. Sutherland G R, Baker E, Callen D F et al 1988 American Journal of Human Genetics 43:331–335
6. Moore M R, Disler P B 1983 Drug-induction of the acute porphyrias. Advances in Drug Reactions and Acute Poisons Review 2:149–189
7. Nordmann Y, Deyback J-C 1990 Human hereditary porphyrias. In: Daley H (ed) Biosynthesis of heme and chlorophylls. McGraw–Hill, New York, p 491–542
8. Elder G H, Smith S G, Smyth S J 1990 Laboratory investigation of the porphyrias. Annals of Clinical Biochemistry 27:395–412
9. Lamoril J, Boulechfar S, de Verneuil H et al 1991 Human erythropoietic protoporphyria: two point mutations in the ferrochelatase gene. Biochemical and Biophysical Research Communications 181:594–599.
10. Chretien S, Dubait A, Beaupain D et al 1988 Alternative transcription and splicing of the human porphobilinogen deaminase gene result either in tissue-specific or in housekeeping expression. Proceedings of the National Academy of Sciences USA 85:6–10
11. Grandchamp B, Nordmann Y 1988 Enzymes of the heme biosynthesis pathway: Recent advances in molecular genetics. Seminars in Hematology 25:303–311
12. Delfau M H, Picat C, De Rooij F et al 1991 Molecular heterogeneity of acute intermittent porphyria: Identification of four additional mutations resulting in the CRIM-negative subtype of the disease. American Journal of Human Genetics 49:421–428
13. Lee J-S, Anvret M 1991 Identification of the most common mutation within the porphobilinogen deaminase gene in Swedish patients with acute intermittent porphyria. Proceedings of the National Academy of Sciences USA 88:10912–10915
14. Llewellyn D H, Scobie G A, Urquhart A J et al 1992 Splice defective mutations of the porphobilinogen, deaminase gene are responsible for acute intermittent porphyria. Netherlands Journal of Medicine 42: A28
15. Koszo F, Elder G H, Roberts A et al 1990 Uroporphyrinogen decarboxylase deficiency in hepatoerythropoietic porphyria: Further evidence for genetic heterogeneity. British Journal of Dermatology 122:365–370
16. Romana M, Grandchamp B, Dubart A et al 1991 Identification of a new mutation responsible for hepatoerythropoietic porphyria 21:225–229
17. Garey J R, Harrison L M, Franklin K F et al 1990 Uroporphyrinogen decarboxylase: A splice site mutation causes the deletion of exon 6 in multiple families with porphyria cutanea tarda. Journal of Clinical Investigation 86:1416–1422
18. Nakahashi Y, Fujita H, Taketani S et al 1992 The molecular defect of ferrochelatase in a patient with erythropoietic protoporphyria. Proceedings of the National Academy of Sciences USA 89:281–285
19. Plewinska M, Thunell S, Holmberg L et al 1991 δ-Amino-levulinate dehydratase deficient porphyria: Identification of the molecular lesions in a severely affected homozygote. American Journal of Human Genetics 49:167–174
20. Boulechfar S, Da Silva V, Deybach J-C et al 1992 Heterogeneity of mutations in the uroporphyrinogen III synthase gene in congenital erythropoietic porphyria. Human Genetics 88:320–324
21. Warner C A, Yoo H-W, Roberts A G, Desnick R J 1992 Congenital erythropoietic porphyria — identification and expression of an exonic mutation in the uroporphrinogen III synthase gene. Journal of Clinical Investigation 89:693–700
22. Brodie M J, Goldberg A 1980 Acute hepatic porphyrias. Clinics in Haematology 9:253–272
23. Bonkowsky H L, Schady W 1982 Neurologic manifestations of acute porphyria. Seminars in Liver Disease 2:108–124
24. Brodie M J, Graham D J M, Goldberg A et al 1978 Thyroid function in acute intermittent porphyria: a neurogenic cause of hyperthyroidism. Hormone and Metabolic Research 10:327–331
25. Mitchell G, Larochelle J, Lambert M et al 1990 Neurologic crises in hereditary tyrosinemia. New England Journal of Medicine 322:432–437
26. Pierach C A, Wierner M K, Cardinal R A et al 1987 Red blood cell porphobilinogen deaminase in the evaluation of acute intermittent porphyria. Journal of the American Medical Association 257:60–61

27. Lee J-S, Anvret M, Lindsten J et al 1988 DNA polymorphisms within the porphobilinogen deaminase gene in two Swedish families with acute intermittent porphyria. Human Genetics 79:379–381
28. Moore M R, McColl K E L 1989 Therapy of the acute porphyrias. Clinical Biochemistry 22:181–188
29. Anderson K E, Spitz I M, Sassa S et al 1984 Prevention of cyclical attacks of acute intermittent porphyria with a long-acting agonist of luteinizing hormone-releasing factor. New England Journal of Medicine 311:643–645
30. Elder G H 1992 Disorders of porphyrin metabolism. In: Soldin S J, Rifai N, Hich J M (eds) The biochemical basis of pediatric disease. American Association for Clinical Chemistry Press, Washington DC, p 475–494
31. Elder G H 1990 Porphyria cutanea tarda: A multifactorial disease. In: Champion R H (ed) Recent advances in dermatology. (Number 8) Churchill Livingstone, Edinburgh, p 55–70
32. O'Reilly K, Snape J, Moore M R 1988 Porphyria cutanea tarda resulting from primary hepatocellular carcinoma. Clinical and Experimental Dermatology 13:44–48
33. Rocchi E, Gilbertini P, Casanelli M et al 1986 Iron removal therapy in porphyria cutanea tarda : phlebotomy versus slow subcutaneous desferrioxamine infusion. British Journal of Dermatology 114:621–629
34. Kushner J P, Barbuto A J, Lee G R 1976 An inherited enzymic defect in porphyria cutanea tarda. Decreased uroporphyrinogen decarboxylase activity. Journal of Clinical Investigation 58:1089–1097
35. Nordmann Y, Deybach J C 1982 Congenital erythropoietic porphyria. Seminars in Liver Disease 2:154–163
36. De Leo V, Poh-Fitzpatrick M, Matthews-Roth M et al 1976 Erythropoietic protoporphyria. 10 years experience. American Journal of Medicine 60:8–22
37. Rank J M, Straka J G, Bloomer J R 1990 Liver in disorders of porphyrin metabolism. Journal of Gastroenterology and Hepatology 5:573–585
38. McColl K E L, Goldberg A 1980 Abnormal porphyrin metabolism in disease other than porphyria. Clinics in Haematology 9:427–444
39. Matthews-Roth M M, Pathak M A, Fitzpatrick T B et al 1974 Beta-carotene as an oral photoprotective agent in erythropoietic protoporphyria. Journal of the American Medical Association 228:1004–1008

10. Collagen disorders

A. C. Nicholls

INTRODUCTION

The collagens constitute the most ubiquitous proteins in the animal kingdom. They comprise the major structural components of diverse connective tissues including skin, bone, tendon, ligament, cornea, cartilage, blood vessel walls, gut, kidney glomeruli, liver and lungs. The physical and mechanical properties necessary for the correct function of these tissues depend upon the formation, with exquisite precision, of large supramolecular structures and their proper interaction with other matrix components such as elastin, laminin, nidogen, fibronectin, proteoglycans and glycoproteins. There is also substantial evidence that collagens play a major role in fetal development. It is hardly surprising, therefore, that a large number of clinical syndromes presenting with a wide variety of symptoms are either known or strongly suspected of being caused by abnormalities of collagenous proteins. We can include in these several osteochondrodysplasias, the various Ehlers–Danlos syndromes, some forms of epidermolysis bullosa, cutis laxa and even more common disorders such as cerebral aneurisms, osteoarthritis and osteoporosis.

Recent years have seen the dawning of a new age of molecular biology, with the advent of the polymerase chain reaction and techniques for identifying subtle DNA abnormalities facilitating rapid progress in the identification of causal mutations and the understanding of the molecular pathology in many of these diseases. One disease, the Marfan syndrome, long suspected of being a collagen disorder, has now been shown to involve defects in another extracellular matrix component (see later).

This chapter reviews the current knowledge of the family of collagen proteins, their genes and biosynthesis and then considers how genetic defects in these proteins cause a number of inherited diseases of connective tissue.

THE COLLAGEN FAMILY OF PROTEINS

Collagen was once defined as a protein that displayed a characteristic X-ray diffraction pattern indicative of a coiled-coil triple helical structure, which had glycine as one-third of the total amino acid residues and which contained two unusual amino acids, hydroxylysine and hydroxyproline. At the time only one protein met these criteria, namely the protein that constituted the major component of skin, tendon and bone. The first evidence for molecular diversity came in 1969 with the discovery that cartilage contained a distinct collagen species:[1] soon after, a third molecular species was identified in fetal skin, blood vessel walls and leiomyomas.[2, 3] Since then the number of proteins included in this family has risen to 14 (Table 10.1) and involves the products of at least 25 different genes. There are other proteins, for example Clq from complement, acetylcholinesterase, conglutinin and surfactant protein that contain so-called collagenous domains but do not participate in supramolecular structures in the extracellular matrix and so are excluded from the collagen family. All collagens are composed of 'collagenous' and 'non-collagenous' domains, the relative proportions of these vary with the collagen type and determine the nature of the supramolecular organization. The 'collagenous' domains have glycine as one-third of the total residues and a high content of imino acids, they also contain the characteristic amino acids, hydroxyproline and hydroxylysine. The primary structure of these domains has a repetitive Gly-X-Y pattern where X is often proline and Y is often hydroxyproline, but can be almost any amino acid. In the native molecule three polypeptide chains, themselves in a polyproline-

Table 10.1 Collagen types, structure, and distribution

Type	Chain Composition	Structure	Distribution
I	$\alpha 1(I)_2\alpha 2(I)$	67 nm banded fibrils	Skin, bone, tendon, lung, ligament, vascular system
I (trimer)	$\alpha 1(I)_3$	67 nm banded fibrils	Embryonic tendon, skin, membranous bones
II	$\alpha 1(II)_3$	67 nm banded fibrils	Hyaline cartilage, intervertebral disc, vitreous humour
III	$\alpha 1(III)_3$	67 nm banded fibrils	Blood vessels, skin, lung, gut
IV	$\alpha 1(IV)_2\alpha 2(IV)$, $\alpha 1(IV)$, $\alpha 2(IV)$, $\alpha 3(IV)\alpha 4(IV)$, $\alpha 5(IV)$	3-D mesh network	Basement membranes
V	$\alpha 1(V)_2\alpha 2(V)$, $\alpha 1(V)\alpha 2(V)\alpha 3(V)$	67 nm banded fibril	Skin, periosteum, placental membranes
VI	$\alpha 1(VI)\alpha 2(VI)\alpha 3(VI)$	100 nm microfibrils	Skin, cartilage, blood vessel intima, placenta
VII	$\alpha 1(VII)_3$	anchoring fibrils	Skin, foetal membranes
VIII	$\alpha 1(VIII)$, $\alpha 2(VIII)$?	hexagonal lattice?	Descemets membrane
IX	$\alpha 1(IX)\alpha 2(IX)\alpha 3(IX)$	fibril associated	Cartilage, vitreous humour
X	$\alpha 1(X)_3$	?	Hypertrophic cartilage
XI	$\alpha 1(XI)\alpha 2(XI)\alpha 3(XI)$? other forms?	67 nm banded fibril	Hyaline cartilage
XII	$\alpha 1(XII)_3$?	fibril associated	Skin
XIII	$\alpha 1(XIII)_3$	?	Skin, intestine, cartilage, muscle
XIV	$\alpha 1(XIV)_3$?	fibril associated	Skin

like helix are coiled about each other to give a triple helical coiled-coil structure or superhelix, rather like a three stranded rope (Fig. 10.1). It is this that produces the characteristic X-ray diffraction pattern seen for the major collagens. In this structure the glycine, which has no α-carbon side-chain, is required to occupy the core of the superhelix. The molecule is stabilized by the formation of interchain hydrogen bonds; in this respect the presence of hydroxyproline is important because it enhances molecular stability by the formation of additional hydrogen bonds through its hydroxyl group (for a detailed description of this structure see Traub & Piez).[4] The triple helical structure thus produced is generally resistant to attack by proteinases but is susceptible to specific proteolytic enzymes called collagenases.

When the three component chains of the molecule are identical it is referred to as a homotrimer and when they are genetically distinct it is termed a heterotrimer.

With knowledge of their molecular structure, the nature of their supramolecular assembly and their gene structure, members of the collagen family have been divided into three distinct subclasses which appear to have evolved separately.

They are:

1. the fibril-forming collagens, types I, II, III, V and XI
2. the non-fibrillar collagens, types IV, VI, VII, VIII, X and XIII

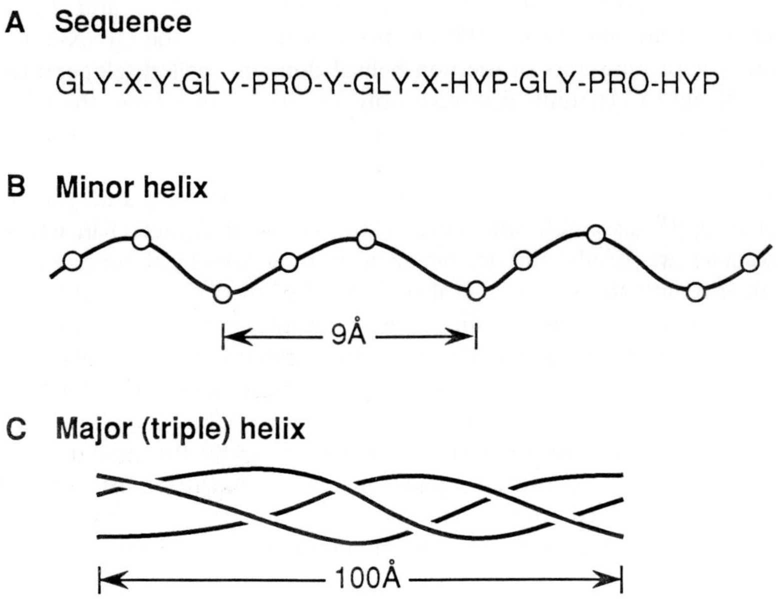

Fig. 10.1 The molecular structure of a typical collagen domain. **A** The repetitive triplet sequence of amino acid residues. **B** The minor helix conformation adopted by individual polypeptide chains. **C** The major helix conformation adopted by the triple stranded molecule.

3. the fibril-associated or FACIT collagens (Fibril Associated Collagens with Interrupted Triple helices), types IX, XII and XIV.

Only a brief description of the individual collagens will be given to demonstrate the molecular diversity. Readers interested in further details are referred to several recent reviews.[5–8]

The fibril-forming collagens

Type I collagen

Type I collagen is the archetypal collagen: it is the most abundant form in the body, constituting approximately 90% of the organic matrix of bone and tendon and 80% of adult skin. It is a major component of cornea, ligament, sclera, heart valves and the annulus fibrosus of the intervertebral disc. It is also present in significant amounts in blood vessel walls, the lung parenchyma, gut, joint capsule and fetal membranes.

The basic molecule is a heterotrimer containing two identical chains designated αl (I) and a third, homologous but gentically distinct chain, α2 (I). As first synthesised the molecule consists of a large central triple helical domain with globular domains at both N- and C-termini. In tissue the molecule is modified by proteolytic scission of the N- and C-terminal domains to produce the mature molecule (see section on Collagen biosynthesis). Each chain of the mature protein contains 1050 residues with 336 residues of glycine, 80–100 residues of hydroxyproline and 110–120 residues of proline. Almost 95% of the sequence is in the Gly-X-Y repeat pattern with remnants of the non-helical domains, called telopeptides, at both N- and C-termini. Although only 15–20 residues long, the telopeptides are critical to the mechanical properties of the tissue for they contain amino acid residues involved in intermolecular cross-linking (see below). These mature molecules, which are some 300 nm long and 1.5 nm in diameter, self-assemble into fibrils (20–2000 nm diameter) in which all molecules are parallel and overlap adjacent molecules by about one-quarter of their length (67 nm or 1 D if molecule length is represented by 4.4 D units)(Fig. 10.2). Between consecutive molecules in the fibril is a small gap of 0.6 D units which, when filled with electron dense stains, gives rise to the characteristic banding pattern in the electron microscope (Fig. 10.2).

The precise manner in which molecules are packed into three-dimensional fibrils and how fibril size is regulated is still the matter of some debate. Recent in vitro experiments[9] have indicated that fibrils grow by a process of nucleated growth, with monomers added to the amino terminal tip to produce longitudinal growth, and filling-in the tips to promote lateral growth.

The diversity of physical properties of major type I collagen-containing tissues, such as skin,tendon, cornea and bone, depends upon the exquisite control of fibril size and organization. For example, the fibrils in tendon

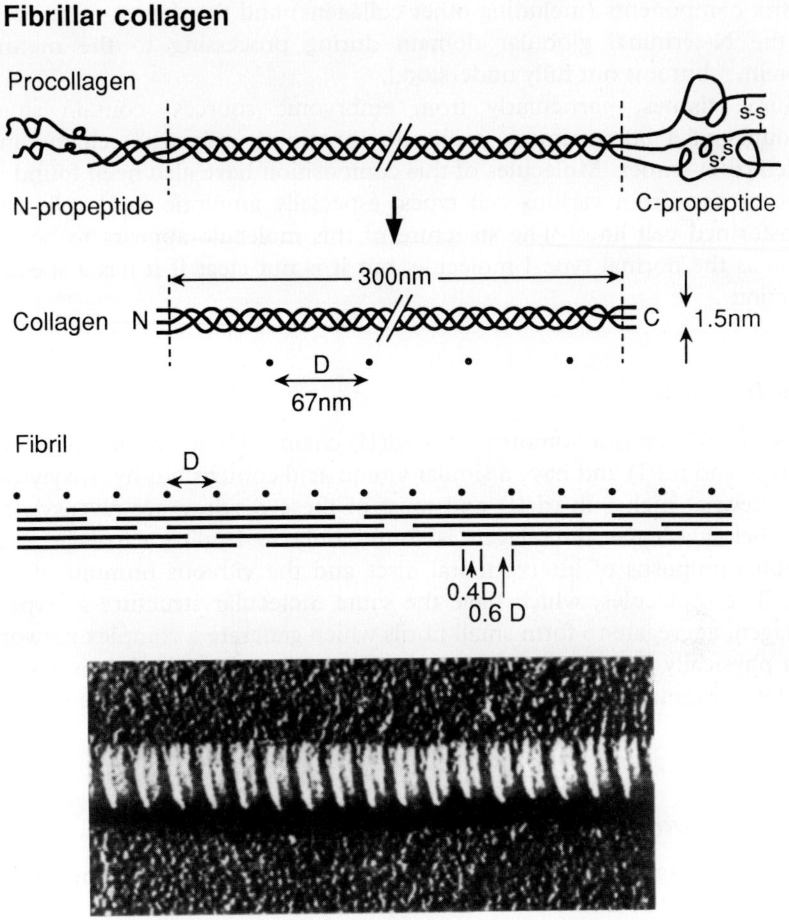

Fig. 10.2 The formation of a fibrillar collagen fibril. The procollagen is converted to collagen by scission of N- and C-terminal propeptides which then assemble into the fibril so that each molecule overlaps its neighbour by 1 D unit (67 nm, 234 amino acid residues, 1 molecule = 4.4 D units) generating 'hole-zones' of 0.6 D and 'overlap-zones' of 0.4 D. This produces the characteristic electron microscopic appearance (bottom).

aggregate into large fibre bundles whose long axes run parallel to the direction of applied stress to produce a tissue with a high tensile strength. The fibres in skin have a more or less random orientation within the matrix, allowing greater flexibility whilst maintaining strength in every direction. In the cornea, however, transparency of the tissue is achieved by having sheets of parallel fibrils, with a precisely controlled, uniformly small diameter, stacked so that the fibril orientation of each sheet is orthogonal to that above and below. In bone the collagen fibrils act as girders reinforcing the mineral deposits. Various hypotheses regarding the mechanism for controlling fibril diameter have been proposed, including interactions with other matrix components (including other collagens) and the degree of removal of the N-terminal globular domain during processing to the mature protein,[10] but it is not fully understood.

Some tissues, particularly from embryonic sources, contain small amounts of a homotrimeric molecule containing only αl(I) chains and called αl(I)-trimer. Molecules of this composition have also been found in supernatants from various cell types, especially amniotic fluid cells and transformed cell lines. The structure of this molecule appears to be the same as the normal type I molecule, but it is not clear if it has a specific function.

Type II collagen

Type II collagen is a homotrimer of αl(II) chains. These are the same size as αl(I) and α2(I) and have a similar amino acid content but hydroxylysine is somewhat higher in αl(II) and most of these residues are glycosylated (see below). Type II collagen is found only in hyaline cartilages, the annulus pulposus of intervertebral discs and the vitreous humour of the eye. The molecules, which have the same molecular structure as type I collagen, aggregate to form small fibrils which generate a complex network that physically entraps the giant proteoglycan complexes and their associated water molecules. This allows the cartilage to withstand large compressive forces.

Type III collagen

Type III collagen is a homotrimer of αl(III) chains and has a similar size and molecular structure to collagen types I and II. It differs from these by having interchain disulphide bonds within the triple-helical domain, a distinction which provides a useful marker in the analysis of pathological conditions. Type III collagen constitutes the major collagenous component of blood vessel walls and fetal skin but has a ubiquitous distribution, being present in varying amounts in almost every tissue containing type I collagen. It is not found in bone and forms only a very minor component of tendon. In skin the relative abundance of type III and type I collagens shows quite dramatic developmental changes. During fetal life type III collagen represents 50% of the total collagens but around parturition this level starts to decline reaching adult levels of 10–15% over the first 10 years of life. During wound healing in adult skin, type III collagen production is stimulated so that initial scar tissue contains almost fetal levels of type III collagen. Normally this returns to adult levels as the scar matures but in hypertrophic scars, for some reason, the type III level remains abnormally high after maturation. These observations suggest type III collagen plays an important developmental role in cutaneous tissues.

Type V collagen

Type V collagen normally occurs as a heterotrimer of two αl(V) and one α2(V) chains[11]; sometimes the stoichiometry of αl(V) and α2(V) and the presence of a third chain, α3(V)[12], suggests alternative combinations, such as $\alpha 1(V)_3$ or αl(V)α2(V)α3(V), are possible. Type V molecules have the same size and structure as those of the fibrillar collagens already described but, unlike these, Type V collagen does not readily form fibrils in vitro. In cell cultures type V collagen appears as a filamentous pericellular network. In tissues there is evidence that it forms heterotypic (mixed) fibrils with type I collagen.[13] Although originally isolated from fetal membranes it has a widespread distribution forming a minor component of such tissues as skin, bone, liver, tendon, cornea, gingiva and muscle.

Type XI collagen

Type XI collagen is a heterotrimer containing 3 distinct α chains, αl(XI) α2(XI)α3(XI), each with a molecular weight of 100 kDa (i.e. containing approximately 1000 amino acids) indicating a molecular structure similar to other fibrillar collagens.[14] It is a minor component of cartilage and has been found in mixed fibrils with type II collagen. Peptide mapping indicates the α3(XI) chain is the product of the same gene as αl(II) with differences in hydroxylysine content. The αl(XI) and α2(XI) chains show a close homology to the αl(V) and α2(V) chains but are distinct gene products. In bone the αl(XI) chain can sometimes associate with αl(V) and α2(V) to form a heterotrimer αl(V)α2(V)αl(XI).[15]

The fibrillar collagens are large proteins, each chain contains more than a 1000 amino acids with substantial intertypic homology. This makes it difficult to obtain recognisable peptide maps with proteolytic enzymes. Fortunately the content of methionine is relatively low and chemical cleavage at these residues with cyanogen bromide gives a small number of manageable polypeptides which can be used for distinguishing and mapping individual chains in normal and pathological conditions.

The non-fibrillar collagens

In contrast to the structural uniformity displayed by the fibrillar collagens the various non-fibrillar collagens have many different molecular structures and generate diverse extracellular matrix aggregates.

Type IV collagen

Type IV collagen is the collagen of basement membranes. The molecules consist of three protein chains MW approximately 140 kDa. The predominant molecular species is $\alpha l(IV)_2\alpha 2(IV)$ but 5 different type IV α chains have been identified. One of these, α5(IV), appears to have a more restricted distribution than the major molecular species, occurring only in the kidney glomerular basement membrane and not in the tubular basement membrane or Bowman's capsule of the same organ.[16]

Type IV collagen molecules comprise three domains, a central collagenous triple-helical domain 350–400 nm long, a large C-terminal globular domain (NCI) and a small N-terminal globular domain (NC2). The amino acid sequences of the collagenous domains have some 20 interruptions of the normal Gly-X-Y pattern; many of these occur in the same position in different chains and probably allow a certain flexibility of the molecule at these points. In tissue, type IV collagen exists as a flexible three-dimensional 'chicken-wire' network (Fig. 10.3A) in which four molecules, two parallel and two antiparallel, associate through interaction of their amino terminal globular domain and an amino terminal segment of the collagenous domain to produce a tightly cross-linked tetramer. The C-terminal globular domain (NCI) then interacts with a like domain of an adjacent molecule and forms intermolecular disulphide bonds.[17]

Type VI collagen

Type VI collagen was first identified in proteolytic extracts of aortic intima and placenta as a high molecular weight disulphide-bonded aggregate which on reduction gave three non-identical short collagen chains, MW 40 –55 kDa. Non-degrading extraction procedures showed that these represented the short (100 nm) triple-helical core of a protein having globular domains at both termini whose individual chains were 160 kDa (αl(VI) and α2(VI)) or 200 kDa (α3(VI)). Amino acid sequences derived from cDNA clones show the collagenous domain has two short interruptions to the Gly-X-Y pattern; the C-terminal globular domain (NCl) comprises two repeats of a 200 residue homologous unit. This is also found once in the N-terminal globular domain (NC2). The NC2 domain of one chain, α3 (VI), is much larger than the others and probably contains several of these repeat units. Alternative splicing of mRNA in the α2 (VI) NCl domain yields two forms of protein, one of which contains only one complete repeat unit. Aggregate forms of this collagen contain dimers of antiparallel molecules which associate laterally to form tetramers stabilised by intermolecular disulphide bonds. These tetramers associate laterally and longitudinally through the globular domains to form a microfibril with a 100 nm periodicity (Fig. 10.3B).[18] Immunofluorescent studies have shown a widespread distribution of the protein in tissues such as skin, aortic media, cartilage, perichondrium, corneal stroma and intervertebral disc, but it is not present in basement membranes.

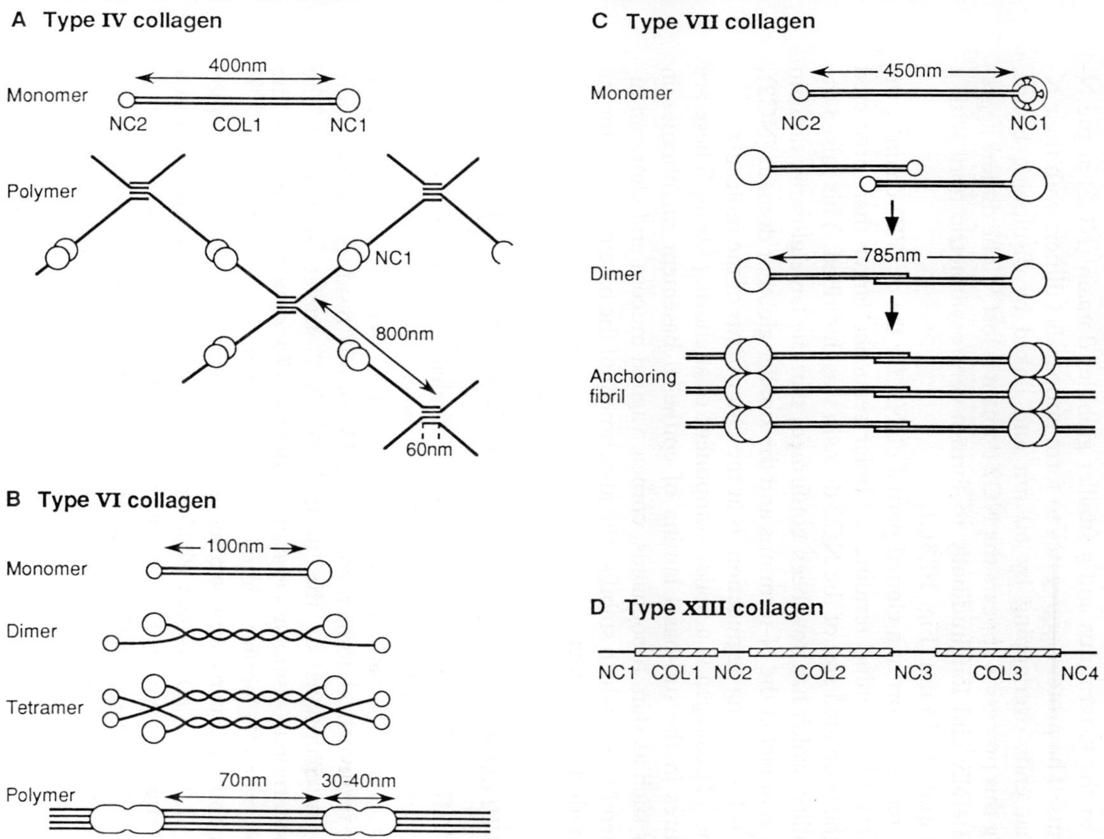

Fig. 10.3 The molecular and supramolecular structures of some non-fibrillar collagens. **A** Type IV collagen and its 'chicken-wire' network. **B** Type VI collagen and the formation of 100 nm microfibrils. **C** Type VII collagen and the formation of anchoring fibrils. **D** The domain structure of type XIII collagen. COL – collagenous domains, NC – non–collagenous domains.

Type VII collagen

Type VII collagen is a homotrimer with a large disulphide-bonded central collagenous domain, approximately 1.5 times the length of that in the fibrillar collagens. Susceptibility to proteinases indicates at least one interruption in the Gly-X-Y sequence of this domain. Each α chain has a 170 kDa triple helical domain, a 150 kDa multidomain globular extension (NCl) at the C-terminus and a smaller globular domain (NC2) at the N-terminus. The protein aggregates to form antiparallel dimers with their N-terminal ends overlapping by 60 nm and linked by disulphide bonds. During this process it appears the NC2 domain is lost.[19] The dimers aggregate laterally and longitudinally to form a centrosymmetric fibril with a repeat unit of 785 nm (Fig. 10.3C).

In a recent report of a cloned partial cDNA for the αl (VII) chain[20], the discovery of an amino terminal globular sequence larger than predicted from the estimated size of the NC2 domain was described. This raised the possibility, which has now been confirmed, that the large globular domain (NCl) is in fact at the N-terminus and the smaller globular domain (NC2), which is lost during aggregation, is at the C-terminus of the molecule.

Type VII collagen is a major component of anchoring fibrils. These are structures in the sub-basal lamina of epithelial basement membranes in tissues such as skin, oesophagus, cornea, vaginal mucosa and chorioamniotic membranes, which stabilise the attachment of the basement membrane to its underlying stroma.

Type VIII collagen

Type VIII collagen is the product of endothelial cell cultures and a major component of Descement's membrane of the cornea. Two distinct α-chain sequences have been identified αl (VIII) and α2 (VIII). Each has a short, central triple-helical domain containing 454 or 457 residues in which there are 8 interruptions of the normal Gly-X-Y triplet sequence. The carboxyterminal globular domain contains 173 amino acids and the aminoterminal globular domain, NC2, contains 117 residues.[21,22] Although both chains are coexpressed by cells and occur in tissue in ratios of 1.5–2.0:1 it is not known whether these represent the components of a heterotrimer or two separate homotrimers. The supramolecular structure of type VIII collagen molecules is not known but it appears to be a major component of the hexagonal lattice of Descement's membrane.

Type X collagen

Type X collagen is a disulphide-bonded homotrimer composed of a 460 residue collagenous domain, a C-terminal globular domain of 170 residues and an N-terminal globular domain of 52 residues, including 18 residues of signal peptide. The collagenous domain has several interruptions in the Gly-X-Y triplet pattern. The protein is the product of hypertrophic chondrocytes and is found around these cells in cartilage undergoing endochondral ossification, but its supramolecular structure is unknown.[23] In molecular structure, amino acid sequence and nucleotide sequence, type X collagen shows close homology to the α-chains of type VIII collagen.

Type XIII collagen

The nature of this protein has been derived solely from cDNA data. It has three collagenous and four non-collagenous domains (Fig. 10.3D). Western blots using antibodies directed against synthetic polypeptides have identified proteins with molecular weights 62 and 67 kDa. Multiple mRNAs are produced by complex alternative splicing involving collagenous domains (COL1 and COL3), non-collagenous domains (NC2) and junctional sequences (COL3, NC4).[24] Northern blot analysis and in situ hybridisation of the mRNA show highest expression in the epidermis and hair follicles of skin, intestinal mucosa, the intertrabecular mesenchyme of bone and the endomysium of striated muscle and cartilage.[25] The supramolecular assembly is unknown.

FACIT collagens

The FACIT collagens (***F**ibril **A**ssociated **C**ollagens with **I**nterrupted **T**riple helices*), i.e. types IX, XII and XIV, do not themselves form supramolecular structures but, as their name implies, are associated with the surface of various fibrillar collagens and may play a major role in mediating fibril size and interactions with other matrix macromolecules.

Type IX collagen

Type IX collagen comprises 5–20% of the total collagen in hyaline cartilage. It is a proteoglycan with a single galactosaminoglycan chain. It contains three distinct polypeptide chains, αl (IX), α2(IX) and α3(IX), intramolecularly disulphide-bonded. The molecule consists of three short triple-helical domains, COL1 (115 residues), COL2 (339 residues) and COL3 (137 amino acids) separated by two short non-collagenous domains NC2 and NC3. The NC3 domain of the α2(IX) has 5 amino acids more than the equivalent region of the α1(IX) or α3(IX) chains and this tends to produce a kink or angle in the molecule (Fig. 10.4A). This is the site of attachment of the glycosaminoglycan chain to the α2(IX) chain. The aminoterminal non-collagenous domain (NC4) of the α1(IX) at 266 residues is much larger than the corresponding domains of the α2(IX) and α3(IX) chains and is highly basic (pI about 10), ideal for interaction with the acidic proteoglycans of the cartilage matrix. Alternative forms of the protein, lacking the α1(IX) NC4 domain, which occur in embryonic cornea and vitreous humour, are generated by using an alternate transcription start site and first exon whilst the rest of the molecule remains the same.[7]

Electron microscopy has shown that type IX collagen is associated in a periodic manner with the surface of type II collagen fibrils. The molecules align with the COL1 and COL2 domains along the surface of the fibril and covalent cross-links are formed. The COL3 and large globular NC4 domain radiate into the matrix.[26]

Type XII collagen

Characterization of type XII collagen is incomplete. It appears to be a disulphide-bonded homotrimer with protein chains of approximately 220 kDa consisting of two short triple-helical segments COL1 (143 residues) and COL2 (152 amino acids) separated by a 43-residue non-collagenous domain. At the C-terminus is a 76-residue globular domain but the bulk of the protein is contained in a large aminoterminal globular domain of 190 kDa with an estimated 1600 amino acid residues.[27] Electron microscopy indicates a molecule with a short (75 nm) triple-helical tail, often with a slight kink, and three 60 nm 'fingers' radiating out from a central globule at one end (Fig. 10.4B). There is considerable sequence homology between the C-terminal triple-helical domains of types XII and IX collagen and between the aminoterminal globular domains, NC4 of type IX, and NC3 of type XII.

Type XII collagen is found in tissues rich in type I collagen such as tendons, ligaments, periosteum and perichondrium, suggesting it may associate with the type I collagen fibrils, in the same way as type IX and type II collagens in cartilage.

Type XIV collagen

A collagen similar to type XII but genetically distinct has been identified in fetal calf tendons and skin.[28] It appears to have at least two short triple-helical domains (10 kDa and 13.5 kDa) and two non-helical domains (NC2 and NC3). The amino acid sequences of the isolated polypeptides shows a clear homology with type XII collagen. This collagen has been designated type XIV.

Two new 190 kDa globular domains derived from collagenous molecules were isolated from fetal bovine skin.[29] The two domains, although identical in size, were immunologically distinct and showed different peptide maps. Western blotting indicated parent molecules of approximately 220 kDa and 300 kDa. Rotary shadowing electron microscopy showed three identical arms (45–55 nm) radiating from a central globule; one form also had small globules at the end of each arm. Monoclonal antibodies showed distinctive and often complementary distributions: in skin one was restricted to the

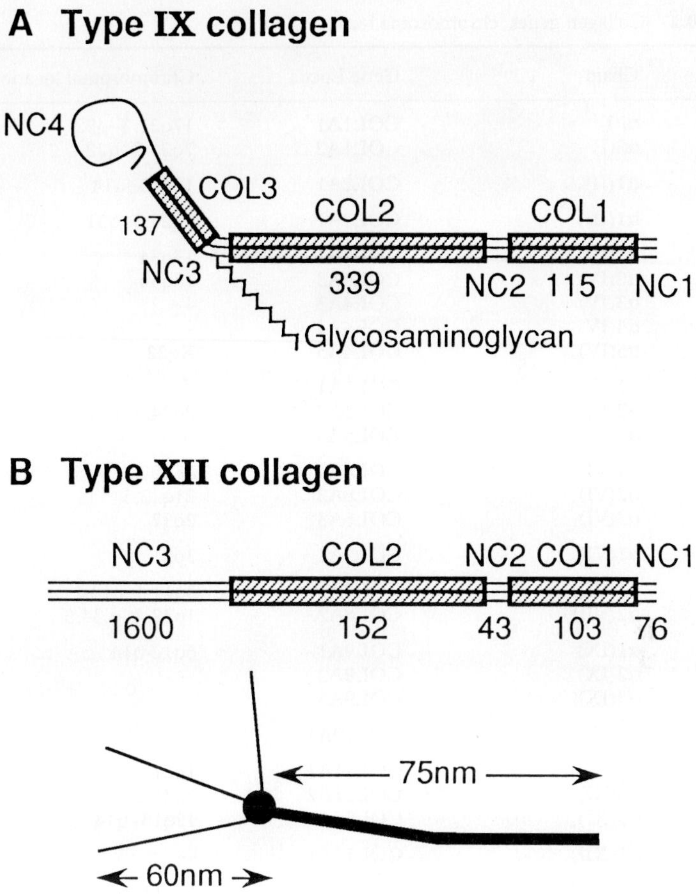

Fig. 10.4 The molecular structure of two FACIT collagens. **A** Type IX collagen with its three 'collagenous' (COL) and four 'non-collagenous' (NC) domains. **B** Type XII collagen with two 'collagenous' and three 'non-collagenous' domains and its appearance on rotary shadowing in the electron microscope. The number of amino acids residues in each domain is shown.

papillary dermis, whilst the other was abundant throughout the reticular dermis but restricted to hair follicles in the papillary dermis. Unlike type XII collagen, both proteins were found in cartilage, one restricted to the articular surface and around blood vessel canals, the other showing a punctate distribution throughout cartilage. These components are assumed to be fragments of a type XII-like collagen.

THE COLLAGEN GENES

The molecular diversity of the collagenous proteins is mirrored by an equal diversity of gene structures suggesting independent evolutionary pathways.

Table 10.2 Collagen genes, chromosome locations

Type	Chain	Gene Locus	Chromosomal location
I	α1(I)	COL1A1	17q21.3–q22
	α2(I)	COL1A2	7q21.3–q22
II	α1(II)	COL2A1	12q13–q14
III	α1(III)	COL3A1	2q24.3–q31
IV	α1(IV)	COL4A1	13q34
	α2(IV)	COL4A2	13q34
	α3(IV)	COL4A3	—
	α4(IV)	COL4A4	—
	α5(IV)	COL4A5	Xq22
V	α1(V)	COL5A1	—
	α2(V)	COL5A2	2q24.3–q31
	α3(V)	COL5A3	—
VI	α1(VI)	COL6A1	21q22.3
	α2(VI)	COL6A2	21q22.3
	α3(VI)	COL6A3	2q37
VII	α1(VII)	COL7A1	3p21
VIII	α1(VIII)	COL8A1	3q11.1–q13.1
	α2(VIII)	COL8A2	1p32.4–p.34.3
IX	α1(IX)	COL9A1	6q12-q14
	α2(IX)	COL9A2	—
	α3(IX)	COL9A3	—
X	α1(X)	COL10A1	—
XI	α1(XI)	COL11A1	1p21
	α2(XI)	COL11A2	6p21.2
	α3(XI)	COL2A1	12q13–q14
XII	α1(XII)	COL12A1	—
XIII	α1(XIII)	COL13A1	10q11–qter

The genes are spread throughout the genome (Table 10.2) with genes for different subunits of heterotrimers usually on different chromosomes. The exceptions to this are the genes for α1(IV) and α2(IV) on chromosome 13 and two genes for type VI collagen chains on chromosome 21. The genes for subunits of two different collagens, α2(V) and α1(III), are clustered with other matrix genes, e.g. elastin and fibronectin, on chromosome 2.

The fibrillar collagen genes

All the fibrillar collagens, types I, II, III, V and XI have a homologous gene structure indicating a common evolution. Although only the genes for the subunits of types I, II and III have been characterised in detail, the information available on the other genes suggests they conform to the same pattern. The genes range in size from 18 to 44 kb and contain 51–54 exons.

The central collagenous domains of each are coded by 44 exons many of which are only 54 bp long, the remainder are either 45 bp, 99 bp, 108 bp or 162 bp (Fig. 10.5). All these exons are multiples of 9 bp and encode a complete set of Gly-X-Y triplets, each exon starting with a full codon for glycine (GGN) and ending with a full codon for the Y amino acid. The frequency of 54 bp exons has led to the suggestion that these genes evolved by amplification of a 54 bp primordial gene with recombination generating other exon sizes. The intron/exon arrangement is highly conserved for all types of fibrillar collagens and across species (both vertebrates and invertebrates) implying their highly ordered supramolecular structure is extremely intolerant of change in this domain.

At either end of the collagenous domain are 'fusion' exons encoding both helical and non-helical sequences. The C-propeptide domain is contained in four exons which are highly conserved among the collagen types; more divergence in gene structure has been allowed for the N-propeptide sequences both in exon size and number (Fig. 10.5).

Non-fibrillar collagen genes

Type IV collagen

The type IV collagen genes appear to be larger than the fibrillar collagen genes. Overlapping genomic clones covering more than 100 kb were required to cover the whole of the human α1(IV) mRNA. They have multiple exons which are not uniform in size, ranging from 27 to 213 bp. Many of these do not conform to the 9 bp motif encoding a complete set of Gly-X-Y triplets. Several have split codons at the 5' or 3' ends, with the loss of the first G of a glycine codon from the beginning of one exon and the addition of that G to the 3' end of the preceding exon. Others contain imperfections in the Gly-X-Y repeat, with the loss of an X or Y codon giving Gly-X-Gly or loss of a glycine codon giving Gly-X-Y-X-Y-Gly. It is probably significant that exons encoding the aminoterminal portion of the triple-helical domain, responsible for intermolecular interaction and tetramer formation, adhere rigidly to the 9 bp rule. Although closely homologous at the amino acid level, the C-termini of the α1(IV) and α2(IV) show considerable differences in exon size and organisation.

The genes for α1(IV) and α2(IV) have an arrangement on chromosome 13 unique among the collagens, for they are arranged head-to-head with coding sequences on opposite strands of DNA, and transcription start sites only 42 bp apart. They appear to use a common promoter and enhancer element.

cDNA and genomic clones for another type IV collagen chain, α5(IV), have recently been isolated. The gene was localized to Xq22, the first collagen gene on the X chromosome, the same region as the X-linked Alport's syndrome (McKusick no. 104200) locus.

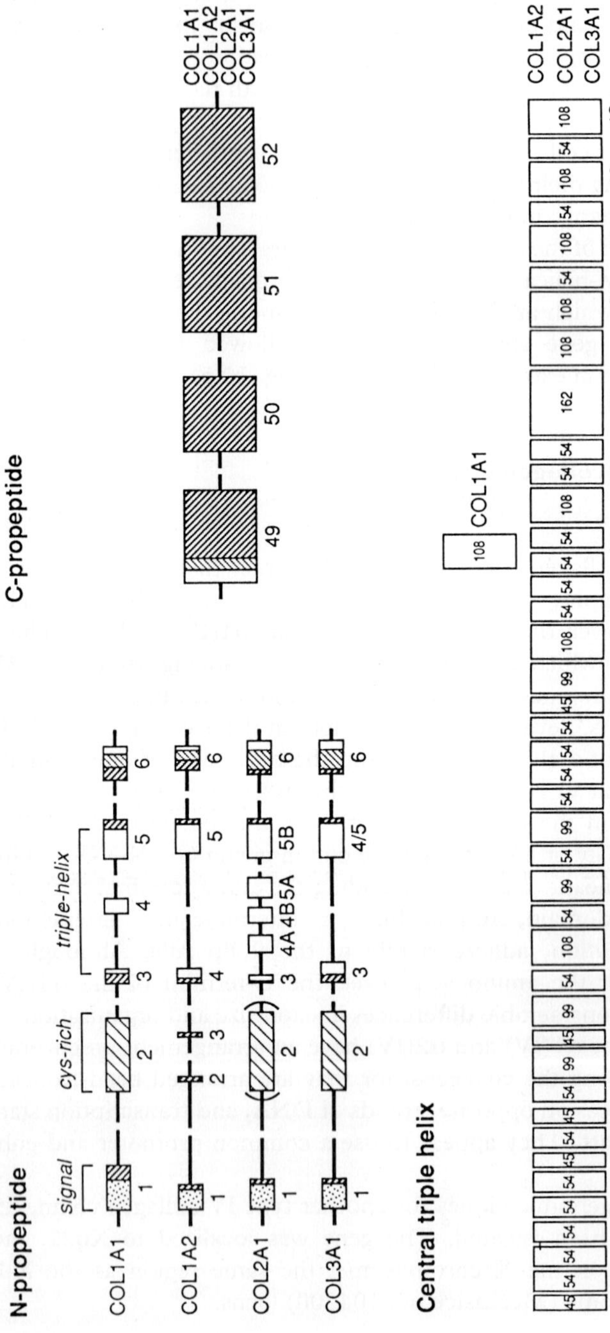

Fig. 10.5 Intron/exon structure of the fibrillar collagen genes. Exons are numbered from the 5' end. Exon 6 marks the transition from N-propeptide to central triple-helical domain. Similarly exon 49 marks the transition from triple helix to C-propeptide. Note that all triple helical exons are multiples of 9 bp, and the large number of 54 bp exons in this domain.

Type XIII collagen

The gene for α1(XIII) is exceptionally large (>130 kb) for an mRNA of only 2.3 kb. It contains 39 exons, 28 of these coding only for triple-helical sequences with sizes ranging from 27 bp to 153 bp. All but 6 of these exons conform to the 9 bp rule; the others have split codons or imperfections in the Gly-X-Y sequence. The gene undergoes complex alternative splicing involving exons in collagenous domains COL1 and COL3, and non-collagenous domains NC2 and NC4.[30]

Type VIII and type X collagens

These two short-chain collagens show considerable structural homology at the protein level and at the gene level (Fig. 10.6). Unlike the other collagens the genes have only a few exons (three for α1(X) and four for α1(VIII)). The whole of the C-terminal globular domain (NC1), the central triple-helical domain (COL1) and part of the aminoterminal globular domain (NC2) are encoded in a single exon of about 2 kb; another exon encodes the remainder of NC2 and the signal peptide, and the other exon(s) code for the 5' untranslated region. The similarity of the gene structures firmly establishes these as members of a discrete subclass of collagens.[22, 31, 32]

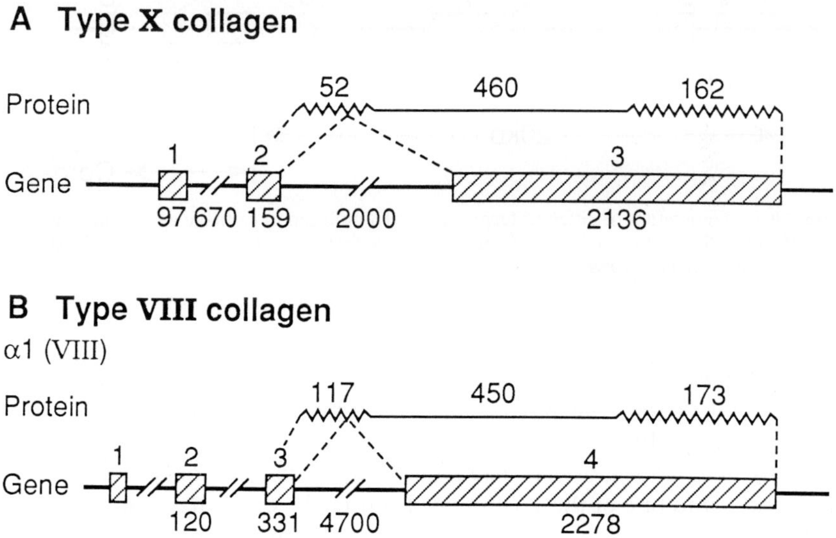

Fig. 10.6 Intron/exon structure of the genes for type X and type VIII collagen showing the close homology between proteins and between genes.

The FACIT collagens

Type IX collagen

Genes coding for α1(IX) and α2(IX) have been cloned and partially characterised. They have a similar intron/exon structure but a large difference in size: 100 kb for α1(IX) and 10 kb for α2(IX). The gene for α2(IX) contains 32 exons. Most exons encoding the triple-helical domains conform to the 9 bp rule; i.e. exons begin with a complete codon for glycine and end with a complete codon for Y. Half of these exons are also 54 bp long. Those exons not conforming to the 9 bp rule either contain interruptions of the triplet amino acid sequence or have split codons at one or both ends. The frequency of 54 bp exons in these genes has led to the hypothesis that this collagen originated from a 54 bp primordial gene, like the fibrillar collagens, but the supramolecular structure allowed for more variation than could be tolerated by fibril-forming molecules.[6]

Some forms of α1(IX) lack the large N-terminal globular domain NC4; cDNA and genomic clones have shown this is due to the use of an alternative promoter and first exon in intron 6, some 20 kb downstream from the normal promoter (Fig. 10.7).[33]

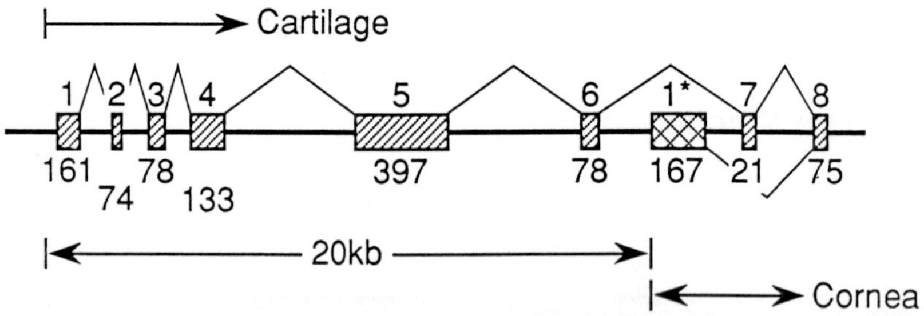

Fig. 10.7 Generation of different forms of type IX collagen in cartilage and cornea by the use of two different promoters producing alternative first exons 1 and 1* some 20 kb apart (After Nishimura et al 1989[33]).

Type XII collagen

The 3' end of the type XII collagen gene has been cloned and 7 exons characterised (Fig. 10.8). Three are fusion exons containing both triple-helical and globular sequences, four contain only collagenous sequences and one of these is 54 bp. Four of the exons have split codons. Although they do not correspond in size, the overall pattern of intron/exon arrangements for this region of type XII is clearly homologous to type IX (Fig. 10.8).[34]

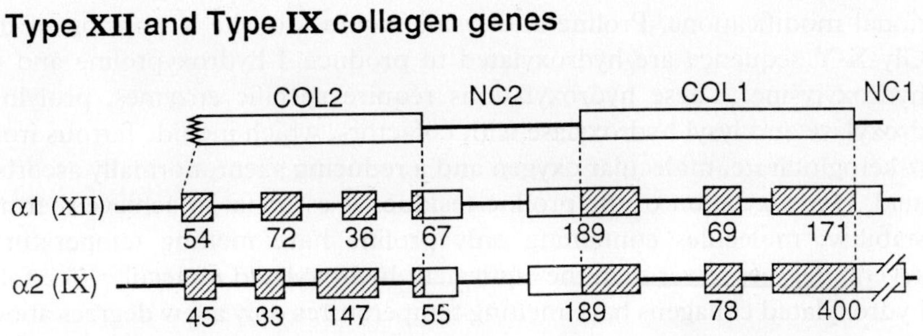

Fig. 10.8 Comparison of the intron/exon structure of type XII and type IX collagen genes showing clear homology (After Gordon et al 1989[34]).

COLLAGEN BIOSYNTHESIS

The biosynthesis of the major fibrillar collagens has been established in some detail. Although the following description refers principally to these proteins it is thought that all collagens follow a similar pathway, specific details varying to suit the nature of the supramolecular structure.

The main steps identified in the biosynthesis of collagens are:

1. gene selection and transcription
2. splicing and processing to mature mRNA
3. translation of mRNA to yield prepro-α-chains
4. cleavage of signal peptide
5. post-translational modification i.e. hydroxylation of specific proline and lysine residues, glycosylation of hydroxylysines, addition of a high mannose oligosaccharide to the C propeptide
6. molecular assembly, disulphide bond formation between C-propeptides (protein disulphide isomerase) and triple helix formation
7. secretion of procollagen
8. cleavage of aminoterminal and carboxyterminal propeptides (procollagen-N-proteinase, procollagen-C-proteinase)
9. supramolecular assembly (e.g. fibril formation)
10. oxidation of specific lysine and hydoxylysine residues (lysyl oxidase) and covalent cross-link formation
11. maturation of cross-links.

Many cells synthesise several collagens simultaneously; the relative amounts are transcriptionally regulated and tissue-specific. The large number of exons in most collagen genes demands a high degree of precision of the splicing machinery to generate fully functional messenger RNA. The mRNAs are translated on membrane-bound polysomes into precursor form preprocollagen chains. These are extruded into the lumen of the rough endoplasmic reticulum where they undergo several post-translational modifications. Proline and lysine residues in the Y position of the Gly-X-Y sequence are hydroxylated to produce 4-hydroxyproline and 5-hydroxylysine. These hydroxylations require specific enzymes, prolylhydroxylase and lysyl hydroxylase with cofactors, which include ferrous iron, α-ketoglutarate, molecular oxygen and a reducing agent, normally ascorbic acid. Hydroxylation of the proline residues is essential to achieve thermal stability: molecules containing only proline have melting temperatures several degrees lower than the equivalent hydroxylated molecule. The fully hydroxylated collagens have melting temperatures only a few degrees above the ambient temperature of the organism.

Some of the hydroxylysine residues are further modified by the sequential addition of galactose and glucose moieties to the hydroxyl group by two specific glycosyl transferases. The degree of post-translational modification of lysine is variable, depending on the collagen type, the tissue and the age of the organism. Embryonic tissues for example are more heavily hydroxylated than the equivalent adult tissue.

These post-translational modifications only occur whilst the chains are in a random coil configuration. Once a triple helix is formed the proteins are no longer substrates for the enzymes. Molecular assembly is initiated by the interaction of the C-propeptides and the formation of interchain disulphide bonds by the enzyme protein disulphide isomerase (which appears to be a subunit of the prolylhydroxylase enzyme). Winding of the triple helix then propagates towards the N-terminus of the molecule.

The completed triple-helical precursor molecule, procollagen, is secreted via the golgi and microtubules into the extracellular space. A substantial proportion (10–30%) of newly synthesised collagen is diverted from this pathway to be degraded intracellularly. The function of this process is not entirely clear, but to some extent it acts as a quality control mechanism since incorporation of destabilising amino acid analogues into the protein, or the presence of a mutation, leads to an increase in the basal rate of degradation.

Once in the extracellular space the N- and C-propeptides of the fibrillar collagens are proteolytically removed by two specific enzymes, procollagen-N-proteinase and procollagen-C-proteinase which cleave all three chains simultaneously. The fibrillar collagen molecules produced by this process then self-assemble into the 'quarter-staggered' fibrils previously described, directed solely by the amino acid sequence. Removal of the N-propeptides may not be complete and may provide one means of controlling fibril size. Non-fibrillar collagens appear to undergo only limited proteolysis of their globular termini, if any.

Molecules are then stabilised within fibrils by the formation of a unique set of covalent intermolecular cross links, initiated by the oxidation of the ε-amino groups of lysines or hydroxylysines in the telopeptides by a copper-requiring enzyme, lysyl oxidase. This produces a terminal aldehyde group (allysine), which then condenses with the ε-amino groups of lysines or hydroxylysines in the helical domain of adjacent molecules to form a Schiff base. If two hydroxylysines are involved in cross-link formation the initial Schiff base can undergo Amadori rearrangement to produce a more stable ketoimine structure (Fig. 10.9A). These cross-links are only intermediate forms and disappear as the tissue matures to form complex cross-links such as the pyridinolines (Fig. 10.9B).

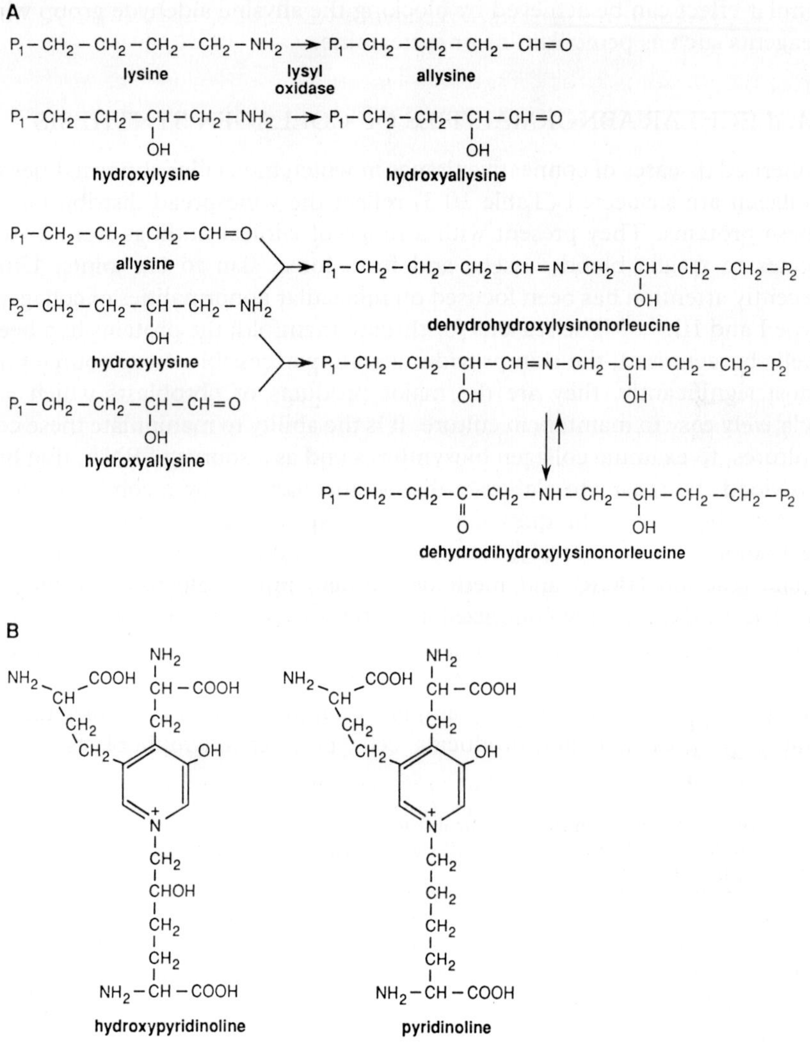

Fig. 10.9 Covalent intermolecular cross-linking of collagens. **A** The formation of bifunctional cross-links. Peptidyl lysine or hydroxylysine is oxidatively deaminated to allysine or hydroxyallysine which then condenses with an hydroxylysine of an adjacent molecule to form Schiff bases, dehydrohydroxylysinonorleucine and dehydrodihydroxylysinonorleucine. The latter can undergo rearrangement and exists predominantly in the keto form. **B** The multifunctional cross-links hydroxypyridinoline and pyridinoline.

The critical importance of cross-linking to the ultimate mechanical integrity of connective tissues is demonstrated by a drug-induced disease called lathyrism. Here, a compound, called β-aminopropionitrile, derived from the seeds of the sweet pea *Lathyrus oderatus*, irreversibly inhibits the enzyme, lysyl oxidase. There is a marked decrease in the tensile strength of the connective tissues, resulting in extreme skin fragility, skeletal deformities and severe blood vessel weakness leading to aneurysms and rupture. A similar effect can be achieved by blocking the allysine aldehyde group with reagents such as penicillamine or cysteamine.

MOLECULAR ABNORMALITIES OF COLLAGEN SYNTHESIS

Inherited diseases of connective tissues in which molecular abnormalities of collagen are suspected (Table 10.3) reflect the widespread distribution of these proteins. They present with a range of clinical findings from brittle bones to fragile blood vessels, and from loose skin to lax joints. Until recently attention has been focused on molecular abnormalities of collagens type I and III.[35, 36] The reasons for this are manifold; the proteins had been well characterised; the skin provides a readily accessible tissue source but, most significantly, they are the major products of fibroblasts which are relatively easy to maintain in culture. It is the ability to manipulate these cell cultures, to examine collagen biosynthesis and as a source of RNA, that has provided the means to elaborate disease mechanisms by a combination of protein chemistry techniques (e.g. peptide mapping) and recombinant DNA technology. More recently, however, the introduction of the polymerase chain reaction (PCR) and methods for detecting single base changes in nucleic acids have revolutionized the study of genetic disorders to such effect that abnormalities of collagens normally expressed in inaccessible tissues, e.g. cartilage and basement membrane, can be studied by direct analysis of genomic DNA, or by amplification of the low level of illegitimate transcripts present in 'non-producing' cell types such as lymphoblasts.

Table 10.3 Inherited connective tissue diseases in which collagens are or may be abnormal. AD – autosomal dominant, AR – autosomal recessive, XLR – X-linked recessive, XLD – X-linked dominant

Disease	Mode of inheritance
Osteogenesis imperfecta (OI)	AD, AR
Ehlers–Danlos syndrome (EDS) (some)	AD, AR, XLR
Chondrodysplasias (some)	AD, AR
Cutis laxa	AD, AR
Occipital Horn syndrome (formerly X-linked Cutis laxa EDS-Type IX)	XLR
Epidermolysis bullosa (some)	AD, AR
Alport's syndrome	XLD
Larsen's syndrome	
Progeria	?AR

Osteogenesis imperfecta (McKusick 166200, 166210, 166220, 259420)

Osteogenesis imperfecta (OI) is undoubtedly the most studied of the collagen disorders. The primary manifestations of OI are multiple fractures and long bone deformity resulting from exceedingly fragile, poorly calcified bones. It is however a systemic disorder and abnormalities of skin, teeth, sclera, heart valves and vasculature are also observed. It is a clinically and genetically heterogeneous group of disorders with a population frequency of about 1 in 10 000. Severity can range from mild disease, with few fractures and minimal long bone deformity, through severe progressively deforming disease, to perinatally lethal disease. Both autosomal dominant and recessive inheritance have been documented.

Many attempts have been made to classify the syndrome clinically. The current standard was proposed by Sillence et al[37] based on phenotypic, radiologic and genetic criteria (Table 10.4). It recognises four major types, but heterogeneity within these groups is evident, and many patients do not meet all the criteria established for any one type. This difficulty in classification is probably a direct result of the diversity of causal mutations in this disorder. All tissues affected in osteogenesis imperfecta contain predominantly type I collagen. In the most severe cases histology shows a marked paucity and disorganization of the collagen in bone. The genes for this protein were therefore prime candidates for the disease locus. The first direct evidence came in 1975 when Penttinen and colleagues[39] showed that cultured skin fibroblasts from an infant with a particularly severe, lethal disease produced abnormally low levels of type I collagen. Subsequent studies[40,41] showed that two forms of $\alpha 1$(I) chain were present in these cultures, one approximately 80 residues shorter than normal. Analysis of genomic DNA from the patient revealed an intron-to-intron deletion of approximately 500 bp resulting in the loss of 3 complete exons from the centre of the triple helical domain. Although the shortened chains could be incorporated into trimeric molecules the mutant protein was unstable, poorly secreted and most was degraded intracellularly. Because there are two $\alpha 1$(I) chains per type I collagen molecule, mutant $\alpha 1$(I) chains can be associated with normal chains in trimers. In a heterozygous state this would mean that only 25% of the molecules would be normal and 75% would contain either 1 or 2 mutant chains (Fig. 10.10). This ability of mutant protein to sequester normal chains into an abnormal molecule, dubbed 'protein suicide', amplifies the effect of the mutation and explains the dominant nature of most collagen mutations.

Such large deletions of genomic DNA are, however, infrequent causes of OI; more subtle mutations are the norm. Many early studies of OI patients recognised that the type I collagen extracted from tissues, or produced by cell cultures, had higher than normal levels of hydroxylysine and glycosy-

Table 10.4 Classification and characteristics of osteogenesis imperfecta (OI) after Sillence[37]. AD – autosomal dominant, AR – autosomal recessive

Type	McKusick no.	Inheritance	Clinical features
I	166200	AD	A Normal stature, blue sclerae, mild deformity, late-onset fractures, deafness, normal teeth
			B As A but with dentinogenesis imperfecta
II	166210	AD (new) AR (?rare)	Perinatally lethal, severe osseous fragility with:
			A Broad crumpled long bones and beaded ribs
			B Broad crumpled long bones, no beading of ribs
			C Thin, deformed long bones, thin beaded ribs
III	259420*	AD (new) AR (uncommon)	Moderately severe to severe osseous fragility, variable scleral colour, severe and progressive deformity of bones
IV	166220	AD	Normal sclerae, mild to moderate long bone deformity, short stature, dentinogenesis imperfecta

*McKusick in 'Mendelian Inheritance in Man' 9th ed[38] classifies OI Type III as a recessive disorder but biochemical studies have shown that most individuals with this phenotype have a dominant disorder

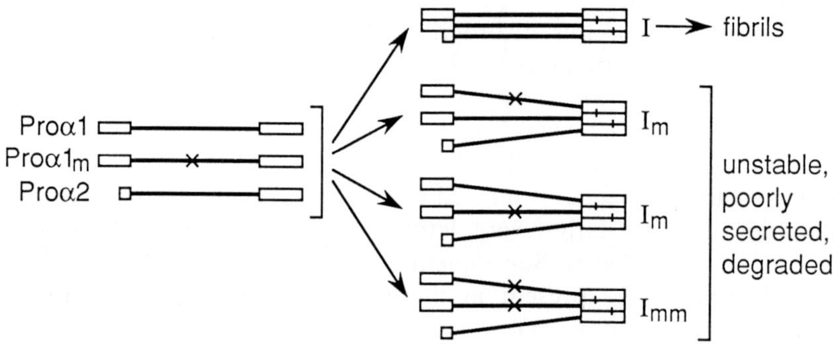

Fig. 10.10 The 'suicide protein' hypothesis showing the dominant effect of mutations in the pro α1(I) chain. Free association of normal and mutant chains leads to 3 out of 4 of the molecules produced being abnormal. (After Williams & Prockop 1983[42]).

lated hydroxylysine. The excessive hydroxylation was variable but did not clearly correlate with disease severity. An explanation of this phenomenon was provided by Bonadio and Byers[43] following a study of several patients with lethal OI. They proposed that the disease was caused by small mutations in the collagen α-chains e.g. amino acid substitutions or small deletions that delayed formation of the triple helix. Thus the protein chains associated as usual through their C-propeptides and initiated triple helix formation but when the mutation was encountered there was an energy barrier to further propagation. The portions of the α-chains on the aminoterminal side of the mutation remained non-triple-helical and therefore substrates for the hydroxylases and glycosylases for a longer time than normal becoming overmodified. When triple helix formation was finally completed, all the chains of the mutant molecule, irrespective of which one(s) carried the mutation, would be overmodified at the aminoterminal side of the mutation. The degree of overmodification would thus vary with the position of the mutation (Fig. 10.11).

Conversely, mapping the onset of overmodification within the molecule would indicate the position of the mutation. Overmodification is readily identified by electrophoresis of the denatured α-chains, because overmodified polypeptides migrate more slowly than normal. In situ cyanogen bromide peptide mapping of the partially resolved components yields tilted bands for overmodified peptides but flat bands for normal peptides (Fig. 10.11). By combining this type of peptide mapping with region-specific PCR amplification, more than 70 mutations have now been identified in OI. They fall into three main classes, amino acid substitutions in the triple-helical domain, exon skips or deletions in the triple helix and mutations affecting the C-terminal, non-helical domain.

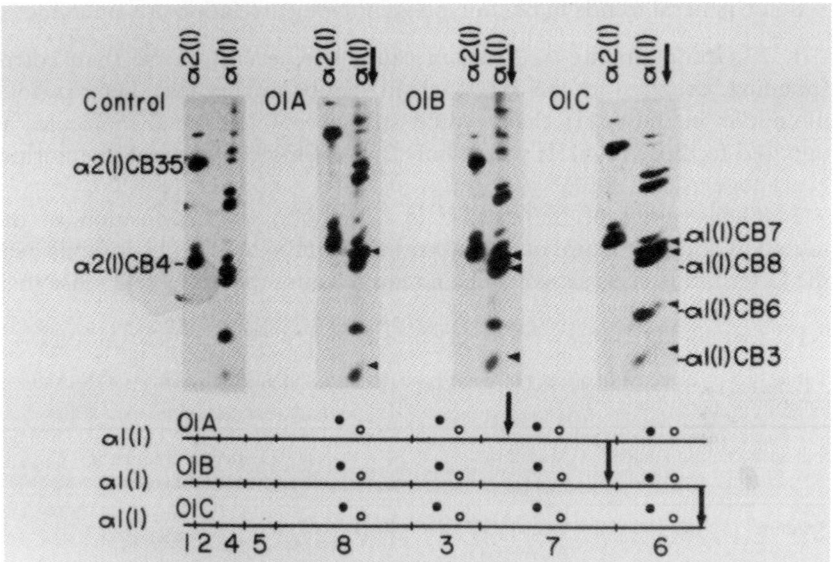

Fig. 10.11 Two-dimensional electrophoretic maps of type I collagen produced by patients with Type II osteogenesis imperfecta (OI). The α-chains have been separated from right to left in the first dimension digested in situ with cyanogen bromide then electrophoresed vertically. Tilting of the bands for individual CB peptides (arrowheads) indicates heterogeneity due to excessive post-translation modification. Three categories of patient are identified (OIA, OIB, OIC) by the CB peptides that are affected. The lower part of the figure gives a schematic representation of the α1(I) chain from each patient. The circles represent the relative migration of normal (open circles) and abnormal (closed circles) peptides, and the arrows indicate probable sites for the mutation in each category of patient that would give rise to the observed patterns. Reproduced with permission from Nature 1985 Bonadio & Byers[43]

Amino acid substitutions in the triple helix

The critical role of the glycine residue in the Gly-X-Y sequence in the formation of the triple helical structure has been underscored by the fact that virtually every disease-causing mutation in this domain has resulted in substitution of this glycine by another amino acid. The bulkier side-chain of the substituting amino acid cannot be comfortably accommodated in the core of the triple helix and hence destabilizes the molecular structure.

Single base changes in the codon for glycine (GGN) can generate the codons for eight amino acids or a stop signal (Table 10.5). From the preferred codon usage for glycine in the cDNA sequence of the α1(I) and α2(I) chains and the known mutation rates the probabilities of each substitution occurring can be calculated (Table 10.5). The glycine substitutions identified at the time of writing are indicated in Fig. 10.12. Glycine → cysteine changes in the α1(I) chain are most common because they are easy to recognize; incorporation of two mutant chains in a molecule leads to the formation of disulphide-bonded dimers. Others such as Gly→ Ala are clearly underrepresented so far.

Some general trends in phenotype–genotype correlation are emerging:

1. Mutations in the α2(I) chain cause less severe disease than corresponding changes in the α1(I) chain, probably because heterozygous mutations in the α2(I) chain would still give 50% normal molecules as opposed to those in α1(I) where only 25% of molecules would be normal (see above).

2. The severity of the disease is a function of the position of the mutation and the nature of the substituting amino acid. Substitutions near the C-terminus of a particular chain tend to cause more severe disease than

Table 10.5 Expected frequency of single base mutations in glycine codons (GGN) and consequent substitutions

Substituted amino acid	Mutation	% Expected frequency in fibrillar collagens
Arginine	CGA CGT CGC CGG AGA AGG	19
Valine	GTA GTT GTC GTG	16
Alanine	GCA GCT GCC GCG	16
Cysteine	TGT TGC	14
Serine	AGT AGC	14
Aspartate	GAT GAC	14
Glutamate	GAA GAG	2.6
Tryptophan	TGG	0.4
Stop	TGA	2.0

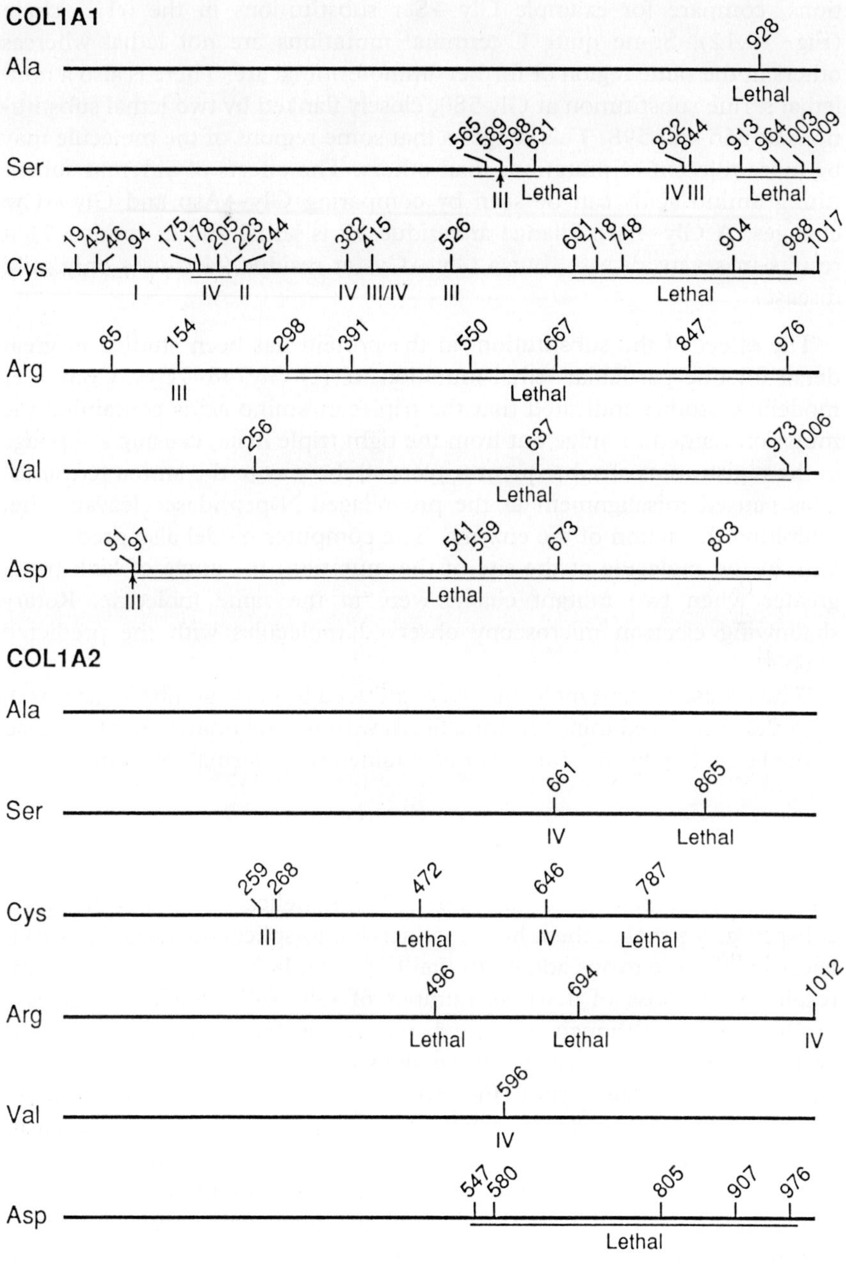

Fig. 10.12 Diagrammatic representation of amino acid substitutions observed in the α1(I), (COL1A1), or α2(1), (COL1A2), chains and the clinical phenotype of patients with osteogenesis imperfecta. Each represents the substitution of a glycine in the Gly-X-Y sequence by the amino acids identified on the left. The Roman numerals refer to the Sillence type of OI for the patient (After Byers et al[35]).

similar changes nearer to the aminoterminus. However there are exceptions, compare for example Gly→Ser substitutions in the α1(I) chain (Fig. 10.12). Some quite C-terminal mutations are not lethal whereas others in the same region or further aminoterminal are. There is also a non-lethal serine substitution at Gly 589, closely flanked by two lethal substitutions at 565 and 598. This suggests that some regions of the molecule may be more tolerant of mutations than others. The effects of different substituting amino acids can be seen by comparing Gly→Asp and Gly→Cys changes. A Gly→Asp change at residue 97 is lethal and at residue 91 it results in severe disease, but a Gly→Cys at residue 94 causes only mild disease.

The effect of the substitution on the protein has been studied in great detail for one particular lethal mutation, α1(I) Gly748→Cys. Computer modelling studies indicated that the triplet of amino acids containing the mutation tended to bulge out from the tight triple helix, causing a slippage in the registration of subsequent triplets all the way to the amino terminus. This caused misalignment at the procollagen-N-peptidase cleavage site, inhibiting the action of the enzyme. The computer model also predicted a kink in the molecule at the site of the mutation, the angle of kink being greater when two mutant chains were in the same molecule. Rotary shadowing electron microscopy observed molecules with the predicted kinks.[44]

When these mutant molecules were induced to undergo fibrillogenesis in vitro they produced thin, dendritic fibrils with several branch points instead of the large, highly structured fibrils obtained with normal molecules.[45]

Exon skips and deletions in the triple-helical domain

The multiexon modular structure of the triple-helical domain of the type I collagen genes makes them highly vulnerable to splicing defects. However, because all these exons adhere to the 9 bp rule, loss of one or more exons results in the loss of a whole number of Gly-X-Y triplets and gives a product which, although shortened, remains in-frame and maintains the critical (Gly-X-Y)n sequence. Exon skips have been identified in patients with various OI phenotypes (Fig. 10.13). They are all the result of point mutations or small genomic deletions that disrupt the 5' or 3' consensus splice site sequences (AG——GTAAGT). Phenotype – genotype correlations of exon skips are complicated. For some mutations affecting the moderately conserved bases the aberrant splicing is only partial and can be affected by external factors like temperature. In other cases the effect of the mutation is modified because abnormally spliced protein never leaves the cell, leaving the extracellular matrix with reduced amounts of normal protein.

Deletions smaller than exons have been described, a 9 bp deletion from

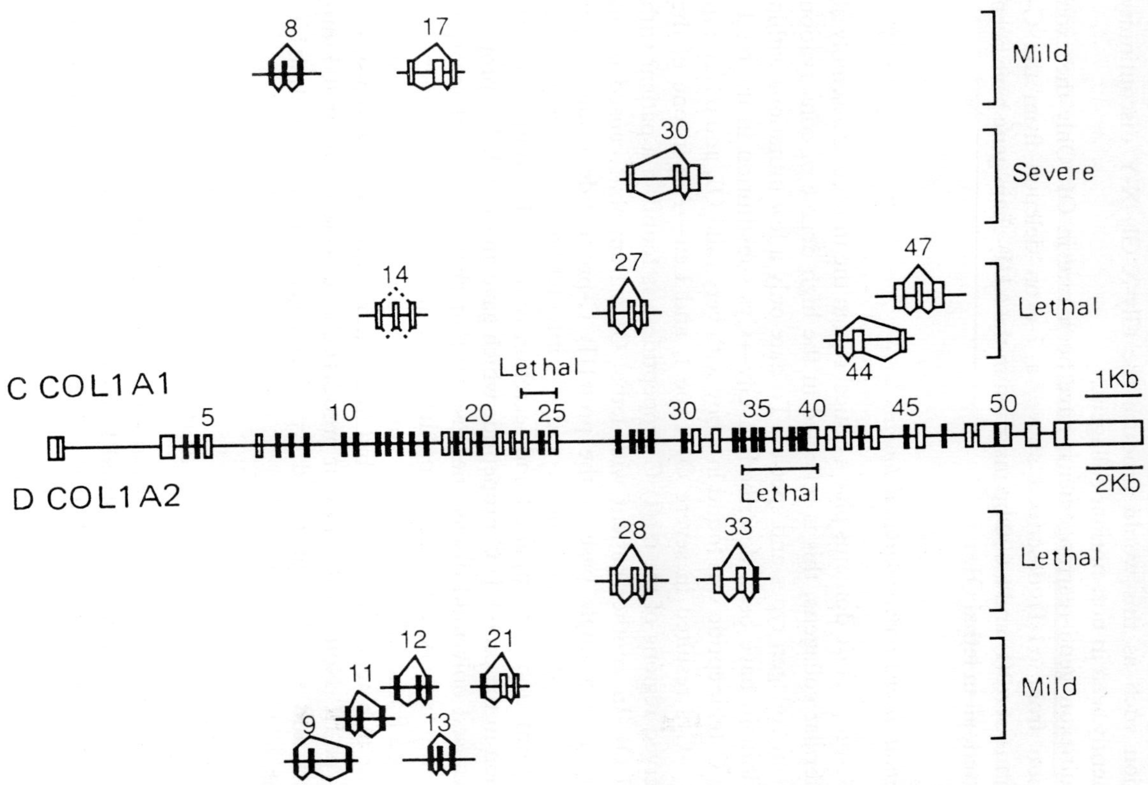

Fig. 10.13 Diagrammatic representation of exon skips in the α1(I) and α2(I) chains observed in patients with osteogenesis imperfecta. (After Byers et al[35]). The numbers indicate the exon skipped in each case.

the α1(I) gene, removing a complete Gly-Ala-Pro triplet between residues 868 and 876 (where there are three such triplets), caused lethal OI in two separate cases. Deletion of a Gly-Pro-Pro triplet from the C-terminus of the α2(I) chain resulted in mild disease. A deletion of 3 bp encoding valine 255 of the α2(I) chain was found in a severe OI patient. A single codon deletion such as this would produce the Gly-X-Gly-X-Y discontinuity frequently seen in non-fibrillar collagens.

Multiexon gene rearrangements have been rare in OI. Only the exon deletion from α1(I) described above, a 7-exon deletion from the C-terminus of α2(I) and a 600 bp insertion in the α1(I) chain gene have been reported, all in lethal OI.

Mutations in the carboxyterminal domain

The C-propeptide domains play a critical role in the molecular assembly of the fibrillar collagens, this is reflected in the high degree of conservation between collagen types and species. To date only a few mutations within this domain have been described. A Gly→Cys substitution in the α1(I) chain C-telopeptide was found in a boy with very mild OI, and α1(I) Trp 1134→Cys resulted in severe OI Type I, and Leu→Arg in one of the conserved regions of the α1(I) C-propeptide was found in a patient with lethal OI. In another patient with lethal OI a frameshift caused by an insertion of a single base in the proα1(I) C-propeptide resulted in a truncated C-propeptide which could still interact with other chains, but helix formation was impaired and secretion reduced. In contrast a 5 bp deletion in the proα1(I) C-propeptide which gave an extended C-propeptide caused only mild disease because mutant chains were not incorporated into trimers. Likewise a 4 bp deletion from the α2(I) C-propeptide, causing a frameshift of the last 37 amino acid residues, was almost asymptomatic in heterozygous parents but in a homozygous child caused severe OI Type III. None of the mutant proα2(I) chains were incorporated into trimers and the child produced type I collagen containing only α1(I) chains.

Mutations that effect a quantitative decrease in type I collagen

Many patients with the mildest form of osteogenesis imperfecta (OI Type I) produce about half the normal levels of an apparently normal type I collagen in cultured cells. This is usually accompanied by a reduction in the steady state level of cytoplasmic mRNA for α1(I). Mutations causing this phenomenon have yet to be identified but could include promoter or enhancer mutations, splicing abnormalities that do not allow unspliced message to leave the nucleus or messenger instability leading to rapid turnover in the cytoplasm. A similar phenotype could be generated at the protein level by a premature stop codon or a structural mutation in the C-propeptide which prevents incorporation of mutant pro α1(I) chains into trimers.

The insertion of a retrovirus into the first intron of the mouse COL1A1 gene shut off transcription of that allele.[46] In the homozygous state this caused death in utero on day 13 due to ruptured blood vessels, but in the heterozygous state the mice had symptoms of mild OI.[47]

The genetics of OI

From pedigree structures it is clear that Sillence types I and IV OI are dominantly inherited, likewise there is substantial molecular evidence that sporadic cases of lethal and severe OI are also the result of de novo heterozygous mutations of collagen genes. However the recurrence of severe or lethal phenotypes in sibs born to clinically normal parents is higher than expected for the de novo mutation rate suggesting that occasionally OI is recessively inherited. To cover this possibility, a recurrence risk of 6% is often quoted in families with normal unrelated parents and 25% to consanguineous parents. However there is increasing evidence that recessive inheritance of OI is rare and restricted to consanguineous families or to isolated populations where there may be a common founder mutation. Only one family with third cousin parents has had recessive inheritance of a collagen mutation clearly demonstrated (the 4 bp deletion from the α2(I) C-propeptide cited above). In the majority of cases affected sibs have been shown to be heterozygous for collagen mutations with one parent who is a gonadal and often somatic mosaic for the mutation. The expression of somatic mosaicism may be so low as to be undetectable in the parent except under the closest scrutiny, in others it may be sufficiently high to manifest as a mild OI phenotype, as in a man with OI Type IV who fathered a child with lethal OI. Both had the same mutation but in the father only 50% of the cells carried the mutation.[48]

OI caused by mutations in non-collagen genes

A large multicentre linkage study, involving families from many populations, demonstrated that dominantly inherited osteogenesis imperfecta always segregated with one of the two genes for type I collagen. Direct analysis of mutations has also implicated these genes in most cases of sporadic OI. However there are some families in the native South African, caucasian and Asian populations, with recessively inherited OI, where the disease shows discordant segregation to both COL1A1 and COL1A2 loci. This suggests that the OI phenotype can be caused by mutations in genes other than the collagens but as yet they have not been identified. In a mouse model with some features of a recessive OI the collagens were normal but a partial deficiency of osteonectin, another bone matrix protein, was observed.

Classification of OI

At the beginning of this section the difficulties in classifying OI on clinical grounds were raised. The reasons for this are now apparent. Mutations causing OI are spread uniformly along the genes; there are no 'hot spots' where clustering of mutations is apparent; nor are particular types of disease restricted to certain areas of the molecule, although it can be said there is a gradient of severity from one end to another. It is also the case that with very few exceptions the mutations described to date are unique to the particular family and have not recurred in unrelated pedigrees. The exceptions so far are α1(I)Gly154 →Arg in OI Type III and α1(I)Gly1003 → Ser in OI Type II and deletion of exon 21 caused by two different splicing abnormalities. Presumably as more mutations are identified coincidence with unrelated previously recorded cases will occur.

The Ehlers–Danlos syndrome

The Ehlers–Danlos syndrome (EDS) is a heterogeneous group of disorders in which the patients present with a velvety soft, fragile skin, a tendency to severe bruising and scarring, hypermobile joints and vascular abnormalities. The variable expression of these clinical signs and the involvement of other tissues or organs has allowed the classification of ten subtypes (Table 10.6). So far the biochemical basis is known in only a few of these types.

Ehlers–Danlos syndrome Type IV (McKusick 130050)

EDS Type IV is the most catastrophic form of the syndrome. Patients present with a remarkably thin, translucent skin showing a prominent venous network. They bruise easily and have such extreme vascular fragility that spontaneous ruptures of large or medium-sized blood vessels, bowel or uterus are often fatal. Some patients also show a prematurely aged appearance of hands and feet (acrogeria). The disease is caused by a defect of type III collagen, as demonstrated by direct biochemical analysis of tissues and cell cultures and segregation analysis with RFLPs for COL3Al. The types of mutation occurring in these patients and their effects on the protein are similar to those described for type I collagen in OI. Point mutations at glycine codons, splicing defects and large deletions have all been identified (Table 10.7) as heterozygous defects. As type III collagen is a homotrimer, sequestration of normal chains by mutant chains in a heterozygous individual will mean that only one in eight molecules will be normal; the remainder will have either one, two or three mutant chains.

Ehlers–Danlos syndrome Type VI (McKusick 225400)

EDS Type VI was the first inherited connective tissue disease to have its molecular basis identified.[49, 50] It is a rare autosomal recessive disorder

Table 10.6 Classification and features of the Ehlers–Danlos syndrome (EDS). AD – autosomal dominant, AR autosomal recessive, XLR – X-linked recessive

Type	Inheritance	Features
EDS I (gravis)	AD	Severe joint hypermobility, skin hyperextensibility, tissue fragility
EDS II (mitis)	AD	Mild–moderate joint laxity, skin hyperextensibility, tissue fragility
EDS III (benign, hypermobile)	AD	Generalized severe joint hypermobility without skeletal deformity, mild tissue fragility, skin hyperextensibility
EDS IV (ecchymotic)	AD	Severe bruising, frequent rupture of large arteries or bowel, low skin hyperextensibility
EDS V	XLR	Marked skin hyperextensibility with variable fragility, minimal joint hypermobility, frequent skeletal deformities
EDS VI (ocular type)	AR	Marked joint hypermobility, mild skin hyperextensibility, severe scoliosis, frequent ocular rupture and retinal detachment
EDS-VII (arthrochalasis multiplex congenita)	AD AR?	Short stature, severe joint laxity, multiple congenital dislocations, moderate skin hyperextensibility, bruising
EDS VIII (periodontitis type)	AD	Mild–moderate joint laxity, severe skin fragility, severe periodontitis with early tooth loss
EDS IX – Vacant		
EDS X	AR?	Mild joint hypermobility easy bruising, petechiae, striae distensae, platelet aggregation defect

Table 10.7 Mutations in the type III collagen gene. EDS – Ehlers–Danlos syndrome

Mutation	Disease
G^{+1} IVS16→A (splicing)	Moderate EDS IV
G^{+1} IVS20→A (splicing)	EDS IV/aneurysms
G^{+5} IVS25→T (splicing)	
G^{+5} IVS27→A (splicing)	EDS IV
G^{+1} IVS41→A (splicing)	EDS IV
G^{+1} IVS42→A (splicing)	Severe EDS IV
Gly619→ Arg	Familial aneurysms
Gly790→Ser	Severe EDS IV
Gly847→Glu	EDS IV
Gly883→Asp	Mild EDS IV
Gly910→Val	EDS IV
27 bp deletion exon 37	Atypical EDS IV
7.5 kb deletion exons 9–24	Severe EDS IV
9 kb deletion exons 34–48	Mild EDS IV
3.3 kb deletion	Severe EDS IV

typified by marked hyperextensibility of the skin, joint laxity, severe kyphoscoliosis and ocular globe fragility. Tissue collagens from affected individuals show a much reduced hydroxylysine content due to a deficiency in the modifying enzyme lysyl hydroxylase and a deficiency of intermolecular cross-linking. Two types of enzyme defect have been identified: a much reduced level of normal enzyme, and a structurally abnormal enzyme with low activity, altered affinity for the ascorbate cofactor and reduced thermal stability. The hydroxylysine deficiency in these patients shows some intertissue variability; the skin for example has virtually no hydroxylysine, bones and tendons slightly more, but cartilage is normally hydroxylated. This raises the interesting possibility that there are tissue-specific or collagen-type specific isoenzymes.

Ehlers–Danlos syndrome Type VII (McKusick 130060, 225410)

Patients with EDS Type VII present with extreme joint laxity, short stature and a soft, mildly hyperextensible but not necessarily fragile skin. Many affected individuals are born with bilateral hip dislocations and subsequently have multiple joint dislocations. All the patients characterised have shown abnormalities in the conversion of type I procollagen to collagen. Initially this was thought to be due to a deficiency of the enzyme procollagen-N-proteinase. However, subsequent studies identified deletions of 24 or 18 amino acids from the αl(I) or α2(I) chains respectively, including the telopeptide and N-proteinase cleavage site. In both COL1A1 and COL1A2 these sequences are encoded by a single exon, exon 6, and the mutations caused aberrant splicing of this exon (Table 10.8). In some cases exon skipping was only partial and sensitive to temperature.

In certain inbred animals, for example cattle, sheep, dogs and Himalayan cats, there is a severe recessive form of the disease, called dermatosporaxis, where the skin fragility is extreme. Here there is a total absence of N-propeptides in the procollagen molecules. These molecules can then only aggregate into thin ribbon-like fibrils, often referred to as hyeroglyphic fibrils, in contrast to the rounded

Table 10.8 Mutations in the seven characterized EDS Type VII patients

Genomic mutation	cDNA	Observation
COL1A1 last nt exon 6 G→A	Skip exon 6, Met → Ile	Partial
COL1A1 last nt exon 6 G→A	Skip exon 6, Met → Ile	Temperature-sensitive
COL1A2 last nt exon 6 G→A	Skip exon 6, Met → Ile	Temperature-sensitive
COL1A2 IVS6 G^{+1} → A	Exon 6 skip	100%
COL1A2 IVS6 G^{+2} → C	Exon 6 skip	
COL1A2 IVS6 G^{+1} → A	Exon 6 skip	100%
COL1A2 IVS6 G^{+1} → A	Exon 6 skip	100%

cross-section of normal collagen fibrils. The abnormality in molecular packing is reflected by an absence of normal intermolecular cross-linking. This form of the disease has now been observed in humans also.

Other Ehlers–Danlos syndromes

The molecular bases of the remaining forms of the Ehlers–Danlos syndrome are unknown. Ultrastructural studies have shown that in many there is abnormal collagen fibrillogenesis, but limited evidence from RFLP linkage analysis has failed to identify any collagen gene as a potential candidate. It is possible that defects in other extracellular matrix components that impinge on fibrillogenesis may cause these diseases. In EDS Type X, for example, there is evidence for a defect in fibronectin.

The Chondrodysplasias

There are more than a 100 recognised disorders of growth plate or cartilage. Cartilage is a complex tissue involving interactions between proteoglycans, glycosaminoglycans and several collagen types (see above). As type II is the major collagenous component of this tissue it has received most attention as the potential candidate gene in these disorders. Linkage analysis of COL2A1 has shown positive segregation in some forms of spondyloepiphyseal dysplasia (SED, McKusick 183900) and in some families with Stickler's syndrome (McKusick 108300) but discordance in others. Linkage to COL2A1 has been excluded in some dominant pedigrees with achondroplasia, multiple epiphyseal dysplasia, hypochondroplasia, pseudoachondroplasia, diaphyseal aclesis and trichorhinophalangeal syndrome.

The identification of causal mutations in these disorders has been frustrated by the restricted expression of the gene, the difficulty of obtaining sufficient tissue for analysis and problems associated with maintaining the chondrocyte phenotype during in vitro culture. Modern techniques have now solved or circumvented many of these problems.

Direct analysis of tissue from patients with achondrogenesis, a lethal short-limbed dwarfism showed reduced amounts of type II collagen and the abnormal presence of type I collagen in cartilage. The type II collagen extracted from the tissue was electrophoretically abnormal suggesting excessive post-translational modification. Similarly, biopsied tissue from patients with different forms of spondyloepiphyseal dysplasia (SED, McKusick 183900) and spondyloepimetaphyseal dysplasia (SEMD, McKusick 183849) contained type II collagen that was overmodified to varying extents. Cyanogen bromide peptide mapping of the mutant protein showed that the overmodified peptides varied from patient to patient in a similar manner to the type I collagen in osteogenesis imperfecta.[51] Further investigations have identified a Gly943 → Ser substitution in one COL2A1 allele of a patient with achondrogenesis; a 390 bp genomic deletion eliminating the 36-residue exon 48; an in-frame tandem duplication of 45 bp within exon 48, and a Gly997→Ser substitution, also in exon 48, in patients with forms of SED. The latter characterization[52] is a landmark for such investigations, for use was made of the power of PCR amplification to amplify the low basal levels of mRNAs for tissue-specific proteins in cells from other tissues, otherwise known as 'illegitimate transcription'. The minute amounts of mRNA for $\alpha 1$(II) produced by fibroblasts and lymphoblastoid cells were amplified to identify this mutation which was subsequently confirmed upon analysis of genomic DNA.

Direct analysis of genomic DNA in a family with Stickler's syndrome (arthrophthalmopathy) identified an Arg732 → stop mutation in one COL2A1 allele. In another family, primary osteoarthritis and a mild chondrodysplasia segregated with one COL2A1 allele. Sequencing of genomic DNA revealed an Arg519 → Cys substitution as the only change from normal. The substitution was subsequently confirmed by biochemical analysis of tissue.

Epidermolysis bullosa

Epidermolysis bullosa (EB) is a group of diseases characterized by traumatically induced blistering of the skin. There is a variable involvement of nails and mucous membranes. EB is separated into three major subtypes depending on the plane of cleavage within the skin. In one type, the dystrophic form (DEB) the skin splits below the lamina densa of the dermoepidermal basement membrane. Autosomal recessive (McKusick 226450, 226500, 226600) and autosomal dominant (McKusick 131700) inheritance occurs, but in both cases there are ultrastructural abnormalities of the anchoring fibril network of the dermoepidermal junction. In severe recessive disease different immunofluorescence studies with antibodies to type VII collagen, the major component of anchoring fibrils, have yielded contrasting results. Some have shown a complete absence of the protein, others that it is present, perhaps in reduced amounts, but not properly assembled into anchoring fibrils, and another that it is retained within the epidermis of these patients. There have also been reports that some, but not all, recessive DEB patients show an increased activity of collagenase (a proteolytic enzyme capable of cleaving within the triple-helical domain of some collagens) and one report that identified increased amounts of stromelysin, another matrix metalloproteinase capable of degrading type VII collagen. These latter studies would suggest a degradative mechanism for the loss of anchoring fibrils in some patients, but there is obvious genetic heterogeneity.

RFLP analysis using the recently cloned cDNA for type VII collagen has shown tight linkage to the milder dominant form of DEB indicating that this form is due to structural abnormalities of the protein.[53]

Cutis laxa (McKusick 123700, 219100)

The primary characteristic of cutis laxa is loose and sagging skin. Inheritance can be autosomal dominant or autosomal recessive. In the dominant form changes are restricted to the dermis, but the recessive form shows more systemic involvement with pulmonary emphysema, hernias and diverticulae of the gastrointestinal and genitourinary tracts as common features. The associated cardiopulmonary complications are often fatal in childhood. The molecular defect(s) of this disease are unknown. Ultrastructurally the skin shows abnormalities of elastic fibres, and quantitative changes in elastin and type VI collagen have been reported in different patients.

The Marfan syndrome (McKusick 154700)

The Marfan syndrome is a heterogeneous group of autosomal dominant disorders in which there are skeletal, cardiovascular and ocular abnormalities. The typical Marfan patient is tall with long arms, fingers and feet (arachnodactyly), pectus deformities of the chest, scoliosis, ectopia lentis and mitral valve prolapse. Dilatation of the ascending aota and aortic dissection are common and life-threatening.

For many years the Marfan syndrome was considered a potential collagen disorder; some of the clinical features are similar to those induced by lathyrism the disease caused by inhibition of lysyl oxidase. Linkage analysis in several large kindreds excluded all the major collagen loci, and use of anonymous DNA probes eventually localized the disease gene to chromosome 15q15–21.[54,55] Coincidentally, immunohistochemical abnormalities were identified in the skin of patients, using antibodies to a novel microfibrillar glycoprotein, fibrillin.[56] Subsequently two genes containing fibrillin-like sequences were cloned, one localized to chromosome 5, the other localized to chromosome 15q12–21, showed tight linkage to the Marfan disease locus[57] and mutations in this gene are being identified.[58]

Other diseases

The Occipital Horn syndrome, which includes patients previously classified as EDS Type IX and X-linked cutis laxa, and Menke's syndrome are both X-linked disorders characterised by lax skin, hypermobile joints, bladder diverticulae and other signs of connective tissue weakness. Both diseases are associated with abnormal copper metabolism which causes a reduced activity of the cross-linking enzyme, lysyl oxidase, for which copper is a cofactor. A similar abnormality of copper transport and lysyl oxidase activity is associated with the X-linked *mottled* locus in mice. Severely affected individuals die prematurely from ruptured arterial aneurysms resulting from the weakness of the uncross-linked tissue.

Alport's syndrome (McKusick 104200) is a dominantly inherited X-linked progressive nephritis, often accompanied by hearing loss and eye lesions. It is characterised by ultrastructural abnormalities of the glomerular basement membrane (GBM) including patchy thickening and thinning with splitting of the lamina densa. The disease locus was mapped to Xq22–24. The gene for the α5(IV) chain was also localized to this region and mutations of this gene have been identified in patients with Alport's syndrome. One, a deletion of about 15 kb, caused the loss of 6 exons; another was a point mutation in the C-terminal non-helical domain (NC –1) that changed a conserved cysteine to serine, and three major gene rearrangements involving large deletions or insertions have been identified.

Implications for more common disorders

Although osteogenesis imperfecta is a relatively rare form of inherited osteopaenia, in its mildest forms there is considerable phenotypic overlap with a much more common form of osteopaenia, osteoporosis. The latter must have many causes, but in some instances there is a clear familial predisposition suggesting an underlying genetic defect. The paradigm of osteogenesis imperfecta would suggest type I collagen genes as good candidates. Indeed there is some support for this hypothesis. A lady with postmenopausal osteoporosis was found to harbour a Gly661→Ser substitution in one α2(I) allele. The heterozygous parents of the patient with the 4 bp deletion in the α2(I) C-propeptide were radiologically osteoporotic, and some mutations near to the amino terminal of the α1(I) or α2(I) chains, e.g. αl(I) Gly19→Cys, α1(I)Gly43→Cys and α2(I) Δ exon 9 deletion, were found in patients with severe premature osteoporosis but minimal signs of osteogenesis imperfecta.

As with type I collagen, the mutations in type III collagen observed so far in EDS Type IV may represent the severe extreme of a spectrum of disorders affecting the vascular system. An α1(III) Gly619→Arg has been found in a patient with familial aortic aneurysms but no other signs of the Ehlers–Danlos syndrome, and there is clear evidence that a proportion of patients with cerebral aneurysms, a common cause of strokes, have decreased synthesis of type III collagen.

CONCLUSION

In the past few years there has been a rapid expansion in our knowledge of the molecular diversity of the collagen gene family although characterisation of some of the latest additions is still incomplete at both protein and gene level. Diseases associated with abnormalities of several collagens have been identified, and the nature of causal mutations established in many cases. We now understand in general terms how mutations in the major collagen genes can affect molecular assembly, molecular stability and supramolecular assembly and these lessons will provide the basis for later studies on the minority collagens. The wide distribution of mutations in type I collagen, leading to osteogenesis imperfecta, has helped explain why this group of disorders has proven so difficult to classify on clinical grounds, and has allowed us to draw up some tentative rules for phenotype–genotype correlation. In the near future it should be possible to do the same for type III collagen mutations.

The identification of mutations in these proteins has been greatly accelerated by the advent of the polymerase chain reaction and by recently developed methods of mismatch analysis. Application of such techniques to other collagens whose expression is restricted to inaccessible tissues should greatly facilitate the identification of mutations in these proteins. The paradigm for this approach has already been established with identification of a type II collagen mutation using fibroblast and lymphoblastoid cultures. In vitro mutagenesis of cloned genes and the generation of transgenic animals should provide further insight into structure–function relationships, and enable us to identify candidate diseases for those collagen genes for which none exists at present.

REFERENCES

1. Miller E J, Matukas V J 1969 Chick cartilage collagen: a new type of αl chain not present in bone or skin of the species. Proceedings of the National Academy of Sciences USA 64:1264–1268
2. Chung E, Miller E J 1974 Collagen polymorphism: characterization of molecules with the chain composition $\alpha l(III)_3$ in human tissues. Science 183:1200–1201
3. Epstein E M 1974 $\alpha l(III)_3$ Human skin collagen. Release by pepsin digestion and preponderance in fetal life. Journal of Biological Chemistry 249:3225–3231
4. Traub W, Piez K A 1971 The chemistry and structure of collagen. Advances in Protein Chemistry 25:243–352
5. Bornstein P, Sage H 1980 Structurally distinct collagen types. Annual Reviews of Biochemistry 49:957–1003
6. Vuorio E, de Crombrugghe B 1990 The family of collagen genes. Annual Reviews of Biochemistry 59:837–872
7. Shaw L M, Olsen B R 1991 FACIT collagens: diverse molecular bridges in extracellular matrices. Trends in Biological Science 16:191–194
8. Van der Rest M, Garrone R 1991 Collagen family of proteins. FASEB Journal 5:2814–2823
9. Kadler K E, Hojima Y, Prockop D J 1990 Collagen fibrils in vitro grow from pointed tips in the C- to N-terminal direction. Biochemical Journal 268:339–343
10. Chapman J A 1989 The regulation of size and form in the assembly of collagen fibrils in vivo. Biopolymers 28:1367–13892, 2201–2205
11. Burgeson R E, El Adli F A, Kaitila I, Hollister D W 1976 Fetal membrane collagens: identification of two new collagen alpha chains. Proceedings of the National Academy of Sciences USA 73:2579–2583
12. Brown R A, Shuttleworth C A, Weiss J B 1978 Three new α-chains of collagen from a non-basement membrane source. Biochemical and Biophysical Research Communications 80:866–872
13. Birk D E, Fitch J M, Babiarz J P, Linsenmeyer T F 1988 Collagen type I and V are present in the same fibril in the avian corneal stroma. Journal of Cell Biology 106:999–1008
14. Burgeson R E, Hollister D W 1979 Collagen heterogeneity in human cartilage:

identification of several new collagen chains. Biochemical and Biophysical Research Communications 87:1124–1131
15. Niyibizi C, Eyre D R 1989 Identification of the cartilage αl(XI) chain in type V collagen from bovine bone. FEBS Letters 242:314–318
16. Hostikka S L, Eddy R L, Byers M G, Höyhtyä M, Shows T B, Tryggvason K 1990 Identification of a distinct type IV collagen α chain with restricted kidney distribution and assignment of its gene to the locus of X chromosome linked Alport Syndrome. Proceedings of the National Academy of Sciences USA 87:1606–1610
17. Timpl R, Wiedeman H, van Delden V, Furthmayr H, Kühn K 1981 A network model for the organization of type IV collagen molecules in basement membranes. European Journal of Biochemistry 120:203–211
18. Furthmayr H, Wiedemann H, Timpl R, Odermatt E, Engel J 1983 Electron microscopical approach to a structural model of intima collagen. Biochemical Journal 211:303–311
19. Lunstrum G P, Kuo H-J, Rosenbaum L M, Keene D R, Glanville R W, Sakai L Y, Burgeson R E 1987 Anchoring fibrils contain the carboxyl-terminal globular domain of type VII procollagen but lack the amino-terminal globular domain. Journal of Biological Chemistry 262:13706–13712
20. Parente M G, Chung L C, Ryynänen J et al 1991 Human type VII collagen : cDNA cloning and chromosomal mapping of the gene. Proceedings of the National Academy of Sciences USA 88:6931–6935
21. Yamaguchi N, Benya P D, van der Rest M, Ninomiya Y 1989 The cloning and sequencing of α1(VIII) collagen cDNAs demonstrate that type VIII collagen is a short chain collagen and contains triple-helical and carboxyl-terminal non-triple-helical domains similar to those of type X collagen. Journal of Biological Chemistry 264:16022–16029
22. Muragaki Y, Jacenko O, Apte S, Mattei M G, Ninomiya Y, Olsen B R 1991 The α2(VIII) collagen gene – a novel member of the short chain collagen family located on the human chromosome 1. Journal of Biological Chemistry 266:7721–7727
23. Schmid T M, Linsenmeyer T F 1985 Immunohistochemical localization of short chain cartilage collagen (type X) in avian tissues. Journal of Cell Biology 100:598–605
24. Pihlajaniemi T, Tamminen M 1990 The αl chain of type XIII collagen consists of three collagenous and four non-collagenous domains and its primary transcript undergoes complex alternative splicing. Journal of Biological Chemistry 265:16922–16928
25. Sandberg M, Tamminen M, Hirvonen H, Vuorio E, Pihlajaniemi T 1989 Expression of mRNAs coding for the αl chain of type XIII collagen in human fetal tissues: Comparison with expression of mRNAs for collagen types I, II and III. Journal of Cell Biology 109:1371–1379
26. Vaughan L, Mendler M, Huber S, Bruckner P, Winterhalter K H, Irwin M I, Mayne R 1988 D-Periodic distribution of collagen type IX along cartilage fibrils. Journal of Cell Biology 106:991–997
27. Dublet B, Oh S, Sugrue S P, Gordon M K, Gerecke D R, Olsen B R, van der Rest M 1989 The structure of avian type XII collagen. αl(XII) chains contain 190 kDA non-triple helical amino terminal domains and form homotrimeric molecules. Journal of Biological Chemistry 264:13150–13156
28. Dublet B, van der Rest M 1991 Type XIV collagen, a new homotrimeric molecule extracted from fetal bovine skin and tendon, with a triple helical disulphide-bonded domain homologous to type IX and type XII collagens. Journal of Biological Chemistry 266:6853–6858
29. Lunstrum G P, Morris N P, McDonagh A M, Keene D R, Burgeson R E 1991 Identification and partial characterization of two type XII-like collagen molecules. Journal of cell Biology 113:963-969
30. Tikka L, Elomaa O, Pihlajaniemi T, Tryggvason K 1991 Human αl(XIII) collagen gene. Multiple forms of the gene transcripts are generated through complex alternative splicing of several short exons. Journal of Biological Chemistry 266:17713–17719
31. LuValle P, Ninomiya Y, Rosenblum N D, Olsen B R 1988 The type X collagen gene. Intron sequences split the 5'-untranslated region and separate the coding regions for the non-collagenous amino-terminal and triple helical domains. Journal of Biological Chemistry 263:18378–18385
32. Yamaguchi N, Mayne R, Ninomiya Y 1991 The α1(VIII) collagen gene is homologous

to the α1(X) collagen gene and contains a large exon encoding the entire triple helical and carboxyl-terminal non-triple helical domains of the αl(VIII) polypeptide. Journal of Biological Chemistry 266:4508–4513
33. Nishimura I, Muragaki Y, Olsen B R 1989 Tissue specific forms of type IX collagen-proteoglycan arise from the use of two widely separated promoters. Journal of Biological Chemistry 264:20033–20041
34. Gordon M K, Gerecke D R, Dublet B, van der Rest M, Olsen B R 1989 Type XII collagen. A large multidomain molecule with partial homology to type IX collagen. Journal of Biological Chemistry 264:19772–19778
35. Byers P H, Wallis G A, Willing M C 1991 Osteogenesis imperfecta translation of mutation to phenotype. Journal of Medical Genetics. 28:433–442
36. Kuivaniemi H, Tromp G, Prockop D J 1991 Mutations in collagen genes: causes of rare and some common diseases in humans. FASEB Journal 5:2052–2061
37. Sillence D O, Senn A, Danks D M 1979 Genetic heterogeneity in osteogenesis imperfecta. Journal of Medical Genetics 16:101–116
38. McKusick V A 1990 Mendelian inheritance in man, 9th edn. Johns Hopkins University Press, Baltimore
39. Penttinen R P, Lichtenstein J R, Martin G R, McKusick V A 1975 Abnormal collagen metabolism in cultured cells in osteogenesis imperfecta. Proceedings of the National Academy of Sciences USA. 72:586–589
40. Barsh G S, Roush C N, Bonadio J, Byers P H, Gelinas R E 1985 Intron-mediated recombination may cause a deletion in an αl type I collagen chain in a lethal form of osteogenesis inperfecta. Proceedings of the National Academy of Sciences USA 82:2870–2874
41. Chu M-L, Gargiulo V, Williams C J, Ramirez F 1985 Multiexon deletion in an osteogenesis imperfecta variant with increased type III collagen mRNA. Journal of Biological Chemistry 260:691–694
42. Williams C J Prockop D J 1983 Synthesis and processing of a Type 1 procollagen containing shortened proα(I) chains by fibroblasts from a patient with osteogenesis imperfecta. Journal of Biological Chemistry 258:5915–5921
43. Bonadio J, Byers P H 1985 Subtle structural alterations in the chains of type I procollagen produce osteogenesis imperfecta type II. Nature 316:363–366
44. Vogel B E, Doelz R, Kadler K E, Hojima Y, Engel J, Prockop D J 1988 A substitution of cysteine for glycine 748 of the α1 chain produces a kink at this site in the procollagen I molecule and an altered N-proteinase cleavage site over 225 nm away. Journal of Biological Chemistry 263:19249–19255
45. Kadler K E, Torre-Blanco A, Adachi E, Vogel B E, Hojima Y, Prockop D J 1991 A type I collagen with substitution of a cysteine for glycine 748 in the α1(I) chain copolymerizes with normal type I collagen and can generate fractal-like structures. Biochemistry 30:5081–5088
46. Schnieke A, Harbers K, Jaenisch R 1983 Embryonic lethal mutation in mice induced by retrovirus insertion into α(I) collagen gene. Nature 304:315–320
47. Bonadio J, Saunders T L, Tsai E et al 1990 Transgenic mouse model of the mild dominant form osteogenesis imperfecta. Proceedings of the National Academy of Sciences USA 87:7145–7149
48. Wallis G A, Starman B J, Zinn A B, Byers P H 1990 Variable expression of osteogenesis imperfecta in a nuclear family is explained by somatic mosaicism for a lethal point mutation in the α1(I) gene (COL1A1)of type I collagen in a parent. American Journal of Human Genetics 46:1034–1040
49. Pinnell S R, Krane S M, Kenzora J E, Glimcher M J 1972 A heritable disorder of connective tissue: hydroxylysine-deficient collagen disease. New England Journal of Medicine 866:1013–1020
50. Krane S M, Pinnell S R, Erbe R W 1972 Lysyl-protocollagen hydroxylase deficiency in fibroblasts from siblings with hydroxylysine-deficient collagen. Proceedings of the National Academy of Sciences USA 69:2899–2903
51. Murray L W, Bautista J, James P L, Rimoin D C 1989 Type II collagen defects in the chondrodysplasias. I. Spondyloepiphyseal dysplasias. American Journal of Human Genetics 45:5–15
52. Chan D, Cole W G 1991 Low basal transcription of genes for tissue specific collagens by fibroblasts and lymphoblastoid cells. Application to the characterization of a glycine 997

to serine substitution in α1(II) collagen chains of a patient with spondyloepiphysial dysplasia. Journal of Biological Chemistry 266:12487–12494
53. Ryynänen M, Knowlton R G, Parente M G, Chung L C, Chu M L, Uitto J 1991 Human type VII collagen. Genetic linkage of the gene (COL7A1) on chromosome 3 to dominant dystrophic epidermolysis bullosa. American Journal of Human Genetic 49:797–803
54. Kainulainen K, Pulkkinen L, Savolainen A, Kaitila I, Peltonen L 1990 Location on chromosome 15 of the gene defect causing Marfan syndrome. New England Journal of Medicine 323:935–939
55. Dietz H C, Pyeritz R E, Hall B D et al 1991 The Marfan syndrome locus: confirmation of assignment to chromosome 15 and identification of tightly linked markers at 15q15–q21.3. Genomics 9:355–361
56. Godfrey M, Menashe V, Weleber R G et al 1990 Cosegregation of elastin associated microfibrillar abnormalities with the Marfan phenotype in families. American Journal of Human Genetics 46:652–660
57. Lee B, Godfrey M, Vitale E et al 1991 Linkage of Marfan syndrome and a phenotypically related disorder to two different fibrillar genes. Nature 352:330–334
58. Dietz H C, Cutting G R, Pyeritz R E et al 1991 Marfan syndrome caused by a recurrent de novo missense mutation in the fibrillin gene. Nature 352:337–339

11. Inherited disorders of steroid biosynthesis

G. M. Addison

INTRODUCTION

The inherited diseases of steroid hormone biosynthesis constitute a large and important group of the inherited metabolic disorders. Biosynthesis of steroid hormones takes place in the adrenal cortex, gonads and placenta; other tissues are involved, however, in both the production of some active steroid metabolites, e.g. dihydrotestosterone from testosterone in the skin, and in the biochemical inactivation, degradation and excretion of the steroids. Inherited disorders of both steroid synthesis and peripheral metabolism have been described.

Physiologically, steroid hormones are divided into three groups, representing glucocorticoid, mineralocorticoid or sex hormone activity, each with specific actions, control, etc., though this distinction is by no means absolute. Inherited diseases resulting in impaired steroid biosynthesis are caused by the absence or altered properties of one of the enzymes in the biosynthetic pathways. As a result there is an accumulation of precursor molecules and often increased activity in alternative pathways of steroid metabolism. The biological activity of the precursor molecules, the increased synthesis of other steroids and the antagonism that can occur between different steroids produce a complex situation in which, for example, a primary defect in the synthesis of cortisol can present clinically as a disturbance of sexual differentiation.

A complete understanding of the clinical and pathological aspects of inborn errors of steroid biosynthesis requires a comprehensive knowledge of the anatomy, biochemistry and physiology of steroid hormone metabolism in fetal and postnatal life, and also of the process of sexual differentiation. Because steroid hormones are involved in the sexual development of the fetus, disorders of steroid synthesis frequently give rise to abnormal sexual development. Detailed reviews have been published elsewhere[1–5]; for the purposes of this chapter only an essential outline will be given. Emphasis will be given to the adrenal cortex since this gland is involved in the synthesis of all three types of steroid and is the major organ involved in inherited disorders of steroid biosynthesis.

THE ADRENAL CORTEX

The adrenal cortex develops from mesodermal tissue beginning in the sixth week of life. By the 20th week there are two distinct zones; an inner fetal zone which constitutes the bulk of the gland and a thin subcapsular zone of small lipid-containing cells termed the adult zone. The adult zone increases in size throughout the remainder of pregnancy and constitutes about 20% of the gland at birth. Postnatally the fetal cortex rapidly degenerates. The steroid biosynthetic activity of the fetal adrenal varies throughout pregnancy but one important function is as an integral part of the fetoplacental unit in the synthesis of oestriol (see later).

During the immediate postnatal period there are considerable structural and biochemical changes. The adrenal develops the classical three zones, the glomerulosa, fasciculata and reticularis. In the infant the glomerulosa is a continuous subcapsular band but in the adult it is usually broken up into discrete islets. The glomerulosa is the site of synthesis of aldosterone while the glucocorticoid and adrenal sex steroid hormones are synthesized in the fasciculata and the reticularis.

The blood supply to the adrenal is complex: three separate arteries join to form a subcapsular plexus from which a few twigs go direct to the adrenal medulla. Capillaries pass downwards through the fasciculata into a capillary network in the reticularis which drains in turn into a single central adrenal vein. It has been suggested that this vascular arrangement has some function in controlling steroid biosynthesis and, in particular, the synthesis of androgens in the reticularis.[6]

STEROID STRUCTURE

All naturally occurring steroids are based on a 4-ring structure, the cyclopentanoperhydrophenanthrene nucleus (Fig. 11.1) and its derivatives of which the largest is cholesterol. The numbering of the carbon atoms of the steroid nucleus is particularly important since the enzymes of steroid

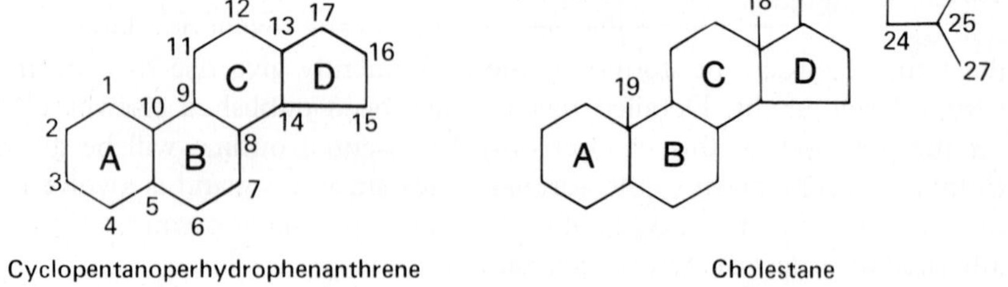

Fig. 11.1 The steroid nucleus, showing numbering of the carbon atoms.

Table 11.1 Steroid nomenclature

Common name	IUPAC nomenclature
Cholesterol	cholest-5-en-3β-ol
Pregnenolone	3β-hydroxypregn-5-en-20-one
Progesterone	pregn-4-ene-3,20-dione
17-Hydroxypregnenolone	3β,17α-dihydroxypregn-5-en-20-one
17-Hydroxyprogesterone	17α-hydroxypregn-4-ene-3,20-dione
11-Deoxycortisol	17α,21-dihydroxypregn-4-ene-3,20-dione
11-Deoxycorticosterone (DOC)	21-hydroxypregn-4-ene-3,20-dione
Corticosterone	11β,21-dihydroxypregn-4-ene-3,20-dione
Cortisol	11β,17,21-trihydroxypregn-4-ene-3,20-dione
18-Hydroxycorticosterone	11β,18,21-trihydroxypregn-4-ene-3,20-dione
Aldosterone	11β,21-dihydroxy-18-al-pregn-4-ene-3,20-dione
Dehydroepiandrosterone (DHA)	3β-hydroxyandrost-5-en-17-one
Androstenedione	androst-4-ene-3,17 dione
Testosterone	17β-hydroxyandrost-4-en-3-one
Dihydrotestosterone (DHT)	17β-hydroxy-5α-androstan-3-one
Oestrone	3-hydroxyoestra-1,3,5(10)-trien-17-one
Oestradiol	oestra-1,3,5(10)-triene-3,17-βdiol

metabolism are in part identified by these numbers e.g. 21-hydroxylase. Hydroxyl or other substituents can be orientated towards the reader (α) or away (β). Isomers can occur which radically alter the three-dimensional structure of the steroids and therefore their biological activity.

Steroid nomenclature (IUPAC)[7] is complicated and is based on the various parent nuclei, cholestane (C27), pregnane (C21), androstane (C19) and oestrane (C18). For general purposes the standard IUPAC names are abbreviated. Systematic and abbreviated names of the most important steroids are listed in Table 11.1.

STEROID HORMONE BIOSYNTHESIS[8]

The classical integrated pathway of steroid hormone biosynthesis is presented in Fig. 11.2. There are 13 different enzymic steps in this overall pathway which represents the sum of the pathways in the different steroid synthesizing tissues. However, recent advances in our understanding of the molecular biology and genetics of these enzymes have revolutionised our understanding of steroid biosynthesis. Several of the enzymes belong to the cytochrome P_{450} superfamily[9] and at least two, P_{450}c11 (11β-hydroxylase, 18-hydroxylase and 18-dehydrogenase) and P_{450}c17 (17-hydroxylase and 17–20 lyase) are single peptides with multifunctional properties. At the time of writing this increase in our knowledge concerning the enzymes of steroid biosynthesis has raised more problems than it has solved. The nomenclature used in this chapter for cytochrome P_{450}s and their respective gene loci is the 1991 recommendation of Nerbert and colleagues, and is designed to be compatible with computerized databases.[10]

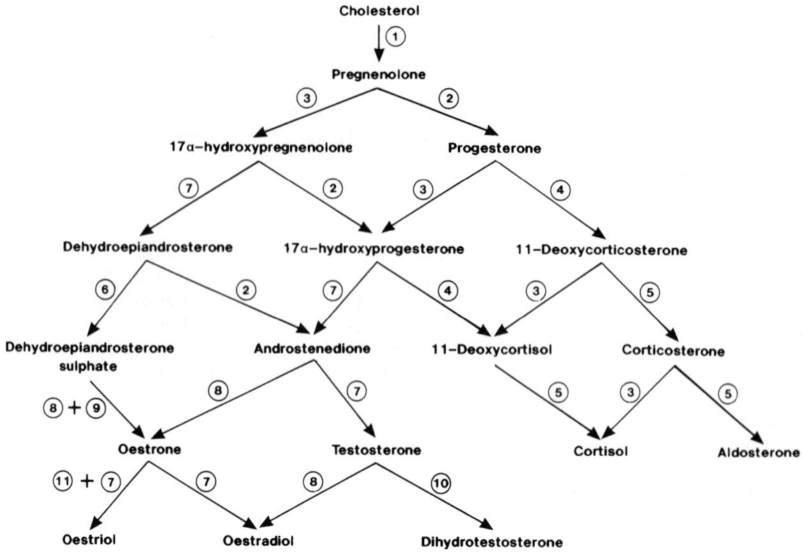

Fig. 11.2 An integrated summary of the biosynthetic pathways of glucocorticoid, mineralocorticoid and sex steroid hormones. The enzymes catalyzing each step are: 1–P_{450}scc; 2–3β-hydroxysteroid dehydrogenase; 3–P_{450}c17; 4–P_{450}c21; 5–P_{450}c11; 6–Steroid sulphotransferase; 7–17β-hydroxysteroid dehydrogenase; 8–P_{450}arom; 9–steroid sulphatase; 10–5α-reductase; 11–16α-hydroxylase.

The pathways shown in Figure 11.2 are idealised and there exist alternative enzymes and possible routes for the metabolism of individual steroids. The role of these other pathways is unclear in the normal human and their activity is usually very low. Activity of the alternative metabolic pathways can be considerably increased in pathological conditions and this accounts for many of the unusual steroids produced in the inborn errors of steroid metabolism.

The properties of the enzymes of steroid hormone biosynthesis are summarised in Table 11.2. For a number of the steroidogenic enzymes there are two copies of the gene. The second gene for P_{450}c21, 17β-hydroxysteroid dehydrogenase and probably P_{450}c11 are non-transcribed: the status of the other genes with two copies is less clear.

On the other hand there exists a considerable body of physiological and biochemical evidence for the existence of multiple isoenzymes.[13] These isoenzymes are found in different or even the same tissues and have specificity for particular groups of steroids. The existence of isoenzymes has been used as one explanation for both clinical heterogeneity and unusual steroid patterns in blood and urine. However, if isoenzymes do exist they must result from tissue-specific promoters, differential transcription and/or post-transcriptional or post-translational modification.

An alternative hypothesis has been proposed to the classical steroid

Table 11.2 Properties of steroid biosynthetic enzymes

Enzyme	Activity	E. C. number	Mol. Wt.	Cellular Localization	Gene	Chromasomal Localization	Gene copies	Exons
P_{450}scc	20,22-desmolase	1.14.15.6	850 000[1]	Mitochondria	*CYP11A1*	15q23–q24	1	9
3β-Hydroxysteroid dehydrogenase	3β-hydroxysteroid dehydrogenase $\Delta^{5,4}$-isomerase	1.1.1.145 5.3.3.1	41 000/ 77 000[2]	Mitochondria and microsomes	*HSDB3*	1p11–p13	2	—
P_{450}c17	17α-hydroxylase 17,20-lyase	1.14.99.9 4.1.2.30	57 000	Microsomes	*CYP17*	10q24–q25	1	8
P_{450}c21	21-hydroxylase	1.14.99.10	55 000	Microsomes	*CYP21*	6p21.3	2	10
P_{450}c11	11β-hydroxylase 18-hydroxylase 18-dehydrogenase	1.14.15.4 1.14.15.5 —	47 000	Mitochondria	*CYP21B1*	8q22	2	9
17β-Hydroxysteroid dehydrogenase	17β-hydroxysteroid dehydrogenase	1.1.1.64	36 000/ 68 000[2]	Microsomes	*h17β-HSD*	17q11–q21	2	6
P_{450}arom	aromatase	—	55 000	Microsomes	*CYP19*	15q21.1	2	10
5α-Reductase	5α-reductase	—	29 500	Microsomes	—	—	(1)	—
Steroid sulpho-transferase	steroid sulpho-transferase	2.8.2.2/4	34,500	Microsomes	—	—	—	—
P_{450}c16	16α-hydroxylase	—	—	Microsomes	—	—	—	—

[1]16 unit oligomer; [2]dimer

biosynthetic pathways in an attempt to explain some observations which are difficult to reconcile with this model. The key element of this hypothesis is that steroid hormones are synthesised normally in a continuous process in biosynthetic units termed 'hormonads'[11]; these hormonads contain all the enzymes, cofactors etc., required to produce a specific steroid. An objection to this hypothesis, namely that the different enzymes are localised in different subcellular fractions (see Table 11.2), has been addressed,[12] though explanations are required for the appearance of biosynthetic intermediates and their metabolites in plasma and urine.

Steroids are synthesised from cholesterol which is usually exogenous; alternatively cholesterol can be synthesised de novo from acetate. Cholesterol is converted to pregnenolone by the enzyme P_{450}scc (cholesterol 20,22-desmolase) with the loss of a 6-carbon side-chain. The action of various hydroxylases, dehydrogenases (reductases), lyases and cyclases (aromatase) converts pregnenolone to the active steroid hormones.

The synthesis of cortisol can proceed along two pathways. In the Δ^4 pathway pregnenolone is first converted to progesterone by the action of 3β-hydroxysteroid dehydrogenase:Δ^{5-4}oxosteroid isomerase (3β-HSD), and then to 17α-hydroxyprogesterone (17OHP). In the alternate Δ^5 pathway the steps are reversed with a 17α-hydroxypregnenolone being formed first and then being converted to 17OHP. In humans the Δ^5 pathway is the route for steroid synthesis since human P_{450}c17 uses 17α-hydroxypregnenolone as its substrate. Further hydroxylation at positions 21 and 11 produce cortisol.

Aldosterone synthesis, which occurs exclusively in the zona glomerulosa, proceeds along the Δ^4 pathway to progesterone and 11-deoxycorticosterone; the hydroxylation at position 21 prevents any action of 17 α-hydroxylase. Following 11β-hydroxylation the C18 methyl group is converted to an aldehyde in a two-step procedure. The first step is 18-hydroxylation to form 18-hydroxycorticosterone; the second step is possibly a dehydrogenase, or alternatively a second hydroxylation and spontaneous or enzymatic dehydration. Only the second step is exclusive to the zona glomerulosa[13]; 18-hydroxycorticosterone can be produced in the zona reticularis and fasciculata.

The major pathway of androgen biosynthesis is via the Δ^4 pathway to 17α-hydroxypregnenolone which is converted to deyhdroepiandrosterone (DHA) by P_{450}c17 (C21 → C19). Testosterone is produced from DHA by the action of 3β-HSD and 17α-hydroxysteroid dehydrogenase. Conversion of testosterone to dihydrotestosterone (DHT) occurs in the testis and also peripherally, the latter accounting for a substantial percentage of circulating DHT in the adult male. The conversion of testosterone to DHT is essential for androgenic activity in certain tissues. Testosterone does not appear to be synthesised in the adrenal under normal circumstances, but the adrenal steroids can give rise to testosterone indirectly by the peripheral conversion of androstenedione.

Oestrogen synthesis has a unique step in which the A ring is aromatised and the C19 carbon is lost (C19–C18). The reaction requires molecular oxygen, NADPH and three sequential hydroxylations, the first two being on the C19 methyl group and the third at C2, followed by a final non-enzymic loss of a water molecule. Androstenedione and testosterone are converted to oestrone and oestradiol-17β respectively. Oestriol is formed by the action of P_{450}c16 (16α-hydroxylase).

The P_{450} enzymes require a redox system to function. P_{450}scc and P_{450}c11 are mitochondrial enzymes where the NADPH-dependent redox system is made up of an iron-sulphur protein, adrenodoxin and a flavoprotein, adrenodoxin reductase. The microsomal P_{450} redox system is a non-specific flavoprotein enzyme, NADPH cytochrome P_{450} reductase.

The three major steroid-producing organs all possess the initial steps of steroid biosynthesis. Tissue-specific steroid production results from the differential expression of genes e.g. ovary and testis lack P_{450}c11 and P_{450}c21 and therefore cannot synthesise glucocorticoids or mineralocorticoids.

Control of steroid biosynthesis

The main regulator of adrenal glucocorticoid and sex hormone biosynthesis is ACTH which acts early in the biosynthetic pathway at the conversion of cholesterol to pregnenolone. A separate adrenal androgen-stimulating hormone has been postulated but there is little evidence to support this hypothesis.[14] ACTH can be detected in the fetus by the 12th week of life and plays a critical role in the development of the adrenal cortex.

ACTH has both acute and chronic effects; both are initiated by the binding of ACTH to a specific receptor on the adrenal cortical cells and are mediated by a second messenger, cyclic AMP. The acute effect results in a rapid increase in hormone production as a result of enhanced binding of cholesterol to P_{450}scc. Other acute effects include increased hydrolysis of cholesterol esters and transport of cholesterol into mitochondria. The overall result is a rapid secretion of cortisol. Chronic effects of ACTH result from not only the induction of steroid biosynthetic enzymes, as evidenced by increased P_{450} mRNAs, but also the increased synthesis of enzymes and proteins involved in electron transfer from cytochrome P_{450}, adrenodoxin, adrenodoxin reductase and NADPH-cytochrome P_{450} reductase.

ACTH is also involved in the control of adrenal mass. Excess ACTH leads to hyperplasia, while absence of the hormone results in adrenal atrophy. This action of ACTH appears to be mediated by insulin-like growth factor 2 (IGF2) via a paracrine effect. A number of other growth factors and bioactive molecules have been demonstrated in vitro to have significant negative and positive effects on steroidogenesis and it is postulated that they may play a role in vivo through paracrine or autocrine effects.[15] These include IGF1, prostaglandin E_2, transforming growth factor beta 1 and angiotensin II. High physiological concentrations of insulin have been shown to have a specific effect on adrenal androgen synthesis by inhibition of 17,20-lyase.[16] The concentration of insulin is affected in turn by counter regulatory hormones such as cortisol, and thus secondary changes in steroid biosynthesis may result from biosynthetic defects which reduce the production of cortisol.

The regulation of ACTH release is complex and the principal points are shown in Fig. 11.3. Secretion of ACTH shows a circadian rhythm with high levels of ACTH (and cortisol) secretion during the early morning

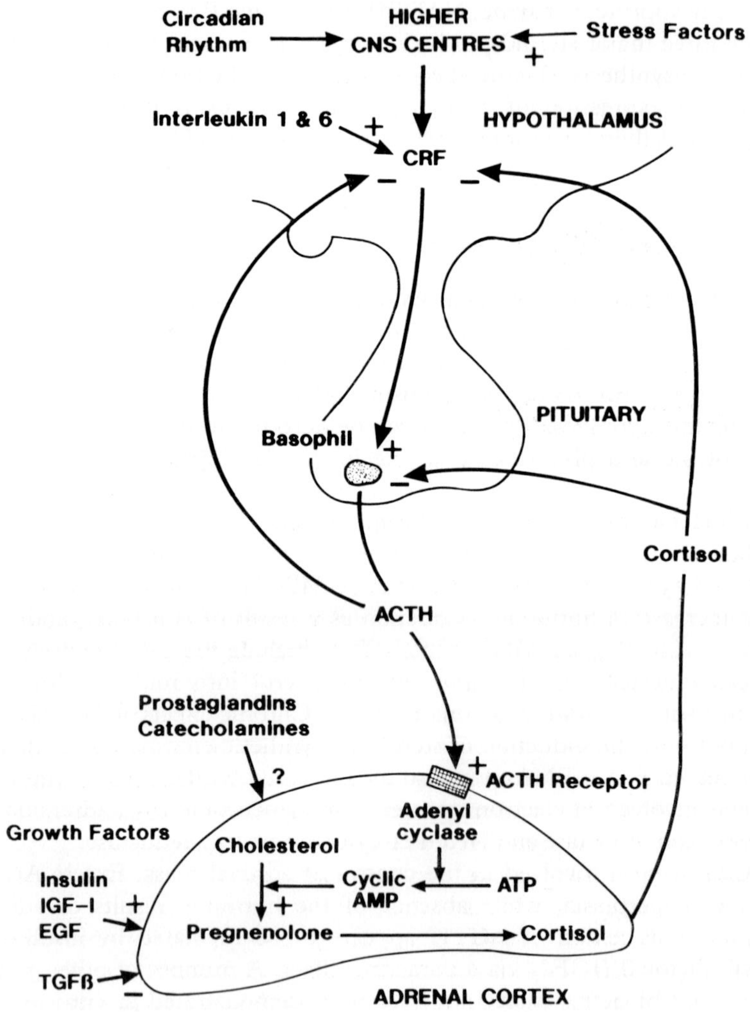

Fig. 11.3 Diagramatic representation of control mechanisms of ACTH release and cortisol biosynthesis.

which then fall gradually throughout the day. Circadian rhythm is established within the first few weeks and months after birth.[17] ACTH secretion is in turn controlled by the release of corticotrophin-releasing factor (CRF) produced in the hypothalamus. CRF release is influenced by many different factors of which stress is a component and which will override circadian rhythm and other inhibitors of ACTH release.

Cortisol has a classical feedback effect on ACTH release; an increase in plasma cortisol concentration will cause a rapid fall in ACTH secretion. In those inborn errors of steroid metabolism which reduce cortisol synthesis, this feedback control mechanism is activated, ACTH secretion is increased and its secretion becomes continuous. This gives rise to glandular hyperplasia and to increased synthesis of cortisol precursors and other metabolites. The glandular hyperplasia occurs in utero and patients with these disorders have congenital adrenal hyperplasia (CAH), but not all steroid biosynthetic defects give rise to CAH. The signs and symptoms of patients with CAH are produced by the lack of cortisol and by other steroid metabolites which, if they are androgenic, can affect sexual differentiation in utero. Maternal ACTH will not cross the placenta but maternal corticosteroid will do so, though in insufficient quantity to effectively reduce ACTH secretion in fetuses with CAH.

The three major factors involved in the control of aldosterone secretion are sodium, potassium and the renin–angiotensin system (Fig. 11.4). The role of ACTH remains controversial in normal individuals, but it is probably of minor importance, while catecholamines, prostaglandins and serotonin may also regulate aldosterone secretion. ACTH may have a more important role in aldosterone regulation in patients with the salt-losing types of CAH.[18] The relationship between aldosterone and the renin–angiotensin system is a negative feedback loop; a fall in aldosterone giving rise to sodium loss and hence a release of renin from the kidney and production of angiotensin II which directly stimulates the cells of the zona glomerulosa to synthesise aldosterone. This feedback mechanism is very sensitive and disorders of steroid biosynthesis which give rise to a loss of body sodium will be accompanied by high renin levels.

It has been proposed that the mass of the individual adrenal zones, and in particular their width, is involved in the control of steroid biosynthesis.[6] This control mechanism relies on the vascular arrangement of the adrenal which can allow the establishment of a metabolic gradient, particularly of steroids, and on the fact that the adrenal cell is pluripotential. Evidence from the study of adrenal cell division and death, and from cell culture experiments, suggests that cells produced in the zona glomerulosa migrate, as they age, through the fasciculata to the reticularis. During this migration they will synthesise in turn mineralocorticoid, glucocorticoid and adrenal androgen, depending on the influence of the immediate environment. It is also probable that the adrenal medulla and the adrenergic nervous system may play a role in the control of steroid biosynthesis.[19]

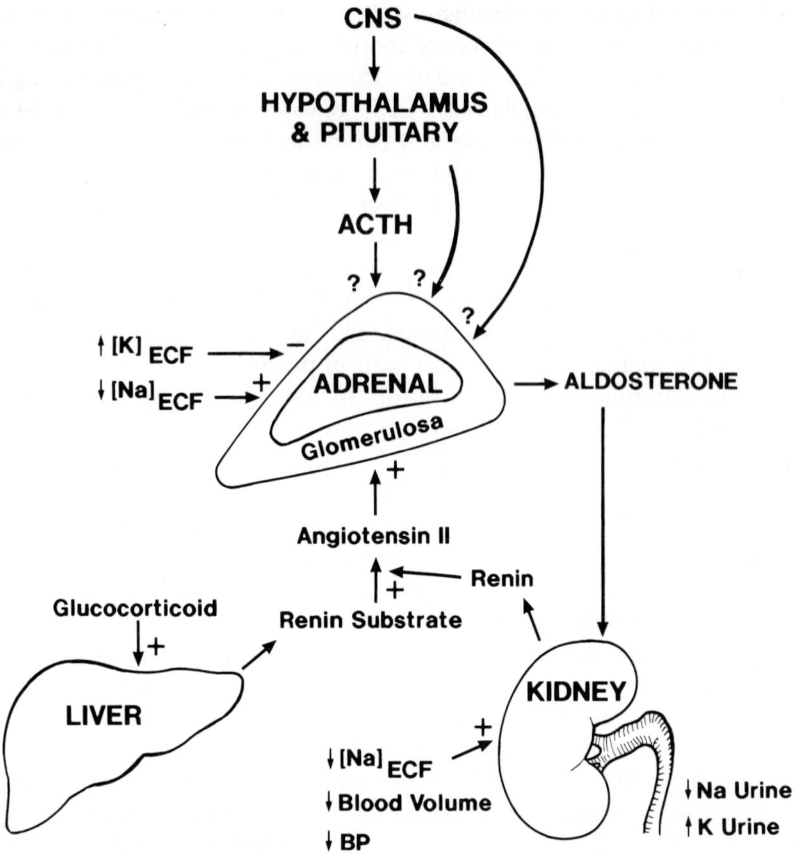

Fig. 11.4 Control of aldosterone biosynthesis and secretion.

Steroid production in the testis and ovary is controlled by follicle-stimulating hormone (FSH) and luteinising hormone (LH), again through specific receptors and a cyclic AMP second messenger. Disturbances of these control mechanisms have not been widely reported in inborn errors of steroid biosynthesis.

THE IMMUNE SYSTEM AND THE ADRENAL CORTEX

There is a complex interaction between the immune system and the biosynthesis and actions of the glucocorticoids.[20] Interleukin-1 is a potent stimulus of ACTH release and acts through CRF. The immune system is also capable of producing extrapituitary ACTH and related peptides. On the other hand glucocorticoids are immunosuppressive and amongst other such actions inhibit interleukin-1 synthesis. The role and functions of the immune system in the pathology of inborn errors of steroid biosynthesis do not appear to have been investigated so far.

THE FETOPLACENTAL UNIT (Fig. 11.5)

In the pregnant state the oestrogens, oestrone, oestradiol and particularly oestriol, are produced in large quantities; the pathway of oestriol synthesis is different from the adult adrenal or ovary. The fetus is deficient in 3β-HSD and thus cannot convert pregnenolone to progesterone. The placenta can carry out this conversion and supply progesterone to the fetal adrenal which can metabolize it to DHA-sulphate. This in turn is returned to the placenta where a sulphatase enzyme is present together with the enzymes to convert DHA to oestrone and oestriol. The fetal liver is capable of converting the DHA-sulphate to 16α-hydroxy-DHA-sulphate which can be further metabolized in the placenta to oestriol. The contribution of maternal adrenal gland to the fetoplacental unit is not clear but DHA-sulphate from the mother can be metabolized in the placenta.

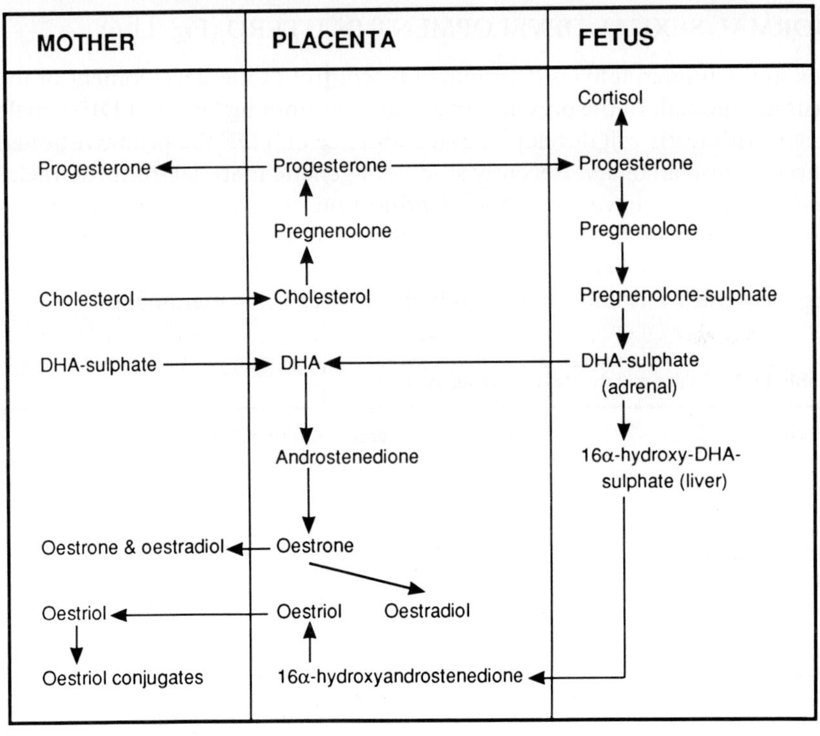

Fig. 11.5 The fetoplacental unit. DHA–dihydroepiandrosterone.

CATABOLISM AND EXCRETION OF STEROIDS

Steroids are catabolized mainly in the liver but additional metabolism of steroids can occur in other tissues.[21] There is some evidence that the adrenal gland itself may also be involved in the catabolism of some steroids, particularly oestrogens. The products of catabolism are excreted in the urine; some products of androgen and oestrogen catabolism are excreted in the bile and undergo enterohepatic circulation, the significance of which is not known.

A number of steps are involved in steroid catabolism, these include reduction, oxidation, hydroxylation, side-chain cleavage and conjugation, usually to form glucuronides or sulphates. A large number of steroid metabolites are produced from one steroid hormone; the major metabolites of cortisol are shown in Table 11.3. Separation of these metabolites by chemical means is difficult and time-consuming and they have been measured by techniques which measure groups of steroids with a particular chemical structure. More specific analysis of urine with gas-chromatographic techniques is the method of choice in the investigation of disorders of steroid biosynthesis, particularly as the chromatographic techniques allow identification of unusual steroids.

NORMAL SEXUAL DEVELOPMENT IN UTERO (Fig. 11.6)

Sex in the human fetus is determined by control of the development of the primitive gonad. In the presence of a testis determining factor (TDF) a male infant with testis will develop[22]; in the absence of TDF the primitive gonad develops into an ovary. Recently studies of genetic material from XX males and XY females have led to the identification of a gene, SRY (*S*ex-determining *R*egion of the *Y*), which has emerged as a strong candidate gene for the production of TDF.[23] The SRY gene is located in the pseudoautosomal region of the Y chromosome and is highly conserved in mammals.

Table 11.3 Major metabolites of cortisol in urine

Metabolite	Average excretion (%)	
Cortisol	1.7	C21
Cortisone	1.7	
Tetrahydrocortisol	17.0	
Allotetrahydrocortisol	9.0	
Tetrahydrocortisone	27.5	
20β-Cortol	9.8	
20α-Cortolone	11.3	
20β-Cortolone	10.3	
11-Oxoaetiocholanolone	3.1	C19
11β-Hydroxyaetiocholanolone	3.9	
11β-Hydroxyandrosterone	1.0	
Others	3.7	

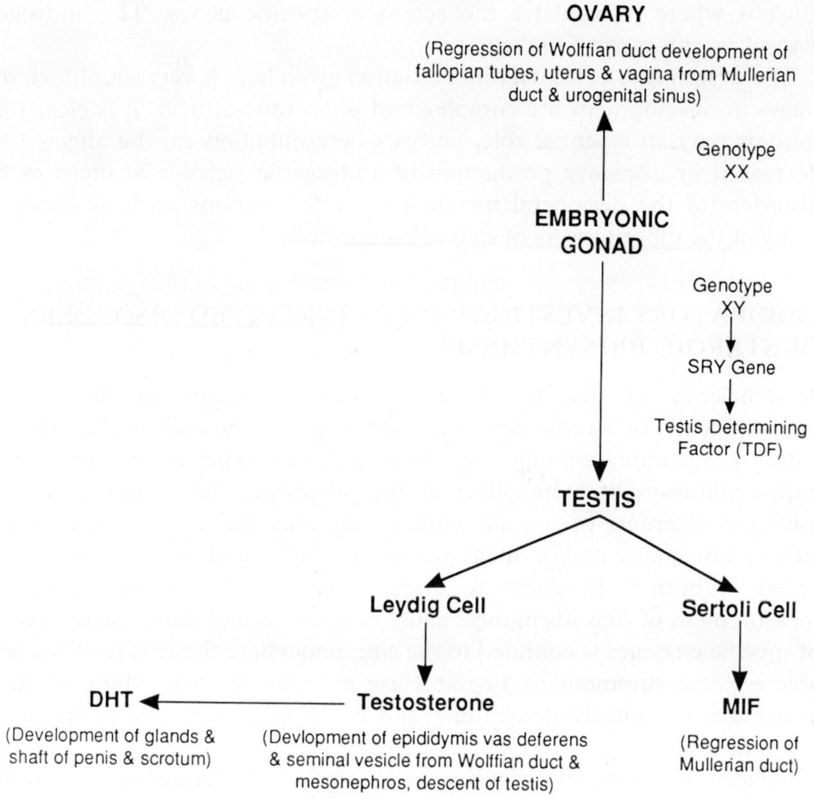

Fig. 11.6 The development and differentiation of the gonad and internal and external genitalia. MIF–Mullerian duct inhibiting factor, DHT–dihydrotestosterone.

The internal genitalia are derived from the Mullerian and Wolffian ducts. This time-critical process depends entirely on the presence of testosterone and the glycoprotein hormone Mullerian duct-inhibiting factor (MIF) produced by the Leydig and Sertoli cells, respectively, of the testis. In the male fetus MIF causes degeneration of Mullerian structures and subsequently the Wolffian duct develops into the epididymis, vas deferens, seminal vesicles and ejaculatory ducts under the influence of testosterone. This action of testosterone does not require its conversion to DHT. Female development occurs in the absence of MIF and testosterone. The major part of the Wolffian duct degenerates while the Mullerian structures become the fallopian tubes, uterus and upper part of the vagina.

The external genitalia develop from the genital tubercle, urethral fold and labioscrotal swelling. In the male these become the glans and shaft of the penis, urethra and scrotum. The process depends on testosterone but in this case conversion to DHT by 5α-reductase is essential for androgen action. The DHT binds to a cytosolic receptor and is then transfered to the nucleus where it regulates the action of specific genes. The androgen cytosol receptors are X-linked.

The description of sexual differentiation given here is very simplified; the stages in development are complex and often time-critical. It is clear that steroids play an essential role, and sex determination can be affected by decreased or excessive production of androgenic steroids in utero or by disorders of the peripheral metabolism of testosterone such as occur in many of the inborn errors of steroid biosynthesis.

LABORATORY INVESTIGATION OF INHERITED DISORDERS OF STEROID BIOSYNTHESIS

A deficiency of activity of any particular enzyme in the steroid pathway leads to a reduction in the formation of the end-product of that pathway, accumulation of intermediates and increasing activity in the alternative pathways of metabolism of the precursors. The investigation of inherited disorders of steroid synthesis requires the measurement of the steroid hormones and/or their precursors and metabolites in urine and blood or both.[24] Response to therapy can also be monitored by the measurement of steroids in these same body fluids and also in saliva. Assay of specific enzymes is confined to the situation where tissue is readily available e.g. measurement of 5α-reductase in a skin biopsy. Many of these assays are technically demanding and are best carried out in specialist laboratories.

Collection of urine is a non-invasive technique, potentially highly useful in paediatric practice but with a number of problems which limit its usefulness. Despite its seeming simplicity, 24-hour urine collections are frequently incorrectly performed, even in hospital. Collections are particularly difficult in neonates when they may be complicated by the existence of abnormal genitalia. Episodic secretion, e.g. circadian rhythms, are masked by 24-hour urine collection, while random collections may be misleading, depending on whether they include or exclude periods of excessive steroid excretion. Urine measurements in the first few days of life are further complicated by the major changes in adrenal function that are occurring at this time, which results in a highly variable pattern of steroid excretion and can give rise to both false positive and negative diagnoses. Urine spot tests such as the 11-oxygenation index, which rely on the ratio of different types of steroids, have not proved universally successful in overcoming this problem. Other factors which can influence measurements of steroids in urine include hepatic and renal function and drugs.

Radioimmunoassay has brought the analysis of specific steroids in plasma, urine and other body fluids within the capacity of many laboratories. These assays lead to improvements in the understanding of the pathophysiology of disorders of steroid metabolism and in diagnosis and monitoring of therapy. However, production of antibodies with high specificity to steroid molecules is difficult; cross-reaction with closely related precursors may cause significant errors and misdiagnoses. Furthermore, even with specific assays, problems arise in the neonatal period as patients with identical disorders can show considerable variations in plasma steroid concentrations and these can also change markedly in the first few weeks of life.[25] High concentrations of 17OHP have been found in sick premature infants without adrenal disease; these concentrations were comparable to those found in patients with P_{450}c21 deficiency.

Dynamic tests of adrenal or gonadal function are sometimes helpful in establishing the diagnosis. ACTH stimulation is useful if the patient has already been treated with cortisol for urgent reasons and a human chorionic gonadotropin (HCG) stimulation test can assist in the investigation of abnormalities of androgen synthesis and metabolism. Other investigations that may be required to clarify the diagnosis include chromosome analysis and radiology of the urogenital tract.

A summary of the patterns of steroids and their metabolites found in the plasma and urine of patients with inborn errors of steroid biosynthesis is given in Table 11.4.

CLASSIFICATION OF INHERITED DISORDERS OF STEROID BIOSYNTHESIS

An ideal classification of steroid biosynthetic disorders awaits the resolution of a number of biochemical and clinical conundrums. The identification of the specific genes and enzymes involved and an understanding of the clinical variability would suggest that the classification should be essentially based on the gene, qualified where necessary by the major organ involvement and by clinical type (Table 11.5). The dominance of the adrenal gland in the current classifications should not be allowed to overshadow the fact that, so far, it appears that the same genes are expressed in the common pathways of all steroid-synthesising organs.

CLINICAL PRESENTATION

Inherited disorders of steroid metabolism can present in a variety of different ways (Table 11.6). The majority of cases are diagnosed in the neonatal period, early infancy or at puberty but an increasing number of patients, particularly with P_{450}c21 deficiency, are being diagnosed in adult life during investigation of female hirsutism or on the basis of HLA typing and DNA studies in affected families (see later). Occasionally patients remain undiagnosed until very late in life. With increasing sophistication of diagnostic methods more patients are being described with presentations differing from the classical descriptions of these defects.

Table 11.4 ACTH, renin, steroid hormones and their metabolites in plasma and urine in the individual disorders of steroid biosynthesis

Deficient enzyme	Increased in plasma	Decreased in plasma	Increased in urine	Decreased in urine
P_{450}scc (20,22-demolase)	ACTH Renin	Cortisol Aldosterone Testosterone		Oxosteroids Oxogenic steroids Pregnanetriol
3β-Hydroxysteroid dehydrogenase	ACTH Renin Pregnenolone 17α-Hydroxypregnenolone DHA	17α-Hydroxyprogesterone Cortisol Aldosterone Testosterone	Oxosteroids(±) Pregnanetriol	Oxogenic steroids
P_{450}c17 (17α-hydroxylase, 17,20-lyase)	ACTH(±) Pregnenolone Progesterone 11-Deoxycorticosterone Corticosterone	Renin 17α-Hydroxyprogesterone Cortisol Testosterone	Pregnanediol	Oxosteroids(±) Pregnanetriol
P_{450}c21 (21-hydroxylase)	ACTH Renin(±) 17α-Hydroxyprogesterone 21-Deoxycortisol DHA Androstenedione Testosterone	Cortisol Aldosterone(±)	Oxosteroids Pregnanetriol Pregnanetriolone 17α-hydroxypregnanolone	Tetrahydrocortisol Cortolone

Table 11.4 *contd*

Deficient enzyme	Increased in plasma	Decreased in plasma	Increased in urine	Decreased in urine
$P_{450}c11$ (11β-hydroxylase)	ACTH 11-Deoxycortisol 11-Deoxycorticosterone Andostenedione Testosterone	Renin Cortisol Aldosterone	Oxosteroids Tetrahydro-11-deoxycortisol Tetrahydro-11-deoxycorticosterone	Tetrahydrocortisol
(Corticosterone methyl oxidase Type I)	Renin	Aldosterone	Corticosterone metabolites	Tetrahydroaldosterone
(Corticosterone methyl oxidase Type II)	Renin	Aldosterone	Corticosterone metabolites Tetrahydro-11-dehydro-18-hydroxycorticosterone	Tetrahydroaldosterone
17β-Hydroxysteroid dehydrogenase	Androstenedione Androstenedione:Testosterone ratio	Testosterone(±) Dihydrotestosterone(±)	Oxosteroids(±)	
5α-Reductase	Testosterone	Dihydrotestosterone		

Table 11.5 Classification of inhertited disorders of steroid biosynthesis

Deficiency disorder	McKusick number	McKusick CAH classification
P_{450}scc	201710	I
3β-Hydroxysteroid Δ-5,4 isomerase	201810	II
P_{450}c17	202110	V
17α-hydroxylase		
17,20-lyase		
combined 17α-hydroxylase, 17,20-lyase		
P_{450}c21	201910	III
P_{450}c11		
11-hydroxylase	202010	IV
corticosterone methyl oxidase Type I	203400	
corticosterone methyl oxidase Type II	203410/124080	
17β-Hydroxysteroid dehydrogenase	264300	
5α-Reductase	264600	
P_{450}arom overactivity	107910	

Table 11.6 Main clinical presentation of inherited disorders of steroid biosynthesis at different ages

Age	Clinical presentation
Prenatal	Elevated or reduced concentrations of specific steroids in amniotic fluid
Neonatal	Ambiguous genitalia Hyponatraemia with renal salt loss Failure to thrive and associated symptoms
Infancy	Hypertension Hyponatraemia
Childhood and adolescence	Virilisation Hirsutism Precocious puberty Delayed puberty Primary amenorrhoea Gynaecomastia Tall stature
Adulthood	Hirsutism Menstrual disturbances Infertility Family history HLA typing

The signs and symptoms of the different disorders (Table 11.7) reflect both the reduction in the activity of the normal steroid hormones and the biological activity of the accumulated precursors and other steroids. Thus the presentation of a defect late in the pathway of cortisol synthesis e.g.

Table 11.7 Main clinical features of the individual inherited disorders of steroid biosynthesis

	Ambiguous genitalia					
Deficient enzyme	Male	Female	Salt loss	Hypertension	Pubertal development	Postnatal virilisation
P_{450}scc (20,22-demolase)	+	–	+	–	Absent, needs induction	–
3β-Hydroxysteroid dehydrogenase	±	±	+	–	May need induction	–
P_{450}c17						
(17α-Hydroxylase)	+	–	–	+	Absent, needs induction	–
(17,20-lyase)	+	–	–	–	Absent, needs induction	–
P_{450}c21 (21-Hydroxylase)	–	+	±	–	Early or normal	+ if undertreated
P450c11						
(11β-Hydroxylase)	–	±	–	±	Early or normal	+ if undertreated
(Corticosterone methyl oxidase Type I)	–	–	+	–	Normal	–
(Corticosterone methyl oxidase Type II)	–	–	+	–	Normal	–
17β-Hydroxysteroid dehydrogenase	+	–	–	–	Normal age: female-to-male gender change	–
5α-Reductase	+	–	–	–	Normal age: variable virilisation	–

21-hydroxylase deficiency can present primarily as a disorder of sexual differentiation due to excess androgen production during fetal development, and the signs and symptoms of cortisol deficiency can be minimal or absent. It follows that the definitive diagnosis of the type of steroid biosynthetic defect is dependent on the results of laboratory investigations.

Two presentations in the neonatal period produce particularly urgent diagnostic problems; these are salt loss with hyponatraemia, and ambiguous genitalia. The differential diagnosis for both are summarised in the lists below; for each there are a large number of other aetiologies which are not disorders of steroid biosynthesis.

Hyponatraemia in the neonate and in early infancy

1. Inadequate intake of sodium
   a. Low sodium milk
   b. Intravenous therapy

2. Increased water intake
   Intravenous therapy

3. Increased net sodium loss
   a. Gastrointestinal
      (i) Diarrhoea
      (ii) Fistulae
   b. Renal
      (i) Anatomical kidney abnormalities
      (ii) Obstructive uropathy
      (iii) Renal tubular disorders
      (iv) Pseudohypoaldosteronism
   c. Mineralocorticoid underactivity
      (i) Congenital adrenal hypoplasia
      (ii) $P_{450}c21$ (21-hydroxylase) deficiency
      (iii) $P_{450}c11$ (11β-hydroxylase) deficiency
      (iv) 3β-hydroxysteroid dehydrogenase deficiency
      (v) $P_{450}scc$ (20,22-desmolase) deficiency
      (vi) $P_{450}c11$ (corticosterone methyl oxidase deficiency Types I and II)

4. Miscellaneous
   a. Syndrome of inappropriate ADH secretion
   b. Bartter's syndrome
   c. Familial hyporeninaemic hypoaldosteronism

Ambiguous genitalia at birth:

1. Genetic females (karyotype 46XX)
   a. Increased endogenous fetal androgen production
      (i) P_{450}c21 (21-hydroxylase) deficiency
      (ii) P_{450}c11 (11β-hydroxylase) deficiency
      (iii) 3β-hydroxysteroid dehydrogenase deficiency
      (iv) Androgen-secreting tumour
   b. Exogenous androgens
      (i) Maternal injection of progestins or androgens in pregnancy (iatrogenic)
      (ii) Maternal androgen-secreting tumour
      (iii) Maternal P_{450}c21 deficiency
   c. Non-hormonal female pseudohermaphroditism
      (i) Urogenital malformations
      (ii) Prominent clitoris of prematurity
      (iii) Associated with dysmorphic syndromes

2. Genetic males (karyotype 46XY)
   a. Decreased fetal androgen biosynthesis
      (i) P_{450}scc (20,22-desmolase) deficiency
      (ii) 3β-hydroxysteroid dehydrogenase deficiency
      (iii) P_{450}c17 (17,20-lyase) deficiency
      (iv) P_{450}c17 (17α-hydroxylase) deficiency
      (v) 17β-hydroxysteroid dehydrogenase deficiency
      (vi) Leydig cell unresponsiveness to HCG and LH
   b. Defective peripheral androgen metabolism
      (i) 5α-reductase deficiency
      (ii) Androgen receptor and postreceptor defects (complete and incomplete testicular feminisation)
   c. Exogenous maternal oestrogen
      Maternal injection (iatrogenic)
   d. Non hormonal male pseudohermaphroditism
      Urogenital malformations
   e. Deficient synthesis or action of MIF

3. Chromosome abnormalities
   Genetic mosaics
   46XY/45X
   46XY/46XX

Treatment

Treatment of hyponatraemia due to a lack of mineralocorticoid activity is relatively simple and life-saving. In the case of ambiguous genitalia the need to reach a decision on the sex for rearing the child is often not treated with the urgency it deserves. It is, however, extremely important for the parents that the child has a definite sex assigned to it in order for the child to be accepted by them and their relatives.

INDIVIDUAL DISORDERS OF STEROID BIOSYNTHESIS

P_{450}scc (cholesterol 20,22-desmolase) deficiency

The conversion of cholesterol to pregnenolone is the initial step in the synthesis of all types of steroids. Patients present in early infancy with severe adrenal crisis. In the first reports of this disorder patients rarely survived infancy but more recently series with survival rates of over 70% have been recorded.[26] Males have ambiguous genitalia, usually severe with complete feminisation, and it is likely that the enzyme deficiency is present in all steroid-synthesising tissues.

The condition is very rare but cases are probably missed because of a neonatal death. At postmortem the adrenal cells are enlarged and filled with lipid-staining material consisting of cholesterol and cholesterol esters. The mode of inheritance is autosomal recessive. Approximately half of all reported cases are from Japan.

The action of P_{450}scc involves three steps, 20S-hydroxylase, 22R-hydroxlase and 20R,22R-lyase which are catalysed by a single enzyme. Different variants of this disorder are theoretically possible from defects in the three steps. Where biochemical investigation has been performed, reduction in cortisol, aldosterone and the urinary metabolites of the sex hormones have been found. Some patients have been described with evidence of some testosterone biosynthesis and male internal genitalia.

The primary sequence of human P_{450}scc has been reported[27] and the gene localized to chromosome 15q23–24[28] but as yet no specific abnormalities have been identified.

It is possible that a similar clinical picture of multiple steroid deficiencies could occur as the result of deficiencies in the associated mitochondrial or microsomal P_{450} reductase systems. One patient has been described who had biochemical changes of P_{450}c17 and P_{450}c21 deficiency[29]. This was explained on the basis of a defect of microsomal steroid P_{450} oxidoreductase, but direct evidence for this was not obtained.

3-Hydroxysteroid dehydrogenase:$\Delta^{5,4}$ oxosteroid isomerase deficiency

The conversion of Δ^5 to Δ^4 steroids is catalysed by 3β-hydroxysteroid dehydrogenase:$\Delta^{5,4}$oxosteroid dehydrogenase (3β-HSD). There is evidence for isoenzymes[3, 30] of 3β-HSD with different specificities for C21 or C19 steroids. The gene in the different organs, adrenal, gonad and liver is almost certainly under different and specific regulation and this, together with the existence of partial deficiencies, is a possible explanation of the varying clinical and biochemical presentations of these cases.

Clinically the patients present with disturbances of electrolyte and water balance and ambiguous genitalia. The severity of hyponatraemia is variable, some cases appear to produce no cortisol or aldosterone and are resistant to treatment, usually dying early. Other cases appear to be able to synthesise small amounts of cortisol and aldosterone and respond more favourably to therapy. Patients with apparently normal mineralocorticoid production, and who do not have salt loss, have also been described. Milder cases can present in late childhood, in puberty and even in adulthood. In the male a variable degree of masculinisation of the external genitalia is found, possibly reflecting different amounts of residual testosterone production or to the action of DHA, a weak androgen which is produced in excess. This latter steroid is probably the cause of the mild masculinisation of females with 3β-HSD deficiency. The disorder is inherited in an autosomal recessive manner.

Contrary to what might be predicted from the biosynthetic pathway progesterone and 17OHP are often elevated in 3β-HSD deficiency, though to a much lower extent than the equivalent steroids pregnenolone and 17-hydroxypregnenolone.

Pregnanetriol, the main urine metabolite of 17OHP, may be increased in the urine and it is obvious that simplistic investigation of these patients with measurement of plasma 17OHP and/or urine pregnanetriol can lead to the mistaken diagnosis of P_{450}c21 deficiency. Hence it is mandatory in all cases of suspected steroid biosynthetic disorders to obtain estimations of several different steroids, and to do repeated investigations where necessary.

Purification of 3β-HSD has shown that the dehydrogenase and isomerase copurify and the functions are performed by a single polypeptide, possibly as a dimer. Studies of the pH optima of the two activities has suggested the involvement of different amino acids. The microsomal and mitochondrial enzymes of the placenta appear identical. No molecular biological evidence of isoenzymes has been described and the physiological and experimental existence of isoenzymes requires explanation.

cDNA for 3βHSD has been isolated and used to deduce the amino acid sequence and localize the gene to the p13 band of chromosome 1. No genetic abnormalities have so far been identified.

P_{450}c17 (17α-hydroxylase and 17,20-lyase) deficiency

These two disorders, previously treated as separate and said to have recessive and X-linked inheritance respectively, are caused by abnormalities of the single-chain polypeptide enzyme P_{450}c17 which has a single active site[31]. Patients with 17α-hydroxylase, 17,20-lyase and combined 17α-hydroxylase/17,20-lyase deficiencies have been described as well as patients with partial deficiencies. 17α-Hydroxylation must occur before the loss of the 2-carbon side-chain and it is almost certain that deficiency of 17,20-lyase is always combined with 17α-hydroxylase deficiency. The differentiation between the combined and 17α-hydroxylase defect based on clinical examination or laboratory investigation is frequently very difficult.

$P_{450}c17$ converts the C21 steroids to 17OHP and 17α–hydroxy-pregnenolone stepwise to androstenedione and dehydroepiandrosterone respectively. Males with $P_{450}c17$ deficiency present with ambiguous genitalia which is frequently severe: females present with delayed puberty or primary amennorhoea. Hypertension can be the presenting symptom and is the result of the increased secretion of steroids with mineralocorticoid activity which also causes a hypokalaemic alkalosis.

Diagnosis is established on the basis of decreased urinary excretion of metabolites of 17OHP and the failure of ACTH and/or HCG to induce increases in plasma androstenedione and dehydroepiandrosterone concentrations. In heterozygotes there is an exaggerated progesterone response to ACTH and in some males at least, elevated basal 17OHP which does not respond to ACTH, suggesting testicular origin and partial enzyme deficiency.

One unusual feature found in $P_{450}c17$ deficiency is the combination of low levels of aldosterone and renin together with high levels of the aldosterone precursor 18-hydroxycorticosterone. Renin and aldosterone secretion are suppressed by the sodium retention and hypokalaemia caused by 11-deoxycorticosterone. The elevated 18-hydroxycorticosterone at first seems to suggest a separate defect in the zona glomerulosa, but there is evidence for the production of this steroid by $P_{450}c11$ in the other adrenocortical zones under the influence of ACTH. Glucocorticoid therapy suppresses the release of ACTH and results in reduction in the secretion of 11-deoxycorticosterone, corticosterone and 18-hydroxycorticosterone, while renin and aldosterone secretion are normalised.

The 17,20-lyase variety of $P_{450}c17$ deficiency constitutes about 10% of this group of disorders. The patients have the signs and symptoms of low sex steroids but cortisol biosynthesis is normal. Urinary metabolites of 17α-hydroxylated steroids are increased.

Since 17-hydroxylated C21 steroids are produced in and secreted by the adrenal, a mechanism must exist which allows the release of these steroids before the action of the 17,20-lyase. In vitro studies with testicular $P_{450}c17$ have suggested that in the presence of excess substrate $P_{450}c17$ produces mainly 17-hydroxylated C21 steroids rather than androgens. It has also been shown that increased activity of microsomal cytochrome P_{450} reductase, producing increased reducing equivalents, results in a greater relative activity of 17,20-lyase and hence favours androgen production.

The *CYP17* gene is located on chromosome 10 and the disorder is clearly recessive. Nine different genetic defects have so far been identified in patients with $P_{450}c17$ deficiency.[31] Two involve small duplications. In the first, there is a 4-base-pair duplication in exon 8 which alters the reading frame of the C-terminal 26 amino acids resulting in an inactive protein. This defect was found in two unrelated Mennonite families in Canada and a second defect involving reduplication, this time of 7 base pairs in exon 2, has been described in Japan. This latter reduplication results in a premature stop codon and the synthesis of an inactive protein. Three further defects described are non-sense mutations causing premature termination. Point mutations $Ser^{106} \rightarrow$ Pro and $Pro^{342} \rightarrow$ Thr resulting in total loss of enzyme activity and $Arg^{496} \rightarrow$ Cys causing partial deficiency have been found. The ninth genetic lesion is a 3 bp deletion of a Phe codon.

P_{450}c21 (21-hydroxylase) deficiency

P_{450}c21 deficiency is one of the most common inborn errors of metabolism and is found at a much higher frequency than all the other disorders of steroid biosynthesis. There are several different clinical presentations covering the entire age range, although the majority of cases are diagnosed in infancy. In the neonatal period female patients classically present with viralisation with or without associated salt loss; male patients at this age present with salt loss. Patients with salt loss can also present later in infancy and breast feeding has been shown to delay the clinical presentation of neonates with salt loss despite biochemical evidence of severe hyponatraemia. Other patients who appear normal at birth present with virilisation or precocious puberty in childhood. A late onset 'non-classical' form presents with acne, hirsutism, menstrual disturbances and infertility in the adult female. A number of asymptomatic individuals with the biochemical stigmata have been discovered on the basis of HLA typing (see later). All forms are inherited in an autosomal recessive mode.

The frequency of the neonatal form of P_{450}c21 deficiency appears variable. In caucasian communities the prevalence in the more recent surveys lies between 1:5000 and 1:15 000 births; this gives a gene frequency of between 1:35 and 1:61. Very high prevalences have been reported among the Yupik Inuit in Alaska with a frequency of 1:500 and in other Alaskan Inuits at a frequency of 1:1500. The proportion of patients with salt loss is approximately 66%[32], although in the Yupik Inuit all cases appear to have salt loss. Information on the frequency of the non-classical type is less certain but estimates of gene frequencies between 1:18 and 1:67 have been derived from studies of hirsute women.

The current approach to diagnosis relies heavily on the measurement of basal plasma 17OHP and, less frequently, androstenedione. ACTH stimulation tests are additionally helpful. There are a number of problems associated with reliance on single measurements[25] with both false positive and false negative results. This is particularly important when the investigation is undertaken early in patients who present with ambiguous genitalia, when the probability of a false negative diagnosis is more frequent.

The CYP21 gene

In the mid 1970s a linkage was established between 21-hydroxylase deficiency and HLA (human leucocyte antigen) type. The complex of HLA genes is found on the short arm of chromosome 6 and it consists of an ordered number of loci which have a large number of alleles. By studying a large number of families with 21-hydroxylase deficiency the gene responsible, *CYP21*, was localised amongst the Class III genes which are found between the Class I genes (HLA types A, B and C) towards the telomere and the Class II genes (HLA types DP, DQ and DR) towards the centromere[33, 34] (Fig. 11.7).

The Class III genes include those for the second and fourth complement components (C2, C4) and the properdin factor B (Bf). A number of HLA haplotypes have been associated with different clinical presentations of $P_{450}c21$ deficiency. HLA haplotype A3-Bw47-DR7 is found in much greater frequency in patients with salt-wasting classical disease, while HLA haplotype B14(Bw65)-DR1 is correlated with the non-classical form.

Further mapping of the Class III loci on chromosome 6 showed that both *CYP21* and the adjacent C4 genes were reduplicated to give 4 genes in the order:

centomere . . . . *CYP21B*-C4B-*CYP21A*-C4A . . . telomere

The two *CYP21* genes are between 97 and 98% homologous, while the C4 genes are more than 99% homologous. Only the *CYP21B* gene is active, the *CYP21A* gene is a pseudogene and contains several missense mutations

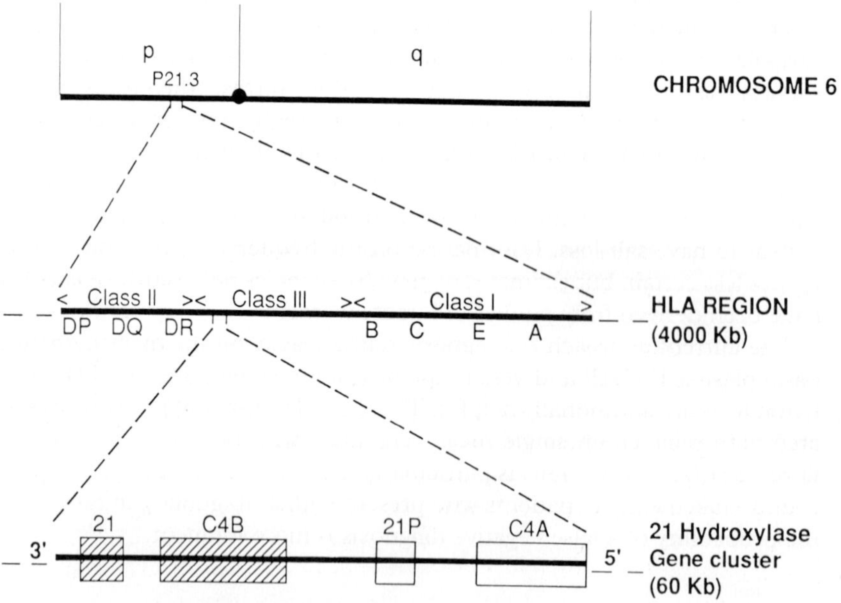

Fig. 11.7 Map of human chromosome 6 showing the human leucocyte antigen (HLA) gene cluster and the location of the gene for $P_{450}c21$ within Class III. The active gene *CYP21* (21) and pseudogene *CYP21P* (21P) are shown in relationship to the reduplicated complement genes C4B and C4A.

as well as base pair deletions (exon 8), base pair insertions (exon 3) and a non-sense mutation. Recently the *CYP21* genes have been renamed: the active gene is now called *CYP21* and the pseudogene *CYP21P*.

One consequence of the arrangement of the duplicated *CYP21* and C4 genes and their very high degree of homology is that during meiosis unequal cross-over events are more likely to occur in this area of the chromosome due to mispairing of the two chromosome 6s. This can result in a gamete with a chromosome 6 in which the genetic defect could be either a complete deletion of the active *CYP21* gene, or several copies of active and/or pseudogene, or in which a combination of *CYP21* and *CYP21P* has occurred. The latter is termed gene conversion. The results of gene conversion can be a gene which is clearly a rearrangement of the two genes but in some cases, due to the high degree of homology between *CYP21* and *CYP21P*, gene conversion can be misinterpreted as simple mutations or small deletions or insertions. This problem led to some confusion in early studies of the frequency of the different types of genetic defects in $P_{450}c21$ deficiency.[33, 34]

Studies of the relative contribution of the different genetic defects have been complicated in part by the relatively small numbers of patients reported in each series, and possibly by population variation. Gene deletion of all or most of *CYP21* is reported in 20–50% of patients by various groups. Major gene conversion of *CYP21* to *CYP21P* is found in an additional 10%. The remaining defects so far identified are due to mutations and small deletions in both introns and exons many, if not all, of which are found in the normal *CYP21P* gene sequence. This fact has been used to suggest that all genetic defects in $P_{450}c21$ deficiency are due to deletions and major or minor gene conversions. In favour of this hypothesis is the fact that some of the individual mutations are strongly linked to particular HLA haplotypes. One particularly common mutation is a $C \rightarrow G$ change in intron 2 which alters RNA splicing. The result of this is a frameshift in exon 3, the production of a stop codon and the production of an inactive protein approximately 20% of the length of $P_{450}c21$.

Attempts to relate the various genetic defects of *CYP21* to the phenotypic disease have only been partly successful.[33] There are a number of identified *CYP21* alleles and patients will usually be heterozygotes for these alleles rather than being homozygous for a single gene defect. This will give rise to several possible phenotypes dependent, at least in part, on residual 21-hydroxylase activity.

If the patient has a combination of chromosomes with gene deletion, major gene conversion or deleterious mutations producing an inactive protein, the salt-wasting type is almost certain to be present. Patients with the simple virilising phenotype may have at least one allele with a less severe genetic defect but cases with two severe defects are reported. The non-classical form of the disease is strongly associated with a $G \rightarrow T$ mutation in exon 7 which results in a Val $\rightarrow$ Leu substitution, but this mutation has also been reported in patients with salt-wasting.

It is probably oversimplistic to try to link specific genotypes to specific phenotypic gene expression. Variability of the disease in HLA identical siblings has been recorded and it is almost certain that there are other as yet unrecognized factors which modify the expression of the *CYP21* gene in vivo.

Salt wasting versus simple virilization

One problem which remains unresolved despite our recent knowledge of the *CYP21* gene is why some patients with 21-hydroxylase deficiency and two severe gene defects have salt wasting and others do not. It is not too difficult to accept that where there is some residual 21-hydroxylase activity then this could be sufficient for effective mineralocorticoid biosynthesis. In the absence of any active $P_{450}c21$ it would be expected that neither glucorticoids or mineralocorticoids would be produced. However, patients with severe forms of $P_{450}c21$ deficiency frequently produce some, but insufficient, cortisol in response to the high concentrations of endogenous or exogenous ACTH, suggesting some 21-hydroxylase activity. A patient has also been reported in whom the genetic defects were a gene deletion and major gene conversion and who could yet produce adequate quantities of aldosterone.[35]

Where does this 21-hydroxylase activity come from? One possibility is that, in the presence of excess 17OHP or other precursors, another adrenal P_{450} with the required properties but not *CYP21* becomes expressed or, alternatively, one of the other existing steroid hydroxylase P_{450}s could behave as a 21-hydroxylase. A second hypothesis involves a hepatic enzyme similar to that found in the rabbit, with 21-hydroxylase and $\Delta^{5,4}$ oxosteroid isomerase activities capable of converting progesterone to deoxycorticosterone, which can act as a mineralocorticoid or be shuttled to the adrenal to be converted to aldosterone. This enzyme has so far not been shown to be active in human liver. Published evidence favours the adrenal as the source of the necessary 21-hydroxylase but is not conclusive.

Also of interest is the amelioration of salt loss with age in many patients.[36] This could be due to an increase in adrenal mass, which is required to reach a critical size. The mass of the adrenal does have some affect on the type of steroid synthesised (see above) so this could be one possible explanation. However, the mechanism whereby changes in mass could overcome absence of essential enzymes has not been explained.

P_{450}c11 (11β-hydroxylase, corticosterone methyl oxidase Types I and II) deficiency

The P_{450} enzyme coded by the *CYP11B* gene has multiple actions; these include 11β-hydroxylation and 18-hydroxylation and dehydrogenation. The disorders caused by deficiencies of these enzymic activities cause two types of disorder. The former can be difficult to distinguish clinically from $P_{450}c21$ deficiency and results from 11β-hydroxylase deficiency. Reduction or loss of the activity affecting the C18 carbon of the steroid nucleus primarily cause symptoms of mineralocorticoid deficiency. Because of this marked clinical difference the two types of disorder will be treated separately.

11β-Hydroxylase deficiency

$P_{450}c11$ (11β-hydroxylase) catalyses the conversion of 11-deoxycortisol and 11-deoxycorticosterone to cortisol and corticosterone respectively. There is considerable biochemical evidence for the existence of several isoenzymes of 11β-hydroxylase with different specificities[3] and that, in particular, the two reactions above are catalysed by different isoenzymes. As yet the relationship of these 'isoenzymes' to *CYP11B* remains to be elucidated. The complex, and as yet not clearly defined, nature of 11β-hydroxylase activity is one possible explanation for the variable clinical and biochemical presentation of patients with 11β-hydroxylase deficiency.[37]

Though the second most common inborn error of steroid biosynthesis, 11β-hydroxylase deficiency was believed to occur in only 5% of cases, studies have suggested, however, that the disorder is more frequent[37], and may account for up to 15% of cases. A higher incidence has been observed in Jews from North Africa and Turkey. The mode of inheritance of 11β-hydroxylase deficiency is autosomal recessive.

The classical presentation in females is with severe ambiguous genitalia and hypertension, and in males with pseudoprecocious puberty or hypertension. In more recent cases the ambiguous genitalia in females has varied between mild clitoral hypertrophy to extreme masculinisation with a penile urethra and fused labioscrotal folds. Some females presenting later in life do not have abnormal genitalia. Hypertension is not universally present and can be absent in patients with the more severe forms of androgen excess. Hypokalaemia is present in a minority of patients. Other presenting symptoms described in patients with 11β-hydroxylase deficiency include tall stature in both sexes, hirsutism and oligo- or amenorrhoea. Hyperpigmentation is a common but variable finding.

The biochemical diagnosis of 11β-hydroxylase deficiency depends on the finding of increased deoxycortisol in plasma and/or its metabolite tetrahydrodeoxycortisol in urine. The urine metabolite may take 3–4 weeks to appear in large quantities.[38] When patients were divided into clinically classical (severe) and mild groups it was shown that tetrahydrodeoxycortisol was much lower in the latter, and the tetrahydro metabolite of deoxycorticosterone was increased in the urine from the classical patients but absent from the mild group. In response to ACTH there was no increase in the excretion of either of these two steroid metabolites in the classical cases, suggesting that the adrenal glands in these patients were already maximally stimulated by endogenous ACTH. On the other hand, while all the mild patients responded to ACTH with an increased excretion of tetrahydrodeoxycortisol, a subgroup did not show any rise in the excretion of tetrahydrodeoxycorticosterone. These findings indicate that the milder cases appear to have an incomplete defect and that at least two types of defect occur. In one the 11-hydroxylation of both 17-hydroxy- and 17-deoxy- steroids is affected, while in the other only the 11-hydroxylation of 17-hydroxy- steroids is involved (11-deoxycortisol to cortisol).[37]

Investigation of obligate heterozygotes of 11β-hydroxylase deficiency reveals no biochemical abnormality in response to ACTH, and it is unlikely that the milder variants represent the heterozygous state.

The cause of the hypertension in these patients remains to be elucidated. It has been postulated that increased plasma concentrations of deoxycorticosterone gave rise to hypertension, but patients with high concentrations of this steroid have been reported as being normotensive, while severely hypertensive patients with very mild elevation of plasma deoxycorticosterone have been found. Hypertension may present for the first time in later childhood. Nearly all patients with 11β-hydroxylase deficiency have evidence of volume expansion with low plasma renin and aldosterone, even though hypertension is absent. Treatment with glucocorticoids reduces ACTH stimulation of the adrenal cortex, blood pressure falls in hypertensive patients and plasma renin rises. The renin activity in treated patients is significantly increased above controls either on a salt-restricted or normal diet. Moderate salt loss occurs on sodium restriction and patients treated with glucocorticoids are at potential risk in other situations which disturb sodium balance.[39] It has been proposed that the mineralocorticoid causing hypertension could be 18-hydroxy,11-deoxycorticosterone because of the relationship between 18 and 11-hydroxylation.

Aldosterone biosynthetic defects

Classically the conversion of corticosterone to aldosterone was believed to be a two-stage procedure involving 18-hydroxylation followed by dehydrogenation. On the other hand Ulick[40] has produced evidence that two hydroxylation steps are involved, catalysed by a catechol methyl oxidase enzyme. This produces 18-dihydrocorticosterone which is converted to aldosterone by the loss of water. Nomenclature for the inherited disorders of aldosterone biosynthesis depends on which of these two pathways is used. Alternative names used in the literature are 18-hydroxylase and 18-dehydrogenase deficiency or corticosterone methyl oxidase deficiency Types I and II (CMOD Type I and CMOD Type II). The latter is now preferred.

The clinical presentation of the two varieties of CMOD are essentially the same. Patients present with failure to thrive, dehydration, hyponatraemia and hyperkalaemia. A few patients can present later in childhood with failure to grow and/or postural hypotension. Family studies have revealed asymptomatic patients, while in others the symptoms may be transitory. In CMOD Type I, patients may present with intermittent pyrexia.

The diagnosis depends to a large extent on the elimination of other causes of hyponatraemia (see p. 440), and in particular other steroid biosynthetic disorders which cause salt wasting. Resistance to the action of aldosterone (pseudohypoaldosteronism) must also be excluded. Clinically helpful distinguishing features are absence of virilisation or other signs of androgen excess, normal blood pressure and the absence of pigmentation.

Biochemically the diagnosis depends on the measurement of plasma aldosterone concentration and renin activity and urinary metabolites of aldosterone, its precursors deoxycorticosterone and corticosterone and their 18-hydroxy-derivatives.[41] Plasma aldosterone concentrations may be low or normal in the presence of increased plasma renin activity. Interpretation of the urinary steroid patterns in these cases is complicated by variations in metabolism due to age and disturbances of sodium homeostasis. Thus, excretion patterns may be different in sodium replete and deplete states. The main findings are decreased tetrahydroaldosterone and increases in various corticosterone metabolites. It has been suggested that tetrahydro,18-hydroxy,11-dehydrocorticosterone is useful in distinguishing the two types of CMOD but this remains to be proven. CMOD can be distinguished from pseudohypoaldosteronism by the increased excretion of tetrahydroaldosterone in the latter disorder.

Both types of CMOD are inherited as autosomal recessive disorders with both males and females affected. There is a considerable difference in incidence; CMOD Type I is very rare, while CMOD Type II is more frequent with a particularly high incidence in Iranian Jews.

The CYP11B gene

Mapping of the *CYP11B* gene to chromosome 8q22 and subsequent studies have shown the existence to two linked homologous genes[42] (cf *CYP21*). These have been called *CYP11B1* and *CYP11B2* and are 95% homologous in the coding regions. The *CYP11B2* gene has not been shown to be transcribed in humans and there are differences in the 5' flanking regions of the two genes which may account for this.

The existence of the two genes has given rise to the hypothesis that two isoenzymes can be synthesised, one involved in the 17-hydroxy-pathway and the other in the 17-deoxy-pathway. The absence of mRNA transcript for human *CYP11B2* appears to rule this out. In the rat two types of P_{450}c11 have been identified: P_{450}c11A, found in all three adrenal zones, has both 11- and 18-hydroxylase activities; P_{450}c11B found only in the rat glomerulosa has 18-hydroxylase and dehydrogenase activities. The regulation of the respective mRNAs is as one would expect if P_{450}c11A was involved in glucocorticoid biosynthesis and P_{450}c11B in mineralocorticoid, i.e. aldosterone, synthesis.

To date only one mutation in *CYP11B1* linked to 11β-hydroxylase deficiency has been recorded. This is a single point mutation which results in the conversion of Arg448, which is highly conserved in eukaryotic P_{450}s, to histidine (CGC→CAC), and has been described in Jews of Moroccan origin.[43] With *CYP21*, all point mutations so far identified appear to be the result of gene conversions (see above); on the other hand the Arg → His mutation does not occur in the *CYP11B2* gene and thus appears to have arisen de novo.

Studies of the genetics of CMOD Type II have produced conflicting evidence that the *Msp*1 restriction site in or near the *CYP11B1* gene is the site of a mutation related to or causing the disease. Further studies are required to elucidate the genetic basis of aldosterone biosynthetic defects.

17β-Hydroxysteroid dehydrogenase deficiency

The conversion of androstenedione and oestrone to testosterone and oestradiol respectively is catalysed by the enzyme 17β-hydroxysteroid dehydrogenase. Deficiency of this enzyme is a very rare disorder which presents with male pseudohermaphroditism. The gonadal enzyme only appears to be affected, since peripheral conversion of androstenedione to testosterone is still present. The diagnosis can be made on the basis of an elevated androstenedione:testosterone ratio. In infants an HCG stimulation test will show a much greater rise in androstenedione than testosterone.

Genital virilisation occurs at puberty in the majority of patients, which could be due to the androgen activity of androstenedione or its peripheral conversion to testosterone. In some patients there is a change in gender role from female to male. Gynaecomastia is found in a minority of cases. Inheritance is probably autosomal recessive.

17βHSD is distributed widely in many tissues. Two genes *h17β-HSDI* and *h17β-HSDII* exist in tandem, located at chromosome 17q12. The two genes are 89% homologous. The active gene is *h17β-HSDII*; a premature stop codon is found in *h17β-HSDI* resulting in a truncated message.[44]

5α-Reductase deficiency

For testosterone to exert some of its biological actions, reduction of the 4–5 double bond in the A-ring of the steroid nucleus by the enzyme 5α-reductase is required, to produce dihydrotestosterone (DHT). In females DHT is essentially derived from the peripheral conversion of testosterone and androstenedione, whereas in adult males 50% of circulating DHT is produced in the testis. In the fetus and neonate the relative contribution of testis and peripheral testosterone conversion is not known. DHT is required for the normal formation of male external genitalia and in 5α-reductase deficiency male neonates will present with pseudohermaphroditism.

Clinically the patients have female external genitalia with clitoral hypertrophy and normal male internal genitalia with testes, epididymes etc. A vaginal pouch may be present. (A similar clinical picture is produced by deficiency of the intracellular receptor protein which is required for DHT action.)

Cases of 5α-reductase deficiency which are less severely feminised, with hypospadias and even normal male external genitalia, have been reported suggesting the possibility of partial deficiencies. At puberty patients show a variable degree of masculinisation; in some cases virilisation is so complete that the patients, reared as females, convert to a male gender role. Female breast development is absent.[45]

In plasma, normal or high concentrations of testosterone are present, with a low plasma DHT and increased plasma testosteron:DHT ratio. The urine shows a reduction in the excretion of 5α-metabolites. In children an HCG stimulation test may be required to demonstrate these changes. Direct measurement of 5α-reductase is possible in skin biopsies from the genital area or fibroblasts grown from them. Studies have shown more than one type of defect; the majority of patients have much reduced enzyme activity, whereas other cases appear to have an unstable enzyme present in normal quantity or reduced to approximately 50%. This suggests that 5α-reductase deficiency is a genetically heterogeneous disorder.

The disease is inherited as an autosomal recessive with a particularly high frequency in the Dominican Republic where it has been extensively studied. Further clusters have been described from Papua New Guinea and Turkey. In the latter cohort the male pseudohermaphrodites also had 17-hydroxysteroid dehydrogenase deficiency.

Sufficient cases are known for investigation of heterozygotes of both sexes and homozygous affected females. No evidence of any endocrinological abnormality of development or reproduction has been found.

5α-Reductase has not yet been purified, nor has the gene been identified and mapped.

THERAPY

The therapy of disorders of steroid biosynthesis can be divided into two distinct stages; the management of the neonatal presentation with ambiguous genitalia and/or salt loss and the subsequent endocrinological, surgical and psychological management of these patients and others presenting with signs and symptoms later in life.

When patients present with salt loss, treatment with intravenous saline and mineralocorticoid replacement is urgently required to re-establish normal plasma volume and sodium homeostasis. A blood sample should be taken prior to treatment with glucocorticoids for the measurement of plasma steroid concentrations and, in addition, a random or, where possible, a timed collection of urine should be obtained. If this is not done, or additional investigations are required, then abnormal steroid metabolism can be revealed on stimulation of the adrenal cortex with exogenous ACTH even while the patient is being given glucocorticoid.

The management of ambiguous genitalia depends on several factors including the specific diagnosis, genotypic sex and degree of genital ambiguity. There is an urgent need for a full evaluation since correctly treated females with $P_{450}c21$ (21-hydroxylase) and $P_{450}c11$ (11β-hydroxylase) deficiencies, accounting for the great majority of cases, can attain normal adulthood with full reproductive capacity. Male patients with severe degrees of feminisation are probably best reared as females after appropriate surgical correction but it should be remembered that patients with 5α-reductase deficiency and 17α-hydroxysteroid dehydrogenase deficiency can undergo successful female-to-male conversion at puberty without medical interference.

The long-term endocrinological management involves replacement of the missing steroids and the suppression of the production of other steroids and unwanted effects. Several different glucocorticoids have been used but the best one, and the optimum dosage regime, are still a matter of debate. The logical approach would appear to be to use exogenous cortisol to mimic the natural circadian rhythm. However, cortisol has a relatively short half-life in vivo and may not suppress ACTH secretion unless given in large doses or several times during the day. Large doses of cortisol cause stunting of growth and Cushingoid features to develop. Longer-acting synthetic glucocorticoids may therefore be more effective. Aldosterone is relatively insoluble and mineralocorticoid replacement is usually with 9α-fluorohydrocortisone (fludrocortisone) though occasionally deoxycorticosterone acetate (DOCA) in depot form may be required.

Assessment of the efficacy of gluco- and mineralocorticoid replacement is complicated by the close interrelationship of the two groups of steroids and their control. There is a need to ensure that replacement steroids are given neither in inadequate nor excessive amounts. Glucocorticoid activity has been assessed by the measurement of urinary ketosteroids and pregnanetriol, plasma 17OHP, 17α-hydroxypregnenolone, androstenedione, testosterone and dehydroepiandrosterone and salivary 17OHP, androstenedione and testosterone. There is some dispute as to the value of these biochemical parameters in assessing control, and it has been suggested that clinical evaluation remains the optimum method for monitoring therapy.[46, 47]

Urine measurements are difficult to use in the assessment of overtreatment and give an integrated measure of adrenal activity over the period of collection, usually 24 hours. Single plasma steroid estimations give information relevant only to one point in time. What is required is a method which allows repeated estimation of adrenal activity throughout the 24-hour period and preferably when the patient is in his normal environment. The measurement of steroids in saliva[48] or in dried blood spots collected onto absorbent paper[49] allow this to be done and glucocorticoid replacement to be optimised. The most useful individual steroids to measure in monitoring glucocorticoid replacement in 21-hydroxylase deficiency are 17OHP and androstenedione.

With the development of plasma renin activity measurements it became possible to assess the efficacy of mineralocorticoid therapy. Elevated plasma renin activity was found in salt-losing and non-salt-losing 21-hydroxylase-deficient patients, reflecting reduction in body sodium: suppression of the plasma renin activity to normal levels has been shown to decrease ACTH secretion and improve management of glucocorticoid therapy as well as ensuring adequate sodium balance.[50] It should be noted that the method for the measurement of plasma renin activity (PRA) depends on adequate synthesis of the renin substrate, angiotensinogen. The synthesis of this α_2-macroglobulin by the liver is regulated in part by glucocorticoids and is lowered in adrenal insufficiency. Thus a decrease in PRA can reflect alteration in renin substrate as well as a reduction in renin concentration.[51]

PRENATAL DIAGNOSIS AND TREATMENT

The major function of prenatal diagnosis, in those disorders of steroid biosynthesis for which it is possible, is to allow in utero treatment in order to prevent masculinisation of female fetuses. This is attempted by the administration of the synthetic glucocorticoid dexamethasone which will cross the placenta and suppress the fetal adrenal. As the masculinisation of fetuses takes place almost before it is possible to establish the diagnosis, the approach so far adopted has been to treat all fetuses as soon as pregnancy has been diagnosed and to discontinue treatment where a non-affected or male fetus is identified. This has been principally tried in patients with $P_{450}c21$ deficiency.

Initially diagnosis relied on the measurement of 17OHP in amniotic fluid; subsequently HLA typing of fetal cells was added. These tests were only available when amniocentesis was safe, which was after masculinisation had occurred. In addition a number of false positive cases have been described using this method. DNA analysis, using chorionic villus sampling, can be performed earlier. For DNA analysis and HLA typing to be successful, family studies need to be undertaken, preferably before pregnancy is started.

Results so far suggest that virilisation can be prevented in about 30% of females and reduced significantly in a further 50%.[52,53] Numbers of cases are relatively small and several questions remain unanswered, not least regarding the optimal dose of dexamethasone. It has also been suggested that results could be improved if treatment was started in anticipation of the pregnancy. Monitoring the fetal hypothalamic–pituitary–adrenal axis can be done by measuring maternal urinary oestriol, which should be regularly performed in affected pregnancies.

Prenatal diagnosis of 11β-hydroxylase deficiency is most easily carried out by measuring maternal urinary excretion of tetrahydro-11-deoxycortisol which can be done at approximately 10 weeks gestation. Later 11-dexycortisol can be measured in amniotic fluid. DNA testing and prenatal treatment have not been reported in this disorder.[54]

HETEROZYGOTE DETECTION

Detection of carriers of *CYP21* gene defects has been attempted by various means. In many cases HLA or DNA analysis will yield the required information, but on occasions these tests are not possible or give equivocal results. In these cases a short ACTH test measuring 17OHP and/or other steroids has been used. For the salt-wasting and simple virilising forms of the disease 17OHP:cortisol ratios at 30 or 60 minutes post-ACTH have been reported, but show overlap with the normal population especially with postpubertal females. The 17OHP:deoxycorticosterone ratio, which measures steroid on both the 17-hydroxy- and 17-deoxy- pathways, appears a better discriminant.

Patients with non-classical 21-hydroxylase deficiency can be relatively easily distinguished from heterozygotes using ACTH-stimulated 17OHP concentrations; distinguishing non-classical heterozygotes from normals is difficult due to overlap even when correcting for cortisol.

SCREENING FOR P_{450}C21 (21-HYDROXYLASE) DEFICIENCY

Retrospective analysis of the age and sex of patients with congenital adrenal hyperplasia suggested that, particularly in males, the diagnosis was being missed or delayed leading to increased mortality and morbidity.[55] This observation, coupled with the development of suitable blood spot assays, led a number of centres throughout the world to establish screening programmes for P_{450}c21 deficiency.[56] Nevertheless, screening has not been universally accepted and there are a number of reasons for this. In any one centre the annual incidence of the disorder is relatively small and large series suitable for statistical analysis take a very long time to be accumulated. Therefore, retrospective surveys will not adequately reflect current clinical and laboratory diagnostic practice and their interrelationships which can vary widely depending on local circumstances. In addition there are problems with the blood spot 17OHP assays used which give high numbers of false positive results, especially from premature and low birthweight infants. Despite attempts to improve the predictive value of a positive screening test by the use of a second-stage test, involving pre-extraction of the 17OHP, false positive rates still vary between 4–25 times the true positive rates.

The argument for screening for P_{450}c21 deficiency remains to be resolved and it is perhaps best reserved for places where the disorder has a high prevalence or where easy access to modern paediatric care is compromised.

OTHER INHERITED DISORDERS OF STEROID METABOLISM

An interesting disorder of P_{450}arom (aromatase) has been reported in which there is excessive peripheral conversion of androgen to oestrogen as a consequence of a markedly increased P_{450}arom acitivity. Male patients presented with gynaecomastia and male sexual development at puberty.[57] The pattern of inheritance is male-limited autosomal dominant (*CYP19*, the gene for P_{450}arom is on chromosome 15) and may be due to a defect in the gene itself or the promoter.

A number of other disorders of steroid metabolism are inherited. Some such as the glucocorticoid[58] or androgen[59] receptor defects are clearly disorders of steroid action rather than steroid biosynthesis. Other disorders such as placental sulphatase[60] and 11β-hydroxysteroid dehydrogenase[61] deficiencies are more difficult to classify. These disorders will not be discussed further here.

REFERENCES

1. Munro Neville A, O'Hare M J 1982 The human adrenal cortex. Springer Verlag, Berlin, p 16–34
2. Symington T 1969 Functional pathology of the adrenal gland. E and S Livingstone, Edinburgh, p 5–28
3. Finkelstein M, Shaeffer J M 1979 Inborn errors of steroid biosynthesis. Physiological Reviews 59:353–406
4. Wilson J D, Griffin J C, George F W, Lewis M 1981 The role of gonadal steroids in sexual differentiation. Recent Progress in Hormone Research 37:1–33
5. Saenger P 1984 Abnormal sex differentiation. Journal of Pediatrics 104:1–17
6. Hornsby P J 1985 The regulation of adrenocortical function by control of growth and structure. In: Anderson D C, Winter J (eds) The adrenal cortex. Butterworth, London, p 1–31
7. Briggs M H, Brotherton J 1971 Nomenclature of steroids. In: Steroid biochemistry and pharmacology. Academic Press, London, p 1–22
8. Makin H L (ed) 1984 Biochemistry of the steroid hormones, 2nd edn. Blackwell Scientific Publishers, Oxford
9. Nerbert D W, Gonzalez F J 1987 P_{450} genes: Structure, evolution and regulation. Annual Reviews of Biochemistry 56:945–993
10. Nerbert D W, Nelson D R, Coon M J, Estabrook R W, Feyereisen R, Fujii-Kuriyama Y, Gonzalez F J, Guengerich F P, Gunsalus I C, Johnson E F, Loper J C, Sato R, Waterman M R, Waxman D J 1991 The P_{450} superfamily: Update on new sequences, gene mapping and recommended nomenclature. DNA and Cell Biology 10:1–14
11. Liebermann S, Greenfield N J, Wolfson A 1984 A heuristic proposal for understanding steroidogenic processes. Endocrine Reviews 5:128–148
12. Lieberman S, Prasad V V K 1990 Heterodox notions on pathways of steroidogenesis. Endocrine Reviews 11:469–493

13. Yanagibashi K, Haniu M, Shively, J E, Shen W H, Hall P 1986 The synthesis of aldosterone by the adrenal cortex. Journal of Biological Chemistry 261: 3556–3562
14. Anderson D C 1980 The adrenal androgen-stimulating hormone does not exist. Lancet 2:454–456
15. Reed M J, James V H T 1989 Regulation of steroid synthesis and metabolism by growth factors. Clinical Endocrinology (Oxford) 31:511–525
16. Nestler J E, McClanahan M A, Clore J N, Blackard W G 1992 Insulin inhibits adrenal 17,20- lyase activity in man. Journal of Clinical Endocrinology and Metabolism 74:362–367
17. Price D A, Close G C, Fielding B 1983 Age of appearance of circadian rhythm in salivary cortisol values in infancy. Archives of Disease in Childhood 58:454–456
18. Biglieri E G, Wajcheenberg B L, Malerbi D A, Okada H, Leme C E, Kater C E 1981 The zonal origins of the mineralocorticoid hormones in the 21-hydroxylation deficiency congenital adrenal hyperplasia. Journal of Clinical Endocrinology and Metabolism 53:964–969
19. Weinkove C, Anderson D C 1985 Interaction between adrenal cortex and medulla. In: Anderson D C, Winter J (eds) The adrenal cortex. Butterworth, London, p 208–234
20. Bateman A, Singh A, Kral T, Solomon S 1989 The immune–hypothalamic–pituitary–adrenal axis. Endocrine Research 10:92–112
21. Paterson R E 1971 Metabolism of the adrenal steroids. In: Christy N P (ed) The human adrenal cortex. Harper and Row, New York, p 87–189
22. McLaren A 1990 What makes a man a man? Nature 346:216–217
23. Berta P, Hawkins J R, Sinclair A H, Taylor A, Griffiths B L, Goodfellow P N, Fellous M 1990 Genetic evidence equating SRY and the testis determining factor. Nature 348:448–450
24. Addison G M, Chard C R, Price D A 1984 Steroid hormone metabolism. In: Hicks J M, Boeckx R L (eds) Pediatric clinical chemistry. W B Saunders, New York, p 240–294
25. De Perretti E, Forest M G 1982 Pitfalls in the etiological diagnosis of congenital adrenal hyperplasia in the early neonatal period. Hormone Research 16:10–22
26. Tanae T, Hashimoto N, Miki Y, Hibi I, Morikawa Y 1988 Clinical studies on eleven patients with congenital lipoid adrenal hyperplasia (Prader's Syndrome). In: Takeda R, Miyamori I (eds) Controversies in disorders of adrenal hormones. Elsevier Science Publishers, Amsterdam, p 193–198
27. Morohashi K, Sogawa K, Omura T, Fijii-Kuriyama Y 1987 Gene structure of human cytochrome P_{450}(SCC), cholesterol desmolase. Journal of Biochemistry 101:879–887
28. Sparkes R S, Klisak I, Miller W L 1991 Regional mapping of genes encoding human steroidogenic enzymes: P_{450}scc to 11q23–q24, adrenodoxin to 11q22, adrenodoxin reductase to 17q24–q25 and P_{450}c17 to 10q24–25. DNA and Cell Biology 10:359–3365
29. Petersen R P, Imperato-McGinley J, Gautier T, Shackleton C 1985 Male pseudohermaphroditism due to multiple defects in steroid-biosynthetic microsomal mixed-function oxidases. New England Journal of Medicine 313:1182–1191
30. Cravioto M del C, Ulloa-Aguirre A, Bermudez J A, Herrera J, Lisker R, Mendez J P, Perez-Palacios G 1986 A new inherited variant of 3β-hydroxysteroid dehydrogenase-isomerase deficiency syndromes: Evidence for the existence of two isoenzymes. Journal of Clinical Endocrinology and Metabolism 63:360–367
31. Yanase T, Simpson E R, Waterman M R 1991 17α-hydroxylase/17,20-lyase deficiency: From clinical investigation to molecular definition. Endocrine Reviews 12:91–108
32. Fife D, Rappaport E B 1983 Prevalence of salt losing among adrenal hyperplasia patients. Clinical Endocrinology (Oxford) 18:259–264
33. Strachan T 1990 Molecular pathology of congenital adrenal hyperplasia. Clinical Endocrinology (Oxford) 32:373–393
34. White P C 1989 Analysis of mutations causing steroid 21-hydroxylase deficiency. Endocrine Research 15:239–256
35. Speiser P W, Agdere L, Ueshiba H, White P C, New M I 1991 Aldosterone synthesis in salt-wasting congenital adrenal hyperplasia with complete absence of adrenal 21-hydroxylase. New England Journal of Medicine 324:145–149
36. New M I, White P C, Pang S, Dupont B, Speiser P W 1989 The adrenal hyperplasias.

In: Scriver O R, Beaudet A L, Sly WS, Valle D (eds) The metabolic basis of inherited disease, 6th edn, McGraw–Hill, New York, Vol 2, p 1881–1917
37. Zachmann M, Tassinari D, Prader A 1983 Clinical and biochemical variability of congenital adrenal hyperplasia due to 11β-hydroxylase deficiency: a study of 25 patients. Journal of Clinical Endocrinology and Metabolism 56:222–229
38. Honour J W, Anderson J M, Shackleton C H L 1983 Difficulties in the diagnosis of congenital adrenal hyperplasia in early infancy: the 11β-hydroxylase defect. Acta Endocrinologica 103:101–109
39. Hochberg Z, Benderly A, Zadik Z 1984 Salt loss in congenital adrenal hyperplasia due to 11β-hydroxylase defect. Archives of Disease in Childhood 59:1092–1094
40. Ulick S 1976 Diagnosis and nomenclature of the disorders of the terminal portion of the aldosterone biosynthetic pathway. Journal of Clinical Endocrinology and Metabolism 43:92–96
41. Honour J W, Dillon M J, Shackleton C H L 1982 Analysis of steroids in urine for differentiation of pseudohypoaldosteronism and aldosterone biosynthetic defects. Journal of Clinical Endocrinology and Metabolism 54:325–331
42. Mornet E, Dupont J, Vitek A, White P C 1989 Characterization of two genes encoding human steroid 11β-hydroxylase (P-45011β). Journal of Biological Chemistry 264:20961–20967
43. White P C, Dupont J, New M I, Leiberman E, Hochberg Z, Rosler A 1991 A mutation in CYP11B1 (Arg-448 → His) associated with steroid 11β-hydroxylase deficiency in Jews of Moroccan origin. Journal of Clinical Investigation 87:1664–1667
44. Luu-The V, Labrie C, Simard J, Lachance Y, Zhao H F, Couet J, Leblanc G, Labrie F 1990 Structure of two in tandem human 17β-hydroxysteroid dehydrogenase genes. Molecular Endocrinology 4:268–275
45. Impertato-McGinley J, Gautier T 1986 Inherited 5α-reductase deficiency in man. Trends in Genetics 2:130–133
46. Hendricks S A, Lippe B M, Kaplan S A, Lavin N, Mayes D 1982 Urinary and serum steroid concentrations in the management of congenital adrenal hyperplasia: lack of physiological correlations. American Journal of Diseases of Children 136:229–232
47. Appan S, Hindmarsh P C, Brook C G D 1989 Monitoring treatment in congenital adrenal hyperplasia. Archives of Disease in Childhood 64:1235–1239
48. Hughes I A, Read G F 1984 Control of congentital adrenal hyperplasia monitored by frequent saliva 17OH-progesterone measurements. Hormone Research 19:77–85
49. Solyom J 1981 Blood spot 17α-hydroxyprogesterone radioimmunoassay in the follow up of congenital adrenal hyperplasia. Clinical Endocrinology (Oxford) 14:547–553
50. Rosler A, Levine L S, Schneider B, Novogroder M, New M I 1977 The interrelationship of sodium balance, plasma renin activity and ACTH in congenital adrenal hyperplasia. Journal of Clinical Endocrinology and Metabolism 45:500–512
51. Rosenthal S M, Reid I A, Kaplan S L, Grumbach M M 1983 Renin substrate depletion in salt losing virilizing adrenal hyperplasia: low plama renin activity despite increased renin concentration. Journal of Pediatrics 102:80–82
52. Speiser P W, Laforgia N, Kato K, Pareira J, Khan R, Yang S Y, Whorwood C, White P C, Elias S, Schriock E, Simpson J L, Taslimi M, Najjar J, May S, Mills G, Crawford C, New M I 1990 First trimester prenatal treatment and molecular genetic diagnosis of congenital adrenal hyperplasia (21-hydroxylase deficiency). Journal of Clinical Endocrinology and Metabolism 70:838–848
53. Forest M G, Betuel H, David M 1989 Prenatal treatment in congenital adrenal hyperplasia due to 21-hydroxylase deficiency: Update 88 of the French multicentric study. Endocrine Research 15:277–301
54. Rosler A, Leiberman E, Rosenmann A, Ben-Uzilio R, Weidemfeld J 1979 Prenatal diagnosis of 11β-hydroxylase deficiency congenital adrenal hyperplasia. Journal of Clinical Endocrinology and Metabolism 49:546–551
55. Lebovitz R M, Pauli R M, Laxova R 1984 Delayed diagnosis in congenital adrenal hyperplasia: need for newborn screening. American Journal of Diseases of Children 138:571–573
56. Pang S, Wallace M A, Hofman L, Thuline H C, Dorche C, Lyon I C T, Dobbins R H, Kling S, Fujieda K, Suwa S 1988 Worldwide experience in newborn screening for congenital adrenal hyperplasia due to 21-hydroxylase deficiency. Pediatrics 81:866–874
57. Berkovitz G D, Guerami A, Brown T R MacDonald P C Migeon C J 1985 Familial

gynecomastia with increased extraglandular aromatization of plasm carbon(19)-steroids. Journal of Clinical Investigation 75:1763–1769
58. Lamberts S W J, Koper J W, Biemond P, den Holder F H, de Jong F H 1992 Cortisol receptor resistance: The variability of its clinical presentation and response to treatment. Journal of Clinical Endocrinology and Metabolism 74:313–321
59. Griffin J E, Wilson J D 1989 The androgen resistance syndromes: 5α-reductase deficiency, testicular feminization and related disorders. In: Scriver C R, Beaudet A L, Sly W S, Valle D (eds) The metabolic basis of inherited disease, 6th end. McGraw–Hill, New York, vol 2, p 1919–1944
60. Shapiro L J 1989 Steroid sulphatase deficiency and X-linked icthyosis. In: Scriver C R, Beaudet A L, Sly W S, Valle D (eds) The metabolic basis of inherited disease, 6th edn. McGraw–Hill, New York, vol 2, p 1945–1964
61. Tannin G M, Agarawal A K, Monder C, New M I, White P C 1991 The human gene for 11β-hydroxysteroid dehydrogenase. Structure, tissue distribution and chromosomal localization. Journal of Biological Chemistry 266:16653–16658

12. Lipid disorders

C. H. Bolton

PLASMA LIPOPROTEINS

General introduction

The lipoproteins of plasma form a complex system for the transport of hydophobic lipids, notably cholesterol esters and triglycerides, in a water-soluble form, between the tissues.

The varying proportions of lipid to protein in these macromolecular complexes produce a wide range of physical properties and the classification and identification of lipoproteins depend on these variations in properties. The most commonly used system of nomenclature is based on hydrated density, though some sources use electrical charge as a basis. By either method lipoproteins naturally fall into four major classes named according to their behaviour in the ultracentrifuge, or on electrophoresis (see Table 12.1).

The bulk of the lipoprotein is made up of a hydrophobic core of cholesterol esters and triglycerides, surrounded by a membrane-like structure containing free cholesterol and phospholipids in which the proteins 'float'. These proteins are known as apolipoproteins or, more simply, apoproteins.

Table 12.1 Properties of lipoproteins

Ultracentrifugal behaviour/ Electrophoretic mobility	Chylomicrons/ Origin	Very low density/pre β	Low density/β	High density/α
% Protein	<2	12	25	50
% Lipid	98	88	75	50
Major lipid	Triglyceride	Triglyceride	cholesterol	cholesterol phospholipid
Major apoprotein	A,C,B48	C,B100,E	B100	A
Major function	Transport of exogenous triglyceride	Transport of endogenous triglyceride	Transport of cholesterol to tissues	Transport of cholesterol from tissues
Origin	Intestine	Intestine and liver	Metabolism of VLDL	Liver and intestine

Table 12.2 Properties and occurrence of the major apoproteins.

Apoprotein	Major lipoprotein fraction	Molecular weight	Function
AI	HDL	28 300	LCAT cofactor
AII	HDL	17 000	Structural protein
B100	VLDL, LDL	513 000	LDL receptor binding
B48	Chylomicrons	265 000	Structural protein and remnant receptor binding
CI	VLDL, HDL	6 331	Not certain
CII	VLDL, HDL	8 837	LPL cofactor
$CIII_{0,1,2}$	VLDL, HDL	8 764	Not certain
$E_{2,3,4}$	VLDL, HDL	33 000	Remnant receptor binding
(a)	LDL, LP(a)	300 – 700 000	Not known

As the proportion of protein increases, so the density of the particle increases. The amount of protein therefore in high density lipoprotein (HDL) is approximately 50% whereas that in chylomicrons is less than 2% (see Table 12.1).

It was originally thought that the apoproteins served only a structural role, stabilising and solubilising the lipid core of the lipoprotein, but it is now known that their functions extend to include enzyme modulation and receptor recognition.

At least 13 human plasma apolipoproteins have been identified and characterised. Many have had their primary structure determined, including apo AI, apo AII, apo B48, apo B100, apo CI, apo CII, apo CIII and apo E. Table 12.2 shows the major apolipoproteins, their occurrence within lipoprotein classes, molecular weights and, where known with certainty, their physiological functions. Several other minor apolipoproteins have been described but their functions are very unclear.

Biosynthesis and metabolism of lipoproteins

Triglyceride-rich lipoproteins

Triglyceride-rich lipoproteins are secreted as chylomicrons and very low density lipoprotein (VLDL) by the small intestine and the liver respectively (Fig. 12.1). The VLDLs, contain apo B100 and the chylomicrons, contain apo B48 (48% of apo B100). After circulation to peripheral tissues they are hydrolysed by the triglyceride hydrolases (EC 3.1.1.3), lipoprotein lipase (EC 3.1.1.34) and hepatic lipase, to give smaller intermediate density lipoproteins (IDLs), which can be further hydrolysed to produce low density lipoproteins (LDLs), and chylomicron remnants.

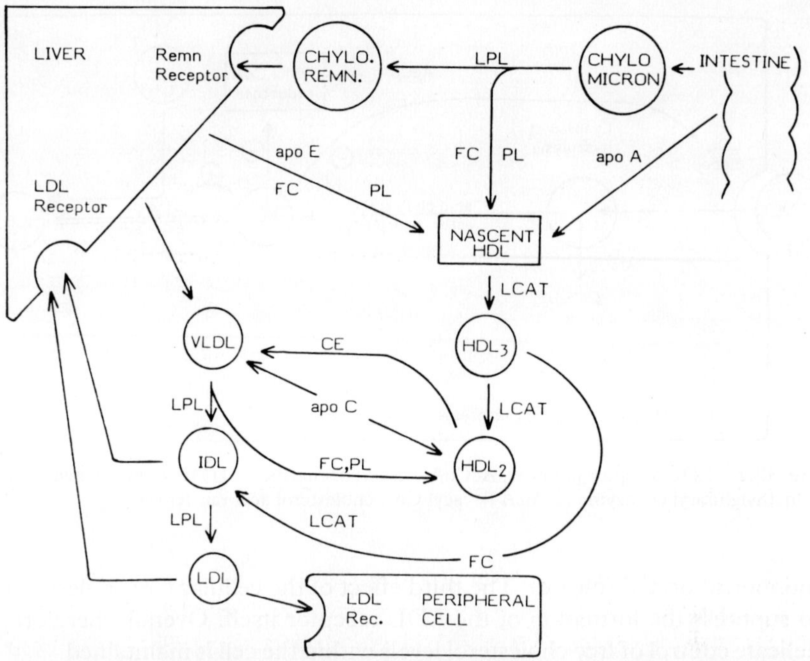

Fig. 12.1 Lipoprotein metabolism, VLDL, LDL, IDL, HDL – Very low, low, intermediate, high density lipoprotein respectively, FC – free cholesterol, PL – phospholipid, CE – cholesterol ester, LCAT – lecithin cholesterol acyltransferase, LPL – lipoprotein lipase, Remn – remnant, Rec. – receptor.

Both of these products, LDL and chylomicron remnants, are removed from the circulation by specific receptor systems. The liver has a receptor for chylomicron remnants which recognises the apo E carried on the surface of the remnant particles. The remnant receptor is therefore often referred to as the E receptor. The high affinity LDL receptor, on the other hand, occurs widely in peripheral cells, such as fibroblasts, endothelial cells, smooth muscle cells and liver cells, and recognises both apo B 100 and apo E. It is therefore called the B,E receptor. Circulating LDL is bound to the cell surface receptor (Fig. 12.2). Endocytosis then takes place and the particle is broken down by lysosomal enzymes, including proteases and an acid lipase, liberating free cholesterol and amino acids. This free cholesterol operates at three levels within the cell. First, it suppresses the activity of 3-hydroxy-3-methylglutaryl coenzyme A reductase (HMG CoA reductase, EC 1.1.1.88) which controls the rate-determining step in cholesterol biosynthesis. Secondly, it stimulates the re-esterification of free cholesterol by activation of the enzyme acyl-CoA:cholesterol acyl transferase (ACAT, EC 2.3.1.26). The overall result of this re-esterification process is to shift the balance of fatty acids in the cholesterol esters from the predominantly polyunsaturated form in the diet (linoleate) to a form more suitable for storage, usually

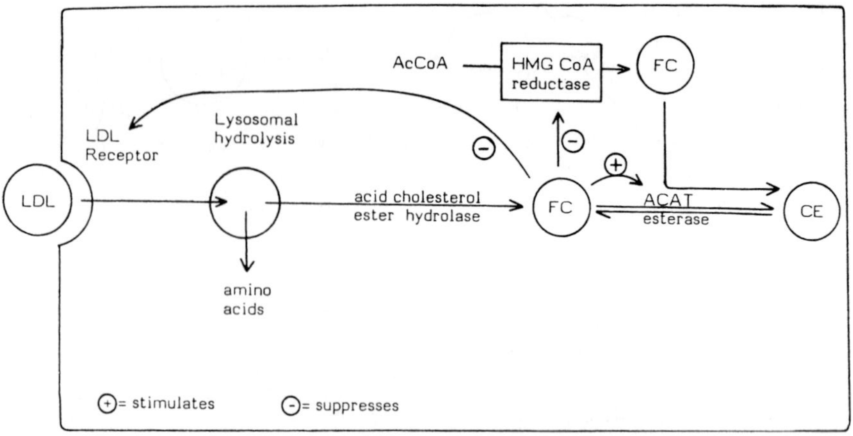

Fig. 12.2 LDL receptor pathway. AcCoA – acetyl coenzyme A, HMG CoA – 3-hydroxy, 3-methylglutaryl coenzyme A, ACAT – acyl CoA cholesterol acyltransferase.

monounsaturated (oleate). The third effect of the cellular free cholesterol is to suppress the formation of the LDL receptor itself. Overall, therefore, a delicate control of free cholesterol levels within the cell is maintained.

It is important to note that apo B48 does not bind to the LDL receptor. It contains only the first 2152 amino acids of apo B100, which excludes the carboxyterminal, receptor-binding domain. This is caused by the insertion of a termination codon at position 6457 of the mRNA resulting from a single C to U substitution. Thus the evidence seems to suggest the separate genetic control of apo B48 and apo B100. This also causes the dietary chylomicron remnants, containing apo B48 with apo E, to be directed to the remnant (E) receptor rather than the LDL (B,E) receptor.[2]

A further apo B100 containing lipoprotein (Lp(a)) occurs in almost all individuals but appears not to be derived by catabolism of triglyceride-rich lipoproteins, but probably by direct hepatic secretion. It contains an additional apoprotein, apo(a), linked via a disulphide bond to apo B100. Its structure is an aberration of the clotting factor plasminogen.[2] Lipoprotein (a) binds to the B,E receptor less avidly than LDL. Its metabolic function is not known with certainty, but it may be that because of the structural similarity of apo(a) to plasminogen, it may have relevance in arterial thrombosis.

High density lipoproteins

The biosynthesis and metabolism of HDL is complicated by the polydispersity of the HDL particle itself (Fig. 2.1) It contains two major subfractions, HDL_2 and HDL_3, differing slightly in size and composition. The lipid and apoprotein components of HDL are derived from the catabolism of both VLDL and chylomicrons, as well as being synthesised directly by both liver and intestine. Hepatic HDL contains mainly apo E, whereas intestinal HDL contains apo A. A further species of HDL is formed in response to prolonged high fat feeding, which is enriched in cholesterol and apo E, and whose density range extends into the LDL region. Its function is a little obscure and it disappears as the diet reverts to normal.

Newly synthesised (nascent) HDL is disc-shaped, and contains no esterified cholesterol. On reaction with the plasma cholesterol-esterifying enzyme, lecithin cholesterol acyltransferase (LCAT, EC 2.3.1.43) the discs are converted into the mature spherical particle, HDL_3, which then acquires apo C, free cholesterol and phospholipid released during lipolysis of triglyceride-rich lipoproteins. The product of this reaction is HDL_2 which in the process releases some of its newly esterified cholesterol and apo C back to triglyceride-rich lipoproteins. This lipid transfer is mediated by one or more lipid transfer proteins.

HDL appears to be involved in reverse cholesterol transport from the peripheral cells to the liver, a process which helps to explain the inverse correlation which exists between HDL-cholesterol concentration and prevalance of premature cardiovascular disease.

Role of apolipoproteins as enzyme regulators

Two of the major enzymes of lipoprotein metabolism, lipoprotein lipase (LPL) and lecithin cholesterol acyltransferase (LCAT) have specific requirements for an apoprotein regulator.

Lipoprotein lipase is the enzyme responsible for the lipolytic breakdown of triglyceride-rich lipoproteins on the endothelial surface. A specific requirement for LPL activity is the presence of apo CII, which is found with the other C apoproteins in chylomicrons, VLDL and also HDL. It has been reported that apo CIII, at least in vitro, inhibits LPL activity but this has not been confirmed in vivo.

LCAT, which catalyses cholesterol esterification in plasma, is only active in the presence of apoprotein AI, one of the major apoproteins of HDL. It has been reported that apo CI also activates LCAT, though it appears to operate through a different mechanism from apo AI. LCAT exists in two forms; αLCAT acts on HDL and βLCAT on VLDL and LDL.

It can be seen therefore that the metabolism of lipoproteins is closely related to the spectrum of apolipoproteins they contain. Previous classifications of lipoprotein disorders have been based almost entirely on the lipid content of the lipoproteins. Although this has served a useful purpose by identifying many of the lipoprotein abnormalities which have been observed, the underlying biochemical problem has frequently remained unsolved. More recent work has shown that much more information can be derived by studying apoprotein abnormalities, many of which occur at the molecular level.

In this chapter therefore, the importance of the apolipoproteins in disorders of lipoprotein metabolism will be stressed wherever possible.

Laboratory investigation of lipoprotein disorders

Some of the techniques required for the analysis of lipoproteins and apoproteins are sophisticated and therefore unlikely to be available in all but the best-equipped clinical laboratories. Many laboratories now, however, are offering more than simple routine lipid assays, and as more reliable standardised methodology becomes available, our knowledge of disease frequency and treatment is likely to improve. Details of analytical procedures are beyond the scope of this article but numerous texts are available which describe the relevant experimental methods.[3–6]

For a full lipoprotein analysis an ultracentrifuge is usually required, though nowadays it is possible to separate most of the lipoproteins by differential precipitation using polyanions etc. This method is commonly employed for the isolation of HDL using heparin, sodium phosphotungstate or dextran sulphate. Having obtained a value for HDL cholesterol, and, provided that the plasma triglyceride level is within normal limits, it is possible to calculate the level of LDL cholesterol from the Friedewald equation[7]:

$$\text{LDL cholesterol (mmol/l)} = \text{Total cholesterol} - \text{HDL cholesterol} - (\text{triglycerides}/2.2)$$

Electrophoresis may be used for the qualitative analysis of whole lipoproteins, and it is mandatory for qualitative analysis of apoproteins. Polyacrylamide gel is the support medium of choice and if this is combined with isoelectric focusing a very powerful tool for the analysis of apoprotein isoforms is available, which in combination with densitometric scanning can produce a semiquantitative analysis of the apoprotein distribution.

For a truly quantitative analysis of apoproteins it is at present necessary to resort to some form of immunoassay. Many methods have been described, including radial immunodiffusion, electroimmunoassay, radioimmunoassay, immunonephelometry and enzyme-linked immunosorbent assay (Table 12.3). All have their relative advantages and disadvantages, but a common factor is that they all require specific antibodies to the desired apoprotein. Many are now commercially available, some in the form of assay kits, but often it is necessary for the laboratory to develop its own antisera. Often, therefore, these assays are available only in laboratories with a strong research interest.

Recent improvements in high performance liquid chromatography (HPLC) and the advent of capillary electrophoresis have increased the scope for non-immunological estimation of apoproteins. At the present time these remain essentially research tools.

The analysis of the lipid content of plasma and lipoproteins is usually less

Table 12.3 Immunological procedures for apoprotein assay

Type of assay	Advantages or disadvantages	Apoproteins assayed	Typical references
Radial immunodiffusion (RID)	Simple, cheap, no automation, small numbers	AI,AII,B,CI	Cheung & Albers 1977[8]
Electroimmunoassay (EIA)	Simple, cheap, no automation, large amount of antibody	AI,AII,B,CI, CII,CIII,E	Curry et al 1978[9]
Radioimmunoassay (RIA)	Very sensitive, specific, large numbers, tedious	AI,AII,B,CII, CIII,E,(a)	Durrington et al 1976[10]
Immunonephelometry (INA)	Large numbers, may be automated, reasonably sensitive, large amount of antibody	AI,AII,B	Rosseneu et al 1981[11]
Enzyme-linked immuno-sorbent assay (ELISA)	Large numbers, may be automated, sensitive, reproducible	AI,B,(a),CII, CIII, E	Alsayed et al 1990[12]

of a problem as most laboratories have efficient working methods for the assay of cholesterol and triglycerides.

The estimation of enzymatic activity for any of the lipid-metabolising enzymes, or the investigation of cell receptor function, are specialised techniques and their availability will therefore be very limited.

Molecular genetics and lipoprotein disorders

The analysis of apolipoprotein genes has increased dramatically in recent years. The genes for most of the human apoproteins have been sequenced and numerous polymorphisms identified, many of which have only marginal clinical significance. Only those mutations which are known to have a direct bearing on disease will be discussed in any detail, in the section relating to that disease. Molecular biological investigations are advancing at an impressive rate, and ultimately the potential for identification of the molecular defect in many lipoprotein disorders will increase, making therapeutic intervention a distinct possibility.

CLASSIFICATION OF LIPOPROTEIN DISORDERS

Most of the well-defined disorders involving lipoproteins can be divided into three groups:

1. defects in an apoprotein involved in synthesis or metabolism of lipoproteins

2. defects in a cell receptor which recognises an apoprotein
3. defects in an enzyme concerned with lipoprotein metabolism.

These disorders are listed in Table 12.4 according to the specific defect and, where known, the type of dyslipoproteinaemia which is most likely to be manifested. In two relatively common inherited disorders, primary hypertriglyceridaemia and combined hyperlipidaemia, the defect is not known with certainty. In Table 12.4 therefore, they are not placed in either of the three main categories. The order of the diseases in Table 12.4 takes no account of their relative incidence, and lipoprotein disorders which arise secondarily to other major metabolic diseases are excluded, even though the profile of lipids generated may be similar, if not identical, to that in primary dyslipoproteinaemias.

There is often a close relationship between lipoproteins and their constituent apoproteins; there can, therefore, often be an overlap of biochemical signs such that the more widely used Fredrickson classification[14,15] (Table 12.5) is unable to identify clearly the underlying metabolic lesion.

Table 12.6 indicates the primary inherited defect which may have to be considered when a major plasma lipid (cholesterol or triglyceride) is found to be abnormal at an initial screen. It has to be emphasised that often more

Table 12.4 Classification of lipoprotein disorders. Type refers to the Fredrickson classification of hyperlipoproteinaemias (Table 12.5).
Numbers in parentheses refer to the McKusick classification of inherited diseases (McKusick[13])

Defect	Localisation	Disorder
Structural	Apoprotein AI	Tangier (205400), Fisheye, apo AI deficiency, apo AI variants, apo AI+CIII deficiency
	Apoprotein B48 +apoprotein B100	Abetalipoproteinaemia (200100), familial hypobetalipoproteinaemia (107730)
	Apoprotein B100	Abetalipoproteinaemia (normotriglyceridaemic)
	Apoprotein B100	Familial defective apoprotein B100
	Apoprotein CII	Chylomicronaemia (apo CII absence), Type I (238600) or Type V(144650)
	Apoprotein E	Type III (107741) or Type V
Receptor	LDL receptor	Familial hypercholesterolaemia Type IIa, (143890, 144400)
	Remnant receptor	Type III
Enzymic	Lipoprotein lipase	Chylomicronaemia Type I
	Hepatic lipase	Type III
	LCAT	LCAT deficiency (245900)
	Cholesterol ester hydrolase	Wolman (278000), cholesterol ester storage disease
	Cholesterol ester transfer protein	CETP deficiency
Unknown		Primary hypertriglyceridaemia (Type IV, 144600 and V)
		Combined hyperlipidaemia, Type IIb (144250)

Table 12.5 Classification of hyperlipoproteinaemias, (Fredrickson et al 1967[14], Beaumont et al 1970[15]). Several lipoprotein disorders have come to be named according to this classification. Although the system leaves much to be desired, it has become a working framework for identifying some of the primary disorders of lipoprotein metabolism. This system will therefore be used for those disorders which fall naturally into one of these categories, whilst accepting that ultimately a more specific definition, identifying the underlying apoprotein or metabolic defect, could be used. The phenotype expressed may arise for a variety of reasons. It is thus a classification of the lipoprotein status of the patient's plasma, rather than the underlying genetic abnormality of the patient.

Lipoprotein abnormality	Phenotype expressed
Raised chylomicrons (chylomicronaemia)	Type I
Raised LDL (hypercholesterolaemia)	Type IIa
Raised LDL and VLDL (combined hyperlipidaemia)	Type IIb
Raised IDL (broad beta disease; beta VLDL)	Type III
Raised VLDL (hypertriglyceridaemia)	Type IV
Raised chylomicrons and VLDL (chylomicronaemia and hypertriglyceridaemia)	Type V

Table 12.6 Relationship between laboratory findings and molecular defect

Laboratory findings	Phenotype	Lipoprotein abnormality	Molecular defect (if known)
Raised cholesterol	Type IIa	LDL, apo B raised	LDL receptor absent or defective
Raised triglycerides	Type I	Chylomicrons raised	LPL or apo CII absent or defective
	Type IV	VLDL raised	?
	Type V	Chylomicrons and VLDL raised	apo CII deficiency
	Fisheye disease	LDL triglycerides raised	α LCAT absent
Raised cholesterol and triglycerides	Type IIb	VLDL and LDL raised	?
	Type III	VLDL raised Apo E2 raised Chylo remnants raised IDL raised	apo E2 homozygosity Remnant receptor defect Hepatic lipase deficient
	Cholesterol ester storage disease	VLDL, LDL raised HDL low	CE hydrolase deficient
	LCAT deficiency	VLDL raised, absence of CE	Absence of LCAT
Decreased cholesterol	Abetalipoproteinaemia	Absence of VLDL, LDL, chylomicrons	Absence of apo B
	Hypobetalipoproteinaemia	Decrease in VLDL, LDL, chylomicrons	Decrease in apo B
	Tangier disease	Absence of HDL	Absence of apo A

than one molecular defect can give expression to a particular lipoprotein phenotype. Because of the rarity of many of these disorders, all more likely causes of a lipid abnormality should first be excluded. The definition of what constitutes an abnormal lipid or lipoprotein concentration is beyond the scope of this article. The influence of age, sex, race, diet, lifestyle, etc. are very significant and the reader is directed to one of the many reviews which cover this subject. All clinical laboratories will have their own definitions of normal ranges.

DEFECTS INVOLVING APOPROTEINS: APOPROTEIN A

Tangier disease (analphalipoproteinaemia)

This rare disorder was first described by Fredrickson in 1961 following its discovery in two inhabitants of Tangier Island, Virginia.

Clinical symptoms

The disease is characterised by the presence of enlarged orange tonsils. Even after tonsillectomy, residual tonsillar tissue may be detected in the pharynx. There is often corneal opacity but without impairment of vision. Hepatosplenomegaly is fairly common, as is peripheral neuropathy. Anaemia (often haemolytic) occurs in many cases and thromocytopenia may be present. The mucosa of the colon and rectum are frequently discoloured.

Histology shows excessive deposition of cholesterol esters in the reticuloendothelial system, particularly in the macrophages and the Schwann cells. This is most evident in the tonsils, bone marrow, intestine, nerves, liver and spleen.

Biochemical signs

Characteristically there is marked plasma hypocholesterolaemia (usually less than 2.6 mmol/l) due to decreased levels of cholesterol esters. Plasma triglycerides may be elevated by the presence of chylomicrons and raised LDL-triglycerides. The most striking feature is, however, the almost complete absence of HDL. The levels of plasma apo AI and apo AII are, as expected, very much reduced to less than 10% of normal values. This is almost certainly due to rapid catabolism of apo AI, apo AII and HDL and a possible slight reduction in synthesis rates of apo AI and apo AII.

Despite the absent HDL fraction, premature atherosclerosis is not considered to be a complication of Tangier disease.

Inheritance and incidence

The disease is autosomally recessive. The symptoms described above are therefore typical of the homozygote. It is extremely rare, and approximately

90% of all recorded cases are of caucasian origin. It is possible that the disease may be more common than it would seem from the small number of cases so far described, since often the symptoms may be mild and may pass unnoticed. The only prominent clinical sign is the enlarged orange tonsil.

Molecular defect and metabolic disorder

It is not known for certain what is the primary cause of the HDL deficiency in Tangier disease. There is no defect in the apo AI gene, and in apo AI structure. It is likely that there is a disorder of intracellular metabolism giving increased levels of triglycerides and cholesterol esters, and rate of phospholipid turnover. There is a small amount of precursor protein resembling pro-apo AI in the HDL infranatant (d > 1.21 g/ml) after ultracentrifugation. This protein is indistinguishable from the pro-apo AI of normal subjects. It is possible that there may be a defect in the proteolysis of pro-apo AI, leading to the absence of apo AI in Tangier plasma. Infusion of labelled normal apo AI and apo AII into Tangier patients has yielded conflicting results. Although the catabolic rate is much greater than normal, it is not clear whether the infused apoproteins can combine to form normal HDL in Tangier subjects.

LCAT activity against both HDL, and VLDL and LDL (α andβ respectively) is present but it is the βLCAT which accounts for all the cholesterol esterification seen in this condition.[16]

Investigation

In the few cases where tonsil changes are not present, differential diagnosis is sometimes necessary to distinguish Tangier disease from, for example, chronic liver disease, biliary cirrhosis, lipid or mucopolysaccharide storage diseases, hypo- and hyperlipoproteinaemias and LCAT deficiency. This can be effectively achieved by histology of liver biopsies or rectal mucosa and by measurement of HDL.

Treatment

No specific treatment is possible. Infusion of normal HDL offers no solution as the half-life of HDL is drastically reduced, and normal apolipoproteins may not be reincorporated into Tangier HDL.

Partial alleviation of symptoms is possible by introducing a low cholesterol diet, thereby reducing the storage of dietary cholesterol as cholesterol esters. A low fat diet is unnecessary as fat transport appears to be normal. If haemolytic anaemia is present, a low carbohydrate diet will reduce the possibility of increased red cell fragility. As diabetes mellitus may develop in old age, weight control is advisable from an early stage.

Hypoalphalipoproteinaemia

This is a rare and heterogeneous condition which includes patients with Tangier disease. Clinical symptoms of Tangier disease are not necessarily apparent. Levels of HDL are approximately half those of normal subjects and the relative amounts of apo AI and apo AII are normal. Confirmation of diagnosis must exclude other possible causes such as obesity, diabetes mellitus, and hypertriglyceridaemia, and by detection of the condition in other family members. In some cases, cardiovascular disease is present.

Apoprotein AI variants

Numerous structural variants of apoprotein AI have been detected by the technique of isoelectric focusing.[17] The clinical consequences of these polymorphisms are not apparent even though in some, e.g. apo AI Milano, there is a marked reduction of HDL level, and in others, e.g. apo AI Giessen, LCAT activity is reduced. Isoelectric focusing will undoubtedly reveal many similar structural variants, whose clinical significance may well remain obscure.

Apoproteins AI and CIII deficiency

This condition, described in 1982, which is symptomatically distinct from Tangier disease, presents with severe premature cardiovascular disease, skin and tendon xanthomas, and corneal opacity. Both apoprotein AI and apoprotein CIII are absent in the homozygotes. HDL levels are low, but LDL is higher than in Tangier disease. In heterozygote family members apo AI and CIII are about half normal levels.

The genes for apo AI and apo CIII are part of the same cluster on chromosome 11 and coded for by opposite DNA strands. In one of the two families described with this condition there was a 7.5 kb insertion in the apo AI gene. In both families the apo CIII gene was indistiguishable from normal. Despite this, because of the linkage, there was no transcription of the gene.

Fish-eye disease

This very rare condition, first described in 1979, presents with dense corneal opacity (resembling boiled fish). There is also marked visual impairment, contrasting with Tangier disease, and atherosclerosis in old age.

Biochemically there is a 90% reduction in plasma HDL – c holesterol, but with normal amounts of total cholesterol. Hypertriglyceridaemia, particularly in the LDL fraction, is present. LCAT activity for VLDL and LDL (βLCAT) is normal but that for HDL (αLCAT) is absent. This explains why cholesterol ester concentrations are normal in spite of the marked deficiency of HDL. Apoproteins AI and AII are reduced to 10–15% of normal values.

DEFECTS INVOLVING APOPROTEINS: APOPROTEIN B

Abetalipoproteinaemia

This disorder was first described in 1950 as the Bassen–Kornzweig syndrome after its discoverers.

Clinical symptoms

Fat malabsorption is present from birth, though jejunal biopsy reveals normal villi, in contrast to coeliac disease. Effects which occur secondarily to malabsorption e.g. anaemia, are present in some children but they can be easily treated. Retinitis pigmentosa and neurological involvement are common.

Biochemical signs

There is a marked plasma hypocholesterolaemia (0.6–3.0 mmol/1), characterised by a lack of all apo B-containing lipoproteins i.e. chylomicrons, VLDL, LDL, both in plasma and intestinal mucosa, the synthesis site of chylomicrons. Plasma triglyceride levels are also characteristically low, usually less than 0.4 mmol/l. The remaining plasma lipids and apoproteins are carried exclusively by the HDL fraction which is present at about half normal concentration. Apo AI and apo AII are correspondingly reduced to about 40% of normal and apo CIII is absent. The phospholipid fraction of HDL is grossly abnormal, with a reduced ratio of lecithin to sphingomyelin and an abnormal fatty acid composition. This results in abnormally shaped red blood cells with spiky projections (acanthocytes).

Inheritance and incidence

Abetalipoproteinaemia is very rare and autosomally recessive. Parents – heterozygotes – are unaffected clinically and have a lipid profile which is not grossly abnormal. It has been reported in several countries but more than 20% of cases are of Jewish origin, and 71% are male though a sex linkage has not been proven. Consanguinity has been shown to be present in about half the cases.

Molecular defect and metabolic disorder

The classical feature of this disease is the complete lack of apoprotein B (both apo B48 and apo B100) in plasma. There are apparently no abnormalities in the apo B gene. Present evidence seems to suggest that apo B is synthesised but that there is a fault in the assembly of the mature lipoprotein.[18]

Cholesterol-feeding experiments in abetalipoproteinaemia have shown that cholesterol absorption is negligible, although sterol excretion is high and bile acid synthesis normal. Whole-body synthesis of cholesterol is however higher than normal, in all probability as a compensatory mechanism for the malabsorption. Diagnosis of abetalipoproteinaemia is dependent on the demonstration of the absence of apoprotein B in plasma by immunoassay.

Treatment

In order to counteract the gastrointestinal symptoms a low fat diet is recommended. The use of medium-chain triglycerides as an alternative calorie source is controversial. Supplements of fat-soluble vitamins A and K are necessary and pharmacologic doses of vitamin E are now thought to be important for the correction of some retinal and neuromuscular abnormalities.

Hypobetalipoproteinaemia

The homozygous form of this disease is clinically and biochemically indistinguishable from abetalipoproteinaemia. However, this variant is incompletely recessive. Heterozygotes have reduced levels of plasma LDL, occasionally overlapping the normal range, with mild clinical signs and symptoms.

Treatment of the heterozygous form is unnecessary, but the homozygote requires similar dietary manipulations to those used for abetalipoproteinaemia.

Normotriglyceridaemic abetalipoproteinaemia

This condition is very rare and represents a variant of classical abetalipoproteinaemia.

The clinical symptoms of the disease are always milder than in typical abetalipoproteinaemia. Biochemically only apo B100 is absent, which means that chylomicron synthesis can take place, though VLDL and LDL are absent. This implies that apo B48 and apo B100 are under separate genetic control and that chylomicron apo B48 is not a precursor of LDL apoprotein B100. The mode of inheritance is unknown.

Chylomicron retention disease

This recently reported disease presents with malabsorption, decreased levels of cholesterol, LDL, apo B and apo AI. Fat-soluble vitamins are also deficient. Chylomicrons do not appear following a fatty meal, though triglycerides in LDL are increased. Large numbers of fat-laden particles are present in enterocytes. This condition appears to be recessively transmitted and distinct from abetalipoproteinaemia and homozygous hypobetalipoproteinaemia. There is probably a defect in the assembly of chylomicrons or in their secretion.

Familial defective apolipoprotein B100

This disorder, first recognised in 1987, presents with symptoms similar to those of familial hypercholesterolaemia. It is autosomally dominant and probably occurs at a frequency of 1:500. A single amino acid mutation of apo B100, glutamine for arginine at residue 3500, causes reduced binding of the modified apoprotein to the LDL high-affinity receptor, which has normal activity in this condition. The mutation can be detected by amplification of a segment of DNA which spans the site in apo B100, followed by hybridisation with probes.

Therapy with HMGCoA reductase inhibitors (statins) will successfully reduce circulating levels of LDL and total plasma cholesterol thereby reducing the symptoms typical of familial hypercholesterolaemia.[19]

Lipoprotein (a) variability

Although there is no specific disease known to be related with certainty to variability in LP(a), the widely differing levels found particularly in caucasians have been related to incidence of cardiovascular disease. Apoprotein (a), the characteristic protein of LP(a) shows marked size heterogeneity which is related to the number of kringles (a particular protein conformation reminiscent of Danish kringle pastry) controlled by the apo(a) gene. Because of the homology between the structure of apo(a) and plasmin there may be a role for apo(a) in a thrombotic pathway, possibly by inhibition of plasmin with the consequent increase in thrombotic risk. The currently available information does not allow us to be in any way dogmatic about its function.[20]

DEFECTS INVOLVING APOPROTEINS: APOPROTEIN CII

Apoprotein CII deficiency

This recently discovered disorder bears some similarities to lipoprotein lipase deficiency and presents mainly with the Type V phenotype.

Clinical symptoms

There is gross plasma lipaemia from an early age, which is often accompanied by lipaemia retinalis, haemolytic anaemia and bouts of acute abdominal pain due to the pancreatitis which often occurs with massive hypertriglyceridaemia. Red cell survival is reduced and diabetes mellitus often develops, which may or may not be insulin-dependent. The lipaemia persists in spite of diabetic control. In the few cases so far described, there is apparently no xanthomata or hepatomegaly, in contrast to lipoprotein lipase deficiency. Little is known of potential clinical complications.

Biochemical signs

Massive hypertriglyceridaemia results from the presence of chylomicrons and elevated levels of VLDL. Electrophoresis or isoelectric focusing of whole plasma or VLDL apoproteins will reveal a complete absence of apoprotein CII. This can be confirmed by immunological tests. The triglyceride-rich lipoproteins from patients will not activate normal lipoprotein lipase, but addition of apo CII by infusion of normal plasma will cause a temporary clearance of lipaemia.

Inheritance and incidence

The disease has an autosomally recessive inheritance. Heterozygotes with 30–50% of normal levels of apo CII, show normal clearance of lipaemia. The number of cases so far described is very small.

Molecular defect and metabolic disorder

The absence of apoprotein CII from the plasma of patients with this disorder can almost certainly be traced to a defect at, or near, the gene coding for apo CII. Studies on fragments of the apo CII molecule have revealed that a short segment of the polypeptide chain (amino acids 55–78) is necessary for the complete activation of lipoprotein lipase. Such fragments may have therapeutic value. A recently discovered mutation has identified a C to G substitution in the third exon of the gene resulting in a stop codon. This terminates the protein at amino acid 36. A highly unstable, non-functional protein is therefore produced. A specific restriction (RsaI) site is lost, and this mutation can be used for diagnosis.[21]

As little as 10% of the normal level of apo CII will restore full lipolytic activity, even in homozygotes.

Treatment

The only suggested treatment to date is a low-fat diet, to alleviate the pancreatitis. Generally subjects live well into middle age in spite of the gross hypertriglyceridaemia.

DEFECTS INVOLVING APOPROTEINS: APOPROTEIN E

Apoprotein E exists in three major isoforms, apo E2, E3 and E4, which are controlled by three alleles at a single genetic locus, thus giving expression to six phenotypes, three homozygous and three heterozygous.[22] Apo E3 and apo E4 are considered to be 'normal' apo E isoforms, and apo E2 'abnormal'.

Apoprotein E2 homozygosity

A total of 1% of the population is homozygous for apo E2 and 1–2% of those present with overt Type III hyperlipoproteinaemia.

Clinical symptoms

The Type III phenotype normally presents with coronary heart disease, peripheral arterial disease, intermittent claudication, xanthomatosis (characteristically yellowish lipid deposits in the palmar creases) and tuberoeruptive xanthomas on the elbows. Other forms of xanthomata and corneal arcus are much less common. Approximately half the patients have hyperuricaemia and abnormal glucose tolerance.

Biochemical signs

The dysbetalipoproteinaemia which usually accompanies apo E2 homozygosity is characterised by the presence of abnormal cholesterol-rich VLDL, showing a broad, β-migrating band on electrophoresis. Ratios of VLDL cholesterol to total triglyceride greater than 0.69 (SI units), or VLDL cholesterol to VLDL triglyceride of over 0.97 are both very good indicators of the condition. The best criterion, however, is apo E2 homozygosity in association with the clinical findings.

Inheritance and incidence

The mode of inheritance of Type III hyperlipoproteinaemia is still not clear though the evidence suggests autosomally dominant transmission. As already mentioned apo E2 homozygosity exists in about 1% of the population, though most of those do not progress to the classical Type III phenotype which probably requires the presence of additional factors producing hyperlipidaemia, or secondary diseases which have the same effect.

Molecular defect and metabolic disorder

The accumulation of β-VLDL in the plasma, characteristic of dysbetalipoproteinaemia and Type III hyperlipoproteinaemia is due to defective removal of chylomicron remnants and IDL. The reason for this lies in the primary structure of the apo E. The three alleles arise following point mutations in the apo E structural gene. Amino acid interchanges take place at positions 112 and 158 of the peptide chain. Thus, in apo E2 two cysteine residues occur at these positions, in apo E3 cysteine is at position 112 and arginine at 158, and in apo E4 arginine occurs at both positions. Apo E2 binds much less avidly to the hepatic remnant receptor than either apo E3 or apo E4. Remnants containing apo E2 therefore are not removed from the circulation for catabolism and therefore accumulate. The defective binding is caused by the cysteine.[23]

Diagnosis and treatment

Apo E2 homozygosity can only be demonstrated with certainty by isoelectric focusing of VLDL proteins. The type III phenotype can be confirmed by clinical findings (particularly the palmar crease xanthomas) coupled with demonstration of the presence of β-VLDL. Type III hyperlipoproteinaemia responds well to dietary modification. Fat restriction with a high polyunsaturated content, low cholesterol and low alcohol will all be beneficial. Lipid-lowering drugs (excluding anion-exchange resins) are usually effective. Cholesterol and triglyceride levels will possibly normalise, but β-VLDL will always persist.

Other aberrations of apoprotein E

In Type V hyperlipoproteinaemia, there is often an increased abundance of individuals with apo E4 (53 compared with 15% in the normal population). It is likely that other genetic disturbances may be required for the full manifestation of the hypertriglyceridaemia characteristic of Type V.

Complete absence of apoprotein E has been shown in one kindred. The clinical picture is that of Type III hyperlipoproteinaemia, i.e. β-VLDL is present due to impaired hepatic removal of remnant particles which lack the ligand for the remnant receptor.

DEFECTS OF RECEPTOR FUNCTION: LDL RECEPTOR

Familial hypercholesterolaemia (FH)

In Fredrickson's classification, this is expressed as the Type IIa phenotype, with characteristically gross elevation of LDL cholesterol concentration and marked clinical signs.

Clinical symptoms

Hypercholesterolaemia is evident within the first year of life. The more frequently found heterozygotes present with arcus corneae and xanthomas during the second decade, and clinical coronary heart disease is evident by the fourth decade. Homozygotes have similar symptoms much earlier, with death ensuing usually before the age of 30 years. Yellow or orange cutaneous xanthomas may even be present at birth, and certainly appear by the fourth year. Tendon xanthomas and arcus, with atheroma, are present during childhood. Virtually all vessels can be affected though coronary vessels are particularly prone, and aortic valve infiltration is common.

Biochemical signs

There is a specific elevation of LDL-cholesterol which causes the total serum cholesterol concentration to be greater than 9 mmol/l in heterozygotes and 15 mmol/l in homozygotes. LDL-cholesterol is twice the normal level in heterozygotes and approximately six times normal in homozygotes. There is apparently no abnormality in composition or structure of the LDL. Thus LDL obtained from a homozygote is metabolised normally when injected into a normal person and will suppress the activity of 3-hydroxy, 3-methylglutaryl (HMG) CoA reductase exactly like normal LDL.

Inheritance and incidence

FH is dominantly transmitted by a single mutant allele. The homozygote is affected much more severely than the heterozygote. The gene is highly penetrant: 90% of all carriers have LDL cholesterol concentrations above the 95 percentile value of the normal population. The gene frequency has been calculated at 1:500 in caucasians in the USA, and as high as 1:200 in London where approximately one person per million is homozygous. The premature death of undiagnosed individuals may explain the apparently small number of homozygotes in relation to the gene frequency. FH is thus one of the most common of the human genetic diseases.

Molecular defect and metabolic disorder

The gene for the LDL-receptor is located on chromosome 19, as also is the gene for apoprotein E–a ligand for the LDL-receptor along with apoprotein B100.

The molecular defect has been described in great detail by Goldstein and Brown and coworkers.[24] There are essentially four groups of mutations which affect the behaviour of the LDL-receptor:

1. Receptor synthesis is eliminated.
2. Transport of the receptor to the cell surface is reduced.
3. Receptors are synthesised with defective ability to bind the LDL protein.
4 Receptors are produced which are unable to internalise the bound LDL.

Within these four main groups there are at least 16 different mutations which have now been located on the gene. Probes for all of these are available. Mutations are found in all the domains of the gene and therefore explain how the various functions relating to the receptor activity are affected.

In the homozygote, receptor function is abolished, thus preventing the binding and/or internalisation of LDL. As a result there is no suppression of HMG CoA reductase activity or activation of ACAT activity within the cell. LDL catabolism can not therefore occur. A massive build-up of LDL in plasma follows, with the resultant risk of its modification and uptake by macrophages, and ultimately premature atherosclerosis.

Heterozygotes have approximately half the amount of receptor activity. LDL accumulation is therefore less severe than in homozygotes.

In all these variations the typical characteristics of familial hypercholesterolaemia will be evident.

Diagnosis

Homozygous FH characteristically has levels of plasma cholesterol in excess of 15 mmol/l. Cutaneous xanthomas and juvenile atherosclerosis are present in childhood. In the heterozygote, simple diagnosis is more difficult, but it is important to ensure that the cause of the hypercholesterolaemia (usually greater than 9 mmol/l) is a raised level of LDL-cholesterol. Tendon xanthomas are frequently but not always present, particularly in younger patients. Vertical transmission of hypercholesterolaemia and xanthomatosis is invariably present in the true familial disorder. It is worth noting that only about one patient in 20 with hypercholesterolaemia has the genuinely familial type. In many symptomatic patients the disease is multifactorial in origin and polygenic in inheritance.

If the specific receptor defect is known, it is possible using the appropriate DNA probes to diagnose FH. Prenatal diagnosis is therefore possible but would be used only in those rare cases when homozygosity is likely. Heterozygosity in the neonate can be diagnosed by measuring the LDL-cholesterol concentration in the cord blood of babies born to known FH gene carriers. It is important to note that general screening is not helpful as most babies with a raised LDL-cholesterol level do not necessarily have FH.

Treatment

Treatment of FH is usually aimed at the reduction of plasma levels of LDL cholesterol which can be done either by stimulation of the receptor or reduction of hepatic synthesis of LDL.

Dietary treatment of FH, or indeed any form of hypercholesterolaemia, consists primarily in reduction of dietary cholesterol and saturated fat, both of which tend to downregulate the LDL-receptor. An increase in polyunsaturated/saturated fat ratio is therefore routinely recommended. It is unlikely, however, that diet alone will have the total desired effect on LDL-cholesterol and some form of pharmacological intervention will be necessary. Clearly this treatment will have little or no effect on homozygous FH patients whose receptor function is non-existent.

Heterozygotes, on the other hand, may respond to a variety of different treatments. The first-line drugs are either the anion-exchange resins, cholestyramine and colestipol, or the HMG CoA reductase inhibitors, simvastatin, lovastatin or pravastatin. Recent work suggests that this latter group is particularly effective in lowering elevated LDL-cholesterol concentrations. A further possible addition to the armoury of treatment is nicotinic acid or one of its derivatives. These drugs may be used in combination for increased effectiveness.[25]

More drastic therapy is necessary for the treatment of homozygous FH. For example, a portocaval shunt or, in some heterozygotes, a partial ileal bypass have had some success. Frequent plasmapheresis has also been shown to be moderately successful on a long-term basis.[26]

Remnant receptor

The hepatic remnant receptor specifically removes from the circulation triglyceride-rich remnant particles, IDL and chylomicron remnants, by recognition of apo E on the particle surface. This receptor has very high affinity for apo E. Its absence or deficiency leads to a marked increase in atherogenic remnant particles and a clinical picture characteristic of Type III hyperlipoproteinaemia.

DEFECTS INVOLVING ENZYME FUNCTION

Lipoprotein lipase deficiency

This disease was first described in 1939 and exhibits the Fredrickson Type I phenotype, with severe fasting chylomicronaemia.

Clinical symptoms

The disease is usually obvious in childhood and is accompanied by epigastric and midabdominal pain. Massive chylomicronaemia is always present following deficient fat absorption. In about half the patients papuloeruptive xanthomas occur in the skin creases or on pressure areas. The liver and spleen are often tender and there is frequent pancreatitis, probably related to the hypertriglyceridaemia. Histology shows foam cells present in bone marrow, spleen and liver, and hepatosplenomegaly occurs often, particularly in periods of high fat intake.

Lipaemia retinalis is frequent and glucose intolerance is rare, in contrast to many other hypertriglyceridaemias. There is no apparent tendency for premature atherosclerosis.

Biochemical signs

There is persistance even in the fasting state of dietary chylomicrons, due to the lack of lipoprotein lipase in the extrahepatic tissues. Apoprotein CII, the cofactor for lipoprotein lipase, is present in its normal concentration. In apoprotein CII deficiency, which also presents with severe chylomicronaemia, either as a Type I or V phenotype, there is a normal level of lipoprotein lipase but with inefficient activation.

Inheritance and incidence

The disease is inherited autosomal recessively and consequently heterozygotes are indistinguishable from normal. It is very rare and has been found in caucasians, Chinese and negroes.

Molecular defect and metabolic disorder

The reason for the low or absent lipoprotein lipase activity on the capillary endothelium is not clear but may be caused by faulty gene expression.

Diagnosis and treatment

Even on a regular diet, there is marked fasting chylomicronaemia. This is particularly evident after standing the plasma overnight in the refrigerator when a creamy layer appears over a clear infranatant. This distinguishes it from Type V, where the creamy layer appears over an opalescent plasma. Levels of triglycerides in plasma can reach 20 mmol/l due solely to the presence of chylomicrons. Cholesterol concentrations are usually normal except in very severe cases. LDL and HDL are usually reduced in concentration and remain so even on treatment.

Dietary treatment is normally restricted to a low-fat (40–60 g/24 h) diet; if calorie supplementation is required, the use of medium-chain triglycerides may be effective since these are absorbed via the portal circulation, not requiring chylomicron synthesis.

As with many hypertriglyceridaemias, it is important to note that this phenotype may arise secondarily to various other diseases e.g. pancreatitis, uncontrolled diabetes, paraproteinaemia etc. but will invariably disappear when the primary cause is successfully treated.

Hepatic lipase deficiency

This enzyme, which is involved in the clearance of triglyceride-rich remnant particles, has functions which are similar to those of lipoprotein lipase but a protein cofactor is not required. Its deficiency produces clinical features characteristic of Type III hyperlipoproteinaemia, with a marked build-up of remnant particles.

Lecithin cholesterol acyltransferase deficiency

Absence of this cholesterol esterifying enzyme from plasma, was first described in 1966 in Norway. It is rare and although it has been recognised in various parts of the world, the greatest proportion of cases occurs in Scandinavia.

Clinical symptoms

Proteinuria occurs early in childhood with renal function deteriorating by middle age in many patients. Corneal opacity is a characteristic of all patients and is typically similar to a severe arcus, with cholesterol crystals being evident under polarising microscopy. Haemolytic anaemia is often present by the third decade. Foam cells are present in bone marrow and in glomerular tissue. Hyperlipidaemia with accelerated atherosclerosis is typical.

Biochemical signs

Elevations in both plasma cholesterol and triglycerides are usual. All lipoproteins are of abnormal composition, largely because of the elevation in free cholesterol and lecithin. Because of the reduced level of esterified cholesterol the LDL and HDL particles are both predominantly disc-shaped and HDL is much reduced in concentration. Most of the total plasma apo AI (usually found in HDL) occurs in the fraction of density greater than 1.21 g/ml, which may relate to the unstable nature of the HDL fraction.

Inheritance and incidence

LCAT deficiency is inherited in an autosomally recessive manner and is caused by a single gene defect. In Western Norway the gene frequency is about 2% and although the disease has been described elsewhere the frequency is much less.

Molecular defect and metabolic disorder

All the biochemical features of this disease are caused by the lack or severe deficiency of LCAT, which normally esterifies free cholesterol in plasma, with the concomitant formation of lysolecithin from lecithin. The normal lipoprotein maturing process which accompanies this, is therefore prevented. The enzyme has been characterised as a glycoprotein with 416 amino acids of molecular weight 63 000. There are at least three different mutations in the gene which probably give rise to different levels of enzyme activity and of protein mass. These produce the varying behaviour which seems to be a feature of the disease.

Treatment

Dietary fat restriction will reduce the elevated levels of LDL cholesterol and may prevent kidney damage. Even so renal transplantation may become necessary but this will have little or no effect on LCAT activity.

Cholesterol ester hydrolase deficiency

A deficiency of acid cholesterol ester hydrolase (EC 3.1.1.13) (see Fig. 12.2) results in two diseases which differ clinically only in degree. Wolman's disease, first described in 1956, is considerably more severe, and is invariably fatal within months of birth. Cholesterol ester storage disease (CESD) is a more benign form of Wolman's disease and can be detected in adulthood.

Clinical symptoms

Both diseases show massive accumulation of lysosomal cholesterol esters and triglycerides. Wolman's disease presents very early with gastrointestinal symptoms, steatorrhea and hepatosplenomegaly. There is marked adrenal calcification and tissue lipid storage which is characteristic. Anaemia develops within 6 weeks of birth and subsequently increases in severity. Foam cells are present in the bone marrow.

The clinical symptoms of CESD are less pronounced than in Wolman's disease. Hepatomegaly occurs with occasional splenomegaly, oesophageal varices and hepatic fibrosis. Premature atherosclerosis is likely.

Biochemical signs

In Wolman's disease, the plasma cholesterol and triglyceride levels are often normal. Hepatic lipids, however, have an elevated content of cholesterol esters.

Inheritance and incidence

Both diseases are inherited in an autosomally recessive manner and are extremely rare. There appears to be an excess of females with CESD, though a sex linkage is not demonstrable.

Molecular defect and metabolic disorder

The major defect is a marked decrease in activity of lysosomal acid cholesterol ester hydrolase in several cells, notably Kupffer cells, liver and spleen macrophages, leucocytes, lymphocytes and fibroblasts. All these cells therefore accumulate vast quantities of cholesterol esters and triglycerides. The enzyme plays a vital role in the breakdown of internalised LDL. Without it there is no formation of free cholesterol to exert its regulating effect on intracellular sterol metabolism. It is believed that Wolman's disease and CESD are two allelic disorders which involve mutations at the gene locus for the hydrolase.

Diagnosis and treatment

Wolman's disease is characteristically accompanied by severe gastrointestinal symptoms and failure to thrive. Radiographic detection of adrenal calcification is strongly suggestive but definitive diagnosis requires the demonstration of lysosomal acid lipase deficiency in lymphocytes or cultured fibroblasts. Prenatal diagnosis of heterozygotes is achieved by the measurement of enzyme levels in cultured amniotic cells or in chorionic villi. The presence of CESD can be confirmed similarly. No therapeutic intervention in either disease is currently believed to be effective.

Cholesterol ester transfer protein deficiency

Recently some cases have been described with a deficiency of cholesterol ester transfer protein (CETP). This was evidenced biochemically by a much increased level of HDL, together with an additional population of small LDL particles. The relationship between this condition and the presence or not of cardiovascular disease is still not clear in spite of the elevated concentrations of the protective HDL. The gene encoding the CETP is on chromosome 16, close to that for LCAT; several restriction fragment length polymorphisms have been identified but their significance clinically is not known.

DISORDERS WITH UNKNOWN PRIMARY DEFECTS

Primary hypertriglyceridaemia

This disease may express the Fredrickson Type IV or Type V phenotype, depending on degree of severity.

Clinical symptoms

The Type IV phenotype, which is milder, has few clinical features. Associations have been noted with obesity, abnormal glucose tolerance, insulin resistance, hyperinsulinism and hyperuricaemia. Premature cardiovascular disease may occur, but xanthomas rarely do. To establish the primary nature of the disorder it is necessary to confirm familial inheritance.

In Type V hyperlipoproteinaemia plasma triglyceride concentrations are grossly elevated. All the above symptoms may be present together with features typical of chylomicronaemia such as eruptive xanthomas, hepatosplenomegaly, abdominal pain (possibly accompanying pancreatitis) and the presence of foam cells in the bone marrow or other organs. Type V rarely occurs in children, which distinguishes it from Type I, and lipoprotein lipase activity is normal.

It is important to note that both forms of hypertriglyceridaemia frequently occur secondarily to other stimuli e.g. diabetes mellitus, alcohol abuse, hormone therapy.

Biochemical signs

Plasma levels of triglycerides are raised in both disorders but considerably more so in Type V. There is no clear cut-off point between the two as chylomicronaemia may often be induced in Type IV patients following high intake of carbohydrates or alcohol. The hypertriglyceridaemia of Type IV is due to VLDL only, whereas that in Type V is also due to chylomicrons. LDL levels in Type V are characteristically low, and in both disorders HDL is reduced.

Inheritance and incidence

Primary hypertriglyceridaemia is inherited in an autosomal dominant fashion though it is not expressed early in life. The heterozygote frequency for Type IV, as determined in the original Seattle study, is 1:100 but the fully expressed Type V disorder is much rarer. The close interrelationship between the two phenotypes means that relatives of Type V cases often show the Type IV pattern.

Molecular defect and metabolic disorder

The primary defect in hypertriglyceridaemia is not known with certainty. The disease is clearly heterogeneous in origin and so it is unlikely that there is a single genetic or metabolic cause. There is strong evidence in support of both an increase in production and a decrease in catabolism of VLDL particles. The additional stimulus to production, or to reduced catabolism, by either exogenous or endogenous factors may often exacerbate a Type IV phenotype into the more severe Type V.

Recent research has suggested that the relative proportions of sialylated to asialylated forms of apoprotein CIII may be relevant to the lipolysis of triglyceride-rich lipoproteins. The importance of this observation is not clear.

Diagnosis and treatment

Hypertriglyceridaemia is characteristic. In Type IV, levels of plasma triglycerides may reach 10 mmol/l with a mean of 5 mmol/l, resulting from an increased VLDL fraction. Diagnosis of the primary disorder is only confirmed if family members are affected. This may only be evident in the third decade.

In Type V hyperlipoproteinaemia the presence of chylomicrons produces much higher levels of triglycerides (usually greater than 11 mmol/l). Cholesterol levels may be slightly raised and it may be necessary to use either ultracentrifugation or electrophoresis to distinguish it from Type III hyperlipidaemia. On the rare occasions when the Type V pattern arises before the age of 20 years it is important to exclude lipoprotein lipase or apo CII deficiencies.

VLDL levels can be reduced by restriction of carbohydrate intake but if chylomicrons are also raised then fat restriction will also be necessary. Additional pharmacological intervention may be required, in the form of fibrate drugs or nicotinic acid and its derivatives.

Combined hyperlipidaemia

This complex disease is phenotypically a Fredrickson Type IIb but other members of the affected family may have very varied lipid profiles. It was first described as a distinct clinical entity in 1973.

Clinical symptoms

Coronary heart disease is very common but is frequently accompanied by obesity, hyperinsulinaemia and abnormal glucose tolerance. Expression of the disease normally occurs in the third decade, though 10–20% of affected children show elevations in plasma lipid levels.

Biochemical signs

There is a modest rise in both cholesterol and triglyceride concentrations in plasma, resulting from increased levels of both VLDL and LDL fractions. Other affected members of the same family may have elevations in either or both of these lipoproteins.

Inheritance and incidence

This disease is transmitted in an autosomally dominant manner with the Type IIb phenotype being common – occurring in about 3% of an apparently healthy London population. In the original description of this disease, 11% of survivors of myocardial infarction under 60 years expressed the Type IIb phenotype. Approximately 20% of patients with the disorder develop premature coronary heart disease. Phenotypic expression often varies within a family, and also within individuals when sampled on different occasions or on different therapy.

Molecular defect and metabolic disorder

The metabolic defect underlying this disorder is probably an overproduction of VLDL apoprotein B in the liver. There is no defect of the LDL-receptor, in contrast to familial hypercholesterolaemia, and there is evidence to suggest that there is no defect in the apo B100 gene. Recent work, however, has identified an association between the disorder and a restriction fragment length polymorphism in the apolipoprotein AI-CIII-AIV gene cluster on chromosome 11.[27] It is likely that in many cases other risk factors may have to be present before the disorder presents with overt coronary disease.

Diagnosis and treatment

In true Type IIb hyperlipoproteinaemia, both cholesterol and triglyceride concentrations are elevated, but family members have to be identified with either of Types IIa, IIb or IV being present, before a diagnosis is confirmed.

Because of the increased risk associated with this disorder, early preventative measures to reduce the elevated lipid fractions are beneficial. Dietary intervention is the first line of attack, using low-cholesterol and low-saturated fat diets, coupled if necessary with lipid-lowering drugs e.g. fibrates.

REFERENCES

1. Brown M S, Goldstein J L 1987 Teaching old dogmas new tricks. Nature 330: 113–114
2. McLean J W, Tomlinson J E, Kuang W-J et al 1987 cDNA sequence of human apolipoprotein (a) is homologous to plasminogen. Nature 330:132–137
3. Havel R J, Eder H A, Bragdon J H 1955 The distribution and chemical composition of ultracentrifugally separated lipoproteins in human serum. Journal of Clinical Investigation 34:1345–1353
4. Burstein M, Legmann P 1982 Lipoprotein precipitation. In Clarkson T B. Kritchevsky D, Pollack O J (eds) Monographs on atherosclerosis. Karger, Basle, vol 2
5. Neuback W, Wieland H, Habernicht A, Muller P, Baggio G, Seidel D 1977 Improved assessment of plasma lipoprotein pattern. III Direct measurement of lipoproteins after gel electrophoresis. Clinical Chemistry 23:1269 – 1300

6. Ghiselli G, Gregg R E, Zech L A, Schaefer E J, Brewer H B Jr 1982 Phenotype study of apolpipoprotein E isoforms in hyperlipoproteinaemia patients. Lancet 2:405–407
7. Friedewald T, Levy R I, Fredrickson D S 1972 Estimation of serum low-density lipoprotein cholesterol without use of the preparative ultracentrifuge. Clinical Chemistry 18:499–502
8. Cheung M C, Albers J J 1977 The measurement of apolipoprotein AI and AII levels in men and women by immunoassay. Journal of Clinical Investigation 60:43–50
9. Curry M D, Gustafson A, Alaupovic P, McConathy W J 1978 Electroimmunoassay, radioimmunoassay and radial immunodiffusion assay evaluated for quantification of human apolipoprotein B in man. Clinical Chemistry 24:280–286
10. Durrington P N, Whicher J T, Warren C, Bolton C H, Hartog M 1976 A comparison of methods for the immunoassay of serum apolipoprotein B in man. Clinica Chimica Acta 71:95–108
11. Rosseneu M, Vercaemst R, Vinaimont M, van Tornout P, Henderson L O, Herbert P N 1981 Quantitative determination of human plasma apolipoprotein AI by immunonephelometry. Clinical Chemistry 27:856–859
12. Alsayed N, Rebourcet R, Chapman J 1990 Concentrations of apoproteins CII, CIII and E in total serum and in the apoprotein B containing lipoproteins determined by a new enzyme-linked immunosorbent assay. Clinical Chemistry 36:2047–22052
13. McKusick V A 1990 Mendelian inheritance in man, 9th edn. Johns Hopkins University Press, Baltimore
14. Fredrickson D S, Levy R I, Lees R S 1967 Fat transport in lipoproteins – an integrated approach to mechanisms and disorders. New England Journal of Medicine 276:36–44, 94–103, 148–156, 215–226, 273–281
15. Beaumont J L, Carlson L A, Cooper G R, Fefjar Z, Fredrickson D S, Strasser T 1970 Classification of hyperlipidaemias and hyperlipoproteinaemias. Bulletin of the World Health Organization 43:891–915
16. Carlson L A, Holmquist L, Assman G 1987 Different substrate specificities of plasma lecithin cholesterol acyltransferase in fisheye disease and Tangier disease. Acta Medica Scandinavica 222:345–350
17. Utermann G, Feussner G, Franceschini G, Haas J, Steinmetz A 1982 Genetic variants of group A apolipoproteins. Rapid methods for screening and characterisation without ultracentrifugation. Journal of Biological Chemistry 257:50–507
18. Menzel H J, Dieplinger H, Lackner C et al 1990 Abetalipoprotenaemia with an apo B100-lipoprotein (a) glycoprotein complex in plasma. Indication for an assembly defect. Journal of Biological Chemistry 265:981–986
19. Illingworth D R, Vakar F, Mahley R W, Weisgraber K H 1992 Hypocholesterolaemic effects of lovastatin in familial defective apolipoprotein B100. Lancet 339:598–600
20. Scott J 1989 Thrombogenesis linked to atherogenesis at last? Nature 341:22–23
21. Crecchio C, Capurso A, Pepe G 1990 Identification of the mutation responsible for a case of plasmatic apolipoprotein CII deficiency (apo CII-Bari). Biochemical and Biophysical Research Communications 168:1118–1127
22. Zannis V I, Breslow J L, Utermann G et al 1982 Proposed nomenclature of apo E isoproteins, apo E genotypes and phenotypes. Journal of Lipid Research 23:911–914
23. Weisgraber K H, Rall S C, Mahley R W 1981 Human apo E apoproteins heterogeneity. Cyteine-arginine interchanges in the amino acid sequence of apo E isoforms. Journal of Biological Chemistry 256:9077–9083
24. Goldstein J L, Brown M S 1985 Progress in understanding the LDL receptor and HMG Coa reductase, two membrane proteins that regulate the plasma cholesterol. Journal of Lipid Research 25:1450–1461
25. Illingworth D R, Bacon S 1989 Treatment of heterozygous familial hypercholesterolaemia with lipid-lowering drugs. Arteriosclerosis 9 (Suppl 1):121–134
26. Thompson G R, Barbir M, Okabayashi K, Trayner I, Larkin S 1989 Plasmapheresis in familial hypercholesterolaemia. Arteriosclerosis 9 (Suppl 1):152–157
27. Wojciechowski A P, Farrall M, Cullen P et al 1991 Familial combined hyperlipidaemia linked to the apolipoprotein AI-CIII-AIV gene cluster on chromosome 11q23–q24. Nature 349:161–164

13. Metal disorders

P. J. Aggett

GENERAL INTRODUCTION

Collectively inherited defects affecting the mechanisms for the absorption, transport, cellular uptake and utilisation, storage and excretion of cations have been described for iron, copper, zinc, magnesium, molybdenum and, possibly, manganese.

IRON

The enterocyte has separate mechanisms for the uptake of haem iron and inorganic iron from the intestinal lumen. Within this cell, haem oxygenase releases the haem iron which thereafter forms a common pool with its inorganic counterpart. The enterocytic uptake and transfer of iron is controlled by the number of receptors at the brush border and by apoferritin which binds and sequesters the metal as ferritin which is lost into the intestinal lumen when the mucosal cell is desquamated. The mucosal content of apoferritin seems to be regulated by the iron content of reticuloendothelial cells in the lamina propria.

After its transfer across the intestinal epithelium, iron is incorporated, as the Fe(III) state, into the glycoprotein transferrin for transport in the circulation to tissues such as the liver and erythroid cells of the bone marrow, where transferrin binds to specific receptors on the cell membranes, and releases its iron either directly or after the entire receptor–transferrin complex has been endocytosed. The iron is incorporated into haem and apoproteins and the residual apotransferrin is extruded and recycled.

Normally, adults contain 4–5 g of iron of which 0.5–1.0 is stored intracellularly in the form of water-soluble ferritin. Denaturation of ferritin by lysosomal enzymes produces the insoluble iron depot haemosiderin; many intermediate degradation products can exist and are particularly evident in tissues with chronic iron overload.

Hereditary (idiopathic, genetic) haemochromatosis (McKusick 235200)

The defect is inherited as an autosomal recessive characteristic.

In hereditary haemochromatosis an excessive amount of iron accumulates in the body 20–40 g, causing extensive tissue damage.[1, 2] The intestinal absorption of iron is inappropriately high for the degree of iron overload; in contrast to individuals with secondary iron overload, the intestinal mucosa and the reticuloendothelial system of patients have a low content of iron and ferritin. The hepatocytic expression of transferrin receptors is low as would be expected for a tissue laden with iron[3]; in contrast, in the gut mucosa there is a failure of homeostatic reduction of iron uptake and, despite iron overload, an inappropiate failure of the mucosal block, leading to increased transfer of iron to the portal circulation.[4] This may reflect a defect in reticuloendothelial regulation of the intestinal absorption of iron. Pathogeneses based on abnormalities of transferrin and its receptors, and of the light and heavy protein subunits of ferritin, seem unlikely since the alleles for these proteins are located on chromosomes 3, 11q and 19q respectively, whereas that for hereditary haemochromatosis is on the short arm of chromosome 6(6p21.3) within 1 centimorgan of the HLA-A locus and it is closely linked with HLA types A3, B7, B14.[2, 5]

The increased burden of iron is distributed throughout the body except for the gut mucosa and reticuloendothelial system. Initially the metal accumulates in ferritin and then in haemosiderin within lysosomes. Subsequent degeneration of these vesicles releases acid hydrolases and iron, which cause proteolytic and oxidative cellular damage.

Clinical features

Any race can be affected although hereditary haemochromatosis is more common in whites of Celtic origin: the gene frequency in whites is approximately 1:20; 0.2 to 0.7% are homozygous and 8–14% are heterozygous.

Among homozygotes, nine times as many men as women present clinically: most do so between 40 and 60 years of age. Presentations in children (see Juvenile haemochromatosis) and in premenopausal women are not unusual. This variability may arise from physiological iron loss in women during their reproductive years; from environmental influences; gene–gene interactions and, possibly, genetic polymorphism. Heterozygotes have increased absorption of iron but if they have no other predisposition to iron overload this is not a significant problem.

The onset of symptoms is insidious. The earliest symptom is a non-specific lassitude, and the condition is seldom diagnosed until other features are recognised. Individuals may present with any combination of the features below. (The figures in parentheses indicate the approximate percentage of patients showing each feature):

- Asymptomatic
- Weakness and lethargy (100)

- Pigmentation (skin, lips, tongue, buccal mucosa, conjunctiva, scars, external genitalia (90)
- Loss of body hair, ichthyosis, dermal atrophy, koilonychia (50)
- Hepatomegaly (95)
- Splenomegaly (50)
- Jaundice (10)
- Hepatocellular carcinoma, cholangiocarcinoma (30)
- Anorexia, lethargy, malaise, confusion, weakness (45)
- Vertigo, loss of auditory acuity, peripheral neuropathy, retinopathy (15)
- Weight loss, vomiting (45)
- Abdominal pain (30)
- Chondrocalcinosis (e.g. knees), bone demineralisation (25–75)
- Chronic arthropathy, 2nd–3rd metacarpal joints and proximal interphalangeal joints, hips (30)
- Cardiomegaly (20–30)
- Cardiomyopathy, ECG changes, dysrhythmias, conduction abnormalities, cardiac failure, constrictive pericarditis
- Diabetes mellitus (60)
- Pituitary damage, testicular atrophy, gynaecomastia (50)
- Loss of libido, impotence, amenorrhoea, hypoparathyroidism, adrenocortical insufficiency, hypothydroidism, low serum somatostatin, hypoprolactinaemia.

Impairment of cellular immunity may also develop.[6]

Skin pigmentation is initially dusky brown and is due to increased melanin production which is more marked on scars, exposed skin and the external genitalia. Later, the skin becomes slate-grey as haemosiderin accumulates in it.

Hepatomegaly is accompanied by increasing hepatocellular necrosis and associated clinical and biochemical indications of hepatic damage. Hepatic fibrosis may progress to frank cirrhosis, and coincident development of portal hypertension leads to an increase in the usually moderate degree of splenomegaly. Cirrhosis and hepatic failure are usually late features.

Chondrocalcinosis may arise from the inhibitory effect of iron on pyrophosphatase activity; as a result pyrophosphate is deposited in articular cartilage. The arthropathy of the hand differs from that of rheumatoid arthritis by the absence of ulnar deviation of the fingers. An atypical hip arthropathy with radiolucency of the femoral head and shearing of the cartilage from the subchondral bone may develop.[7]

Cardiac failure may be a presenting feature in young adults and children. ECG changes include reduced voltage, ventricular ectopics, supraventricular tachycardias and flattened or inverted T-waves. Cardiac arrhythmias are common in alcoholic patients and during early treatment by phlebotomy. Myocardial involvement can be a poor prognostic sign but some problems such as failure and angina pectoris often improve with treatment. Echocardiography can provide evidence of secondary cardiomegaly.

Abdominal pain is common; identified precipitants include ascites, peptic ulceration, pancreatitis, cholecystitis, nephrolithiasis and peritonitis, but a definite cause is seldom found.

Although iron deposits destroy the pancreatic acinar cells, exocrine pancreatic insufficiency is unusual. In contrast two-thirds of cases have reduced secretion of insulin and an impaired glucose tolerance which is exacerbated by hepatic dysfunction. Pituitary damage reduces circulating levels of gonadotrophins which do not respond to exogenous releasing factors.

Diagnosis

Since the clinical manifestations of hereditary haemochromatosis are so protean, early diagnosis depends on a high degree of suspicion and on screening relatives of known cases. The most valuable investigations are those assessing iron overload. The serum iron concentration is elevated above the accepted reference range (10–25 μmol/l), in many cases to over 40 μmol/l. The serum transferrin is more than 60% saturated, with a concomitant fall in iron-binding capacity. Normally serum ferritin concentrations are less than 200 μg/l and 300 μg/l in women and men respectively; in untreated hereditary haemochromatosis values often exceed 1000 μg/l. Occasionally some confusion arises from increased serum ferritin and iron concentrations in patients with secondary iron overload or hepatic necrosis. Conversely, in patients with haemochromatosis, stress, infection and malignancy may lower plasma iron concentrations into the physiological range. If such ambiguities arise when investigating possible cases, it is advisable to repeat these investigations serially (e.g. three times at weekly intervals). Occasionally early iron overload may occur without any increase in the immunodetectable serum ferritin.

If any of these assessments are abnormal a percutaneous needle biopsy of the liver should be taken for histological examination and determination of the iron content. The latter is usually less than 150 μg (2.7 μmol)/100 mg dry weight or 25 μg (0.45 μmol)/100 mg/wet weight of liver, but commonly exceeds 1000 μg/100 mg dry weight in hereditary haemochromatosis. Since the iron content of the liver increases with age, interpretation of the hepatic iron content can be improved, especially in young people, by calculating their hepatic iron/age index (iron μmol/g dry weight, divided by age in years): in homozygotes this index is not less than 1.9[8]. Indirect assessment of iron overload by measuring urinary iron excretion (a diagnostic threshold of 8 mg/24 h urine) after administration of the chelator desferroxamine 500 mg i.m. has been superseded.[1]

On light microscopy, the hepatic parenchyma initially shows periportal accumulation of ferritin and haemosiderin which spreads throughout the lobule as the iron overload increases. Large iron-laden lysosomes appear, the mitochondria and other organelles are usually normal except when excess iron is causing necrosis. Kupffer cells only contain iron in cases with advanced overload. After treatment, liver iron content falls and the lysosomal appearance returns to normal.[9]

Computerised axial tomography may be helpful to assess the iron content of the liver when hepatic biopsy is contraindicated. However the value of MRI to quantify hepatic iron concentration is uncertain.

Other causes of iron overload can usually be distinguished by the clinical history and hepatic histology (e.g. whether or not the Kupffer cells are involved); few produce the degree of overload seen in an untreated patient with idiopathic haemochromatosis.

The causes of secondary iron overload are:

a. Alcoholic liver disease and cirrhosis
b. Ingestion of excessive iron
   1. medicinal
   2. dietary
      fermented beverages with high iron content
c. Post portacaval anastomosis
d. Chronic anaemia
   1. transfusion overload
   2. ineffective erythropoiesis
   3. congenital dyserythropoietic anaemia
   4. sideroblastic anaemias
   5. thalassaemia major, sickle cell anaemia
   6. other haemolytic anaemias, hypoplastic anaemias
f. Porphyria cutanea tarda
g. Transferrin deficiency

Screening

The value of population screening is uncertain; however, a study using a transferrin saturation above 55% and an elevated or increasing serum ferritin concentration as indications for liver biopsy established a prevalence of 0.33% in an asymptomatic population.[10]

As many relatives as possible of known cases should be screened. Since serum values indicative of increased iron burden occur in a quarter of heterozygotes as well as in homozygotes, characterising the HLA haplotypes of the proband and of the family pedigree is particularly valuable in planning further investigations such as liver biopsy. If a relative has no haplotype in common with the patient's then his/her risk of being homozygous for idiopathic haemochromatosis is very small. There is a greater chance that relatives who share a single A or B type with the index case are heterozygous, whereas it is highly likely that those with both A and B types in common with the index case are homozygous for the haemochromatosis gene. However chromosomal recombination can occur, and relatives with HLA haplotypes identical to those of probands do not always have iron overload.

Treatment

The cornerstone of treatment is to reduce the body burden of iron and to minimise acute iron toxicity. The most effective therapy is phlebotomy[11]; about 200–250 mg of iron would be lost with 250 ml of blood. This volume of blood can be withdrawn twice weekly, thereby reducing the iron overload by 20–25 g a year. Since most patients have an overload of about 40 g of iron this treatment would be needed regularly for 2 years. The frequency of venesection may have to be reduced if the patient develops cardiac failure or arrhythmias, which may be induced by hypovolaemia and anaemia. During initial therapy these problems can be exacerbated by mobilisation of tissue iron: they can be minimised by simultaneous administration of chelators such as desferroxamine (4–8 mg slowly iv. per 24 h)[1] or calcium diethylene triamine penta-acetate (DTPA). Although these agents are useful in the management of secondary iron overload, they are unsuitable for routine sole treatment in hereditary haemochromatosis because they cannot induce the loss of iron which is achieved by phlebotomy.

The haemoglobin concentration falls as venesection is initiated; it then usually increases again. With adequate treatment the plasma iron and ferritin concentrations fall gradually and achieve normal levels when the overload has been removed. Serial determinations of haemoglobin to ascertain tolerance of the blood loss, and of serum iron and ferritin to assess residual iron overload, are suitable monitors of treatment. A haemoglobin of 10–11 g/dl, a serum iron of 10 μmol/l and a serum ferritin of less than 200 μg/l, are indications that the iron burden is sufficiently reduced to stop frequent phlebotomy. The frequency of subsequent phlebotomies is adjusted to maintain such iron and ferritin values; most patients need six or fewer venesections annually.

Phlebotomy has considerably improved the prognosis and life expectancy in hereditary haemochromatosis[1,2,12]: it improves glucose tolerance in almost half of patients, but it does not reverse hepatic fibrosis and portal hypertension, hypogonadism, and arthropathy. Before its introduction, patients had a 30% risk of hepatocellular carcinoma and many died from diabetes mellitus, infections, heart failure and liver failure. If adequate treatment is started before the onset of cirrhosis the long-term survival of patients is similar to that of the general population.[12] Persistent cardiomyopathy and hepatic dysfunction indicate a poor prognosis. Survival is indirectly related to the degree of iron overload at diagnosis. Patients with cirrhosis have a worse prognosis and their increased risk of developing hepatocellular carcinoma is not reduced by phlebotomy.[2] HBV immunisation may reduce the risk of malignant transformation. Additionally such patients have an increased risk of neoplasia at other sites such as the rectum, bronchus, pancreas and gallbladder.[2] The onset of malignancy is often heralded by weight loss, fever and a sudden fall in the plasma concentrations of iron and ferritin.

Juvenile haemochromatosis

It is not clear if the presentation of severe iron overload in children is an entity separate from classic hereditary haemochromatosis. In these patients cardiac and endocrine manifestations predominate; liver damage is not severe.[13]

Idiopathic neonatal iron storage disease (neonatal or perinatal haemochromatosis) (McKusick 231100)

In this rare condition of gross iron overload, hepatic haemosiderosis, hepatocellular necrosis and resultant tissue and systemic organ damage develop antenatally in a pattern resembling hereditary haemochromatosis.[14, 15] Most affected children present soon after birth and few survive longer than 4 months of age. Occasionally the onset may be delayed. The babies have intrauterine growth retardation, congenital giant cell hepatitis, sinusoidal fibrosis leading to cirrhosis, and fulminant hepatic failure. Serum iron and ferritin concentrations are usually elevated.

This condition is genetically distinct from hereditary haemochromatosis. First-degree relatives have no increased risk of iron storage disease and there is no clear association with HLA types.[15] It is possible that such iron excess may arise from an intrauterine hepatic insult, as has been suggested by its occurrence in two affected infants and a fetus with giant cell hepatitis delivered to a mother with post-transfusion hepatitis C.

Congenital atransferrinaemia (McKusick 209300)

This very rare entity is inherited as an autosomal recessive defect.[16] Patients present in early childhood with a hypochromic, microcytic and iron-resistant anaemia, a low serum iron with a low iron-binding concentration caused by a very low or absent serum transferrin.

These children also have a systemic iron overload which spares the bone marrow. It is not clear if this overload arises from dietary iron or from that administered in blood transfusions. Intravenous infusions of human transferrin can be beneficial but there are no reports on their extended use.

Other causes of hypotransferrinaemia such as infection, nephrotic syndrome, protein-losing enteropathies, hepatic disease and malignancy can be excluded easily. A similar syndrome arises in autoimmune atransferrinaemia[17], but in this condition gross secondary haemochromatosis is associated with an increased total iron-binding capacity secondary to the incorporation of iron in a circulating immune-complex of transferrin.

Impaired uptake of iron by reticuloendothelial cells (McKusick 206100)

In a brother and sister an iron-resistant hypochromic microcytic anaemia was associated with a high plasma iron concentration and a saturated transferrin or iron binding capacity.[18] Whereas the hepatocytes were laden with iron, the liver and bone marrow reticuloendothelial cells had none. These manifestations may be caused by impaired translocation of iron into the reticuloendothelial cells, secondary to a defect in either the binding of transferrin to the cell membrane receptors or the subsequent translocation of the iron into the cells. An acquired analogous defect with an autoimmune aetiology has been reported in an adult woman.[19]

Microcytic anaemia (hereditary iron-handling disorder, pseudo iron deficiency anaemia) (McKusick 206200)

Three children with a microcytic anaemia in the absence of any obvious cause were found to have malabsorption of iron and an imperfect response to intramuscular iron dextran.[20] It has been proposed that this defect is analogous to an autosomal recessive microcytic anaemia with defective cellular uptake of iron in mk-mk mice.[21] This may represent an abnormality in transferrin receptors.

Iron overload in Africa

In subSaharan Africa, families of index cases with iron overload have a bimodal, rather than a continuous, distribution of transferrin saturation with high saturations accompanied by markedly elevated serum ferritin concentrations. This suggests the presence of a genetic defect, separate from the HLA-linked gene of hereditary haemochromatosis, which causes iron overload independent of high dietary intakes of iron.[22]

COPPER

The daily dietary intake of copper in adults is 1–5 mg. Following its intestinal absorption the metal is transported in the portal circulation bound to albumin and transcuprein, and, to a lesser extent, by free amino acids. These complexes are cleared rapidly by the liver which has a central role in the metabolism of copper. There are at least three discrete hepatic pools of copper; one is that destined for homeostatic secretion in the bile, another comprises the newly synthesised glycoprotein caeruloplasmin and

Table 13.1 Copper-dependent enzyme activities

Enzyme	Activity
Amine oxidases	Amine and polyamine oxidation
Cytochrome-c-oxidase	Mitochondrial oxidative phosphorylation
Dopamine-β-hydrolase	Synthesis of catecholamines
Tyrosinase	Tyrosine – dopa – dopaquinone and melanin
Superoxide dismutase	Cytosolic antioxidant $2O_2^- + 2H^+ \rightarrow H_2O_2 + O_2$
Lysyl oxidase (and related enzymes)	Condensation of amino acids, cross linkages of elastin and collagen
Caeruloplasmin	Multiple oxidase activities, copper transport
Thiol oxidase	Formation of disulphide linkages

the third is a presumed hepatic store of copper. Additionally the liver may contain, as well as its cuproenzymes, a pool of copper associated with a low molecular weight protein called metallothionein. Metallothionein is involved principally with the metabolism of zinc but copper can displace zinc from the protein. Caeruloplasmin is secreted into the systemic circulation where 90–95% of copper is in this form. Caeruloplasmin may have several physiological roles; its oxidase activity facilitates the incorporation of iron into transferrin, and may also serve as a plasma biogenic amine oxidase and as an antioxidant. In addition, since membrane receptors for the endocytosis of caeruloplasmin exist, and because the protein is able to donate copper to apoenzymes, it seems probable that caeruloplasmin has a specific transport role for the element[23]. Some examples of cuproenzyme activities are shown in Table 13.1.

Wilson's disease (hepatolenticular degeneration) (McKusick 277900)

This is a systemic copper toxicosis. Copper initially accumulates in the liver, but then all other tissues become involved.[24, 25] The basic defect is associated with impaired hepatic secretion of copper and defective incorporation of the metal into apocaeruloplasmin. The similarity of systemic and hepatic copper metabolism in Wilson's disease with that in the neonate has stimulated the hypothesis that Wilson's disease is caused by a persistence of the fetal pattern of copper metabolism. A model for this is the guinea pig in which the switch from fetal to adult metabolism of copper occurs at birth.[26] During the last trimester, the fetal hepatic copper increases and is predominantly bound to metallothionein. After birth, as the liver copper declines, copper-metallothionein disappears and copper is associated with functional pools such as superoxide dismutase and with a high molecular weight protein which was absent in the fetus. A similar pattern occurs in humans and interestingly normal human bile contains a high molecular weight copper-containing substance which is absent in patients with Wilson's disease.[27]

The defective allele is on chromosome 13, at distances of 0.4 and 1.2 centimorgans, respectively from D13S31 and D13S59.[28] In contrast the caeruloplasmin gene is located on chromosome 3.

Clinical features and pathogenesis

The incidence of Wilson's disease is estimated to be between 1:200 000 and 1:30 000.[24] The onset of symptoms is variable and the diagnosis is often missed. A chronic insidious presentation is well known and many such patients have had transient icteric episodes which have been attributed to recurrent 'hepatitis'. Another situation when the diagnosis is often overlooked is an acute presentation with haemolysis and hepatic and renal failure secondary to an acute release of free non-caeruloplasmin bound copper from the liver. The precipitants of this acute fulminant presentation are unknown but intercurrent infections or similar stresses may contribute. It is clearly important to consider Wilson's disease in anyone with recurrent jaundice or haemolysis.

The many features of Wilson's disease are shown below:

- Asymptomatic
- Hepatic
  transient hepatitis with intercurrent infections,
  subacute, acute or chronic hepatitis, cryptogenic cirrhosis,
  hepatosplenomegaly, portal hypertension,oesophageal varices,
  pancreatitis, fulminant hepatic failure
- Neurological
  encephalopathy
  clumsiness, deteriorating handwriting and school performance, ataxia,
  fine tremor in limbs and/or tongue, dysarthria, dysphagia, dystonia,
  spasticity, athetosis, muscle spasms,
  coarse flapping tremor at wrists and shoulders,
  peripheral neuropathy, epilepsy (partial or generalised),
  pseudo-bulbar palsy (death),
  'schizophrenia', fatuous drooling facies
  non-specific EEG abnormalities
- Ophthalmic
  Kayser-Fleischer rings, sunflower cataract, strabismus, xerophthalmia,
  impaired visual acuity, pallor of disc,
  night blindness
- Haematological

acute haemolysis, haemolytic anaemia, thrombocytopenia, leucopenia, pancytopenia, coagulopathies, bruising, epistaxes, intravascular coagulation
- Renal
  renal tubular acidosis, concentration defect, amino aciduria, phosphaturia, hypercalcuria, uricosuria, acute renal failure, renal stones, haematuria
- Skeletal
  osteoporosis, patchy osteosclerosis, osteophytes, cysts in long bones, spontaneous fracture, osteomalacia, chondrocalcinosis, osteoarthritis, chondromalacia patellae, osteochondritis dissecans, chondrocalcinosis, arthritis, morning stiffness
- Endocrine
  amenorrhoea, increased incidence of miscarriages, gynaecomastia
- Abdominal pain, colic
- Bacterial peritonitis
- Blue lanulae of finger nails

About 40% of cases present with hepatic features – such patients are usually, but not exclusively, children and young adults; 35% have neurological sequelae, rare but not unknown before adolescence; 12% have endocrine or haematological complications; 10% have neuropsychiatric disease and may have been admitted to psychiatric care before the underlying disorder had been recognised.[29] The insidious and protean manifestations of Wilson's disease are best emphasised by Walshe's aphorism: 'there is no such thing as a typical patient with Wilson's disease'.

All patients have hepatic involvement irrespective of their initial presentation. The youngest reported age of presentation is 4 years, but hepatocellular damage has been detected in an asymptomatic one-year-old sibling of a known case.

In spite of the possible gross neurological disabilities, the patient's intellect is relatively spared until late in the course of the disease and many have a distressing insight into their deterioration. The Kayser–Fleischer rings and sunflower cataracts are caused by the deposition of copper in Descemet's membrane and beneath the lens capsule respectively; both may be detectable only by a slit-lamp microscopic examination. The Kayser–Fleischer rings are brown-green discolorations which appear first at the upper limbus and then in the inferior limbus before they meet bilaterally to encircle the cornea (Fig. 13.1). Rarely only one cornea may be affected. Patients with neurological involvement usually, but not invariably, have Kayser–Fleischer rings but the converse is not true; furthermore these rings are absent in many patients with hepatic involvement, especially those who present with acute hepatic disease. Dysfunction of the nigrostriatal dopaminergic pathway contributes to movement disorders and may persist even after many years of penicillamine treatment.[30]

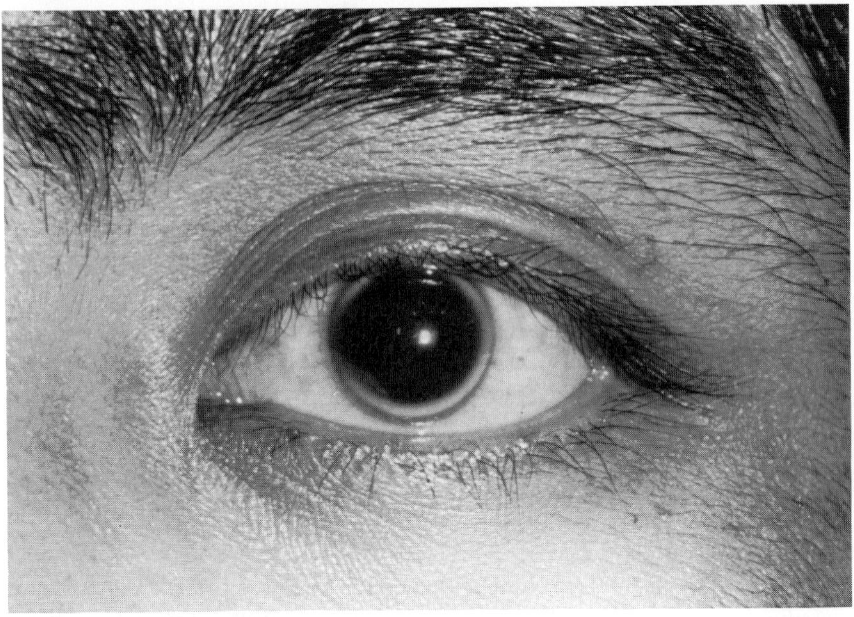

Fig. 13.1 Wilson's disease: Kayser–Fleischer ring. Note that the inferior and superior depositions have met laterally but have not yet fused medially. Reproduced with permission of the Department of Medical Illustration, Unviersity of Aberdeen.

The incidence of epilepsy is ten times that of the general population. Seizures may occur at any time; they often occur shortly after treatment is started. Fortunately they may recede with adequate treatment.[31] Wilson's disease should always be considered in any patient with an occult encephalopathy.

Laboratory findings

In most patients the plasma copper concentration is reduced below 10 μmol/l (reference range 10–25 μmol/l), and is accompanied by hypocaeruloplasminaemia of less than 200 mg/l (reference range 300–400 mg/l). However, in 15% of cases the plasma caeruloplasmin may be in the lower end of the customary reference range. Sometimes subnormal caeruloplasmin concentrations in patients may be elevated into the lower reaches of the healthy range by the acute phase reaction to pregnancy, oestrogen treatment and intercurrent infection or stress. Since in Wilson's disease much of the plasma pool of copper is not bound to caeruloplasmin the urinary excretion of copper is grossly elevated (over 100 μg/24 h compared with usual values of less than 50 μg/24 h).

Percutaneous needle biopsy of the liver is the essential investigation because it enables histological examination of the hepatic parenchyma and, more importantly, direct determination of the tissue content of copper. The histological changes are often non-specific features of hepatocellular degeneration with steatosis, glycogen deposition, ballooned nuclei and pleomorphic mitochondria. Later, piecemeal necrosis, diffuse fibrosis and micronodular cirrhosis with ductular proliferation and mild inflammation develop.[32,33] Oxidative damage reduces the glutathione content and lipofuscin-rich granules may be seen. The lobular distribution of histochemically demonstrable copper in Wilson's disease differs from the more periportal distribution seen in the copper overload of cholestatic sydromes and Indian childhood cirrhosis, but this difference is too non-specific to be diagnostic. In early Wilson's disease copper is distributed diffusely in the hepatocytic cytoplasm and is rarely congregated with cytoplasmic and lysosomal granules. At this stage the metal may be better demonstrated by orcein staining than by rhodamine, but it is important to appreciate that, particularly in young patients, histochemical techniques may not detect excess hepatic copper.[33]

Diagnosis requires an accurate determination of hepatic copper content: usually in Wilson's disease this exceeds 250 μg (3. 9 μmol)/g dry weight compared with normal levels of less than 50 μg (0.8 μmol)/g dry weight.

When hepatic biopsy is contraindicated, or if a suspected patient does not have hypocaeruloplasminaemia, a study of the hepatic uptake and resecretion of radio-copper ^{64}Cu or ^{67}Cu will reflect impaired caeruloplasmin synthesis by showing the failure of radio-copper to reappear in the plasma 4–6 h after its administration.[34] Alternatively, DNA testing could be used instead of liver biopsies in individuals with borderline serum caeruloplasmin levels or in patients with fulminant liver failure.[28]

Other causes of hypocaeruloplasminaemia such as malnutrition, malabsorption, protein-losing enteropathies and proteinuria can be excluded easily. Secondary copper accumulation occurs in cholestasis, primary biliary cirrhosis, and chronic active hepatitis and other conditions which prevent the hepatobiliary excretion of copper. In many of these disorders, microscopically detectable Kayser–Fleischer rings may develop but, apart from Wilson's disease, macroscopic rings have only been reported in a monoclonal gammopathy. Neurological sequelae and basal ganglia lesions secondary in part, at least, to copper overload have developed in chronic cholestatic syndromes, but in these instances plasma copper and caeruloplasmin concentrations are not depressed and plasma and liver copper concentrations seldom approach those of Wilson's disease. In Indian childhood cirrhosis, hepatic copper levels are similar to those of Wilson's disease but these children have normal plasma levels of copper and caeruloplasmin.

One difficult differential diagnosis arises when Wilson's disease presents as fulminant hepatic failure with a rapid onset of icterus, encephalopathy, coagulopathy, renal failure and, as a result of hepatic necrosis, a serum copper which is within the normal range. In these circumstances, the serum caeruloplasmin is uninterpretable. Although these patients will probably have a raised urinary copper, other features, apart from historical clues, which should alert one to the possibility of Wilson's disease are the presence of cirrhosis on biopsy[33] and inappropriately small elevations, if any, in the serum aminotransferase and alkaline phosphatase activities. Values of less than 2.0 for the ratio of alkaline phosphatase:total bilirubin and greater than 4.0 for the aspartate transaminase:alanine transaminase ratio seem to be diagnostic of fulminant hepatic failure due to Wilson's disease[35].

Ancillary investigations will indicate the extent of deranged renal and hepatic function; should help establish the degree of involvement of the myocardium, skeleton, joints and other tissues, and will exclude other possible diagnoses. Cerebral ventricular dilatation, cortical atrophy and degeneration of the basal ganglia can be assessed by computerised axial tomography which can also be used after therapy to monitor the resolution of the basal ganglia lesions. MRI and evoked potentials have shown cerebral lesions, or brain atrophy in all neurologically symptomatic and 44% of asymptomatic patients[36] but there is a poor correlation between MRI findings and clinical neurological symptoms. Prolonged auditory brainstem and somatosensory evoked potentials may reveal a reversible component of the disease that can be a sensitive monitor of treatment efficacy.[37]

To detect asymptomatic homozygotes, all family members, including cousins, of known cases should be screened. The serum caeruloplasmin concentrations of the patient's unaffected parents (i.e. presumed heterozygotes) indicate the serum caeruloplasmin concentrations to expect in the heterozygous kindred. About 10% of heterozygotes have hypocaeruloplasminaemia and anyone with a low caeruloplasmin concentration should be investigated by hepatic biopsy or, less preferably, radiocopper studies. Increasingly polymorphic DNA markers will be available to reliably detect potential Wilson's disease heterozygotes and homozygotes in families at risk; with this approach prenatal diagnosis is also possible.[33] Heterozygotes should not be assumed to be free of any risk of copper toxicosis: heterozygous children have been reported to have hypocaeruloplasminaemia, hypocupraemia, non-specific EEG abnormalities and an increased body burden of copper.[38]

Treatment

The lifelong treatment is aimed at reducing the amount of copper in the body and, if necessary, at preventing the toxic effects of free copper in the tissues and circulation. The most successful agent in this respect has been the chelator D-penicillamine (dimethylcysteine)[24] in daily doses of 0.75–3 g given in three divided doses half an hour before meals. Side-effects are less frequent with D-penicillamine than with mixed D- and L-penicillamine preparations. Patients who present with acute neurological symptoms often become clinically worse when initially treated with penicillamine. The efficacy of penicillamine may arise from its removal of copper from an intermediary ligand, thereby reducing its histotoxicity by enabling it to be excreted in the urine and to induce metallothionein.[39] The efficacy and dosage of chelation therapy can be assessed by monitoring the urinary excretion of copper, which, as a rule of thumb, can be maintained at up to 5 mg of copper per day.

Prolonged use of penicillamine alters the structure of dermal collagen and elastin. Since it can also induce pyridoxine deficiency supplements of this vitamin should be given. Like many other chelators D-penicillamine is non-specific and, as effective de-coppering is achieved, it will chelate other metals, and may, for example, induce zinc deficiency. Normally, however, D-penicillamine therapy is reasonably safe. If side-effects develop, penicillamine can be withdrawn and reintroduced in a reduced dosage; tolerance to gradually increasing doses can be improved by giving prednisolone simultaneously.

If the more serious side-effects of D-penicillamine preclude its continued use, alternative agents are the polyamine chelator trientine (triethylene tetra amine), at a dose of, 0.5–2 g/day[40], unithiol, and ammonium tetrathiomolybdate which is thought to block copper absorption and to form non-toxic complexes with copper systemically. Ammonium tetrathiomolybdate, compared with penicillamine and trientine, may have a more effective decoppering effect[41], and may emerge as an alternative initial therapy.[42]

Large oral doses of zinc (150 mg of elemental zinc per 24 h) are also effective therapy.[43] This has been attributed to zinc inducing the synthesis of metallothionein systemically and in the gut mucosa; this then sequesters copper, prevents its absorption and reduces its systemic toxicity. There is uncertainty about the role of zinc for initial treatment. It may be useful for those with presymptomatic disease and as an adjunct to other maintenance treatment.

Clinical resolution may be slow, neurological abnormalities may take 2 years or more to improve, but the eventual degree of resolution is often rewarding. Kayser–Fleischer rings disappear in the reverse sequence to their development, and there is complete resolution of neurological symptomatology and improvement in the neuropsychiatric manifestations. Hepatic cirrhosis and portal hypertension do not resolve, but hepatocellular carcinoma is rare; resolution of hepatic lesions can be watched, biochemically and by annual or appropriately frequent liver biopsies, to monitor hepatic histology and copper content. Wilsonian chronic active hepatitis, if treated, has a very good prognosis even if cirrhosis is present.[44] With treatment, circulating copper and caeruloplasmin concentrations may actually increase, but usually not to within the physiological range.

The management of a presentation with acute copper toxicity is not easy. Approaches to reducing the free copper in the circulation need to be integrated with the management of any hepatic and renal failure and have included peritoneal dialysis with albumin or D-penicillamine added to the dialysate, intravenous infusions of albumin and plasma exchange. Haemodialysis is less useful. If such interventions and standard supportive treatment are unsuccessful in managing acute or fulminant hepatic failure then hepatic transplantation may have to be considered.[25]

Familial hypocaeruloplasminaemia (McKusick 117700)

An asymptomatic kindred with an autosomal recessive hypocaeruloplasminaemia (i.e. less than 21 mg/l or 23 mg/l in men and women respectively) has been reported[45] in which affected individuals also had low serum copper concentrations but a normal urinary excretion of copper and, most importantly, normal hepatic histology and content of copper.

Menkes' disease (kinky hair disease, trichopoliodystrophy) (McKusick 309400)

Menkes' disease is an X-linked recessive syndrome of overt copper deficiency in which there is a systemic maldistribution of copper.[46] The content of copper in the plasma, brain and liver is greatly reduced whereas that of the kidneys, spleen, pancreas, intestinal mucosa, lung, skin, muscle and, in utero, the placenta are elevated. Most of this excess copper is associated with metallothionein, but since the locus for this protein is on chromosome 16 this phenomenon is probably secondary to the basic metabolic error. The Menkes' gene, which is located in a subregion of band Xq13.2–q13.3 proximal to the PGK1 locus[47], has been isolated and found to code for a protein which is homologous with membrane-bound cation-transporting P type ATPase proteins. Various deletions of the gene have been found, and it is possible that this phenomenon may contribute to the increasingly appreciated heterogeneity of this syndrome.[48]

Affected boys have hypocupraemia, hypocaeruloplasminaemia and low hepatic copper concentrations. These patients have a paradoxical condition of functional copper deficiency in organs which have an abundance of the element. The intestinal absorption of copper is impaired by the retention of the metal in the intestinal mucosa but parenteral copper has no significant therapeutic effect; even though it may increase circulating levels of caeruloplasmin it does not overcome a defect which impairs the incorporation of intracellular copper into cuproenzymes. A consequence of this is that with Menkes' fibroblasts, metallothionein is induced at lower extracellular copper concentrations than with normal cells.[49] Data from a murine model of Menkes' disease suggest that the defect involves a 48 kDa protein.[50]

Clinical features and their pathogeneses[46]

The condition affects all races and has a calculated incidence in western European countries of 1 per 254 000 live-born babies.[51]

The clinical features are summarised below:

- Placid expressionless 'cherubic' face, frontal and occipital bossing, micrognathia, 'cupid's bow' lip, gingival hyperplasia, high arched palate
- Secondary scalp hair and eyebrows: sparse, depigmented, brittle stubbly hair – twisted on long axis (pili torti), irregular calibre (monilethrix), nodelike fracture points (tichorrhexis nodosa)
- Pale skin, non-specific seborrhoeic dermatosis, skin laxity
- Failure to thrive, dysphagia, hiatus hernia, oesophageal reflux, vomiting haematemesis, loose frequent stools, delayed eruption of teeth
- Hypothermia, lethargy, apnoea
- Arterial and venous tortuosity and dilatations, fragmentation of internal elastic lamina, subdural haematomata and intracranial haemorrhages
- Developmental arrest and regression: hypotonia, spasticity with hyperreflexia, focal and generalised epilepsy, retinal degeneration, optic atrophy, blindness, microcysts in pigment epithelium, cataracts
- Inguinal herniae, undescended testes
- Hydroureter and hydronephrosis, urinary reflux, bladder trabeculation and diverticulae
- Skeletal anomalies: wormian bones in skull, periosteal thickening and scorbutic changes, (metaphyseal cupping flared anterior ends of the ribs), delayed skeletal maturation, osteophytes, spurring, osteoporosis, spontaneous fractures, pectus excavatum, clubbed feet.

Most cases present by 2 months of age. Presenting features include the slowing of development and the loss of milestones, such as smiling and social responsiveness, which had already been achieved, convulsions, apnoea, infections and failure to thrive. Although the boys may seem normal at birth, many have non-specific neonatal histories of low Apgar scores, hypotonia, hypothermia, preterm delivery and prolonged jaundice. Initially the hair may be normal but the characteristic changes are usually evident by the time of presentation (Fig. 13.2). During the first 2 weeks of life the plasma concentrations of copper and caeruloplasmin may be normal or elevated; they then fall to levels encountered in normal neonates but, in contradistinction to healthy children, these levels do not show the subsequent normal increase towards the physiological range.

Many of the clinical features can be related to reduced cuproenzyme activities. Low activities and histochemical staining for dopamine-β-hydroxylase and cytochrome-C-oxidase occur in several tissues, including the brain which also has a decreased content of unsaturated fatty acids. Many tissues including muscle, brain and liver exhibit increased lipofuscin and degenerative intracellular changes. Focal cerebral and cerebellar degeneration, with diffuse loss of neurones, non-specific axonal changes and a mitochondrial encephalomyopathy ensue, which may be secondary both to these biochemical abnormalities and to progressive vascular damage. As well as contributing to the vascular changes, defective forma-

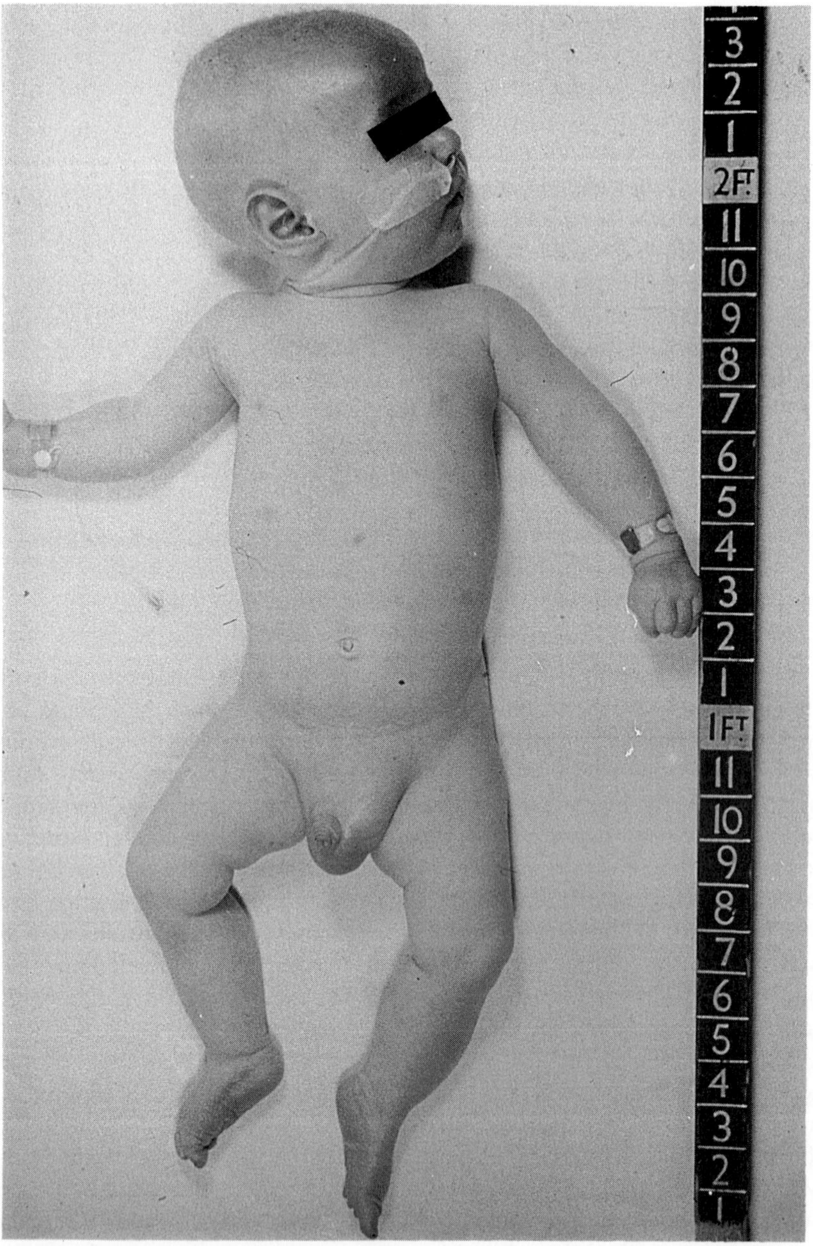

Fig. 13.2 Menkes' disease; this boy has typically abnormal hair, a placid facies and micrognathia. Note also the inguinal hernia, his hypotonic posture and the use of a nasogastric tube to manage the infant's poor feeding. Reproduced with permission of Dr J Wilson, Hospital for Sick Children, London.

tion of connective tissue is responsible for the skeletal, dermal and urogenital tract anomalies and, with prolonged survival, pulmonary emphysema.

The affected hair (Fig. 13.3) has a low copper and pigment content, and an increased content of free sulphydryl groups despite a normal amino acid composition.

If untreated, most patients die by the third year of life. They develop intracranial haemorrhages, increasingly uncontrollable fits, gross failure to thrive and overwhelming infections such as bronchopneumonia, meningitis and septicaemia.

Laboratory investigations

Once Menkes' disease has been suspected on the basis of the clinical picture it can be established by the hypocupraemia (less than 10 μmol/l) and hypocaeruloplasminaemia (less than 20 mg/dl). Further confirmatory investigations can include determination of the abnormally low copper content of a needle biopsy of the liver, the usual range in early infancy being 50–150 μg/g (0.2–2.4 μmol/g) dry weight, and the assessment of the increased uptake and retention in vitro of copper by lymphocyte cultures or fibroblasts.[52]

Radiography and other clinical chemical investigations would demonstrate the presence of skeletal, vascular, urogenital, and biochemical abnormalities. Anaemia and neutropenia do not occur in Menkes' disease although they occur in other forms of copper deficiency.

Prognosis

There is no effective treatment of classic Menkes' disease; parenteral copper salts (e.g. Cu-EDTA, Cu-nitrilotriacetate, and Cu(II)-L-histidine$_2$ complexes) correct the hypocupraemia and hypocaeruloplasminaemia and induce a cupruresis. They also prolong life and modify some features, but, since they do not successfully alter the neurodegenerative changes[53] such treatment has now been generally abandoned. However because the condition has some variability it has been suggested that parenteral copper-histidine supplemented by oral D-penicillamine may be of benefit to early -treated patients with Menkes' disease.[54]

Detection of heterozygotes and antenatal screening

Some heterozygotes for Menkes' disease show evidence of Lyonisation and have some features of the disorder: patchy suntanning may occur in whites and one black mother had areas of depigmented skin. Many heterozygotes have abnormal scalp hair, and altered lymphocytic metabolism of copper. A typical Menkes' syndrome has been described in the sisters of some patients.[47]

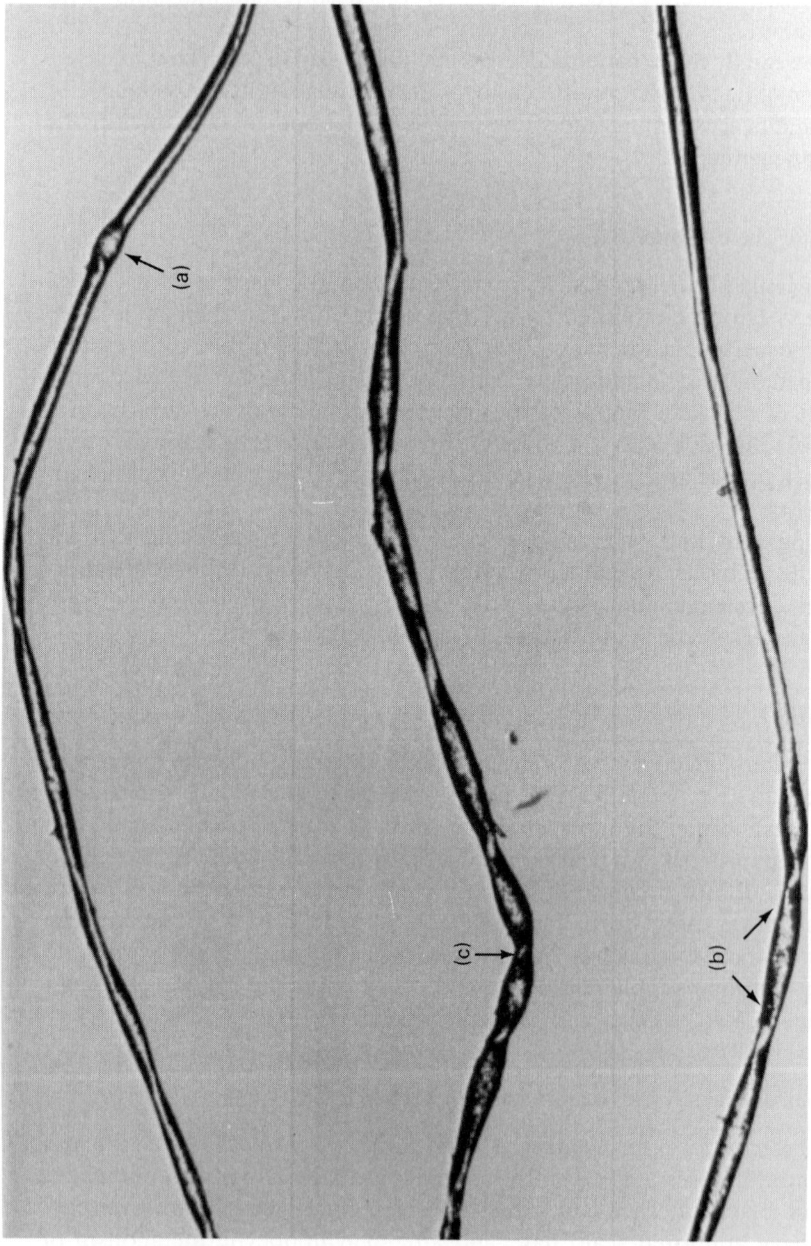

Fig. 13.3 Menkes' disease. Microscopic appearance of the abdominal hair showing; (a) fracture points (trichorexis nodosa); (b) varying calibre (monilethrix), and (c) longitudinal twisting (pili torti). Reproduced with permission of Dr B Lake, Hospital for Sick Children, London.

Antenatal diagnosis in at risk pregnancies is aided by determining the sex of the fetus and, if it is male, by then measuring the uptake and retention of copper in vitro by cultured amniotic fibroblasts.[52] This is a technique which is best referred to a specialist laboratory. The discovery of a high copper content in chorionic villus biopsies may prove to be a more convenient and useful discriminant for antenatal diagnosis.[52] The increased uptake of ^{64}Cu by fibroblasts in culture can also be used to screen for heterozygotes.

Variant forms of the condition have been reported: some severely affected patients have a long survival and some others present later with less severe impairment of growth and intellect, less obvious hair abnormalities, but with neurological defects such as ataxia, choreoathetosis, speech difficulties, hypotonicity of the upper limbs, hyperreflexia of the lower extremities, fine myoclonus of the hands and less severe, but nonetheless typical, abnormal metabolism of copper.[54–56]

Familial benign copper deficiency (McKusick 121270)

A 21-month-old boy presented with failure to thrive, a mild anaemia, fits, and skeletal abnormalities associated with copper deficiency.[57] His development and EEG were normal. His serum caeruloplasmin concentration was normal but his serum copper level was low. He responded to copper supplements. His mother and her brother had hypocupraemia and had some features consistent with copper deficiency. An autosomal dominant form of inheritance has been proposed.

Other neurological abnormalities associated with copper metabolism

Other neurological syndromes have been described in which the aetiological role of altered copper metabolism is less clear than in Wilson's or Menkes' diseases. These include syndromes involving dementia, dysarthria, gait disturbances, involuntary movements, low levels of serum copper and caeruloplasmin, which resemble Wilson's disease but in which copper metabolism was not consistent with that diagnosis.[58–60]

ZINC

Acrodermatitis enteropathica (McKusick 201100)

This rare autosomal recessive condition comprises a systemic zinc deficiency syndrome[61, 62] secondary to a defect in the intestinal absorption of the metal. Systemic handling of zinc appears to be normal as has been supported by the similar zinc contents and uptake by fibroblasts from those with acrodermatitis enteropathica and from normal people.[63]

Clinical features

The clinical features are summarised below:

- Neuropsychiatric: depression, paranoia, apathy, impaired abstract thought, anorexia, cerebellar ataxia, tremor, reversible cerebral atrophy, hoarseness
- Dermatological: periorificial, oral and extensor dermatitis, icthyosis (vesicular-bullous, pustular, hyperkeratotic and acneiform) stomatitis, glossitis paronychia, nail dystrophy, Beau lines, alopecia; hair: fine and brittle, trichonodosis, shaft varying calibre, tapered tips
- Ophthalmological: blepharitis, conjunctivitis, keratopathy, photophobia, corneal opacities, impaired dark adaptation
- Gastrointestinal: loose frequent watery stools, infection, disaccharide intolerance
- Growth retardation, failure to thrive, weight loss
- Recurrent infections: impaired blast response, moniliasis, fungaemia, impaired chemotaxis
- Swelling and pain or tingling in the fingers and feet may precede the rash at these sites.

The protean and relatively non-specific features of acrodermatitis enteropathica arise from the fundamental role of zinc in cellular metabolism. All the major metabolic pathways contain a zinc-dependent enzyme; additionally zinc is involved with nucleic acid and protein synthesis; the regulation of cell division; cytoskeletal function; antioxidant activity; the stabilisation of macromolecules, such as nerve growth factor and of polymers such as presecretory insulin granules, and the association of hormones with receptors both in the nucleus and on the cell membrane. Consequently it is not always possible to ascribe clinical features to the loss of a specific biochemical function. Furthermore, the features of zinc deficiency can be modified by the supply of other nutrients or factors whose metabolism has been deranged. For example, reducing the protein intake ameliorates the neuropsychiatric consequences of zinc deprivation and, in animal models, increased supplies of vitamin E compounds and unsaturated fatty acids correct anomalies resulting from membrane instability and disturbed metabolism of linoleic acid.

Acrodermatitis enteropathica usually presents in infancy. Babies fed on infant formulae develop the syndrome sooner than those fed human breast milk, in whom problems do not appear until solids and alternative formulae are introduced. This difference arises from the better availability for intestinal absorption of zinc in human milk than from the other products, and the benefit persists even if the human milk has been pasteurised.

The earliest recognised feature is the symmetrical, circumorificial, retroauricular and acral dermatitis which may extend to involve the cheeks, trunk and limbs (Figs 13.4 and 13.5). Failure to thrive, anorexia and irritability are the other major presenting features, as was the frequent passage of watery stools until an improved awareness of the condition facilitated earlier diagnosis.

The clinical features deteriorate during infections, physiological stress

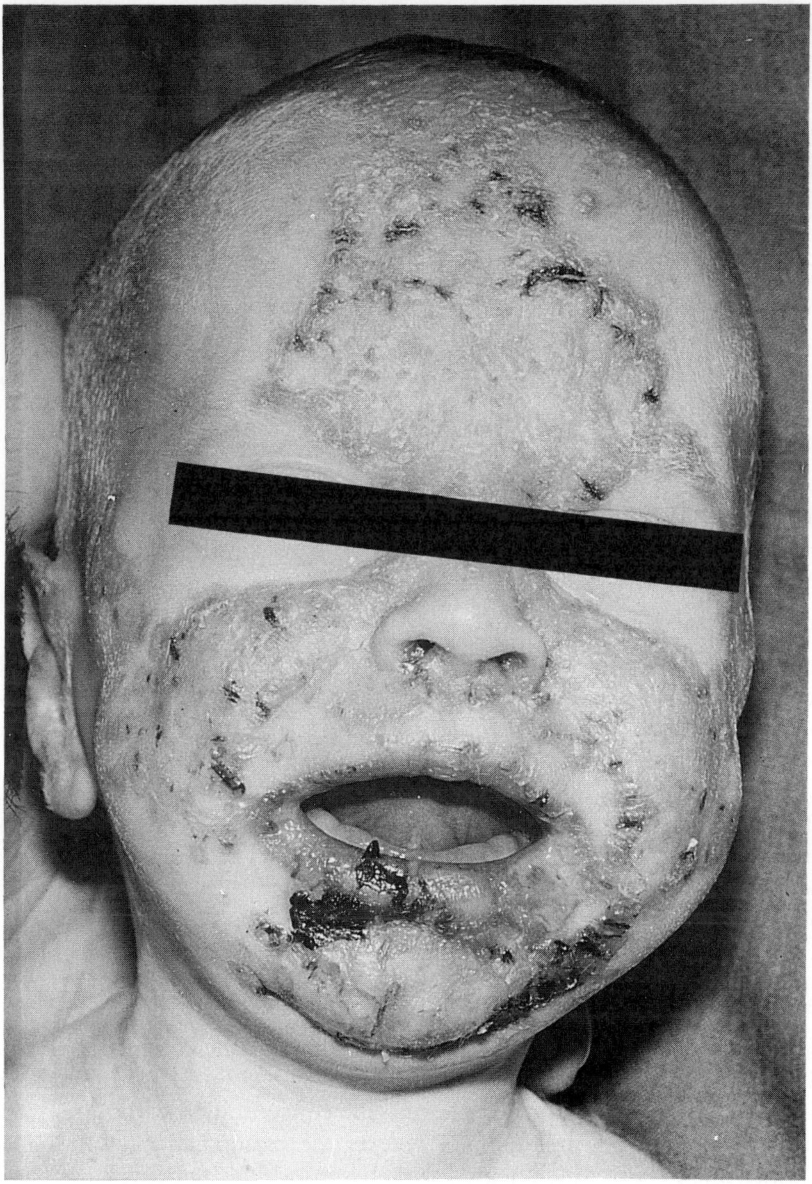

Fig. 13.4 Acrodermatitis enteropathica: this child has a characteristic stomatitis and an extensive symmetrical dermatitis involving the nasolabial folds, the nostrils and the auricles. Reproduced with permission of Dr P Milla

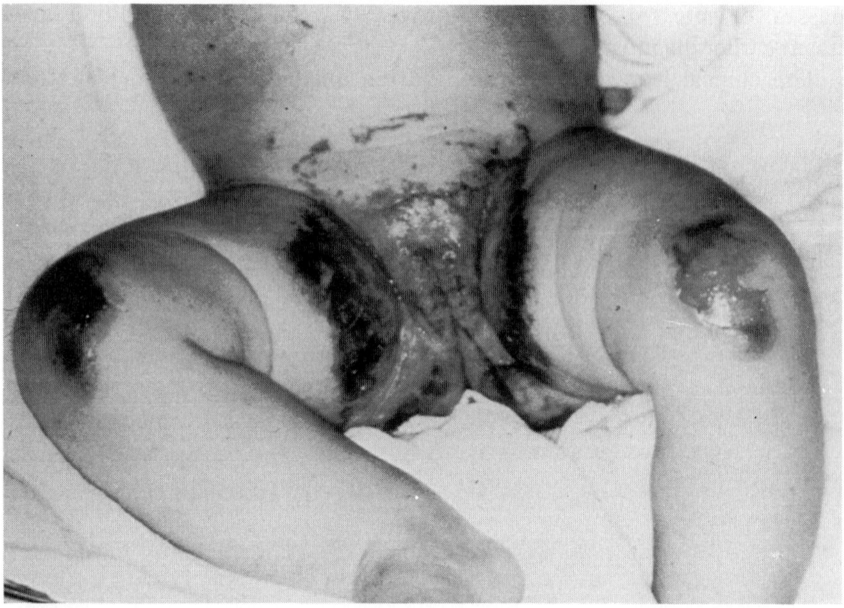

Fig. 13.5 Acrodermatitis enteropathica: severe perineal dermatitis with satellite lesions on the abdomen. The rash has also been precipitated by frictional trauma on both knees. Reproduced with permission of Dr P Milla.

and at times of anabolic demand such as the growth spurts of early childhood, and early puberty. Males are less vulnerable to zinc deficiency after puberty but women may experience relapses during menstruation and pregnancy. The severity of symptoms is variable particularly after the adolescent growth spurt. Some cases present in adolescence or adulthood with chronic skin disorders, neuropsychiatric features or a history of abnormal pregnancies. Miscarriages, congenital skeletal defects and anencephaly have been reported in the pregnancies of affected women but adequate zinc supplementation antenatally and, ideally, before conception obviates this risk.

Laboratory investigations

The major laboratory finding is a reduced plasma zinc concentration, but this is not invariable. Some patients may have clinical features of zinc deficiency in the presence of a plasma zinc concentration within the reference range (9–20 μmol/l). This reflects the maintenance of the small plasma zinc pool by zinc released from tissues which are being catabolised as a consequence of zinc deprivation.

Other biochemical changes, such as low serum alkaline phosphatase activity; raised blood ammonia; hypobetalipoproteinaemia; an altered fatty acid profile in the serum and skin, with reduced 18:1 and 20:4 levels and increased concentrations of 18:2 and trienes, illustrate the diverse metabolic roles of zinc.[64]

Diagnosis

This depends on recognising the clinical features and observing their resolution and later deterioration after the introduction and subsequent withdrawal of oral zinc supplementation. Monitoring the plasma zinc concentrations and the activity of a zinc-dependent enzyme (e.g. alkaline phosphatase) are valuable adjuncts to this approach. Plasma zinc concentrations alone are unreliable markers of zinc deficiency because they are reduced by other pathophysiological stresses and infections. The possibility of finding normal plasma zinc concentrations in symptomatic acrodermatitis enteropathica has been mentioned and it is noteworthy, also, that when zinc therapy starts plasma zinc concentrations may initially fall as newly synthesised body tissue depletes the plasma zinc pool. This paradox, however, resolves when the deficiency is corrected. Hair zinc concentrations are of no value in the diagnosis and management of acrodermatitis enteropathica. In vitro or in vivo zinc absorption tests using radioisotopes (^{65}Zn or ^{69m}Zn) can be used for diagnosis but are not really absolutely necessary: a therapeutic trial with oral zinc for a short period (3–30 μmol zinc/kg per day) is probably as useful.

The differential diagnosis of the skin rash includes psoriasis, familial benign chronic pemphigus, congenital ichthyosiform dermatitis, moniliasis, epidermolysis bullosa, and, in adults, necrolytic migratory erythema. Other important causes of zinc deficiency are protracted malabsorption states in which loss of endogenous zinc may also occur, the use of synthetic diets, and the development of zinc deficiency in ex-preterm neonates. In contrast to acrodermatitis enteropathica the latter infants can become symptomatic whilst being breast fed. Term infants and those on formulae are less often affected. The most convenient means of differentiating these patients from those with acrodermatitis enteropathica is to withdraw the zinc supplementation after 3–6 months and observe the clinical response.

There is no known way of reliably detecting carriers of acrodermatitis enteropathica.

Treatment

Between 35 and 100 mg of elemental zinc per 24 h in divided doses is usually adequate. Zinc sulphate heptahydrate (50 mg, or 0.77 mmol, of elemental zinc in 220 mg) is used commonly but other salts such as the acetate (1 g contains 300 mg, or 4.6 mmol, of zinc) aspartate and gluconate can be used. Effervescent preparations are available and may be more palatable. The dose should be tailored to match the patient's progress;

relatively larger doses are needed during accelerated growth and immediately following initiation of treatment. Whereas male patients may not need continued large doses of zinc after adolescence some supplements are still needed, and women should certainly be advised to maintain their supplements especially if they plan to become pregnant.

Before the pathophysiological role of zinc in acrodermatitis enteropathica was realised chelating agents such as 8-hydroxyquine derivatives were used therapeutically but these are no longer necessary.

With adequate zinc supplements the prognosis of the disorder is excellent but a possible risk of giant squamous cell carcinomas has been proposed.[65]

Familial hyperzincaemia (McKusick 194470)

One pedigree has been reported in which some members inherited, in an autosomal dominant fashion, plasma zinc concentrations up to five times normal (9–20 μmol/l). The additional zinc was associated with plasma albumin and affected individuals were asymptomatic.[66]

MAGNESIUM

Primary hypomagnesaemia (McKusick 248250)

This rare defect may arise from an inability of the intestinal mucosa to absorb magnesium from normal intraluminal concentrations of the metal. However at much higher intraluminal concentrations net intestinal absorption of magnesium is achieved.[67] The occurrence of similar patients in whom primary hypomagnesaemia was associated with renal loss of magnesium and renal tubular dysfunction suggests that there may be an analogous defect in the kidneys.[68] The condition is inherited in an autosomal recessive fashion.

Clinical features[67–69]

Most affected infants were born at term and were apparently healthy during the initial 2–4 weeks of life, after which they became irritable, and developed sleeping and feeding difficulties. Non-specific neurological features then appeared; these progressed through jitteriness and eye-rolling, to hyperreactivity and disturbance and tetany with facial twitching and carpopedal spasm. Not surprisingly, Chvostek's and Trousseau's signs may be positive; generalised convulsions and opisthotonus may then develop. Some infants are hypotonic and areflexic. Other presentations include a protein-losing enteropathy, hyponatraemia and peripheral oedema secondary to the hypomagnesaemia; one child presented with raised intracranial pressure, bulging fontanelles and an increased occipitofrontal circumference. Renal tubular acidosis and hypercalcuria and nephrocalcinosis may occur. If untreated the children deteriorate rapidly, with impaired feeding and increasingly intractable fits resulting in death during infancy.

Laboratory findings

Affected babies are hypocalcaemic and hypomagnesaemic. The latter concentration is reduced markedly and is often less than 0.2 mmol/l (reference range 0.7–1.0 mmol/l). Hypokalaemia and hyponatraemia develop sometimes. Serum inorganic phosphorus concentrations are increased and circulating levels of parathormone are reduced. The hypocalcaemia responds variably to calcium supplements. It may be secondary to impaired secretion of endogenous parathormone or defective end-organ responsiveness or both. Supplements of calcium and parathormone have no effect on the profound hypomagnesaemia. Functional abnormalities are reflected in a grossly but non-specifically abnormal electroencephalogram. Electrocardiographic anomalies which include arrhythmias, prolonged QT intervals, flat and inverted T-waves and U-waves are probably due to the secondary hypocalcaemia and hypokalaemia. Adequate supplements of magnesium rapidly correct all these metabolic anomalies including the renal acidosis.

Diagnosis

Hypomagnesaemia and a favourable clinical and biochemical response to magnesium therapy confirms the diagnosis. Other possible causes of magnesium deficiency such as primary hypoparathyroidism and aldosteronism, excessive urinary loss (including diuretic therapy), malabsorption states and enteropathies, exchange transfusions and magnesium loss secondary to acidosis can be excluded easily. Subsequently the diagnosis of primary hypomagnesaemia rests on the child's continuing dependence on magnesium supplements, inappropriate hypermagnesuria relative to hypomagnesaemia, or on the demonstration of impaired intestinal absorption of the metal.

Treatment

Intramuscular magnesium (0.4–0.75 mmol/kg per 24 h) produces a rapid and gratifying clinical remission. Subsequently oral therapy is adequate, and the dose can be tailored to the clinical response. Supplements providing 1.5–2.0 mmol of elemental magnesium per kg body weight per 24 h may be needed; this is about five times the customary dietary intake. To provide this extra magnesium, magnesium sulphate (4.1 mmol of magnesium in 1 g of $MgSO_47H_2O$) is suitable. Alternative salts include magnesium chloride (4.9 mmol of elemental magnesium in 1 g) and magnesium acetate (4.66 mmol of magnesium in 1 g). Lactate, citrate and hydroxide salts are available also. Although oral supplements correct the clinical, EEG, ECG and most biochemical abnormalities, it is usually difficult to achieve normal serum magnesium concentrations without inducing an undesirable secretory diarrhoea; this is probably an effect of the magnesium itself and it is not ameliorated by using different magnesium salts. The diagnosis and dependence on magnesium supplements can be confirmed by withdrawing the magnesium supplements. Once this has been achieved, affected children will probably need supplements indefinitely.

Hypomagnesaemic tetany (hypomagnesaemia with secondary hypocalcaemia) (McKusick 307600)

This X-linked syndrome resembles the syndrome of primary hypomagnesaemia described above.[70, 71] However the condition has been described in girls and there is a possibility of genetic heterogeneity with X-linked and autosomal forms existing. A translocation defect in one girl suggests that the affected allele might be at Xp22.[71]

MOLYBDENUM

Congenital deficiency of molybdenum-pterin cofactor (McKusick 252150)

A molybdenum-pterin cofactor is required for the activities of sulphite oxidase, aldehyde oxidase, and xanthine dehydrogenase. An autosomal recessively inherited defect in the synthesis of this cofactor leads to impaired metabolism of sulphur amino acids and nucleotides.[72,73] (See p. 88 and p. 305). These patients present as neonates; they have dysmorphic features; feeding difficulties; bilateral dislocation of the lens; hypertonicity or, less commonly, hypotonicity; mental retardation; cerebral and cerebellar atrophy with encephalopathy, and generalised and partial epilepsy. The biochemical anomalies include hypouricaemia, no urinary urothione, xanthinuria, sulphituria, thiosulphaturia and a reduced urinary excretion of inorganic sulphate. The activities of sulphite oxidase activity in fibroblasts from these patients indicates a possible means of prenatal diagnosis.

Studies on fibroblasts from affected patients have identified that this syndrome can be secondary either to inadequate molybdopterin precursor (McKusick 252150) or to a defective converting enzyme (McKusick 252160).[73] No effective management of the disease has been developed and the prognosis is poor.

MANGANESE

Prolidase deficiency (iminodipeptiduria)

A patient with prolidase deficiency also had low red cell arginase activity and a high manganese content in the erythrocytes. It has been proposed that these features could arise from a metabolic defect of manganese metabolism.[74]

REFERENCES

1. Milder M S, Cook J D, Stray S, Finch C A 1980 Idiopathic hemochromatosis, an interim report. Medicine 59:34–49
2. Edwards C Q, Griffen L M, Kushner J P 1990 Southern blood club symposium: an update on selected aspects of hemochromatosis. American Journal of Medical Science 300:245–250
3. Pietrangelo A, Rocchi E, Ferrari A, Ventura E, Cairo G 1991 Regulation of hepatic transferrin, transferrin receptor and ferritin genes in human siderosis. Hepatology 14:1083–1089
4. McClaren G D, Nathanson M H, Jacobs A, Trevett D, Thomson W 1991 Regulation of intestinal iron absorption and mucosal iron kinetics in hereditary hemochromatosis. Journal of Laboratory and Clinical Medicine 117:390–401
5. Edwards C Q, Griffen L M, Dadone M M, Skolnick M H, Kushner J P 1986 Mapping the locus of hereditary haemochromatosis: localisation between HLA-B and HLA-A. American Journal of Human Genetics 38:805–811
6. Bryan C F, Leech S H, Kumar P, Gaumer R, Bozelka B, Morgan J 1991 The immune system in hereditary hemochromatosis: a quantitative and functional assessment of the cellular arm. American Journal of Medical Science 301:55–61
7. Axford J S, Bomford A, Revell P, Watt I, Williams R, Hamilton E B 1991 Hip arthropathy in genetic hemochromatosis. Radiographic and histologic features. Arthritis and Rheumatism 34:357–361.
8. Summers K M, Halliday J W, Powell L W 1990 Identification of hemochromatosis in homozygous subjects by measurement of hepatic iron index. Hepatology 12:20–25
9. Stal P, Glaumann H, Hultcrantz R 1990 Liver cell damage and lysosomal iron storage in patients with idiopathic hemochromatosis. A light and electron microscopic study. Journal of Hepatology 11:172–180
10. Leggett B A, Halliday J W, Brown N N, Bryant S, Powell L W 1990 Prevalence of hemochromatosis amongst asymptomatic Australians. British Journal of Haematology 74:525–530
11. Crosby W H A history of phlebotomy therapy for hemochromatosis. 1991 American Journal of Medical Science 301:28–31
12. Adams P, Speechley M, Kertesz A E 1991 Long-term survival analysis in hereditary hemochromatosis. Gastroenterology 101:368–372
13. Halliday J W 1989 Inherited iron overload. Acta Paediatrica Scandinavica Suppl 361:86–95
14. Barnard J A, Manci E 1991 Idiopathic neonatal iron-storage disease. Gastroenterology 101:1420–1427
15. Dalhoj J, Kiaer H, Wiggers P, Grady R W, Jones R L, Knisely A S 1990 Iron storage disease in parents and sibs of infants with neonatal hemochromatosis: 30-year follow-up. American Journal of Medical Genetics 37:342–345
16. Goya N, Miyazaki S, Kodate S, Ushio B 1972 A family of congenital atransferrinemia. Blood 40:239–245
17. Westerhausen M, Meuret G 1977 Transferrin -immune complex disease. Acta Haematologica 57:96–101
18. Sahadi N T, Nathan D G, Diamond L K 1964 Iron deficiency anaemia associated with an error of iron metabolism in two siblings. Journal of Clinical Investigation 43:510–521

19. Hyman E S 1983 Acquired iron-deficiency anaemia due to impaired iron transport. Lancet 1:91–94
20. Buchanan G R, Sheehan R G 1981 Malabsorption and defective utilisation of iron in three siblings. Journal of Pediatrics 98:723–728
21. Bannerman R M 1981 Of mice, men and microcytes. Journal of Pediatrics 98:960–962
22. Gordeuk V, Mukiibi J, Hasstedt S J et al 1992 Iron overload in Africa. New England Journal of Medicine 326:95–100
23. O'Dell B L 1990 Copper in present knowledge. In : Brown M L (ed) Nutrition. International Life Sciences – Nutrition Foundation, Washington, USA, p 261–267
24. Scheinberg I H, Sternlieb I 1984 Wilson's Disease. W B Saunders, London
25. Sternlieb I 1990 Perspectives on Wilson's disease. Hepatology 12:1234–1239
26. Bingle C D, Srai S K, Epstein O 1990 Developmental changes in hepatic copper proteins in the guinea pig. Journal of Hepatology 10:138–143
27. Iyengar V, Brewer G J, Dick R D, Chung O Y 1988 Studies of cholecystokinin-stimulated biliary secretions reveal a high molecular weight copper-binding substance in normal subjects that is absent in patients with Wilson's disease. Journal of laboratory and Clinical Medicine 111:267–274
28. Farrer L A, Bowcock A M, Hebert J M et al 1991 Predictive testing for Wilson's disease using tightly linked and flanking DNA markers. Neurology 41:992–999
29. Dening T R 1985 Psychiatric aspects of Wilson's disease. British Journal of Psychiatry 147:677–682
30. Snow B J, Bhatt M, Martin W R, Li D, Calne D B 1991 The nigrostriatal dopaminergic pathway in Wilson's disease studied with positron emission tomography. Journal of Neurology Neurosurgery and Psychiatry 54:12–17
31. Dening T R, Berrios G E, Walshe J M 1988 Wilson's disease and epilepsy. Brain 111:1139–1155
32. Goldfisher S, Popper H, Sternlieb I 1980 The significance of variations in the distribution of copper in liver disease. American Journal of Pathology 99:715–730
33. Davies S E, Williams R, Portmann B 1989 Hepatic morphology and histochemistry of Wilson's disease presenting as fulminant hepatic failure:a study of 11 cases. Histopathology 15:385–394
34. Sternlieb I, Scheinberg I H 1979 The role of radiocopper in the diagnosis of Wilson's disease. Gastroenterology 77: 138–142
35. Berman D H, Leventhal R I, Gavaler J S, Cadoff E M, van Thiel D H 1991 Clinical differentiation of fulminant Wilsonian hepatitis from other causes of hepatic failure. Gastroenterology 100:1129–1134
36. Grimm G, Oder W, Prayer L, Ferenci P, Madl C 1990 Evoked potentials in assessment and follow-up of patients with Wilson's disease. Lancet 336:963–964
37. Prayer L, Wimberger D, Kramer J, Grimm G, Oder W, Imhof H 1990 Cranial MRI in Wilson's disease. Neuroradiology 32:211–214
38. Maracek Z, Nevsimalova S 1984 Biochemical and clinical changes in Wilson's disease heterozygotes. Journal of Inherited Metabolic Disease 7:41–45
39. McArdle H J, Kyriakou P, Grimes A, Mercer J F, Danks D M 1990 The effect of D-penicillamine on metallothionein mRNA levels and copper distribution in mouse hepatocytes. Chemico-Biological Interactions 75:315–324
40. Dubois R S, Rodgerson D O, Hambidge K M 1990 Treatment of Wilson's disease with triethylene tetramine hydrochloride (trientine). Journal of Pediatric Gastroenterology and Nutrition 10:77–81
41. McQuaid A, Mason J 1991 A comparison of the effects of penicillamine, trientine, and trithiomolybdate on [35S]-labelled metallothionein in vitro; implications for Wilson's disease therapy. Journal of Inorganic Biochemistry 41:87–92
42. Brewer G J, Dick R D, Yuzbasiyan Gurkin V, Tankanow R, Young A B, Kluin K J 1991 Initial therapy of patients with Wilson's disease with tetrathiomolybdate. Archives of Neurology 48:42–47
43. Veen C, Van den Hamer C J, de Leeuw P W 1991 Zinc sulphate therapy for Wilson's disease after acute deterioration during treatment with low-dose D-penicillamine. Journal of Internal Medicine 229:549–552
44. Schilsky M L, Scheinberg I H, Sternlieb I 1991 Prognosis of Wilsonian chronic active hepatitis. Gastroenterology 100:762–767

45. Edwards C Q, Williams D M, Cartwright G E 1979 Hereditary hypoceruloplasminemia, Clinical Genetics 15:311–316
46. Danks D M, Campbell P E, Stevens B J, Mayne V, Cartwright E 1972 Menkes' kinky hair syndrome: an inherited defect in copper absorption with widespread effects. Pediatrics 50:188–201
47. Verga V, Hall B K, Wang S R, Johnson S, Higgins J V, Glover T W 1991 Localization of the translocation breakpoint in a female with Menkes syndrome to Xq13.2–q13.3 proximal to PGK-1. American Journal of Human Genetics 48:1133–1138
48. Davies K 1993 Cloning the Menkes' disease gene. Nature 361:98
49. Hamer D H 1987 Metallothionein gene regulation in Menkes' syndrome. Archives of Dermatology 123:1384a–1385a
50. Palida F A, Ettinger M J 1991 Identification of proteins involved in intracellular copper metabolism. Low levels of a approximately 48 kDa copper-binding protein in the brindled mouse model of Menkes' disease. Journal of Biological Chemistry 266:4586–4592
51. Tonnesen T, Kleijer W J, Horn N 1991 Incidence of Menkes' disease. Human Genetics 86:408–410
52. Tonnesen T, Horn N, Sondergaard F et al 1987 Experience with first trimester prenatal diagnosis of Menkes' disease. Prenatal Diagnosis 7:497–509
53. Johnsen D E, Coleman L, Poe L 1991 M R of progressive neurodegenerative change in treated Menkes' kinky hair disease. Neuroradiology 33: 181–182
54. Nadal D, Baerlocher K 1988 Menkes' disease: long-term treatment with copper and D-penicillamine. European Journal of Pediatrics 147:621–625
55. Gerdes A M, Tonnesen T, Pergament E et al 1988 Variability in clinical expression of Menkes syndrome. European Journal of Pediatrics 148:132–135
56. Inagaki M, Hashimoto K, Yoshino K et al 1988 Atypical form of Menkes' kinky hair disease with mitochondrial NADH-CoQ reductase deficiency. Neuropediatrics 19:52–55
57. Mehes K, Petrovicz E 1982 Familial benign copper deficiency. Archives of Disease in Childhood 57:716–718
58. Willvonseder R, Goldstein N P, McCall J T, Yoss R E, Tauxe W N 1973 A hereditary disorder with dementia, spastic dysarthria, vertical eye movement paresis, gait disturbance, splenomegaly and abnormal copper metabolism. Neurology 23:1039–1049
59. Godwin-Austen R B, Robinson A, Evans K, Lascelles P T 1978 An unusual neurological disorder of copper metabolism clinically resembling Wilson's disease but biochemically a distinct entity. Journal of Neurological Sciences 39:85–98
60. Ono S, Kurisaki H 1988 An unusual neurological disorder with abnormal copper metabolism.Journal of Neurology 235:397–399
61. Aggett P J 1988 Severe zinc deficiency. In Mills C F (ed) Zinc in Human Biology.Springer-Verlag, London, p 259–280
62. Van Wouwe J P 1989 Clinical and laboratory diagnosis of acrodermatitis enteropathica. European Journal of Pediatrics 149:2–8
63. Ackland M L, Danks D M, McArdle H J 1989 Zinc transport by fibroblasts from patients with acrodermatitis enteropathica. Biology of Trace Elements Research 22:257–263
64. Mack D, Koletzko B, Cunnane S, Cutz E, Griffiths A 1989 Acrodermatitis enteropathica with normal serum zinc levels: diagnostic value of small bowel biopsy and essential fatty acid determination. Gut 30:1426–1429
65. Mori O, Hachisuka H, Kasada M, Kaji H, Sasai Y 1990 Acrodermatitis enteropathica with giant squamous cell carcinomas. Journal of the American Academy of Dermatology 23:1174–1175
66. Failla M L, van der Verdonk M, Morgan W T, Smith J C 1982 Characterisation of zinc binding proteins of plasma in familial hyperzincaemia. Journal of Laboratory and Clinical Medicine 100: 953–952
67. Milla P J, Aggett P J, Wolff O H, Harries J T 1979 Studies in primary hypomagnesaemia: evidence for defective carrier mediated small intestinal transport of magnesium. Gut 20:1028–1033
68. Manz F, Scharer K, Janka P, Lombeck I 1978 Renal magnesium wasting, incomplete tubular acidosis, hypercalcinuria, and nephrocalcinosis in siblings. European Journal of Paediatrics 128:67–79

69. Paunier L, Radde I C, Kooh S U, Cohen P E, Fraser D 1968 Primary hypomagnesaemia with secondary hypocalcaemia in an infant. Pediatrics 41: 385–402
70. Mettey R, Hoppeler A 1982 Les déficits magnésiens de l'enfant. Archives Francais Paediatrie 39:837–844
71. Meyer M, Mattei J F, Viallard J L, Goumy P, Dastague B, Malpuech G 1978 Hypocalcémie magnesodépendante par trouble spécifique de l'absorption du magnésium, associe à une anomalie chromosomique. Revue Francais Endocrinologique Clinique 19:101–108
72. Wadman S K, Duran M, Beemer F A, Cats B P, Johnson J L, Rajagopalan K V, Saudubray J M, Ogier H, Charpentier C, Berger R, Smith G P A, Wilson J, Krywawych S 1983 Absence of hepatic molybdenum cofactor: an inborn error of metabolism leading to a combined deficiency of sulphite oxidase and xanthine dehydrogenase. Journal of Inherited Metabolic Disease 6 Suppl 1:78–83
73. Johnson J L, Wuebbens M M, Mandell R, Shih V E 1989 Molybdenum cofactor biosynthesis in humans: identification of two complementation groups of cofactor-deficient patients and preliminary characterisation of a diffusible molybdopterin precursor. Journal of Clinical Investigation 83: 897–903
74. Lombeck I, Wendel U, Versieck J 1986 Increased manganese content and reduced arginase activity in erythrocytes of a patient with prolidase deficiency (iminodipeptiduria). European Journal of Paediatrics 144:571–573

14. Red cell disorders

A. J. Grimes   N. G. P. Slater

INTRODUCTION

The human, mature red cell is conveniently considered under three main headings: membrane, carbohydrate and associated metabolism and haemoglobin. Whilst it is true that there are innumerable enzyme systems present which are not included in this trio, the majority are not involved in cellular function in the mature cell; rather they are redundant remnants immured within the cell following enucleation and subsequent loss of subcellular fragments in the precursor stage.

Inherited abnormalities are known within each of the three areas; some are common, others are rare; some do not affect red-cell survival while others are associated with haemolytic disease. Often the primary defects are unique to red cells, but sometimes other tissues are affected.

Malaria is still the commonest serious disease affecting humans, and most genetic defects of human red cells are examples of the polymorphic resistance of the cells to the presence of *Plasmodium falciparum*, because the compulsory erythrocytic stage of the parasite requires that it can invade and develop in a compatible environment and this is not available in a red cell carrying a hereditary defect. Resistance to *Plasmodium falciparum* occurs with heterozygous carriers and this has been examined in some detail in the more common single gene hereditary defects, namely glucose-6-phosphate dehydrogenase (G6PD) deficiency, sickle-cell anaemia and the thalassaemias, but also in South-East Asian ovalocytosis. Study was further stimulated following 1976 when a continuous culture technique for the parasite became available which allows in vitro studies to be carried out. Details continue to emerge on the different hazards to malarial parasite growth in genetically abnormal red cells, and these are mentioned under the relevant genetic disorder.

DISORDERS OF THE RED-CELL MEMBRANE

The normal membrane

Red-cell membranes differ from those of other cells in having a one-to-one ratio of protein and lipid; the constituents of these two classes are shown in

Tables 14.1 and 14.2. The carbohydrate component of the membrane is restricted to the integral glycoproteins (see later) with sugar residues obtruding on the extracellular side of the cell and incorporating the blood group antigens.

Table 14.1 Lipids in the human red-cell membrane. (Values expressed as % dry weight of total)

Neutral		Phospholipid		Glycosphingolipid	
		Neutral			
Cholesterol (free)	20	Phosphatidylcholine	20	Globosides	13
Cholesterol (esterified)	2	Sphingomyelin	15	Gangliosides	2
Free fatty acids	2				
		Acidic			
		Phosphatidylethanolamine	16		
		Phosphatidylserine	4		
		Phosphatidate	2		
		Lysolecithin	4		

Table 14.2 Major proteins in the human red cell membrane. (Table based on references 1–3)

	Name	Integral (I)/ peripheral (P)	Molecular Weight ($kD_a \times 10^5$)	Proportion (% total dry weight)
Coomassie Blue stain Band number				
1 } 2	Spectrin	P	2.4; 2.2	25
2.1 } 2.2 } 2.3	Ankyrin	P	2.15; 1.86; 1.6	5
3	Anion transport	I	0.9–1.0	25
4.1	—	P	0.8	4–5
4.2	—	P	0.72	5
5	Actin	P	0.45	4–5
6	GAPD	P	0.35	4–5
PAS stain Band number				
PAS 1 } PAS 2	Glycophorin A	I	0.31 approx.	1.5
PAS 3	Glycophorin B	I	0.23 approx.	0.5
Glycoconnectin	Glycophorin C	I	0.29 approx	0.3

Lipids (Table 14.1)

All red-cell lipid is contained within the membrane. The phospholipids comprise approximately 60% by weight of total lipid, of which some 60% is neutral and the remainder acidic. The major constituents are the phosphatidyl esters of choline, ethanolamine and serine, together with sphingomyelin. These four phospholipids form the planar, hydrophobic bilayer contained in the membrane interior. Free fatty acids, gangliosides, phosphatidate and lysolecithin are present in the membrane only in small amounts. The lipid bilayer is asymmetrical, most of the sphingomyelin and phosphatidylcholine being located on the outer half, with the bulk of phosphatidylethanolamine (about 80%) and all the phosphatidylserine on the cytoplasmic side.

Some 23% of total lipid is cholesterol, almost all of it unesterified. Unlike the phospholipids, it exchanges continuously with its plasma counterpart, and the planar configuration and non-polar character of the molecule allows it to enter the bilayer and remain there, distributed uniformly at a fixed concentration. Its presence affects membrane fluidity: an increase in cholesterol enlarges and a decrease diminishes the surface area of the cell. Such changes have consequences for the cell; removal of enough cholesterol from the membrane will reduce the surface area sufficiently to transform the normal discocyte into a microspherocyte.

Proteins (Table 14.2)

Electrophoresis on SDS polyacrylamide gel consistently reveals some 12 major membrane proteins, many with demonstrable function. They are of two general types, integral and peripheral.[1,2] The former enter or span the membrane, sometimes several times, with a hydrophobic domain contiguous with the lipid bilayer and polar regions at the extremities of the molecule. On the cytoplasmic side these are associated with a cytoskeleton (see below) while on the extracellular face the polar ends carry sugar residues associated with the blood group antigens. The peripheral proteins are located on the cytoplasmic side of the membrane where they are attached to the obtruding integral proteins and polar phospholipid heads of the bilayer to form the cytoskeleton.

Cytoskeleton

The grouping of membrane proteins into peripheral and integral arose from the treatment of membranes with mild non-ionic detergents, which solubilised the lipid bilayer, and integral proteins associated with it, to leave a complex of peripheral proteins having the shape of the red cell. This is the cytoskeleton, a loosely ordered, flexible, two-dimensional network of protein tetramers (spectrin) anchored at specific points on the inner surface of the membrane. This net of filamentous protein gives shape, strength and flexibility to the cell and allows it to recover from short-term configurational changes, such as occur in the microcirculation. However, severe constraints, rigidity because of cell ageing, or congenital or acquired defects of cytoskeletal proteins, can cause permanent abnormalities of cell morphology and possibly a shortening of the cell lifespan.

The major components of the cytoskeleton (Fig. 14.1) are *spectrin* (bands 1 and 2, accounting for approximately two-thirds of cytoskeletal weight), *ankyrin* (band 2.1), band *4.1* and *actin* (band 5). Two spectrin filaments (1 and 2) lie together to form a heterodimer 100 nm long, which is attached at one end to a second heterodimer forming a tetramer which is the major building block. This tetramer has three known functional regions. The first is the contact site of the two ends of the heterodimers which form the tetramer. The second is a tail locality where spectrin is linked with actin, band 4.1 and adducin in a complex that attaches it to the inner wall of the membrane via an integral protein glycophorin C (*glycoconnectin*) and also weakly via phosphatidylserine in the bilipid layer. The third region is a major membrane binding site on the 2-spectrin, some 20 nm from the dimer–dimer contact point, where spectrin links with ankyrin, which is also attached to the integral, trans-membrane anion transporter protein band 3. The two-dimensional configuration of the spectrin network is formed at the 4.1-actin junction by branching, one dimer strand attaching to a strand from a different dimer.

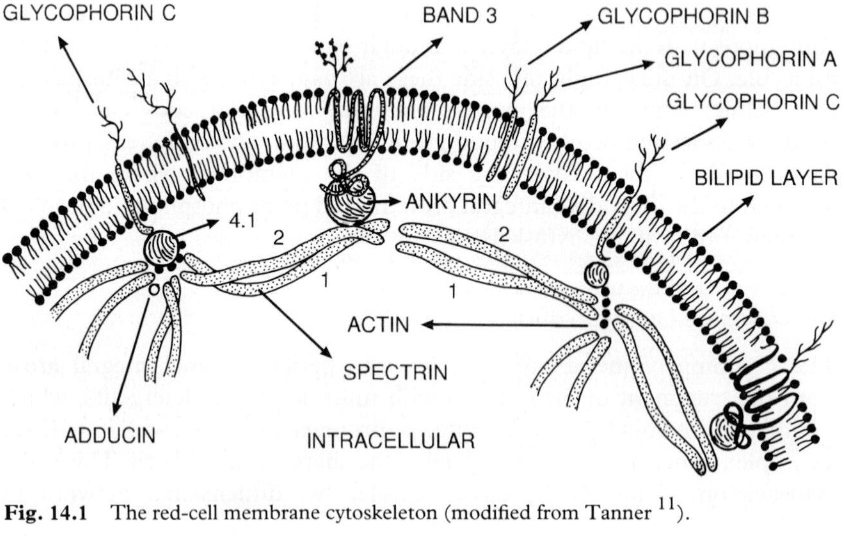

Fig. 14.1 The red-cell membrane cytoskeleton (modified from Tanner [11]).

The abnormal membrane

Hereditary spherocytosis (McKusick 182900)

Hereditary spherocytosis (HS) is transmitted as an autosomal dominant in the majority of cases, although there are a number with recessive inheritance, sometimes with significant haemolysis. HS is the commonest congenital haemolytic anaemia in cases of northern European extraction (about 1 in 5000) although it is not peculiar to any ethnic group. The disorder is more heterogeneous than formerly supposed and it is likely that there are many unreported cases of very mild or asymptomatic HS. Typically, the disorder is associated with a mild to moderate haemolytic anaemia, although occasionally haemolysis may be severe and transfusion-dependent. Moderate splenomegaly occurs and splenectomy, when practicable, resolves the anaemia.

Blood examination reveals the usual features of haemolysis i.e. anaemia, reticulocytosis and raised serum bilirubin; the blood film shows polychromasia, anisocytosis and, particularly, microspherocytes. The fresh blood osmotic fragility curve may indicate fragile cells. Curves made from blood incubated for 24 h are more likely than fresh blood to reveal an abnormality, with a marked shift towards fragile cells. Incubation of sterile, defibrinated blood for 48 h gives abnormal lysis, but with added glucose present this is reduced and may be within the normal range (autohaemolysis test). Dilute suspensions of red cells in acid-buffered glycerol solution undergo more lysis than normal cells (AGLT test). There is currently no single diagnostic test for HS, but those mentioned above, the beneficial effect of splenectomy and a family history will, in the absence of an autoimmune process, furnish a definitive diagnosis.

Early studies to demonstrate biochemical abnormalities in the red cells in HS failed to reveal any defects of glycolysis; the results usually indicated only the presence of a young red-cell population. Interest turned towards the membrane, and first indications that the defect(s) lay here came from demonstrations of membrane instability in vitro, and abnormalities both in monovalent cation transport and the phosphorylation of some membrane proteins. It is now clear that these are secondary to a primary structural defect in the cytoskeleton. The sphering process is gradual: reticulocytes and young red cells in HS have a normal morphology, but congenital membrane instability causes fragments to be lost gradually. As a result the surface area diminishes without loss of intracellular contents, and this yields microspherocytes during cell ageing. The reticuloendothelial system, notably the spleen, hastens spontaneous sphering because splenic sinusoids are a physiologically poor environment for red cells, although normal cells survive multiple transits. In HS the splenic transit time lengthens with increased sphering, the process being aggravated by the unfavourable milieu. The sphered cells may be metabolically and physiologically functional but become rigid and undeformable.

Hereditary elliptocytosis (McKusick 130500 and 130600)

Hereditary elliptocytosis (HE) is a more heterogeneous disorder than HS and has been classified into three types on the basis of cell morphology[3]: *common HE* with a biconcave elliptocyte, *spherocytic HE*, and *stomatocytic elliptocytosis* or *South-East Asian ovalocytosis*.

Common hereditary elliptocytosis. Apart from a few exceptions, HE is inherited as an autosomal dominant. Normal blood contains up to 5% elliptocytes; in patients with HE there can be from 30 to 100% present and the disorder varies from being asymptomatic to displaying severe haemolysis with splenomegaly. The diagnosis is made from the blood film and the finding of autosomal dominant inheritance in the family. The majority of patients with common HE are symptomless, but where haemolysis is severe, perhaps requiring splenectomy, the blood film may show microspherocytes, poikilocytes (tear-drop cells) and red-cell fragments. In general, the degree of elliptocytosis correlates poorly with severity of the disease, and there is variation within patients as well as between them. As in HS, elliptocyte formation is a progressive process, nucleated precursors are round and reticulocytes are notably less ellipsoidal than mature cells.

The presence of elliptocytes in normal blood, and their presence in increased numbers, together with poikilocytosis, in hypochromic, microcytic and megaloblastic anaemias, myelofibrosis and pyruvate kinase deficiency, does not usually confuse a diagnosis of HE, since, in addition to increased elliptocytes in HE, the patient and family history should reveal their long-term persistence on the blood film.

Osmotic fragility in HE is usually normal, unless the condition is severe, or unless poikilocytosis and red-cell fragments, frequently spheroidal, are present. Where there is a mutant spectrin present, as in homozygous, doubly heterozygous and mildly affected heterozygous patients, the elliptocytes, isolated cytoskeletons, and the purified spectrin are all thermolabile. The cells, membranes and cytoskeletons are also mechanically fragile.

As with HS, splenectomy is the routine treatment when haemolysis and gallstones are notable features of the condition.

Spherocytic elliptocytosis. This is a rare form of HE in which the blood film shows thickened elliptocytes as well as spherocytes, and haemolysis is present despite the relatively moderate abnormality in red-cell morphology.

South-East Asian ovalocytosis. This condition, also known as stomatocytic HE, is prevalent in South-East Asia where there is a 30% incidence among some ethnic groups. Clinical haemolysis is not present, although the red cells are abnormally rigid; they are also abnormally resistant to invasion by malarial parasites in vitro, and blood of affected patients has a low parasite count in areas endemic for malaria. It is suggested that the trait has been positively selected because of this resistance and that the membrane abnormality renders the cell less attractive to invasion by the parasite.

The major chemical defect in the cells is a functionally and structurally abnormal cytoplasmic segment of the band 3 protein. As a consequence the binding to ankyrin is too tight and the band 3 protein has reduced lateral mobility.

Hereditary stomatocytosis (McKusick 185000 and 185010)

Stomatocytes are cup- or bowl-shaped in wet preparations; in dried preparations a longitudinal slit can be seen in place of the pallid central area. They can be prepared by chemical manipulation in vitro and occur also in association with malignant disease, thalassaemia minor, alcoholic liver disease, infectious mononucleosis and GSH glutathione peroxidase deficiency. In hereditary stomatocytosis 10–40% of the cells may be stomatocytes, with a reticulocyte count up to 40%.

The primary defect in this disorder is likely to be in the membrane, but earlier studies were much concerned with abnormalities of stomatocytic cation flux. Characteristically, the cells have increased water content (hydrocytosis) and surface area and volume, and marked aberrations in cation content and flux. The intracellular Na^+ can be ten times the normal value, while K^+ is low; the total ($Na^+ + K^+$) is high, which is reflected by the increased cell volume. Net leakage of the two cations is high and, for Na^+, even faster than the high cell content would suggest. Active Na^+/K^+ transport is rapid and the usual coupled transport ratio of $3Na^+$ to $2K^+$ is considerably increased because of the relatively higher active flux of Na^+ over K^+. This increased active flux is accompanied by an increased glucose consumption and, since the active transport mechanism is located within the membrane, it provides some evidence for a membrane abnormality.

Hereditary pyropoikilocytosis (McKusick 266140)

Poikilocytes, or tear-drop cells, are present on blood films in a number of disparate disorders such as iron deficiency, thalassaemia, myelofibrosis and megaloblastic anaemia. They also arise from intravascular damage to cells, as in microangiopathic haemolytic anaemia. The hereditary form of pyropoikilocytosis (HP) is a rare disorder overlapping in certain respects with HE; often one parent, as well as other family members, has mild HE or is asymptomatic but carries the spectrin defect. The cells are thermolabile, as in HE.

Molecular defects of membrane proteins[4]

Since the 1960s, many anaemic patients who had been diagnosed under the general heading of congenital non-spherocytic haemolytic anaemia have since been categorised as suffering from specific red-cell enzymopathies. This became possible with the advent of enzyme assay techniques. In a similar way, those congenital anaemias currently diagnosed on morpholog-

Table 14.3 Known hereditary membrane abnormalities

Spectrin deficiency	
Mild to moderate	Mild or typical hereditary spherocytosis (HS)
Severe	Autosomal recessive HS or hereditary pyropoikilocytosis (HP)
Spectrin (1) defects	
Inadequate tetramer formation	Mild to moderate hereditary elliptocytosis (HP) (HE)
	Asymptomatic HP
Decrease of spectrin (1)	Severe HE
Spectrin (2) defects	
Inadequate tetramer formation	Mild to moderate HE
Defective spectrin-ankyrin link	Mild HE
Defective spectrin-4.1 link	HS (autosomal dominant)
Ankyrin deficiency	
Mild decrease	Mild or typical HS
Severe decrease	Atypical severe HS
4.1 Defect	
Deficiency	Severe HE with spheroelliptocytes
Abnormal 4.1	Mild HE or asymptomatic
Glycophorin C deficiency	Mild HE
4.2 Deficiency	
Partial or complete	HS (autosomal recessive)
Increased ankyrin affinity	South-East Asian ovalocytosis

ical grounds as hereditary spherocytosis, elliptocytosis, pyropoikilocytosis, ovalocytosis, etc. will no doubt be categorised according to the specific molecular defects of the cytoskeleton. Current information on the known membrane abnormalities is tabulated in Table 14.3.

DISORDERS OF THE EMBDEN–MEYERHOF PATHWAY (EMP)

The normal pathway

This pathway (Fig. 14.2) consumes 1–2 mmols glucose per litre of packed red cells per hour at 37°C in normal, human red cells. This is the sole substrate needed by the cell and among the intermediates produced, five are essential for red-cell function and viability (Table 14.4). This low rate of glycolysis is dependent on the tidal flow of plasma glucose, which is always adequate even in acute hypoglycaemia. Plasma glucose passes across the cell by facilitated diffusion, a rapid process which requires a carrier but no energy, and the intracellular level, similar to the plasma level when expressed in terms of cell or plasma water, does not affect the rate of consumption by the cells, A detailed account of carbohydrate metabolism of human red cells is available.[5]

ATP. This nucleotide is required in several reactions in addition to its role in glycolysis. Its most studied function is to provide the energy to

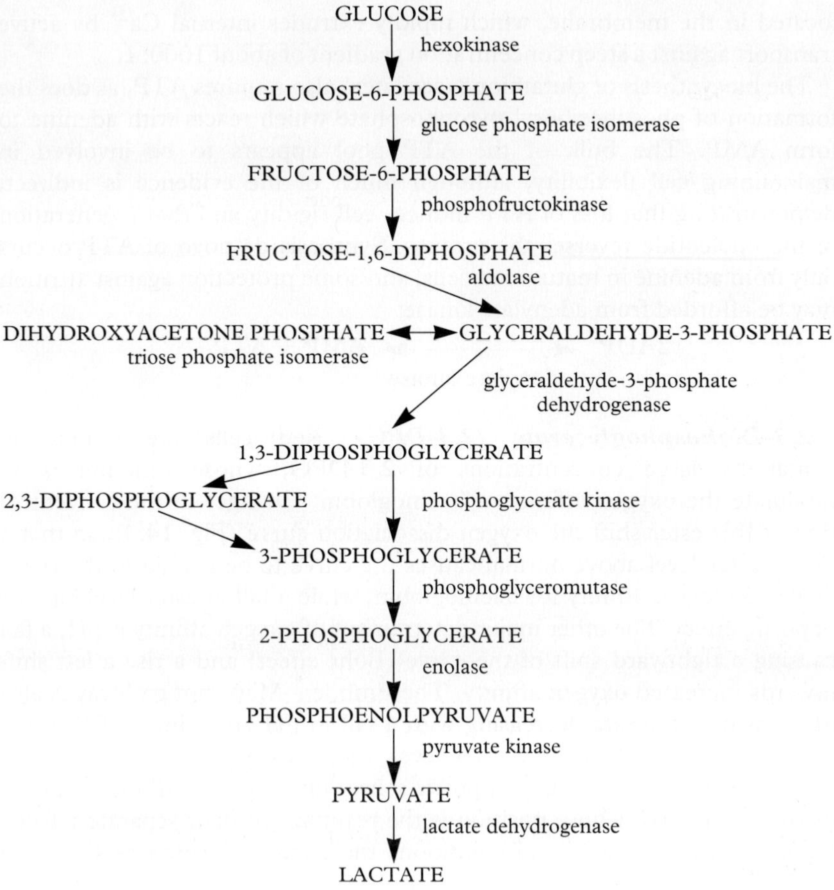

Fig. 14.2 The Embden – Meyerhof pathway (EMP).

Table 14.4 Concentration of key red-cell intermediates. Values refer to mmol/l packed cells

ATP	0.8–1.4
2,3-DPG	3.0–4.0
GSH	2.2
NAD^+ +(H)	0.03–0.07
$NADP^+$ +(H)	0.045

maintain active Na^+ and K^+ transport: the membrane-sited sodium pump, which transfers these cations, relatively slowly through the membrane bidirectionally (Na^+ out, K^+ in) in the ratio of 3: 2, by a mechanism similar to that operating in other cells. However, calculation reveals that only some 20% of the nucleotide is used in this process; the quantitative deployment of the remainder is unclear. Some ATP is required in the calcium pump, also located in the membrane, which rapidly extrudes internal Ca^{2+} by active transport against a steep concentration gradient of about 1000: 1.

The biosynthesis of glutathione (see later) also requires ATP, as does the formation of phosphoribosyl pyrophosphate which reacts with adenine to form AMP. The bulk of the ATP pool appears to be involved in maintaining cell flexibility, although much of the evidence is indirect, demonstrating that loss of ATP induces cell rigidity and that regeneration of the nucleotide reverses the process. Synthesis de novo of ATP occurs only from adenine in mature red cells, and some protection against attrition may be afforded from adenylate kinase:

$$2\text{ADP} \underset{\text{adenylate kinase}}{\longleftrightarrow} \text{AMP} + \text{ATP}$$

2,3-Diphosphoglycerate (2,3-DPG). Red cells are unique in containing large concentrations of 2,3-DPG, whose function is to modulate the oxygen affinity of haemoglobin. Changes in the concentration of this ester shift the oxygen dissociation curve (Fig. 14.3), so that a rise in ester level above normal causes the curve to be shifted to the right, lowering oxygen affinity for haemoglobin, while a fall in ester level has the opposite effect. The other major determinant of oxygen affinity is pH, a fall causing a rightward shift of the curve (Bohr effect) and a rise a left shift towards increased oxygen affinity. The Embden–Meyerhof pathway is also pH sensitive, the rate decreasing with a fall in pH and, since a fall in the glycolytic rate decreases the ester level, these two variables of ester level and intracellular pH work in opposite senses upon oxygen affinity to give a dissociation curve whose position is the resultant of their separate effects. Under normal physiological conditions the curve is located as shown in Figure 14.3. The curve shifts to abnormal positions in a number of situations: acid–base disturbances; conditions of abnormal 2,3-DPG levels as in anaemia, hypoxia and congenital glycolytic deficiency; and in some haemoglobinopathies in which the affinity for the ester is abnormal.

NAD^+/NADH. This coenzyme functions at two sites in the cell: as well as its role in the Embden–Meyerhof pathway, it is involved with NADH-linked methaemoglobin reductase, which is the most important of four pathways for the reduction of methaemoglobin.

Glutathione and $NADP^+$/NADPH are both associated with the second glycolytic pathway in the cell, the pentose phosphate pathway which is described later.

The abnormal pathway

Demonstrations of low activity have been recorded for each of the enzymes of the Embden–Meyerhof pathway in red cells, with the exception of phosphoglycerate mutase, and each, with the exception of lactate dehydrogenase, is associated with a congenital non-spherocytic haemolytic

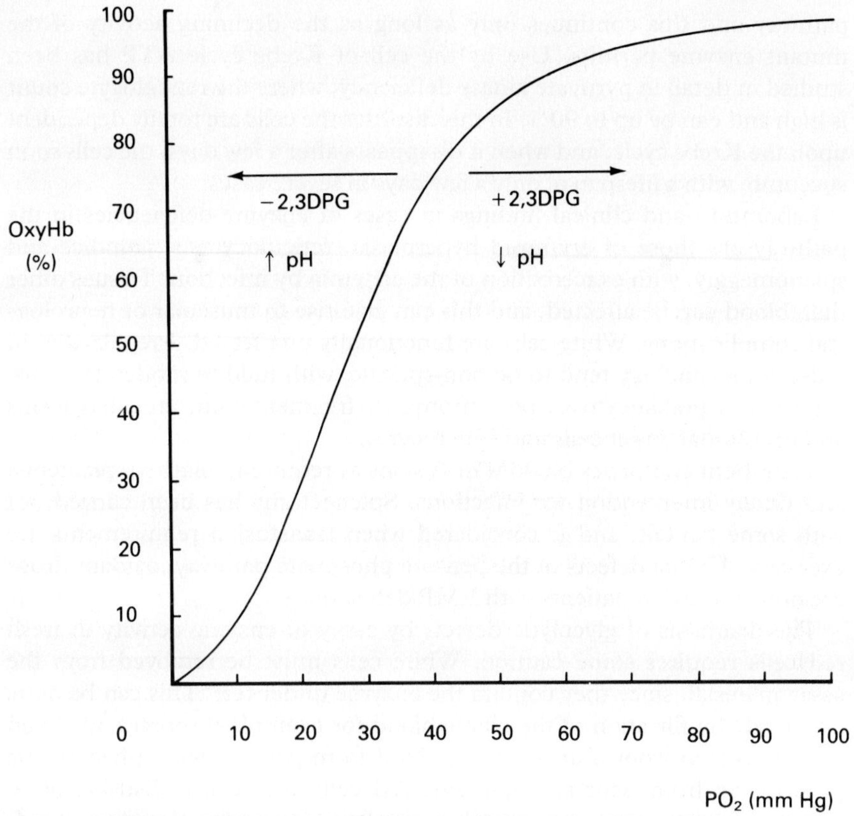

Fig. 14.3 Normal oxygen dissociation curve. (2,3 DPG: 2,3-diphosphoglycerate.)

anaemia. These diseases are rare, and even the commonest, pyruvate kinase deficiency, has been reported in only some 300 cases.

All deficiencies so far reported are due to a mutant enzyme, present in near-normal concentration in young cells. The mutant may be unstable, so that the activity declines with abnormal rapidity with cell age, or it may have abnormal kinetics; it may also have both characteristics. The diagnostic feature is a subnormal activity in the tested white-cell-free blood sample, which indicates a glycolytic block that results in a shortened red-cell life span and a haemolytic anaemia whose severity depends upon the cellular activity of the mutant enzyme. The young red-cell population present in any haemolytic anaemia is associated with a high reticulocyte count, and these young circulating cells contain vestigial Krebs cycle activity which fades with disappearance of the mitochondria during the few days of maturation, before red cells become morphologically indistinguishable from mature cells. While Krebs cycle activity persists, supplementary ATP is available, and this continues until the cell matures and the Krebs cycle fades away. The cell then depends upon the ATP generated in the Embden–Meyerhof pathway and this continues only as long as the declining activity of the mutant enzyme permits. Use by the cell of Krebs cycle ATP has been studied in detail in pyruvate kinase deficiency, where the reticulocyte count is high and can be up to 90%. In this disorder the cells are totally dependent upon the Krebs cycle, and when it disappears after a few days, the cells soon succumb, with a lifespan of only a few days in severe cases.

Laboratory and clinical findings in cases of enzyme deficiencies in the pathway are those of erythroid hyperplasia, reticulocytosis, jaundice and splenomegaly, with exacerbation of the anaemia by infection. Tissues other than blood can be affected, and this can give rise to muscular or neurological complications. White cells are functionally unaffected. Irregularities in red-cell morphology tend to be non-specific, with mild to moderate anisocytosis and poikilocytosis, polychromasia, fragmentation, crenated forms and occasional target cells and spherocytes.

Treatment comprises blood transfusions as required, folate supplements, and timely intervention for infections. Splenectomy has been carried out with some benefit, and is considered when transfusion requirements are excessive. Unlike defects of the pentose phosphate pathway, oxidant drugs are not a hazard in patients with EMP deficiencies.

The diagnosis of glycolytic defects by assay of enzyme activity in fresh red cells requires some caution. White cells must be removed from the assay material, since they contain the enzyme under test. This can be done effectively by filtration of the whole blood for example through boiled and washed cotton wool. Furthermore, blood from patients with a haemolytic process, or from neonates, contains red cells whose age distribution is skewed towards young cells and these contain higher activities of most red-cell enzymes than do older cells, so that a partial deficiency may be masked, giving values within the normal range. If the mutant enzyme activity is low, as in homozygotes, there is usually no problem in diagnosis. The difficulty presented by partially lowered activity can be resolved in several ways:

1. some family members may be affected but have no haemolytic accompaniment
2. the enzyme under test can be assayed against another normal but cell-age related enzyme
3. data can be accumulated on the activity of the enzyme under test in normal, young red-cell populations
4. fractionation of the test blood sample into older and younger cells by centrifugation may give a rate of decline of activity which is different from that in a normal, young red-cell sample.

Enzymes and variants of the Embden–Meyerhof pathway

Hexokinase (McKusick 235700)

Hexokinase in normal red cells has the lowest capacity of the EMP enzymes; it has been called the glycolytic pacemaker, since its decay with cell age reflects that of glucose consumption in a rate-limiting manner. In young red cells the activity is tenfold or more that of old cells and, like most other Embden–Meyerhof pathway enzymes, it follows a biphasic curve of decline in activity with time. Loss of the early high capacity has been shown to be due to proteolysis of HK1, the isozyme present in most other tissues. There is also evidence of a second isozyme, HKR, in reticulocytes with activity and kinetic properties similar to HK1, but with a short half-life and under separate genetic control.

Hexokinase deficiency was first described in 1964 in three patients with Fanconi's syndrome without haemolytic anaemia, in whom the disorder may have been caused by chromosome breaks. Since then hereditary deficiency of the enzyme has been reported as the primary defect, associated with haemolytic anaemia, in some 12 patients. Activity of the enzyme was within or below the normal range, but actually low by comparison with normal, reticulocyte-rich blood. The disorder is typically autosomal recessive. In several of the cases glucose consumption was lower than anticipated for the young red-cell population present. Intermediates downstream of the block are depressed; the low level of 2,3-diphosphoglycerate increases the oxygen affinity of haemoglobin and patients are less active physically than would be expected for their degree of anaemia.

This defect highlights a further diagnostic problem applicable to some other enzyme defects. When a variant has a high K_m value, assay of the enzyme with the excess substrate usually present may yield a normal result. At a lower and more physiological substrate concentration the deficiency may be revealed. In default of establishing the K_m, red-cell enzymes should be assayed at both high and low substrate levels.[6]

Glucose phosphate isomerase (McKusick 172400)

The decay in activity of this enzyme in normal red cells is graphically a biphasic curve with a steep fall followed by a slow one, and a half-life ($t_{1/2}$) of about 159 days. One isozymic form is present in young cells, but ageing causes a chemical change to give two components with different charge. The secondary isozyme is more heat-stable.

A number of cases of glucose phosphate isomerase deficiency are known, many not associated with haemolytic anaemia which is the only clinical disorder recognised in this deficiency; where anaemia does occur it may be mild or severe. Osmotic fragility is near normal, with increased autohaemolysis only slightly reduced in the presence of glucose. A decrease in white cell and plasma activity is a common feature. The deficiency is autosomal recessive; about half of affected subjects are homozygotes, the remainder compound heterozygotes. Many of the variants have been characterised electrophoretically, by K_m values or pH activity curves.

Variants with low activity are thermolabile. The glucose-6-phosphate concentration is raised in red cells while fructose-6-phosphate is near normal. Activity of the pentose phosphate pathway is normal but recycling is notably restricted. ATP is low or normal.

Phosphofructokinase (McKusick 171850 and 232800)

This enzyme is an important regulator of red-cell glycolysis and is sensitive to a number of effectors. The normal enzyme is a tetramer with three different subunits, M in muscle, L in liver and F in fibroblasts, platelets, lymphocytes, kidney and brain (see Introduction, p. 9). Red cells contain L and M subunits in approximately similar amounts with the five possible isozymes of L and M.

A red-cell and muscle deficiency of the enzyme (Type VII glycogen storage disease) is reported in three Japanese siblings with clinical histories compatible with muscle phosphorylase deficiency (McArdle's disease) and evidence of a haemolytic anaemia. Red cells contained about 50% normal phosphofructokinase activity and the muscle component M was missing. In another patient whose red cells contained 60% of normal activity, there was an associated haemolytic anaemia but a normal muscle enzyme activity and no muscular abnormality. Presumably the L subunit was affected in the red cells. Despite haemolysis, the osmotic fragility, authohaemolysis, red-cell K^+, Na^+ and Na^+ flux, together with lactate production, were all normal. The patient's mother and maternal grandmother showed similar low phosphofructokinase activity but without haemolysis. Following these initial reports, other cases have been described; 29 cases of muscle phosphofructokinase deficiency were recorded by 1986, and in 22 in whom it was measured, red-cell activity of the enzyme was also reduced (17–60% normal). Six cases are known with a lowered red-cell but normal muscle activity of the enzyme (L subunit disorder).

Both glucose-6-phosphate and fructose-6-phosphate levels are increased in red cells in phosphofructokinase deficiency, as is 2,3-diphosphoglycerate, and it is suggested that the first two intermediates stimulate activity of the pentose phosphate pathway, thereby increasing phosphoribosylpyrophosphate, purine and pyrimidine production, a notion that arose from the finding of hyperuricaemia and gout in a patient. Muscle glycogen storage is also increased.

Hereditary phosphofructokinase deficiency, in association with a haemolytic anaemia, is also recognised in Springer spaniels.

Aldolase (McKusick 103580)

Some four cases have been described, one in a mentally handicapped child with a mild haemolytic anaemia. The parents were first cousins with normal red-cell activity of the enzyme. The red-cell enzyme is designated A while B, which is located in liver, kidney cortex and small intestine, is deficient in hereditary fructose intolerance (p. 53). Thus, red-cell aldolase activity is normal in fructose intolerance and red cells cannot be used to diagnose the disorder. In one of the cases of red-cell aldolase deficiency, in which lymphocytes contained about 30% normal activity, enzyme A has been cloned from cultured lymphoblasts and the variant shown to contain a single amino acid substitution of aspartate by glycine.

Glyceraldehyde-3-phosphate dehydrogenase (McKusick 138400)

Few cases of this disorder are known. In one, with red-cell glyceraldehyde-3-phosphate dehydrogenase activity only 20–30% normal, the disorder was accompanied by a compensated haemolytic anaemia; in others with 50% deficiency of enzyme activity there was no anaemia. A large family is described in whom the deficiency is accompanied by hereditary spherocytosis. This is of interest since in this disorder there is a membrane defect and glyceraldehyde-3-phosphate dehydrogenase is a membrane-sited enzyme attached electrostatically to band 3 protein.

Triose phosphate isomerase (McKusick 190450)

In humans this enzyme is a dimer of identical subunits encoded by a single locus on chromosome 24. A deficiency of the enzyme is reported in some 22 children from seven unrelated families, and all but one have died in infancy from neurological dysfunction, haemolytic anaemia and susceptibility to infection. In the first reported case a child had a chronic haemolytic anaemia and progressive muscular disorder; red-cell activity of the enzyme in a surviving child, also with haemolytic anaemia, was 10% of normal. Both parents showed intermediate heterozygote values without associated haemolysis. The authors[7] later reported another child, similar to the first and with both parents heterozygotes; the two families were thought to be related. In another family[8] the heterozygous mother of a homozygous child was diagnosed from fetal red cells during a second pregnancy as carrying a heterozygote fetus; the child was delivered and subsequently survived. Inheritance of the deficiency follows an autosomal recessive pattern, and in the few cases examined the enzyme is a thermolabile mutant with an aspartate residue in place of glutamate.

Where red-cell intermediates have been measured, high glucose consumption has been found even after correction for the young cell population present. The pentose phosphate pathway is adequate, ATP normal or somewhat low, and dihydroxyacetone phosphate inordinately high. Fructose-1,6-diphosphate and glyceraldehyde-3-phosphate are also increased. It has been suggested that since dihydroxyacetone phosphate is not metabolised further in red cells, the high levels may be toxic.

2,3-Diphosphoglycerate mutase (McKusick 222800)

Activity of this enzyme is found only in red cells, where it has three functions. It catalyses both the formation and the degradation of 2,3-diphosphoglycerate; that is it acts as both a mutase and a phosphatase. In addition, it acts as a phosphoglyceromutase, although the conversion of 3- to 2-phosphoglycerate is catalysed also by a specific mutase. The cDNAs for both enzymes have been cloned, and the genes for the 2,3-phosphoglycerate mutase and the 3-phosphoglycerate mutase reside on chromosome 7 and 10 respectively.

Several cases of deficiency of this enzyme, with activities around 50% of normal, are reported in association with a haemolytic anaemia, usually with a low 2,3-diphosphoglycerate level. A complete deficiency accompanied by negligible 2,3-diphoshoglycerate is also reported in a man with compensatory polycythaemia due to the increased haemoglobin oxygen affinity, but without haemolysis.[9]

Phosphoglycerokinase (McKusick 261700)

Moderate deficiency with haemolytic anaemia was first described in 1968, since when a number of cases have been reported and a sex-linked basis of transmission established. White cells can also be affected. Red-cell ATP levels are said to be low and 2,3-diphosphoglycerate high, while pyruvate and lactate production are normal. Female heterozygotes have two red-cell populations, one normal and the other enzyme deficient.

Pyruvate kinase (McKusick 266200)

Mammalian tissue contains four isozymes of pyruvate kinase: M_1 (muscle, heart and brain), M_2 (kidney, muscle, heart and brain), L (liver) and R (red cells). The red-cell isoenzyme R (or L^1) is immunologically and kinetically indistinguishable from the major liver enzyme and both have low activity in pyruvate kinase deficiency. In erythroid precursors the M_2 isozyme is present and L formation occurs following a decrease in the M-type. The red-cell enzyme R (L^1) then undergoes proteolysis in the maturing red cell, from the tetramer (${L^1}_4$) present in erythroblasts, to a heterotetramer $L_2{L^1}_2$. The gene for the L-type enzyme is located on chromosome 1. Other blood cells contain the M-type isozyme.

Deficiency of this enzyme is the commonest of the Embden–Meyerhof pathway enzyme defects and over 300 cases are recorded. Heterozygotes have intermediate values in red-cell activity, usually with a normal blood film and no signs of haemolysis. Homozygotes show a marked reduction of red-cell activity (5–40% normal) with an associated non-spherocytic haemolytic anaemia of mild to marked severity. The reticulocyte count increases notably following splenectomy but the anaemia is only marginally improved. In severe cases the blood film shows bizarre crenation of many red cells. Red cells and and reticulocytes are poorly flexible.

Both parents of severely affected patients have intermediate deficiency, as do all progeny of a grossly deficient parent. This, together with the occurrence of consanguinity, indicates an autosomal inheritance. Different mutants show marked differences in electrophoretic mobility, kinetic properties, catalytic activity and stability. In patients with severe haemolysis the enzyme is thermally unstable, with decreased affinity for its substrate phosphoenol pyruvate, decreased activation by fructose 1,6-diphosphate and increased inhibition by ATP. However, the exact nature of the molecular defect remains unknown.

In pyruvate kinase deficiency, as in the other red-cell glycolytic enzymopathies associated with haemolysis, there are related abnormalities. Most frequently reported is the elevated 2, 3-diphosphoglycerate arising from the block distal to the formation of this ester. Other esters formed after the pyruvate kinase step are also raised, but the high diphosphoglycerate level is notable because of the high concentration normally present and also because of its effect upon the O_2 dissociation curve. This is to shift the curve to the right and consequently confer upon the patient an increased oxygen availability and a wellbeing not usually associated with the degree of anaemia present. Red-cell ATP is low or low-normal and the amount measured is the sum of that produced from the restricted Embden–Meyerhof pathway together with that arising from the fading Krebs cycle present in the reticulocytes. The cycle disappears after a few days and red cells are then dependent on anaerobic glycolysis; this is inadequate and the cells rapidly become senescent. The total NAD^+ + NADH level is low, although the NAD^+/NADH ratio is normal. Glucose consumption is near the normal range but low after correction for the young red-cell population present. Pentose phosphate pathway activity is somewhat depressed relative to that of the Embden–Meyerhof pathway.

Lactate dehydrogenase (McKusick 150100)

One case of red-cell deficiency is reported in an elderly diabetic Japanese male with no other haematological abnormality. Normal red cells contain four tetrameric isozymes of the enzyme made up from heart (H) and muscle (M) subunits. The four isozymes H_4: H_3 M_1: H_2 M_2: H_1 M_3 are normally present in the ratio 39:40:20:1, respectively; in the patient's red cells only the M isozyme was present with an activity about 5% of normal. Fructose-1,6-diphosphate, dihydroxyacetone phosphate and glyceraldehyde-3-phosphate levels were raised but whole blood pyruvate was normal and lactate low. Although dihydroxyacetone phosphate was raised ten times above the normal value, there was no apparent effect on the cells, in contrast to the suggested effect of this ester in triose phosphate isomerase deficiency (see earlier). A brother and five offspring of the propositus had red-cell LDH activity around 50% of the mean normal with a 50% lack of H_4.

DISORDERS OF THE PENTOSE PHOSPHATE PATHWAY

Under normal conditions this pathway is responsible for only some 2% of consumed glucose in mature, human red cells but it can be stimulated up to about 40-fold under the influence of an electron acceptor such as methylene blue. The pathway is a shunt, and two of its products, glyceraldehyde-3-phosphate and fructose-6-phosphate, are intermediates of the main anaerobic pathway (Fig. 14.4). The purpose of the shunt is twofold, providing ribose-5-phosphate which is involved in the limited purine metabolism of red cells, together with reducing potential to counter the oxidative assault to which red cells are subjected.

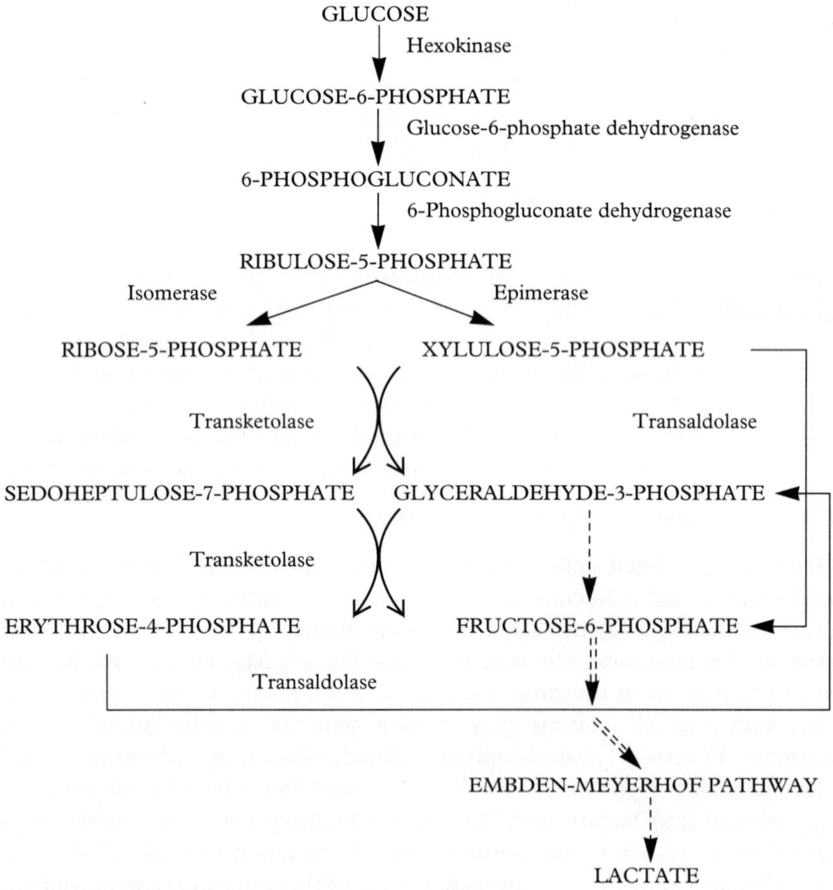

Fig. 14.4 The pentose phosphate pathway.

Purine metabolism

The ribose-5-phosphate (R5P) produced in the pentose phosphate pathway is a reactant in the formation of 5-phosphoribosyl-α-1-pyrophosphate (PRPP) from ATP:

$$\text{R5P} + \text{ATP} \xrightarrow[\text{synthetase}]{\text{PRPP}} \text{PRPP} + \text{AMP}$$

PRPP is involved in two types of reactions. It combines with L-glutamine as a preliminary step in purine ring synthesis, a reaction which does not occur in mature red cells; and also with adenine to form adenylic acid (AMP), a reaction catalysed by adenine phosphoribosyltransferase:

$$\text{PRPP} + \text{adenine} \xrightarrow[\text{adenine phosphoribosyltransferase}]{} \text{AMP} + \text{P}_i$$

This reaction is part of the purine salvage pathway and both reactants are present in red cells in low concentration (adenine 0.6 μM, PRPP 3.4 μM); their significance is not clear although red cells may be a general carrier for adenine. Both are elevated in Lesch–Nyhan syndrome (the severe form of hypoxanthine-guanine phosphoribosyltransferase (HPRT) deficiency (Ch. 8), as is the activity of adenine phosphoribosyltransferase. Megaloblastic marrow changes are seen in this condition and patients may have low serum folate and mild anaemia.

AMP arises in red cells from the two reactions above, from spontaneous ATP breakdown, and also via the adenylate kinase reaction:

$$\text{2ADP} \xrightarrow[\text{adenylate kinase}]{} \text{AMP} + \text{ATP}$$

Adenylate kinase provides a route to top up the ATP level where undue degradation to ADP may have occurred. The enzyme appears to be important in red cells, since a deficiency (McKusick 201600) is usually, although not invariably, accompanied by diminished red-cell survival with a non-spherocytic haemolytic anaemia. In one report of this rare disorder the defect coexisted with G6PD deficiency in an Arab family in whom both parents and six of nine offspring had a partial deficiency but were haematologically normal, while two siblings had severe deficiency of the enzyme accompanied by haemolytic anaemia; the ninth child was deceased. Total adenine nucleotides (AMP + ADP + ATP) were increased only in accord with the young red cell population present while the diphosphate was somewhat raised in relation to total nucleotide.

Adenylate kinase has three isozymes, AK_1, AK_2 and AK_3, and AK_1 is present in red cells. Both alleles have been cloned from the DNA of a deficient patient with haemolytic anaemia, and a substitution of arginine by tryptophan has been demonstrated.

Adenosine deaminase catalyses the deamination of adenosine or 2'-deoxyadenosine to inosine or 2'-deoxyinosine. Congenital deficiency of the enzyme is described in some 50 families in association with combined immunodeficiency, which arises through disturbed purine nucleoside metabolism in B and T lymphocytes. The disorder is inherited in an autosomal recessive manner. A decreased activity in the red cells of two patients with severely impaired cellular immunity was associated with a normal red-cell lifespan. Furthermore, a number of cases are known of complete red-cell adenosine deaminase deficiency without impaired cellular immunity. The disorder is described in detail in Chapter 8.

Markedly increased red-cell activity of adenosine deaminase with haemolytic anaemia is reported in some families. The overproduction appears to be tissue-specific, white cells and skin fibroblasts being normal.

Pyrimidine metabolism

The metabolism of pyrimidine in mature red cells is little understood although its relevance is apparent from the haemolytic anaemia associated with pyrimidine-5'-nucleotidase deficiency. This deficiency, described further in Chapter 8, is inherited in an autosomal recessive manner and is the third commonest cause of non-spherocytic haemolytic anaemia. It is notable for the prominent basophilic stippling in the red cells, reminiscent of lead poisoning. Red-cell pyrimidine nucleotides and glutathione are greatly increased. Pyridine-5'-nucleotidase activity is also reduced in lead poisoning and in β-thalassaemia minor.

Reducing capacity in red cells

Lacking the ability to synthesise protein or lipid, mature red cells cannot replace material damaged through oxidation, and the associated reactions linked to the pentose phosphate pathway are intended to prevent or reverse oxidative deterioration (Fig. 14.5).

The targets for oxidation in red cells are lipids, protein -SH groups and Fe^{2+} in haem. Lipids are maintained in status quo essentially through the presence of dietary vitamin E. Protein thiol groups are protected by glutathione (GSH) which is present in red cells in high concentration (approximately 2 mM), with less than 1% of the total in the ineffective oxidised dimer state (GSSG). GSH which becomes oxidised is reconverted to the reduced state by the action of NADPH-dependent GSH reductase. GSH plays other roles: as a cofactor for glyoxalase, whose function in red cells is uncertain; as the prosthetic group for glyceraldehyde-3-phosphate dehydrogenase; in the detoxication of certain foreign hydrocarbons, and in

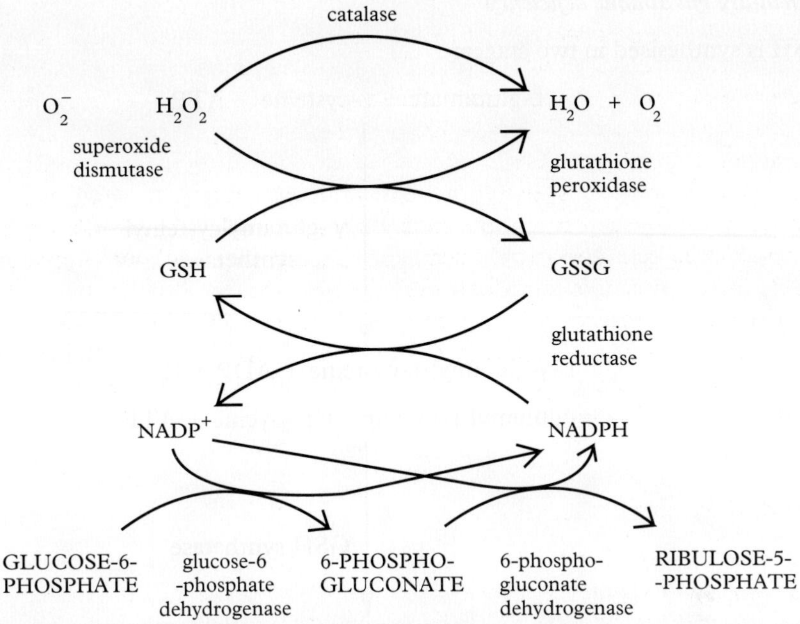

Fig. 14.5 Reactions associated with the pentose phosphate pathway.

the decomposition of H_2O_2 which is catalysed by GSH peroxidase. GSH is synthesised de novo with a $t_{1/2}$ in mature red cells of approximately 3 days; the rate of synthesis is modified by the known ability of oxidised GSH (GSSG) to leak from red cells.

Abnormal GSH levels occur in a number of different clinical conditions. High values are found in pyrimidine-5^1-nucleotidase deficiency, in the acquired disorders of iron deficiency, hypothyroidism and in some patients with lymphoma, myelofibrosis and acute and chronic leukaemia. Elevated levels are also found in the blood of normal neonates. Low levels of the tripeptide are found notably in GSH deficiency but also in G6PD and GSH reductase deficiency, renal and liver failure, hyperthyroidism, stomatocytosis and unstable haemoglobinopathy (see later). Low red-cell GSH levels arise through inadequate synthesis (congenital GSH deficiency), inadequate regeneration (GSH reductase and G6PD deficiency) or immoderate oxidative activity (exogenous oxidative assault). Regardless of the mechanism by which a markedly low level occurs, it is accompanied by haemolysis of the cells, although, as in stomatocytosis and the unstable haemoglobinopathies, it may not be the primary cause.

Hereditary glutathione deficiency

GSH is synthesised in two stages:

1. L-glutamate + L-cysteine + ATP

$$\downarrow \text{ γ -glutamylcysteinyl synthetase}$$

L-γ-glutamyl-L-cysteine + ADP + P_i

2. L-γ-glutamyl-L-cysteine + L-glycine + ATP

$$\downarrow \text{ GSH synthetase}$$

GSH + ADP + P_1

Both enzymes are present in red cells, but the other components comprising the γ-glutamyl cycle (Ch. 4) are not known to be present. Inherited GSH deficiency is a rare disorder accompanied by haemolytic anaemia, and arises from defects in either of the two synthetic enzymes. The notable features of γ-glutamylcysteine synthetase deficiency (McKusick 230450), in addition to haemolysis, are neuromuscular degeneration and aminoaciduria. GSH synthetase deficiency appears to occur in two forms; one as a mild disorder (McKusick 231900) affecting red cells only, with haemolytic anaemia as the sole clinical feature. The second form is more severe, and the haemolytic anaemia is accompanied by metabolic acidosis, abnormal CNS function and excessive 5-oxoprolinuria with a number of tissues involved (see Chapter 3).

Glutathione reductase (GR)

Low red-cell activity of this enzyme is well recorded, but almost all cases have arisen from low dietary riboflavin which depletes the enzyme of its flavin cofactor. In the inherited form the deficiency (McKusick 138300) is rare, the mode of inheritance uncertain and the condition not associated with any haematological disorder.

Acquired deficiency, arising from riboflavin insufficiency, is associated with a variety of haematological abnormalities – non-spherocytic haemolytic anaemia, pancytopenia, leukopenia, thrombocytopenia, acute leukaemia, haemophilia B, homozygous Hbc disease and α-thalassaemia, and it has repeatedly been shown both in vivo and in vitro that supplementation with riboflavin or FAD restores low GSH reductase activity to normal. Elevated levels of red-cell activity occur in cases of high dietary riboflavin and nicotinic acid, and also in uraemia, cirrhosis, diabetes mellitus and gout.

Glutathione peroxidase

The decomposition of H_2O_2 in red cells is catalysed both by glutathione peroxidase and catalase. The former reaction is more effective with low levels of peroxide, while catalase activity preponderates in the presence of high levels. That glutathione peroxidase is vital and the more important of the two for cell survival seems clear from the haemolytic anaemia which arises from its deficiency; catalase deficiency is without any haematological consequences. Glutathione peroxidase is specific for GSH but will reduce a number of peroxides other than H_2O_2. The enzyme is unusual in lacking haem or flavin as a prosthetic group and in containing selenium; the enzyme in red cells shows a direct correlation with the plasma selenium.

Low glutathione peroxidase activity occurs in the red cells of premature and full-term neonates and is one cause of their sensitivity to oxidative assault. The deficiency is temporary; activities reach adult levels after some 6 months postnatally. The few known cases of hereditary deficiency are associated with haemolysis (McKusick 231700). Acquired deficiency is associated with march haemoglobinuria, disseminated intravascular coagulation with red-cell fragmentation, acanthocytosis and iron-deficiency anaemia. Ethnic differences are reported within normal individuals, Jews having lower values than North European non-Jews. It is the variety of conditions under which low values occur that has complicated the demonstration of truly inherited glutathione peroxidase deficiency as well as its mode of inheritance.

Catalase

Inherited red-cell catalase deficiency (McKusick 115500) is a rare defect affecting Japanese and Swiss people. The mutant enzymes are structurally different in the two groups and whilst neither is associated with any haematological disorder, affected Japanese also have oral gangrene. In the latter group the disorder follows an autosomal recessive pattern; red cells of heterozygotes contain around 50% normal catalase activity while homozygotes give values of only 0–3% normal. Nasal, marrow and liver catalase is also abnormal and the Japanese mutant appears to be more stable than that in affected Swiss. Swiss homozygotes yield 0–1.3% of normal red-cell activity whilst heterozygotes have 60–85%. It is unclear why only Japanese mutants show clinical features of the disorder. The consequence to red cells of containing either mutant is an inability to decompose high levels of

H_2O_2. It has been shown with the Swiss mutant that the pentose phosphate pathway is slightly stimulated, a consequence of its dependence upon glutathione peroxidase for peroxide degradation; nevertheless this route appears to be adequate even when acatalasic red cells are exposed to doses of primaquine, provoking a haemolytic response in G6PD-deficiency.

Glucose-6-phosphate dehydrogenase (G6PD) (McKusick 305900)

The purpose of the pentose phosphate pathway in red cells is to maintain GSH in the reduced state and to provide ribose-5-phosphate (see below). G6PD is the first enzyme in the pathway and its activity is maintained by three factors: availability of glucose-6-phosphate, and the levels of $NADP^+$ and of NADPH. In the resting state the coenzyme is almost completely reduced and G6PD operates at a low rate; inhibition of the enzyme by NADPH is reversible and the activity of G6PD depends upon the $NADPH/NADP^+$ ratio. The enzyme is made up of identical units (mol. wt. about 59 kDa) and functions in dimeric or tetrameric form depending upon pH. The complete sequence of amino acids for G6PD is known both from protein sequencing, which suggests 513 residues, and from isolation and characterisation of cDNA and of genomic clones for G6PD, which yields 515 amino acids. The gene comprises 13 exons and 12 introns, covering some 18 kilobase pairs.[10]

Approximately 400 variants of the normal human enzyme (G6PD B) are known and deficiency of the enzyme, that is a low activity, is the commonest of the red-cell enzymopathies, affecting some 400 million people worldwide. In some of the rare cases the variant is particularly unstable and the very low activity of the enzyme is associated with a chronic non-spherocytic haemolytic anaemia; the majority of variants display only moderately low activity in intact cells and give rise to haemolytic episodes only after ingestion of certain oxidative drugs, fava beans, or with some infections or metabolic acidosis. Variants have been arranged for convenience into five groups[10] (see Table 14.5) depending upon maximum G6PD activity determined in fresh haemolysates. Of the large number of variants, 98% of cases carry either G6PD A- (African variant, primaquine sensitivity) or the G6PD Mediterranean (favism) variant. All other affected cases carrying a rarer variant. An exception is G6PD Canton which is relatively common.

In addition to the normal enzyme G6PD B, peptide mapping of both G6PD A+ and Hektoen shows both to have a single amino acid substitution. More recently, molecular analysis of several other variants has been undertaken, showing single nucleotide substitutions in all variants except three.

Genetic features. The G6PD locus is at the end of the long arm of the X chromosome, close to the loci for haemophilia, colour-blindness and adrenoleukodystrophy. Affected G6PD-deficient males are hemizygotes

Table 14.5 Classification of G6PD variants. See Beutler[10] for further details

Group	Symptoms	Variants	Activity (% of normal)	Examples
1	Chronic haemolysis	47	0–35 (mean 9)	Oklahoma Chicago Boston Tokyo
2	Usually no haemolysis	37	0–10 (mean 4)	Mediterranean Ferrara Taiwan
3	Moderate to mild deficiency	36	7–75 (mean 27)	A- Canton
4	Mild or no deficiency	19	6–105 (mean 103)	B+ A+ Baltimore
5	Increased activity	1	400	Hektoen

while females are heterozygotes; because of random inactivation of one or other of the two female X chromosomes early in embryological development (Lyon hypothesis, see Ch.1), females heterozygous for G6PD deficiency produce two populations of red cells, one enzyme-deficient and the other normal. Total red-cell G6PD activities in blood samples are intermediate in value, and vary in different patients between normal and male hemizygous levels, the exact values depending upon the proportion of normal to deficient cells in the blood sample. It also follows from gene inactivation, that normal males and females have red-cell G6PD activities within a common normal range.

Mechanism of haemolysis In G6PD deficiency, the essential shortcoming is the inability of the red cell to cope with oxidative attack from endogenous and exogenous sources. Haemolytic drugs are exogenous agents which, either directly or via their metabolites, produce reactants such as H_2O_2 and free radicals, which provoke in red cells the observed symptoms of oxidative damage, that is, the presence of Heinz bodies, methaemoglobin, sulphaemoglobin, red-cell fragmentation and the features of intravascular haemolysis. Damage also occurs to the membrane and intracellular enzymes.

The consequences to normal red cells of oxidation are that GSH reacts to protect and reverse -SH group oxidation, being converted in the process to the inactive dimer GSSG. This dimer is also formed through the action of GSH peroxidase when it catalyses the degradation of H_2O_2. GSSG is readily reduced to GSH by the action of GSH reductase, which requires NADPH as coenzyme, converting it to $NADP^+$. $NADP^+$ is a stimulus to the pentose phosphate pathway whose activity can increase some 40-fold in normal red cells, and the maintenance of GSH levels is assured provided the oxidative assault does not swamp the system. A second target for oxidation is the ferrous iron in the haem groups of haemoglobin (see later); this oxidation can also be reversed through the action of both NADH- and NADPH-linked methaemoglobin reductase, as well from a small but unpredictable direct reduction by GSH and ascorbate. In G6PD deficiency, methaemoglobin formation takes place following drug action but is not a marked feature since the old cells contain more methaemoglobin and are destroyed preferentially by the oxidative assault.

The problem in G6PD deficiency is that although the cells have an only slightly lowered GSH content, once this is consumed during an oxidative assault there is no mechanism for its adequate replenishment. With most variants the pentose phosphate pathway can be stimulated to some extent, but this depends upon the activity of the variant, and stimulation is usually inadequate to replace and maintain the GSH consumed. The ability of red cells to synthesise replacement GSH de novo is quite insufficient in this situation.

Subjects in group 1 (Table 14.5) are made up of a considerable variety of rare variants. They have a chronic non-spherocytic haemolytic anaemia in the absence of exogenous agents, a consequence of the low activity of an unstable variant in their red cells, and they are at particular risk from oxidative drugs. They differ also from the two common variants in that tissues other than white cells and eye lens are affected (see below). The measured activity in a blood sample from any individual, abnormal or normal, is a mean value because young cells have a higher, and old cells a lower, activity of most enzymes. With group 1 patients this is critical because the low values in old cells are insufficient to maintain the pentose phosphate pathway and protect the cells against the endogenous oxidative assault to which all red cells are prey. The other groups have variants with higher mean values for G6PD activity, and since these patients do not have a haemolytic anaemia under normal conditions, the activities are presumably adequate to cope with normal oxidative stress. However, with an exogeneous oxidative attack, as from certain drugs given in therapeutic doses, all variants (except group 5) are susceptible and the severity of the haemolytic crisis depends upon the ability of the cells to marshal their principal detoxication mechanism. Clearly, the level of administered drug also determines the degree of red-cell destruction, and very high doses would destroy even normal red cells if their protective mechanisms were swamped.

American male negro volunteers with G6PD deficiency have been carefully studied after therapeutic doses (30 mg base per 24 h) of the antimalarial primaquine, and the sequence of haematological events is well documented. Evidence of haemolysis is apparent within 3 days of receiving the drug; an acute phase follows, lasting 8–12 days, when the haemoglobin reaches a minimum and clinical jaundice is evident. The urine contains excess urobilin and haemoglobinuria may be present. By the tenth day recovery is evident and a reticulocyte peak occurs at around 14 days. The haemoglobin level rises to near normal at 28 or more days. With continued drug ingestion at the same dose the degree of haemolysis settles to a steady state; if the drug is stopped the haematological state reverts to the pre-dose condition, but if drug dosage is increased then haemolysis also increases and is maintained with continuing ingestion of the drug at this more severe level. Thus, the haemolytic anaemia arising from drugs is self-limiting, and this arises because old and more sensitive cells are preferentially destroyed, so that a younger cohort appears with increased G6PD activities; increasing the dosage renders the older cells of the younger cohort vulnerable.

Other haemolytic drugs differ in their potency but produce a similar overall haematological sequence.

Haemolytic agents. A large number of drugs have been implicated as haemolytic agents in G6PD deficiency, but for most of them either there has been no confirmation of toxicity, or an infection for which the drug was prescribed was itself the haemolytic precipitant. Drugs and chemicals regarded as haemolytic in G6PD deficiency are shown in Table 14.6.

Haemolytic episodes in G6PD deficiency arising from infections rather than from drugs are well established. Haemolysis tends to be mild, although it may be severe and recovery slow because marrow depression accompanies the infection. Haemolysis is common in bacterial pneumonia, viral hepatitis and typhoid fever, and in infection with salmonella, *Escherichia coli* proteus, staphylococci, β-haemolytic streptococci and rickettsiae.

Diabetic acidosis may also provoke haemolysis in G6PD-deficient individuals. The pentose phosphate pathway is not pH-sensitive although

Table 14.6 Drugs and chemicals implicated as haemolytic in G6PD deficiency

Acetanilide
Methylene blue
Naphthalene (lavatory deodorant, mothballs)
Nalidixic acid (Mictral, Negram, Uriben)
Niridazole (Ambilhar)
Nitrofurantoin (Furadantin, Furan, Berkfurin, Macrodantin, Ceduran, Urantoin)
Pamaquine (Plasmoquine)
Pentaquine
Primaquine
Sulphanilamide (Rhinamid)
Sulphacetamide (Albucid, Bleph-10 Liquifilm, Ocusol, Cortucid, Sulfaped, Isoptocetamide, Sultrin)
Sulphapyridine (M & B 693)
Sulphamethoxazole (Gantanol, Bactrim, Septrin, Cotrimox, Comox, Fectrim, Laratrim, Co-trimoxazole)
Thiazosulphone (Promizole)
Toluidine blue
Trinitrotoluene

the first intermediate of the pathway, glucose-6-phosphate, is also an intermediate in the main anaerobic pathway whose activity falls with decreasing pH. However, glucose-6-phosphate increases with pH fall and so the mechanism is unclear.

Both the African (A−) and Mediterranean variants are oxidant-drug sensitive, but the very low activity of the latter variant renders it more drug-sensitive than the A−, in particular to fava beans (see below) which do not affect individuals with the A− variant.

G6PD and malaria. Many studies have shown that G6PD deficiency confers protection against falciparum malaria, and that this advantage accounts for the large-scale distribution of the disorder. However, the correlation is geographically variable and better where favism exists. Malarial parasites can invade G6PD-deficient cells normally but maturation is impaired. How inherited disorders of red cells present an unsatisfactory environment to the developing parasite is a complex problem currently under active study. The host red cell undergoes considerable change during parasite growth with, for example, a fall in intracellular pH and ATP, increased Ca^{2+} permeability and an unbalanced monovalent cation content. Membrane changes are also observed. Metabolites produced by parasites require detoxication, and in G6PD deficiency there is an inability to respond to oxidative stress, so that, if G6PD activity is low as in the group 2 variants (Table 14.5), neither parasite nor red cell may survive.

Neonatal jaundice. Red-cell G6PD activity is above normal in the red cells of normal neonates, although they are at risk for the first few months of life because their red cells contain low levels of GSH peroxidase, NADH methaemoglobin reductase, catalase and possibly vitamin E; this sensitivity increases with prematurity. In the absence of undue oxidative stress, related haematological problems do not arise, and the sensitivity disappears at around 3 months of life when a new population of red cells has turned over with adult enzyme activities.

Neonates with G6PD deficiency are at a particular risk from oxidative haemolysis and there is the possibility of neonatal jaundice, whose severity depends upon the variant enzyme in the red cells. Thus, deficient Mediterranean, Thai and Chinese neonates have a high incidence of jaundice. Oddly, American infants with the A-variant are not unduly affected, but Nigerian infants with the same variant carry a high risk.

The African variant (*G6PD A*−) (McKusick 305900.0002)

The discovery of G6PD deficiency in 1956 was the outcome of studies of the haematological effects on American negroes (that is, of African stock) of the antimalarial primaquine, a drug harmless to normal patients in therapeutic doses, but provoking an acute, self-limiting haemolytic attack in some 11% of male negroes; these affected cases were later shown to be G6PD-deficient. An associated red-cell abnormality was a somewhat low red-cell GSH. The incidence among affected female heterozygotes was about 3%.

Electrophoresis elicited that 70% of normal American male negroes carry the common and normal B+ enzyme in their red cells, while the remainder have a second A+ variant which has a near-normal activity. In the A+ variant aspartate replaces asparagine, and this confers increased electrophoretic mobility on A+ (110 compared with 100 for B+). It was the absence of a discernible A+ band in affected male negroes that caused them to be designated as A−. Normal African females are also B+ or A+, but some are both, while affected heterozygotes are A–/A+, A–/B+ or homozygous A−.

The enzymic activities of the B+, A+ and A– variants are 100, 90 and 8–20% respectively, but their kinetic properties are similar (Table 14.7). The low activity of the A− variant is not due to impaired synthesis; activity in red-cell precursors and reticulocytes is normal, but the enzyme appears somewhat unstable, with fewer active molecules present in mature cells.

In addition to red cells, the eye lens has a reduced G6PD activity in affected negroes, a consequence of the similar and limited cell metabolism in the two tissues. Whole-body studies have indicated that the mean basal metabolic rate may be less than normal in affected negroes, suggesting that other tissues are involved. However, other tissues can synthesise protein to offset an increased degradation of the enzyme, and, for example, G6PD in the white cells of affected negroes has the same characteristics as the red-cell enzyme but a near-normal activity, presumably because replacement of degraded enzyme takes place. Platelet G6PD activity is also low in G6PD-deficienct negroes.

The intermediate values found in red-cell samples from affected females can be a problem in the event of the need for diagnosis during a haemolytic crisis, because the enlarged young red-cell population containing increased

Table 14.7 Some characteristics of common G6PD variants

Variant	Mobility	Activity	Heat stability	pH curve	K_m (μM)	
					G6P	NADP$^+$
B+	100	100	Normal	Normal	50–70	2.9–4.4
A+	110	80–100	Normal	Normal	50–70	2.9–4.4
A–	110	8–20	Normal	Normal	50–70	2.9–4.4
Mediterranean (favism)	100	0–7	Labile	Biphasic	19–26	1.2–1.6
Canton	105	4–24	Labile	Biphasic	18–36	—

G6PD activity of both variants may give assay values which mask a deficiency. Standard assays measure enzyme activity in the overall red-cell sample and will not reveal the deficiency, which can be observed only with a cytochemical technique. Alternatively, family studies may reveal the diagnosis, or fresh blood may be tested after the crisis when the cell population has resumed its usual age distribution.

The Mediterranean variant (*Favism, Baghdad spring fever*) (McKusick 305900.0006)

This is the second common mutant, and the haemolytic crises following ingestion by affected individuals of fresh fava beans (*vicia faba*) have long been recognised. Amongst his other activities, Pythagoras founded a religion based upon some 15 tenets, of which one forbade the eating of beans. The term favism appeared at the turn of the century, but the mechanism of the acute haemolytic episodes was not appreciated until a Meditteranean variant was demonstrated. The mutant is prevalent in all countries bordering on the Mediterranean basin and in the Middle East, but with a markedly non-uniform distribution, a consequence of both static and mobile populations and the diverse ethnic origins of the inhabitants. Favism also occurs in Taiwan and southern China, where fava beans are eaten and group 2 variants occur (Table 14.4). In the Mediterranean littoral, collected data from a number of surveys show, for example, that 6.6% of some 16 000 Greeks tested and 8% of approximately 15 000 people in polyethnic Israel were G6PD-deficient; but the latter value masks wide differences between ethnic groups within Israel. The incidence in central Italy is low, as in Iran (0.7%), but in Sardinia the overall value is 17%.

The Mediterranean variant is structurally different from the A− enzyme; red-cell activity in affected males is only 0–7% and it follows that they are more drug-sensitive than A− individuals, and to a wider range of haemolytic agents. Their low red-cell activity can also explain the sensitivity to fava beans, since A− Africans are not affected. It is suggested by many authors that the presence of the Mediterranean variant is a necessary but not sufficient condition for favism, and that other factors, genetic and environmental, are involved. Allergy to fava bean pollen is not now regarded as a factor, and the increased potency of the bean when fresh and containing effective levels of toxic agent(s) is explicable, but the mechanism of increased tolerance to the bean with subject age, and the failure of the majority of individuals with the Mediteranean variant to develop favism are not clear.

The period between bean ingestion and advent of haemolytic crisis varies with the type, potency, culinary state and amount of beans eaten, as well as gastric and intestinal transit time and activity; signs of impending crisis are nevertheless present within 48 h. Cases are on record of the toxic factor(s) being passed to breast-fed infants, and Iranian folklore discourages mothers from eating beans for 6 weeks following delivery.

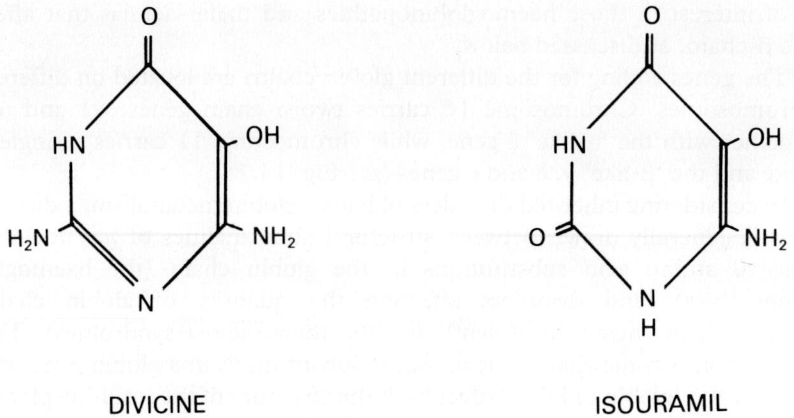

Fig. 14.6 Structures of divicine and isouramil.

Fresh fava beans contain several glycosides, and recent studies implicate the two pyrimidine aglycones divicine and isouramil as effective haemolytic agents (Fig. 14.6). They both have reducing properties and can react with O_2 to form H_2O_2, the oxidised pyrimidines can then react with GSH to reform divicine and isouramil. The net result is a catalytic cycle in which GSH is oxidised by molecular O_2. These pyrimidines have been shown to oxidise GSH, increase methaemoglobin, decrease deformability and cause membrane damage in red cells in vitro to a greater extent with the Mediterranean than with the normal B+ variant.

Whilst favism is confined to the Mediterranean littoral and the Far East, isolated cases are reported in Britain in patients without apparent foreign ancestry who have eaten fava beans.

DISORDERS OF HAEMOGLOBIN

Abnormalities of haem synthesis are considered in Chapter 9. In the present chapter, quantitative and qualitative disorders of globin synthesis are described.

Globin synthesis. Globin is a tetramer consisting of two α- or α-like and two β- or β-like chains. In adult life the major globin present in red cells in most individuals is $\alpha_2\ \beta_2$ (HbA), with a minor component of $\alpha_2\ \delta_2$ (HbA2). During embryonic and fetal life, other haemoglobins are synthesized: Hb Gower 1 ($\zeta_2\ \epsilon_2$), Gower 2 ($\alpha_2\ \epsilon_2$) and Portland ($\alpha_2\epsilon_2$) in the embryo, followed by fetal haemoglobin, HbF ($\alpha_2\gamma_2$) in the fetus and newborn. Synthesis of γ-chains and hence of HbF ceases gradually over the first few months of extrauterine life, alongside a gradual increase in β-chain synthesis. Hence disorders of β-globin metabolism do not become clinically apparent until a few months after birth. The mechanism that determines the cessation of γ-chain synthesis in favour of β-chains (the 'switch') is of interest in those haemoglobinopathies and thalassaemias that affect the β-chain, as discussed below.

The genes coding for the different globin chains are located on different chromosomes. Chromosome 16 carries two α-chain genes, α1 and α2, together with the 'α-like' ζ gene, while chromosome 11 carries a single β gene and the 'β-like' γ, δ and ϵ genes (see Fig. 14.7).

In considering inherited disorders of haemoglobin metabolism, a distinction is generally drawn between structural abnormalities of haemoglobin due to amino acid substitutions in the globin chain (the haemoglobinopathies), and disorders affecting the quantity of globin chains produced, or their rate of synthesis (the thalassaemia syndromes). This distinction is somewhat artificial. Some substitutions in a globin gene (e.g. that for the -globin of HbE) affect both the structure of the resulting globin, and its rate of synthesis, and, additionally, its intracellular survival: poor survival implying deficient haemoglobinisation of mature red cells. Such combined quantitative and qualitative defects of haemoglobin are often termed *thalassaemic haemoglobinopathies*.[17] For simplicity, however, the distinction between the two main types of disorder is largely adhered to in the description that follows.

Haemoglobinopathies (McKusick 141900)

Of the many variants of HbA, only a few are associated with haematological disorders; the most important of these are HbS, HbC and HbE, the HbM group, unstable haemoglobins, and haemoglobins with abnormal oxygen affinity. The structure and function of normal haemoglobin have been considered elsewhere (see, for example, Huehns 1982[12]).

HbS, (Sickle cell syndromes)

In haemoglobin S, valine replaces glutamate as the sixth amino acid of the β-chain; this alters the electrical charge on the molecule, giving a slower electrophoretic mobility, by which it can be identified. The abnormality is due to a single base substitution in the β-chain gene. In the homozygous form, sickle-cell disease, an abnormal gene is inherited from each parent, whereas in the mild heterozygous form, sickle-cell trait, a single abnormal gene is inherited. The disorder occurs primarily in negro populations, with a low incidence in the Mediterranean area, southern Arabia and India.

Hbs does not appear at birth, but becomes demonstrable during the first few months of life when the abnormal β-chains begin to be synthesised. In sickle-cell disease the anaemia is usually severe, with variable haemolysis. Reticulocyte counts vary from 10 to 20%, with notable polychromasia and some punctate basophilia.

Howell–Jolly bodies and siderocytes may be present, with normoblasts in severe cases. The tendency of red cells to sickle in vivo produces a range of

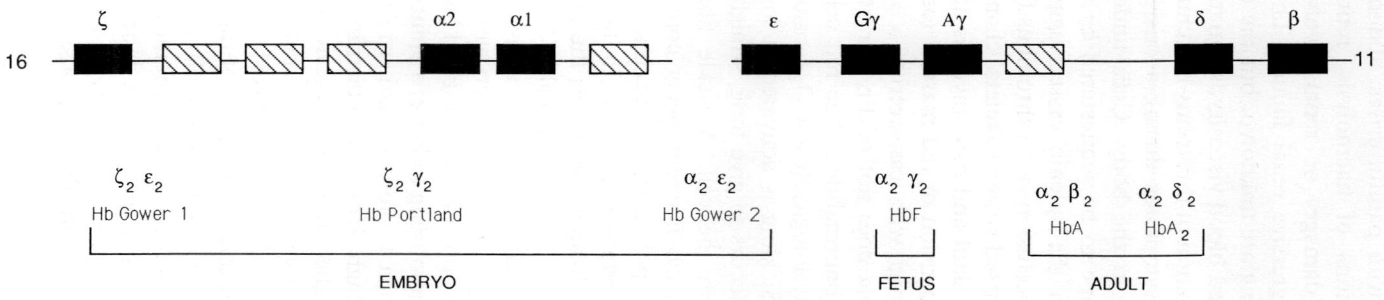

Fig. 14.7 The α-and β-globin gene clusters. Active genes are labelled with their Greek letters. Silent pseudogenes for globin chains are shown hatched and unlabelled. The different types of haemoglobin molecules formed during development are shown below. (Adapted from Weatherall et al [14]).

clinical symptoms together with painful crises: abdominal, bone or joint pain, leg ulcers, exacerbations of haemolysis, retinal and pulmonary lesions, priapism, hepatic damage, or renal involvement which may provoke haematuria or progressive renal failure. The conditions which initiate a bout of local sickling are unknown, but the event is followed by red-cell aggregation, increased blood viscosity, stagnation and anoxia with further sickling and the formation of thrombus-like clumps.

The diversity of clinical symptoms during a crisis arises because the event may occur anywhere in the body. Cells undergoing sickling are sufficiently abnormal in shape to be sequestered by the spleen, and the adverse environment within the splenic vessels aggravates the sickling process. Repeated vascular occlusions with thrombus formation eventually produce a shrunken and fibrosed spleen. Skeletal changes also occur, with periosteal thickening in the skull and osteomyelitis at sites of ischaemia. Bone deformities due to expansion of red marrow (as seen in the thalassaemias) may also occur, though with less severity.

In sickle-cell trait, anaemia does not occur, nor are there usually any clinical or haematological abnormalities. The red cells contain 20–45% HbS, but sickle only at unphysiologically low O_2 tensions.

The sickling process. Sickling is activated at low O_2 tension when aggregation of deoxy-HbS occurs to give long, straight fibres which form parallel bundles and deform the cell. A sickle fibre comprises seven filaments plaited together, each filament being composed of two linear threads of molecules. Further polymerisation occurs only if the cell content of deoxy-Hbs is above a certain minimum. In homozygotes the HbS content is 80–100%, and with such high levels the cells will sickle within the normal range of O_2 tension. The red cells also contain HbA_2 and HbF in concentrations that vary from individual to individual and from cell to cell, and so the degree of sickling varies between patients. Haemoglobin in the oxy- state is uninvolved in polymerisation. Fetal haemoglobin (HbF) is more effective than HbA in inhibiting sickling, a point of relevance both in infants and in populations such as those of southern Arabia where the HbF content of red cells may be high. HbF is also distributed non-uniformly in red cells, and those with a higher content will survive longer.

Sickling in vivo occurs mainly in the venous circulation and is reversed in the arterial circulation. Cells which remain sickled cannot negotiate the capillaries and are destroyed; this is one cause of the haemolytic anaemia. Sickled cells contain spicules which may break off, resulting in loss of cells or in membrane changes which increase membrane fragility; membrane damage can also arise from precipitation of HbS on the cytoplasmic surface.

Repeated sickling–unsickling further damages the membrane and produces stiffening which leads eventually to irreversibly sickled cells (ISC); these are a major cause of haemolysis since they do not survive long, especially while the spleen still functions. Direct evidence that the membrane is abnormal in sickled cells is given by increased Na^+ and K^+ flux, with net loss of K^+ over Na^+ to give cell dehydration. Lactate production is increased in vitro, with a fall in intracellular pH. The red cells in sickle-cell disease have an increased Ca^{2+} content and increased permeability to this cation on sickling, which may contribute to their increased rigidity.

The mixed sickle-cell syndromes. Inheritance of HbS from one parent and a second β-chain abnormality from the other leads to a spectrum of mixed syndromes, characterised by sickling of varying degrees of severity. The combination of HbS with a β-thalassaemia gene (HbS/β-thal) can produce a syndrome clinically indistinguishable from homozygous sickle-cell disease: if the β-thalassaemia gene suppresses β-globin production only partially the condition may be much milder, with a higher haemoglobin level and less frequent sickling crises. Coinheritance of a HbS and HbC gene (see below) is also very common, since the two genes exist in the same populations. HbS/C disease is a sickle-cell syndrome in which again the haemoglobin level is higher and (in many cases) sickling is less common. However, the higher haemoglobin is not an advantage, since blood viscosity is higher and sickling attacks can be more catastrophic. Pregnancy and labour, and surgical operations, represent the greatest risk to such patients. Sickling in the retinal vessels is also particularly common in this condition.

Malaria and HbS. In heterozygotes (HbA/S), the presence of HbS protects against the successful development of malarial parasites at the erythrocytic stage, and probably also later when the modified host red cell has adhered to endothelial cells in the deep vasculature. This resistance of HbS-containing cells to the presence of malarial parasites involves several intracellular events whose practical significance is not currently clear, but the parasite can induce sickling which accelerates removal of the infected cell from the circulation, the so-called 'suicidal infection'. Also, the formation of HbS polymers is part of the sickling process and these may be detrimental to the parasite. It is possible that when infected red cells later develop their protruberances on the cell surface and adhere to endothelial cells, the schizogony phase, sickling occurs which puts the cell at further risk.

Haemoglobin C

Like HbS, this results from a single amino acid substitution at position 6 in the β-chain: glutamate is replaced by lysine. The main importance of this variant is in its interaction with haemoglobin S to produce a sickle-cell syndrome (see above). Homozygous HbC gives rise to a mild haemolytic anaemia with prominent target cells; intraerythrocytic haemoglobin crystals form and cause increased red-cell rigidity with a shortened lifespan. Heterozygous HbC is of no clinical importance.

Haemoglobin E

This is the second most common abnormal haemoglobin in the world, and occurs at high frequency in South-East Asian populations. A single nucleotide substitution is responsible, leading to incorporation of lysine instead of glutamate at position 26 of the β-chain. In addition to being chemically abnormal, the haemoglobin is produced at an abnormally slow rate and has a shortened intracellular survival; this likens it to a thalassaemic condition and it is more fully discussed below under β-thalassaemia. Homozygous HbE gives rise to a mild microcytic anaemia, often with a haemolytic element (raised reticulocytes and splenomegaly). The heterozygous condition is of no clinical significance.

Methaemoglobin and HbM

The loss of an electron from haem Fe II converts haemoglobin (FeII) into methaemoglobin(FeIII) (MetHb) whose ferric iron has no oxygen-carrying capacity. MetHb is formed continuously in normal red cells in vivo at a slow rate, but the level in fresh, whole blood is maintained at about 1% by the several reducing systems in the cell, particularly NADH-linked methaemoglobin reductase (diaphorase). High levels of MetHb can arise in only three ways: induction by chemical agents including drugs, inherited diaphorase deficiency, or the presence of a haemoglobin variant (of the HbM group).

MetHb is not itself associated with haemolysis; the main symptom of methaemoglobinaemia is cyanosis through inadequate oxygen carriage. This is present when MetHb reaches 10–20% of total haemoglobin, although such a level is tolerated clinically without ill effects. At around 40% MetHb, symptoms of fatigue, dizziness, headaches, exertional dyspnoea and tachycardia may be present and at about 60% stupor occurs; levels of MetHb above 70% are lethal.

When methaemoglobinaemia arises through the action upon red cells of chemicals or drugs, there is usually concomitant oxidative damage to the cell and so haemolysis may be an accompaniment. An exception is nitrite, which at sufficient concentration will give rise to MetHb but without causing haemolysis. MetHb accumulates if mechanisms for reducing it are absent, as in diaphorase deficiency. Apart from the accumulation of MetHb, there are no other abnormalities apparent in this deficiency, which is one of the two inherited red-cell disorders that are treatable (the other being hereditary spherocytosis, see earlier). Either ascorbate (500 mg/24 h orally) or, more effectively and certainly more dramatically, methylene blue (100–300 mg/24 h orally), will maintain MetHb at a normal low level. The former acts by direct chemical reduction of MetHb, the latter by acting as an electron acceptor to NADPH, stimulating the pentose phosphate pathway to turn the coenzyme over at a faster rate and make NADPH more available for NADPH-linked MetHb reductase.

There are several variants of the HbM group (e.g. HbM Boston, Hyde Park, Milwaukee, Saskatoon and Iwate). In each of these an amino acid replacement affects the binding of haem FeII to histidine. In four of the variants histidine itself is replaced by tyrosine, while in HbM Milwaukee substitution of glutamate for valine in the β-chain haem pocket results in bonding of the glutamate γ-COOH group with FeIII. As a consequence the iron in these variants is locked into the FeIII state and cannot be reduced by the systems which normally convert MetHb to Hb. Other HbM variants are described but not fully characterised. In some, the red-cell lifespan is shortened but other abnormalities are not described and the only clinical symptom is cyanosis. Affected patients are heterozygotes with 10–25% of their haemoglobin in the FeIII state.

The distinction between MetHb and HbM is made from their absorption spectra. MetHb has a characteristic peak at 630 nm while the HbMs have an identifiable peak at lower wavelengths; in addition, some variants display differences in the 500–600 nm region. HbM can also be identified electrophoretically.

The unstable haemoglobins

This group of variants (e.g. Hb Shepherds Bush, Zürich), earlier called the congenital Heinz-body anaemias, has in common an inherent instability of the haemoglobin molecule which results in spontaneous intracellular degradation to yield Heinz bodies. These are seen in methyl-violet stained red cells only from splenectomised patients, because the spleen can extract intracellular particles without sequestering the cells. Affected subjects have a non-spherocytic haemolytic anaemia: cells in which insoluble haemoglobin breakdown products are formed undergo irreversible damage with shortening of the cell lifespan. This process is hastened by auto-oxidation of the haemoglobin, yielding oxidants that cause further membrane damage.

Unstable haemoglobins can be demonstrated by starch gel or polyacrylamide electrophoresis, or by exploiting the instability of the haemoglobin. Tests which depend upon the lability of the haemoglobin molecule involve heating buffered haemolysates at 50°C, or at 37°C in the presence of isopropanol, or simply shaking, and noting precipitation of the unstable haemoglobin; HbA can withstand such treatment and remains in solution. The precipitated material consists primarily of the unstable globin containing decreased amounts of haem. Otherwise, fresh cells can be incubated for 24 h when they produce abnormal amounts of inclusion bodies and MetHb. Variants differ both in their stability and intracellular concentration, and this is reflected in the severity of the haemolytic anaemia, which varies between patients from mild to severe. Blood films show polychromasia, anisocytosis, hypochromia and often punctate basophilia. The oxygen affinity of the haemoglobin varies between variants, and some patients excrete dark urine due to the presence of dipyrrolic metabolites of degraded haem.

For the most part, the defect in unstable variants lies at the α–β interface or within the haem pocket; this increases the flexibility and unfolding of the globin. Breakdown of unstable haemoglobin variants occurs generally through loss of haem groups, which further destabilises the globin moiety and decreases its solubility.[13] Dissociation of the molecule into separate α- and β-chains can occur, and also a subunit can be weakened by distortion. Depending upon the variant, some or all of these reactions may occur. Breakdown of the unstable haemoglobin is probably initiated by MetHb formation which leads to insoluble hemichrome (dimer) production, and -SH groups become inactive through mixed disulphide formation with GSH. The loss of GSH, but particularly the presence of insoluble degradation products, damages the cell membrane and shortens its lifespan. A further hazard to the cells is their sensitivity to oxidant drugs or viral infections.

The unstable haemoglobins described above are rare, and arise from single amino acid substitutions in globin chains. A much commoner unstable haemoglobin is HbH, a β-globin tetramer which occurs in α-thalassaemia.

The thalassaemia syndromes (McKusick 273500)

The common feature of this group of disorders is an inherited abnormality in the rate of synthesis of one or other globin chain, directly resulting in a reduction in normal haemoglobin production. The poorly haemoglobinized red cells are microcytic and hypochromic. In addition, the imbalance between α- and β-chain production leads to accumulation of excess unpaired α- or β-chains. These are unstable, and give rise to a variable haemolytic element leading to intramedullary death of red cell precursors, or to haemolysis of circulating red cells. Haemolysis is probably more important than underproduction in causing anaemia. The symptoms common to many thalassaemic syndromes include anaemia, haemolytic jaundice, splenomegaly, and abnormal skeletal development due to a gross expansion of the haemopoietic marrow.

A genetic abnormality causing a thalassaemic picture may occur in association with an inherited haemoglobinopathy; such mixed disorders are common, and give rise to a wide variety of clinical syndromes (see below). Extensive reviews of the genetics and clinical features of the thalassaemias are available.[14–16]

The primary defect in thalassaemia is in the DNA sequence, but it can be expressed at any stage of protein biosynthesis. There are marked differences in this respect between α- and β-thalassaemias.

α-Thalassaemia

The great majority (over 95%) of known α-thalassaemia genes represent deletions of one or both α-globin genes on chromosome 16. Deletion of a single gene is paradoxically designated as α-thalassaemia 2, and deletion of both as α-thalassaemia 1. The α-thalassaemia 2 gene is common in the Mediterranean area, the Middle East, India, South East Asia, Indonesia and the South Pacific, and also very common in negroes of African origin. In the heterozygous state, the deletion means that the individual lacks one out of four α-chain genes; the defect is clinically insignificant, and such individuals are described as 'silent carriers' of α-thalassaemia 2 trait. They may show borderline low values for mean cell haemoglobin (MCH) and mean cell volume (MCV), or no abnormality at all. Homozygosity for the character, with a lack of two out of the four α-globin genes, produces α-thalassaemia trait; affected individuals are usually clinically normal, but show a reduced MCV of about 70 fl, a reduced MCH, a raised red cell count, and often mild anaemia.

The α-thalassaemia 1 deletion, involving loss of both α-globin genes on a single chromosome, can produce more severe clinical conditions. This deletion occurs in the Mediterranean area, South-East Asia, the Philippines and elsewhere, but is extremely rare in negroes. Heterozygosity for the double deletion plus a normal chromosome 16 produces a clinical picture indistinguishable from that seen in homozygotes for the α-thalassaemia 2 deletion (see above).

A double heterozygote for the α-thalassaemia 1 and α-thalassaemia 2 deletions, who lacks three of the four α-globin genes, suffers from a relatively severe form of α-thalassaemia known as HbH disease. In this condition HbA production is only 25% of normal; excess γ-chains accumulate during fetal life, and excess β-chains postnatally. Both these chains, when produced in relative excess, form tetramers and their presence is a diagnostic feature: the γ_4 tetramer is Hb Barts and the β_4 tetramer HbH. Both are ineffective for oxygen carriage, unstable in solution and tend to precipitate, causing haemolysis. The instability of HbH arises from the presence of two additional and accessible-SH groups on the β-chain, rendering it abnormally sensitive to oxidation. The precipitated haemoglobin gives rise to inclusions in the red cells, which can be detected in splenectomised patients (as in the case of the other unstable haemoglobins, see above). In unsplenectomised patients, inclusions can be formed in vitro by incubation of fresh red cells with a redox dye, brilliant cresyl blue. The relative concentration of the β_4 tetramer in red cells varies between 5 and 40%.

The combination of haemolysis due to HbH precipitation, with underproduction of haemoglobin, generally gives rise to a fairly severe anaemia, often with bone deformities and splenomegaly, but not requiring transfusion. This is the clinical picture of so-called *thalassaemia intermedia.*

However, there is wide variation in the clinical severity of HbH disease, with some patients being able to lead almost normal lives, while in others the anaemia is severe enough to necessitate regular transfusion. (Some of this variation can be accounted for by the fact that the two α-chain genes on one chromosome produce globin chains at unequal rates, and genetic defects affecting the more active gene tend to be more severe.[15]

Homozygosity for the severe α-thalassaemia 1 deletion implies loss of all four α-globin genes. This is lethal in utero: the fetus dies with severe anaemia and hydrops, the red cells showing accumulation of β_4-chains (Hb Barts). The condition is called Barts hydrops.

Genetic lesions resulting in α-thalassaemic states can also occur without deletion of the α-globin gene. Most are rare; one that is relatively common in South-East Asia is Hb Constant Spring. This results from a mutation in the normal termination codon for α-globin, leading to continued translation of the DNA and the production of an abnormally elongated globin chain. This is produced at a much reduced rate and also is unstable, so its effect is equivalent to that of the α-thalassaemia 2 deletion.

β-Thalassaemia

Each chromosome 11 carries only a single β-globin gene. Hence, in principle, β-thalassaemia can exist in two degrees of severity: the heterozygous state (β-thalassaemia minor) and the homozygous (β-thalassaemia major). β-Thalassaemia genes are common throughout the 'thalassaemia belt' embracing the Mediterranean, Middle East, Africa, India, South-East Asia and Indonesia.

Clinically, β-thalassaemia minor is a mild condition with haemoglobin only slightly lower than normal, with microcytic hypochromic red cells but no other clinical abnormality. An increased relative concentration of the minor haemoglobin component HbA2 ($\alpha_2\, \gamma_2$) is a diagnostic feature.

β-Thalassaemia major implies total or near-total inability to synthesize β-globin chains. This is of no significance during intrauterine life (in contrast to α-chain defects) since at this stage the predominant non-α globin chain is the γ-chain of HbF. Thus β-thalassaemia major becomes clinically apparent some months after birth, when γ-chain production ceases. Anaemia then becomes progressively more severe, reaching a degree that necessitates transfusion to preserve life.

The genetic basis of β-thalassaemia is very varied. Deletion of a whole β-globin gene is very rare. Most β-thalassaemia genes affect one or other stage in the transfer of information from DNA to protein. There are mutations associated with premature mRNA chain termination (non-sense mutants), frameshifts, abnormal capping or splicing of mRNA, or interference with translation of mRNA[16]. Although over 90 different mutations have been identified, any given population is likely to show only a few of these. Functionally, there is an important distinction between mutations that completely abolish β-globin production by the affected chromosome (β^0 type) and those that allow some residual production (β^+ type). There is a wide variety in the severity of the different β-thalassaemic alleles; this accounts for the clinical syndrome of β-thalassaemia intermedia, which may occur in homozygotes or double heterozygotes for the milder variants. At the other extreme, some variants can produce the picture of thalassaemia intermedia in the heterozygote, generally through the production of a highly unstable β-globin.[16]

δ-Globin abnormalities

δ-Globin is an analogue of β-globin, and the genes for the two proteins lie close together (see Fig. 14.7). The syndrome of δβ-thalassaemia (associated in the homozygous state with failure to produce any β- or δ-chains at all, the only haemoglobin produced being HbF), is caused by a large deletion spanning the whole β-globin locus and a large part of that for δ-globin. A less extensive deletion, affecting the 3' half of the δ gene and the 5' half of the β gene, results in the production of Hb Lepore, a compound of α-chains with hybrid δβ-chains. The deletion results from mispairing of similar sites on the δ and β genes during crossing-over in meiosis, and produces a hybrid globin with the 5' end of the δ chain and the 3' end of the β-chain. Because of the ineffective production of the hybrid chains and consequent α /non-α chain imbalance, Hb Lepore is clinically similar to β-thalassaemia in both heterozygotes and homozygotes; compound heterozygotes for Hb Lepore and β-thalassaemia have the phenotype of β-thalassaemia major.

Another type of deletion affecting the δ and β genes is associated with the benign condition of *hereditary persistence of fetal haemoglobin* (HPFH). Here the deletion of both δ and β genes appears to bring enhancer sequences into the vicinity of the intact γ genes, preventing the normal switch-off of γ-chain production. In the homozygous state, therefore, this condition is associated with production of greatly increased amounts of HbF, with no HbA or A_2 but no anaemia. Other genetic variants of HPFH exist in which point mutations in promoter or enhancer sequences for γ-globin result in continued excess production of these chains, without impairment of HbA production.

Hybrid conditions

The thalassaemic syndromes and the haemoglobinopathies occur with a very similar geographical distribution, and it is not surprising that mixed conditions occur commonly.

Interaction of a β-thalassaemia gene with the gene for HbS produces the syndrome of HbS/β-thalassaemia, which is discussed above under Sickle cell syndromes.

Interaction of α-with β-thalassaemic genes gives rise to relatively milder thalassaemic conditions, because the imbalance in production of the two globin chains is alleviated. Thus, for example, homozygous β-thalassaemia associated with heterozygous α-thalassaemia 1 produces a thalassaemia of only intermediate severity.

A second important interaction, of frequent occurrence in the Far East, is that between HbE and β-thalassaemia. The gene for HbE (see above, under haemoglobin E) contains a single nucleotide substitution which activates a cryptic RNA splice site, leading to alternate splicing of mRNA with the production of a structurally abnormal mRNA molecule that cannot be translated. Alternate splicing affects about half the mRNA produced by the gene, greatly reducing the rate of globin synthesis. In addition, the HbE molecule is less stable than HbA and undergoes intracellular precipitation. As a result, compound heterozygotes for HbE and β-thalassaemia have the phenotype of β-thalassaemia major or intermedia.[17] (Homozygous HbE and HbE trait are described above under Haemoglobinopathies).

Diagnostic methods in the thalassaemias

Basic diagnosis of a thalassaemic condition depends on a blood count and blood film examination, showing microcytosis and hypochromia (confirmed by the MCV and MCH), with characteristic morphological abnormalities including schistocytes, target cells, and in severe cases nucleated erythroblasts in the circulation. In β-thalassaemia minor, the HbA2 is raised. In α-thalassaemia trait (two deletions out of four) there may be no additional abnormality; occasionally some HbH is detectable by cytochemical staining with brilliant cresyl blue. In HbH disease, abundant HbH precipitates are seen by this technique, and HbH can also be detected electrophoretically.

The diagnosis can be refined by globin chain synthesis studies. A variety of recombinant DNA techniques can be used to pinpoint the exact genetic defect. These include Southern blotting, hybridization with specific oligonucleotide DNA probes, and the use of linkage markers. Such techniques are of particular value in genetic counselling and antenatal diagnosis. The subject has been reviewed.[14]

Treatment of the thalassaemias is symptomatic and is based on blood transfusion, with subcutaneous desferrioxamine (Desferal) to chelate iron and reduce the inevitable iron loading that results both from transfusion and from the increased iron absorption present in these conditions. Iron overload causes endocrine abnormalities including poor growth, delayed or failed puberty, infertility, diabetes mellitus etc. In more advanced cases, involvement of hepatic and cardiac tissue causes fatal organ failure. With optimal iron chelation therapy, most patients survive into middle age and many may be normally fertile. Some patients require splenectomy, usually because splenomegaly interferes with their transfusion response. The only curative treatment available today is bone marrow transplantation, which has a high success rate when undertaken early, before iron overload has caused tissue damage, and when donor and recipient are well matched.

A number of experimental approaches hold promise for the future. Drugs may be used to inhibit or reverse the switch mechanism that stops HbF production (of relevance in β-globin abnormalities only); hydroxyurea is partially effective in this respect, but has not been shown to be clinically useful. More sophisticated forms of genetic engineering would be aimed at inserting normal globin genes into haemopoietic precursors. On the more immediate practical level, availability of an oral iron-chelating agent would be of enormous value, and a number of candidate compounds are under evaluation.

REFERENCES

1. Lux S E 1983 Disorders of the red cell skeleton: hereditary spherocytosis and hereditary elliptocytosis. In: Stanbury J B, Wyngaarden J B, Fredrickson D S, Goldstein J L, Brown M S (eds) The metabolic basis of inherited disease, 5th edn. McGraw-Hill, New York, p 1573–1605
2. Fairbanks G, Steck T L, Wallach D F H 1971 Electrophoretic analysis of the major polypeptides of the human erythrocyte membrane. Biochemistry 10:2606–2617
3. Palek J, Lux S E 1983 Red cell membrane skeletal defects in hereditary and acquired hemolytic anemias. Seminars in Hematology 20:189–224
4. Palek J, Lambert S 1990 Genetics of red cell membrane protein. Seminars in Hematology 27:290–332
5. Grimes A J 1980 Human red cell metabolism. Blackwell Scientific Publications, Oxford
6. Beutler E, Blume K G, Kaplan J C, Lohr G W, Ramot B, Valentine W N 1977 International Committee for Standardisation in Haematology: recommended methods for red-cell enzyme analysis. British Journal of Haematology 35:331–340
7. Schneider A S, Valentine W N, Baughan M A, Paglia D E, Shore N A, Heins H L 1965 Triosephosphate isomerase deficiency. A multi-system inherited enzyme disorder. Clinical and genetic aspects. In: Beutler E (ed) Hereditary disorders of erythrocyte metabolism. Grune and Stratton, New York, p 265.
8. Bellingham A J, Lestas A N, Williams A H P, Nicolaides K H 1989 Prenatal diagnosis of a red-cell enzymopathy: triose phosphate isomerase deficiency. Lancet 2:419–421.
9. Rosa R, Prehu M, Beuzard Y, Rosa J 1987 The first case of a complete deficiency of diphosphoglycerate mutase in human erythrocytes. Journal of Clinical Investigation 62:907–915
10. Beutler E 1987 Glucose-6-phosphate dehydrogenase deficiency. In: Hemolytic anemia in disorders of red cell metabolism. Plenum Medical, New York, p 23–167.
11. Tanner M J A 1983 Erythrocyte membrane structure and function. In: Malaria and the red cell. CIBA Foundation symposium No 94, Pitman, London, p 3–23
12. Huehns E R 1982 The structure and function of haemoglobin: clinical disorders due to abnormal haemoglobin structure. In: Hardisty R M, Weatherall D J (eds) Blood and its disorders, 2nd edn. Blackwell Scientific Publications, Oxford, p 323–400
13. Winterbourn C C 1990 Oxidative denaturation in congenital hemolytic anemias: the unstable haemoglobins. Seminars in Hematology 27:41–50
14. Weatherall D J, Clegg J B, Higgs D R et al 1989 The hemoglobinopathies. In: Scriver C R, Beaudet A L, Sly W S (eds) The metabolic basis of inherited disease, 6th edn. New York, McGraw–Hill, p. 2281–2339

15. Liebhaber S A 1989 α-Thalassemia. Hemoglobin 13:685–731
16. Kazazian H H, Dowling C E, Boehm C D, Warren T C, Economou E P, Katz J, Stylianos E A 1990 Gene defects in β-thalassemia and their prenatal diagnosis. Annals of the New York Academy of Sciences ('6th Cooley's Anemia Symposium' issue), 612:1–14
17. Adams J G, Coleman M B 1990 Structural hemoglobin variants that produce the phenotype of thalassemia. Seminars in Hematology 27:229–238

Index

The Inherited metabolic diseases.

$110.00

DATE			